Dellmann's
Textbook of Veterinary Histology

Dellmann's
Textbook of Veterinary Histology

Seventh Edition

Edited by

Marxa L. Figueiredo, PhD
Department of Basic Medical Sciences
Purdue University
West Lafayette, Indiana

John J. Turek, PhD
Department of Basic Medical Sciences
Purdue University
West Lafayette, Indiana

WILEY

Published by John Wiley & Sons, Inc., Hoboken, New Jersey.
Published simultaneously in Canada.

Library of Congress Cataloging-in-Publication Data:
Names: Figueiredo, Marxa, 1977– editor. | Turek, John J., 1952– editor.
Title: Dellmann's textbook of veterinary histology / [edited by] Marxa Figueiredo, John J. Turek.
Other titles: Textbook of veterinary histology
Description: Seventh edition. | Hoboken, New Jersey : Wiley-Blackwell, [2025] | Includes bibliographical references and index.
Identifiers: LCCN 2024047938 (print) | LCCN 2024047939 (ebook) | ISBN 9781394196678 (hardback) | ISBN 9781394196685 (adobe pdf) | ISBN 9781394196708 (epub)
Subjects: MESH: Histology | Anatomy, Veterinary | Histological Techniques–veterinary
Classification: LCC SF757.3 (print) | LCC SF757.3 (ebook) | NLM SF 757.3 | DDC 636.089/1–dc23/eng/20250321
LC record available at https://lccn.loc.gov/2024047938
LC ebook record available at https://lccn.loc.gov/2024047939

Cover Design: Wiley
Cover Images: Courtesy of Marxa L. Figueiredo and John J. Turek

Set in 9.5/12.5pt STIX Two Text by Straive, Pondicherry, India

Printed in Singapore
M125236_010425

Dedicated to

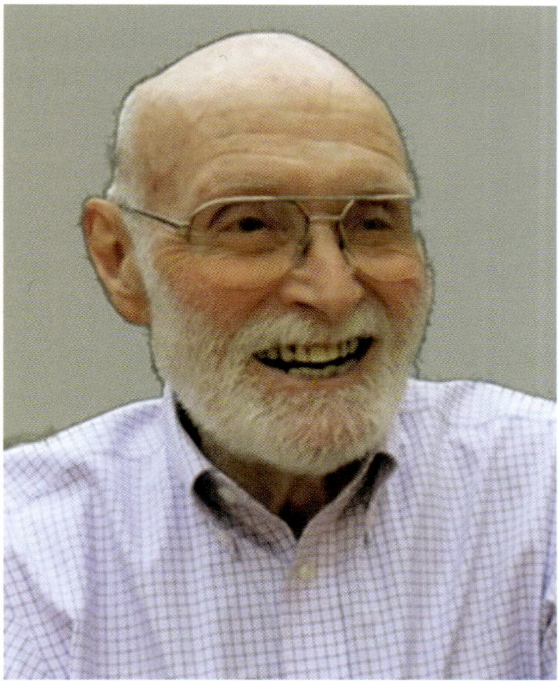

H.-Dieter Dellmann, Docteur-Vétérinaire, Habil.

Contents

Contributors

Elikplimi K. Asem, DVM, PhD
Professor
Department of Basic Medical Sciences
Purdue University College of Veterinary Medicine
West Lafayette, Indiana

Estela Bevilacqua, PhD
Professor
Lab for Maternal–Fetal Interactions and Placenta Research
Department of Cellular and Developmental Biology
Institute of Biomedical Sciences
University of São Paulo
São Paulo, SP, Brazil

Ji-Ming Feng, PhD
Associate Professor
Department of Comparative Biomedical Sciences
School of Veterinary Medicine
Louisiana State University
Baton Rouge, Louisiana

Marxa L. Figueiredo, PhD
Associate Professor
Department of Basic Medical Sciences
Purdue University College of Veterinary Medicine
West Lafayette, Indiana

Carlos E. Fonseca Alves, DVM, MSc, PhD
Associate Professor, Universidade Paulista-UNIP, Bauru
Laboratory of Cancer Immunopathology and Biology
Department of Veterinary Surgery and Anesthesiology and
School of Veterinary Medicine and Animal Science
São Paulo State University-UNESP
Botucatu, SP, Brazil

Karl Klisch, PhD
Division of Veterinary Anatomy
Vetsuisse Faculty
Länggass-Strasse 120
University of Bern
Bern, Switzerland

Craig McGowan, PhD
Associate Professor
Department of Clinical Integrative Anatomical Sciences
Keck School of Medicine
University of Southern California
Los Angeles, California

Joanne B. Messick, VMD, PhD, Dip. ACVP
Professor
Department of Comparative Pathobiology
Purdue University College of Veterinary Medicine
West Lafayette, Indiana

Nancy A. Monteiro-Riviere, PhD, ATS
Distinguished University Professor Emeritus and
Regents Distinguished Professor of Toxicology
Kansas State University, Manhattan, Kansas

and

Professor Emeritus of Investigative Dermatology and Toxicology
Center for Chemical Toxicology Research
North Carolina State University
Raleigh, North Carolina

Olalekan M. Ogundele, PhD
Associate Professor
Anatomy and Neuroscience
Department of Comparative Biomedical Sciences
School of Veterinary Medicine
Louisiana State University
Baton Rouge, Louisiana

Cornelia W. Peterson, DVM, PhD, DACVP
Assistant Professor of Anatomic Pathology
Department of Comparative Pathobiology
Tufts University Cummings School of Veterinary Medicine
North Grafton, Massachusetts

Charles G. Plopper, PhD
Professor Emeritus
Department of Anatomy
Physiology and Cell Biology
School of Veterinary Medicine
University of California
Davis, California

Christopher Premanandan, DVM, PhD, DACVP, DACT
Professor
Department of Veterinary Biosciences
The Ohio State University
Columbus, Ohio

Charles McLean Press, BSc (Vet.), BVSc, PhD
Professor
Department of Preclinical Sciences and Pathology
Faculty of Veterinary Medicine
Norwegian University of Life Sciences
Ås, Norway

John J. Turek, PhD
Professor
Department of Basic Medical Sciences
Purdue University College of Veterinary Medicine
West Lafayette, Indiana

Preface

The publication of the seventh edition of the *Textbook of Veterinary Histology* marks nearly half a century since H.-Dieter Dellmann and Esther M. Brown first brought this book to veterinary students, histology instructors, and other biologists in 1976. Dr Dellmann continued this book through five English editions. The textbook has also been reprinted in Spanish, Japanese, Italian, Indonesian, Portuguese, and Korean editions for international veterinary students. Dr Dellmann's dedication and contribution to veterinary histology has been perpetuated ever since by a varied editorial team, and his name is honored in the title of this edition.

The current version of this textbook has been adapted as a teaching tool not only for veterinary students but also for graduate students and other histologists training in fields related to veterinary medicine. The text and images for this edition have been updated with the most current information available at the time of publication.

With the retirement of Dr Dellmann, Dr J. A. Eurell and Dr B. Frappier contributed as editors for the sixth edition. We are thankful for their outstanding contributions, many of which have been maintained in the seventh edition. We also extend our thanks to the contributors of the sixth edition who did not participate in this edition; their work is greatly appreciated and has informed our updates. The former contributors whose chapters were updated in the seventh edition include: *Donald R Adams, Ourania M Andrisani, Alvin Beitz, Martin Bergmann, Vibeke Dantzer, EJ Ehrhart, Jo Ann Eurell, Thomas F Fletcher, Brian L Frappier, Ralph E Hamor, Ronald L Hullinger, Thor Landsverk, Lars-Inge Larsson, Rudolf Leiser, Johanna Plendl, Janis Priedkalns, David C Van Sickle, Jill W Verlander,* and *Karl-Heinz Wrobel*. Returning contributors include *Charles G Plopper, Charles McLean Press, Joanne Messick*, and *Nancy A Monteiro-Riviere*. New contributors for the seventh edition include, along with the editors, *Elikplimi Asem, Estela Bevillaqua, Ji-Ming Feng, Carlos Eduardo Alves Fonseca, Karl Klisch, Craig McGowan, Olalekan Ogundele, Cornelia Peterson*, and *Christopher Premanandan*. Their highly diverse expertise has made this project possible. At Purdue University, the editors offer appreciation and thanks to Dr Laurie Jaeger for expert advice, as well as for supporting the editorial team to make the seventh edition a reality.

We recently learned that Dr Dellmann passed away in the Fall of 2023. Dr. Dellmann received his Diploma in Veterinary Medicine from the École Nationale Vétérinaire d'Alfort, France, in 1954. He then completed his postgraduate studies at Ludwig-Maximilians University in Munich, Germany, in 1961, where he received his PhD in Veterinary Medicine. He taught Veterinary Anatomy and Microscopic Anatomy at Iowa State University for over 21 years. He was named Clarence Harley Covault Distinguished Professor and was also an elected member of the French National Academy of Veterinary Medicine. It is said that Dr Dellmann's favorite line from an aria in Beethoven's Fidelio was, "*I have done my duty*." This indeed holds true, and he shall remain a highly respected histologist who made significant contributions to veterinary medicine. We honor him and are thankful for all his contributions to the field. He will be forever missed by the histology community.

We also regrettably finish this work in the absence of our dear colleague, Dr Russell P. Main, whom we had planned to have as part of our editorial team. Dr Main's work focused on comparative skeletal mechanics, bone histomorphology, and growth among major tetrapod groups. He was a faculty member at Purdue University in the College of Veterinary Medicine and the Weldon School of Biomedical Engineering from 2011 to 2023. Dr Main served tirelessly as a dedicated scientist, teacher, and mentor. He will be missed by the histology community at Purdue University and beyond.

Finally, we are deeply appreciative of Dr W. E. Haensly and Dr J. Eurell for their contributions to the sixth edition, including their many outstanding images, a significant portion of which we have retained in the seventh edition.

We are pleased to present this updated work for the benefit of veterinary students, graduate students, and histologists working in fields related to veterinary medicine for years to come.

Marxa L. Figueiredo
John J. Turek
West Lafayette, Indiana

About the Companion Website

This book is accompanied by a companion website:

www.wiley.com/go/figueiredo/vethistology7e

The website includes Figure PPTs

1

Cytology

Ji-Ming Feng

CHAPTER MENU

General Overview

The cell is the smallest unit of life, and all living matter (**protoplasm**) is composed of cells. Cells possess the unique abilities to replicate and to create energy from inanimate matter, which are qualities that characterize life itself. Many living creatures are unicellular (i.e., consist of a single cell), but higher. organisms are comprised of a multiplicity of cells that specialize in different functions including absorption, digestion, and excretion.

In primitive **prokaryotic** cells, such as bacteria, there is little organization of the many molecules needed for the life processes. In contrast, in **eukaryotic** organisms, the genetic material is organized within a nucleus (karyon), and many other processes have become confined to membrane-bounded **organelles**. This **compartmentation** prevents the unordered mixing of different biochemical pathways, thus allowing for more sophisticated cellular functions. The compartmentation also allows the cells to increase in size by ordered delivery of membrane-delimited molecules to their

Dellmann's Textbook of Veterinary Histology, Seventh Edition. Edited by Marxa L. Figueiredo and John J. Turek.

Companion website: www.wiley.com/go/figueiredo/vethistology7e

appropriate destinations. Thus, bacteria only reach 1 to 5 μm in size, while most eukaryotic cells range between 5 and 50 μm.

Eukaryotic cell structure and function thus depend upon membranes and membrane-enclosed structures. The cell itself is delimited by the **cell membrane**. The **cytoplasm** consists of organelles, inclusions, and cytoskeletal components, enclosed in a semi-viscous liquid, the **cytosol** (Fig. 1-1). The study of the structural components of the cell is referred to as **cytology**, while the study of the integration of cells to form tissues and organs is referred to as **histology**. Such integration involves three different components: the cells themselves, the **extracellular matrix (ECM)**, and **tissue fluids**. The ECM components are synthesized by cells and are present in different proportions in different tissues. Tissue fluids transport nutrients, hormones, gases, and waste products to and from the cells.

Many parts of the cell can be studied using the light microscope, which allows the maximal resolution of structures down to 0.2 μm in diameter at magnifications up to 1000 to 1500 times. However, many cellular structures are smaller, requiring the use of an electron microscope, offering much better resolution (down to 0.1 nm) and higher magnifications (up to ×400,000).

In most cases, it is necessary to stain cells and tissues to increase their contrast in light or electron microscopy. A common light microscopy stain is a combination of the dyes hematoxylin and eosin (H&E), which stain nuclei blue and cytoplasm pink, respectively. When negative molecular groups bind positively charged (basic) dyes (such as derivatives of hematoxylin), the stained structures are described as **basophilic**. In contrast, basic components (such as hemoglobin in mature red blood cells) attract positively charged (acidic) dyes such as eosin and are termed **acidophilic**. Electron-absorbing heavy metal ions serve as stains for electron microscopy. These stains show little chemical specificity but impart contrast to cellular structures. In contrast, histochemistry allows the localization of specific molecules by the use of antibodies tagged with labels that are detectable in the light or electron microscope (immunohistochemistry). Antibodies are often labeled with fluorescent dyes for observation in fluorescence microscopes. Enzyme histochemistry utilizes enzyme substrates that produce colored or electron-dense reaction products that precipitate at the site of enzyme activity. The study of living cells requires the use of special optical methods (phase contrast or interference contrast microscopy), which enhance contrast of different cell components. Additionally, living cells can be stained with vital dyes that make it possible to follow fluorescent proteins expressed by genetically manipulated living cells.

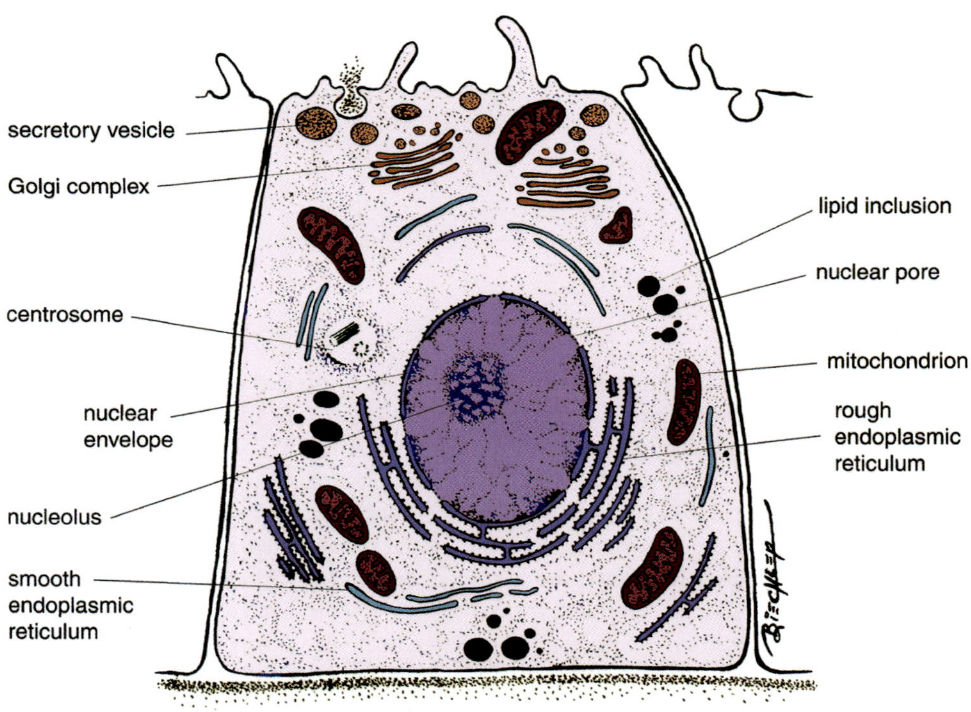

Figure 1-1 Schematic drawing of the general organization of an epithelial cell.

Cell Membrane

The **cell membrane** (plasmalemma) encloses the cell and forms its boundary with the surrounding environment. The internal milieu of the cell must be kept constant, so the cell membrane is involved in the active and passive transport of ions, water, oxygen, carbon dioxide, nutrients, and secretory and excretory products. The cell membrane is also involved in anchoring the cell to surrounding structures, as well as participating in signaling and recognition events. This structure is sometimes referred to as a **unit membrane**, which follows the theory that all biologic membranes share the same structure.

The cell membrane is 8 to 10 nm thick and exhibits a characteristic trilaminar structure in electron micrographs (Fig. 1-2). This structure consists of an outer and inner electron-dense lamina separated by an electron-lucent layer. Biochemically, the cell membrane is primarily composed of **phospholipids**, which have hydrophilic heads and hydrophobic tails. The phospholipids form a bilayer in the membrane, with the hydrophobic tails oriented inward and the hydrophilic heads facing outward and toward the cytosol (Fig. 1-3). Such arrangement of the phospholipids has been correlated to the trilaminar structure, with the polar heads and associated proteins making up the electron-dense laminae and the hydrophobic tails forming the electron-lucent layer. The bilayer also contains other lipids, such as cholesterol, which helps maintain membrane fluidity and stability, and carbohydrate-containing glycolipids, which play roles in cell recognition and signaling.

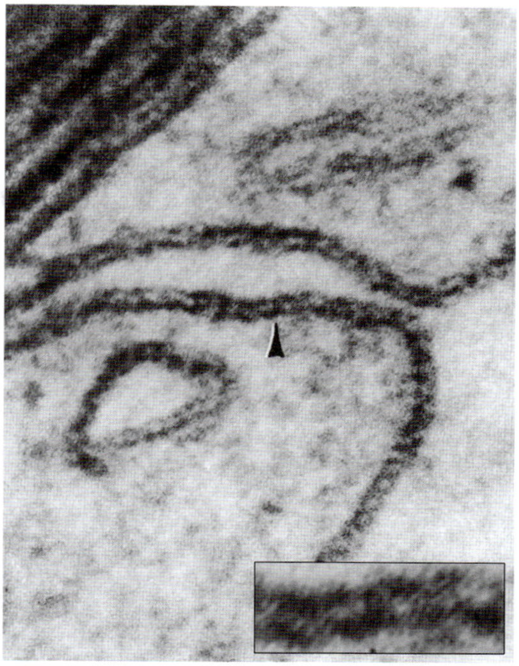

Figure 1-2 Electron micrograph of the plasma membrane (arrowhead) (×415,000) at the mesaxon of a neurolemmocyte (myelin-forming cell) with the inset (lower right) to show its trilaminar structure.

Proteins associated with the cell membrane are either inserted into the phospholipid bilayer (**integral proteins**) or attached to its inner or outer surfaces (**peripheral proteins**). **Transmembrane proteins** are integral proteins that span the entire thickness of the lipid bilayer. A fluid mosaic is created by transmembrane proteins, which can diffuse laterally in the lipid bilayer. However, protein diffusion is often restricted by cytoskeletal components, cell junctions, and specialized membrane substructures known as lipid rafts. **Lipid rafts** are regions of the membrane with high concentrations of cholesterol and sphingolipids, which decrease the fluidity of the lipid bilayer. Some lipid rafts contain proteins called caveolins, which facilitate the reorganization of the membrane into pear-shaped invaginations known as **caveolae**. These caveolae participate in various cellular processes, and specific ligands such as albumin, folic acid, and alkaline phosphatase are internalized via caveolae. In addition, caveolae are a pathway for cellular entry of pathogens such as polyoma virus and type 1 fimbriated bacteria (strains of *Escherichia coli*).

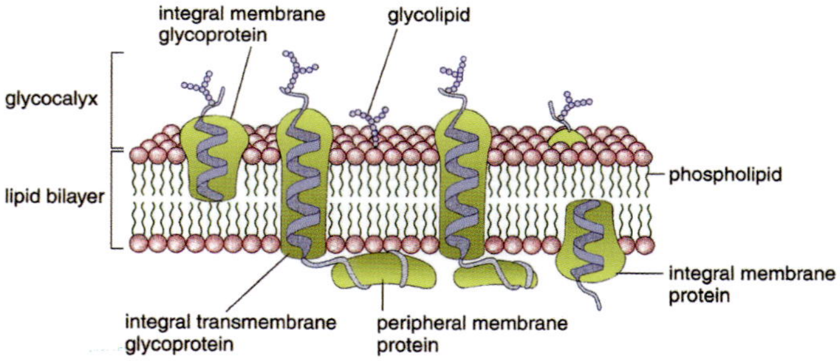

Figure 1-3 Schematic drawing of the organization of the cell membrane.

Some integral membrane proteins attach to oligosaccharides, forming glycoproteins, while others attach to larger polysaccharides known as glycosaminoglycans, forming proteoglycans. Both oligosaccharides and glycosaminoglycans are present on the external surface of the cell membrane. Together with the carbohydrate portion of glycolipids, they form a carbohydrate-rich external cell coat, the **glycocalyx**. The glycocalyx is involved in many important functions relating to cell recognition, signaling, and mechanical protection. For example, blood group antigens are part of the glycocalyx of blood cells. The glycocalyx can be visualized by histochemical staining techniques such as the periodic-acid-Schiff (PAS) method or with labeled lectins, proteins that bind to specific carbohydrate structures. The cell membrane is asymmetrical with respect to its distribution of membrane proteins, the glycocalyx, and phospholipids. This asymmetry is essential for various cellular processes, including cell signaling, membrane trafficking, and cell-to-cell interactions.

Some **transmembrane proteins** are involved in cell-to-cell or cell-to-matrix interactions, while others act as carriers or channels that transport substances such as ions and glucose across the membrane. Still, other transmembrane proteins serve as **receptors** that transmit signals from outside the cell to the inside. Certain hormones, including steroid hormones, can pass through the plasmalemma and bind directly to intracellular receptors. Most hormones, growth factors, and neurotransmitters are either too large or too hydrophilic to pass through the cell membrane, and therefore use transmembrane proteins as receptors. Binding of these molecules to the extracellular region of such receptors evokes intracellular activation of the so-called **second messengers**, such as cyclic adenosine monophosphate. Second messengers are intracellular molecules that relay the extracellular message to the interior of the cell, triggering a cascade of cellular responses.

Nucleus

The shape, structure, and position of the nucleus vary considerably between cell types, and these characteristics are useful for cell identification. For example, lymphocytes typically have a round nucleus, while granulocytes have a lobulated nucleus. The **nucleus** is centrally located in many cell types, but in others, it is displaced to the periphery (e.g., fat cells and skeletal muscle cells). Most cells have a single nucleus, but some, like osteoclasts, possess multiple nuclei. Multinucleated cells may originate from either the fusion of mononuclear cells or incomplete division. Mature mammalian red blood cells, on the other hand, lack a nucleus.

Nuclear Envelope

The nucleus is enclosed by a **nuclear envelope**, which contains nuclear pores that control the flow of materials between the nucleus and the cytoplasm. The nuclear envelope is composed of double-unit membranes separated by a narrow (25 to 70 nm) **perinuclear space** (Fig. 1-4). The outer membrane is often studded with ribosomes and may be continuous with the rough endoplasmic reticulum (Fig. 1-4). On the inside of the inner membrane, the **nuclear lamina** is present. The nuclear lamina is an interwoven meshwork of specialized intermediate filaments called **lamins** that provide the nucleus with mechanical strength. Circular **nuclear pores** are interspersed at intervals throughout the nuclear envelope.

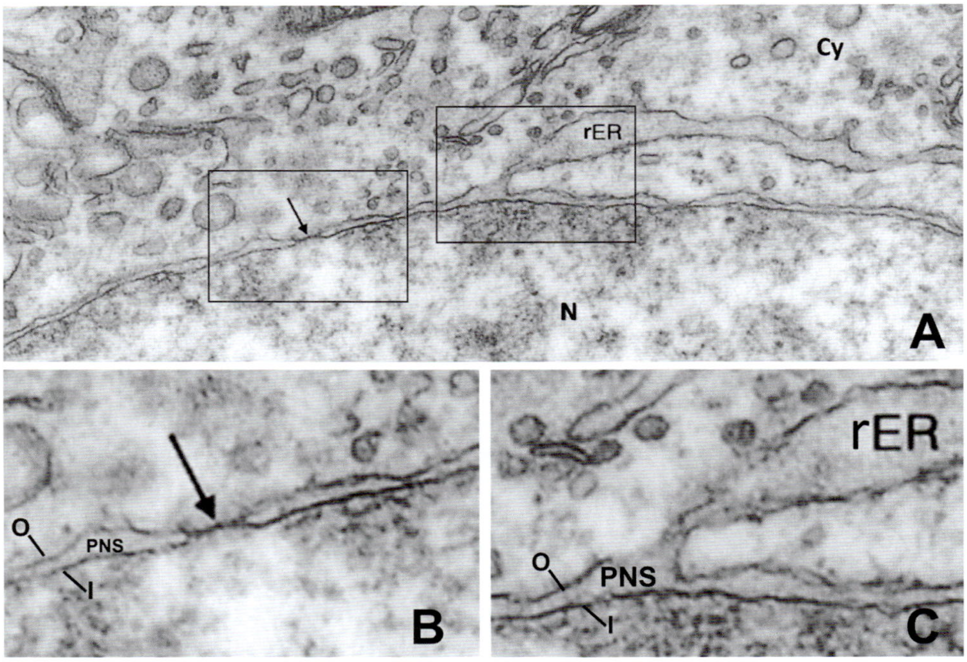

Figure 1-4 **A.** Electron micrograph of a part of the nucleus (N) and cytoplasm (Cy) of a neurohypophysial glial cell (×67,000). **B.** The nuclear envelope, pierced by nuclear pores (arrow), consists of double-unit membranes separated by a narrow perinuclear space (PNS). **C.** The perinuclear space between the inner (I) and outer (O) nuclear membranes is continuous with a cisterna of the rough endoplasmic reticulum (rER).

Materials pass through these pores in a manner strictly controlled by proteins of the nuclear pore complex. Small molecules and ions can pass the pores via simple diffusion. However, large molecules (e.g., proteins) over 11 nm in size must use a highly selective transport process to shuttle through the nuclear pores. Signal sequences of macromolecules to be transported need be recognized by the receptor sites of the nuclear pore complex. The bidirectional traffic of macromolecules between the nucleus and the cytoplasm is mediated by the specific groups of proteins: (a) **exportins** that transport macromolecules (e.g., ribonucleic acid [RNA]) from the nucleus to the cytoplasm and (b) **importins** that transport cargo (e.g., protein subunits of ribosomes) from the cytoplasm to the nucleus. In this way, protein synthesis is restricted to the cytoplasm, while permitting the nucleus to process and refine the precursor messenger RNAs without risking their translation into proteins during processing (e.g., the alternative splicing of pre-mRNAs to remove the noncoding intron segments).

Chromatin and Chromosome

Chromatin refers to deoxyribonucleic acid (DNA), complexed with proteins, of which the basic **histones** form the quantitatively most important part and are involved in chromatin packing. Nonhistone proteins refer to proteins that are also involved in chromatin packing and protection or that participate in regulation of DNA duplication, transcription, and repair.

In specimens stained with hematoxylin or other basic dyes, the nucleus exhibits areas of intense staining referred to as **heterochromatin**. Heterochromatin often occurs at the periphery of the nucleus, attached to the nuclear lamina, and consists of condensed DNA. Additionally, the nucleus contains lightly stained **euchromatin** that represents uncoiled DNA accessible for transcription into RNA. Ultrastructurally, heterochromatin appears as electron-dense granular masses, while euchromatin appears as electron-lucent masses. The proportion of heterochromatin to euchromatin varies between cells and is often an identifying feature (Fig. 1-5).

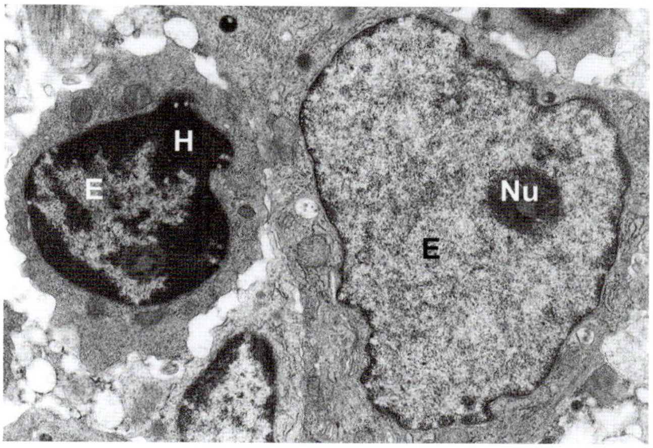

Figure 1-5 Electron micrograph of a lymphocyte (left) with more electron-dense heterochromatin (H) in the periphery, while a reticular cell (right) shows more electron-lucent euchromatin (E). A nucleolus (Nu) is present in the nucleus of the reticular cell (×10,000).

Chromatin is packed by coiling at several levels of organization. The basic unit is the **nucleosome**, formed from 200 base pairs of double-stranded DNA complexed with several histones. The exact number of base pairs involved is species variable. **Nucleosomes** are separated by shorter sequences of double-stranded **DNA**, approximately 50 base pairs in length. Even during transcription, euchromatin is composed of nucleosomes and internucleosomal strands, while transcriptionally inactive heterochromatin is further coiled. Heterochromatin is characterized by 30-nm **chromatin fibers** consisting of spirals of coiled nucleosomes. Even more elaborate coiling and structuring of chromatin occurs in conjunction with mitosis or meiosis, resulting in recognizable **chromosomes**.

In all cells of female individuals, one of the two X chromosomes is permanently inactivated and does not participate in transcription. The inactive X chromosome is recognizable in epithelial cells from the oral cavity as a single granule called **sex chromatin** (Barr body). In neutrophils, the sex chromatin takes the form of a drumstick-like appendage to the nucleus (Fig. 1-6). These structures have been used for gender testing in the past, but today, in situ hybridization techniques using labeled DNA probes that

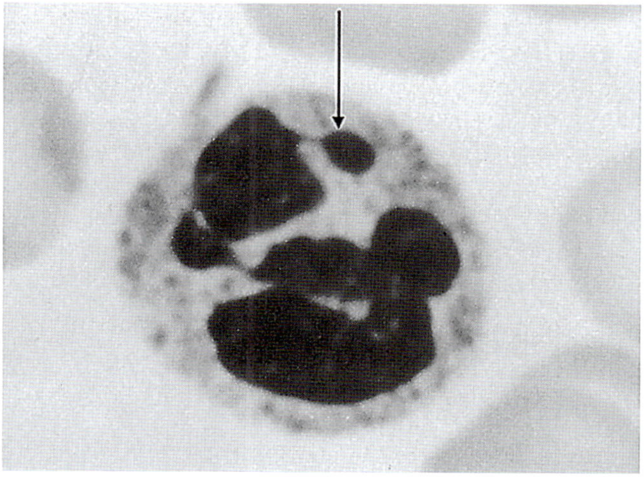

Figure 1-6 Sex chromatin (Barr body, arrow) is visible in the nucleus of a neutrophil from a female (×3800).

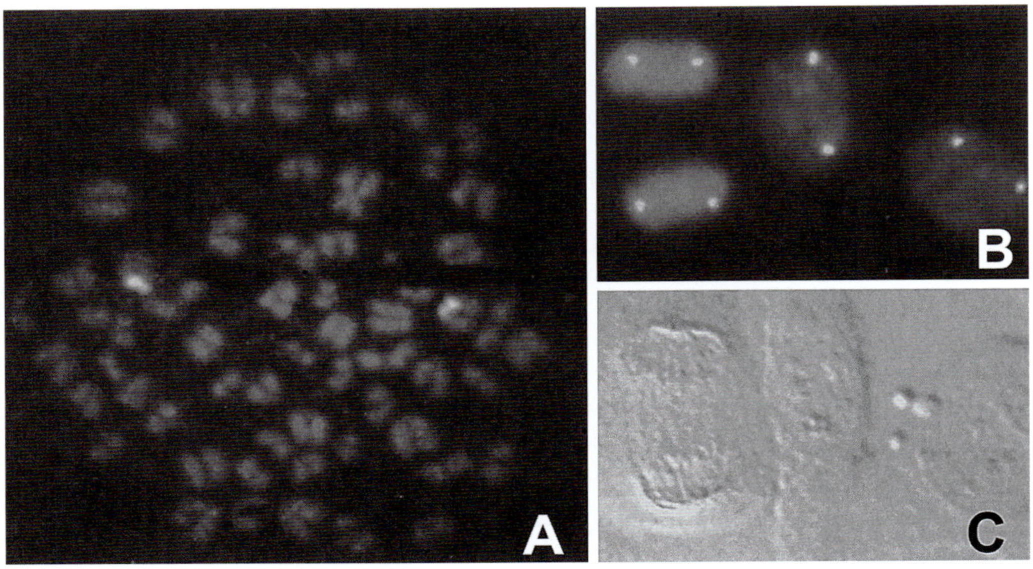

Figure 1-7 Bovine chromosome pair 7 is identified by their intense (white) fluorescence using in situ hybridization on spread metaphase chromosomes **(A)**, cultured bovine endothelial cells observed in fluorescence **(B)**, and in interference contrast to highlight morphologic details **(C)**. DNA has been gently counterstained with a more weakly fluorescent dye. In panels **B** and **C**, note the presence of a dividing cell (anaphase; left), in which the two pairs of chromosome 7 are being divided between the two daughter cells. In panels **B** and **C**, also note the presence of two interphase cells (right), each containing two fluorescent dots corresponding to two copies of chromosome 7. This approach facilitates the determination of chromosome numbers easily even in interphase cells, eliminating the need for lengthy preparation of metaphase chromosomes (×2000).

specifically bind to X chromosomes are preferred. The formula for genetic information encoded in DNA is written using four letters representing the bases adenine (A), guanine (G), thymine (T), and cytosine (C). The sequence of these bases determines the information encoded in genes of DNA, and this information is passed on (transcribed) to RNA.

Hybridization refers to the unique sequence of bases of the applied probe that binds to the complementary sequence of nucleotides in the DNA being investigated (A binds to T and G to C). This technique affords a high degree of specificity, and the probe can be labeled with a variety of substances that are detectable by either light or electron microscopy. Probes that are complementary to specific chromosome regions or genes can be used for prenatal diagnosis of hereditary diseases (Fig. 1-7).

Nucleolus

The **nucleolus** is a spherical structure suspended in the nuclear matrix and is involved in the production of ribosomes. At the light microscopic level, a nucleolus ranges up to 1 μm in diameter and usually stains with basic dyes such as hematoxylin, depending on its RNA content (Fig. 1-8A). The number of nucleoli is determined by the number of active **nucleolar organizing regions** (NORs), which are chromosomal regions responsible for encoding **ribosomal RNA** (rRNA). Normally, there are fewer nucleoli than NORs because either some NORs are inactivated or several fuse to form one nucleolus. At the electron microscopic level, the nucleolus is a dense nonmembrane-bounded structure (Fig. 1-8B) with areas of varying electron density. A **granular component** representing maturing ribosomal subunits is often prominent. **Fibrillar components** representing NOR DNA and transcribed rRNA are also observed.

Nucleoplasm and Nuclear Matrix

All other morphologically indiscernible materials in nucleus are collectively called nucleoplasm. It consists of various types of RNAs (such as transfer RNA [tRNA], rRNA, and mRNA), enzymes, variable-sized ribonucleoprotein particles (RNPs), and the nuclear matrix. RNPs are involved in mRNA splicing. The **nuclear matrix** refers to filamentous material remaining after enzymatic digestion and extraction of the nucleus, which is somewhat analogous to the cell cytoskeleton but far more dynamic. The nuclear matrix is believed to be important for positioning chromosomes in the nucleus in a pattern resembling that observed during mitotic cell division.

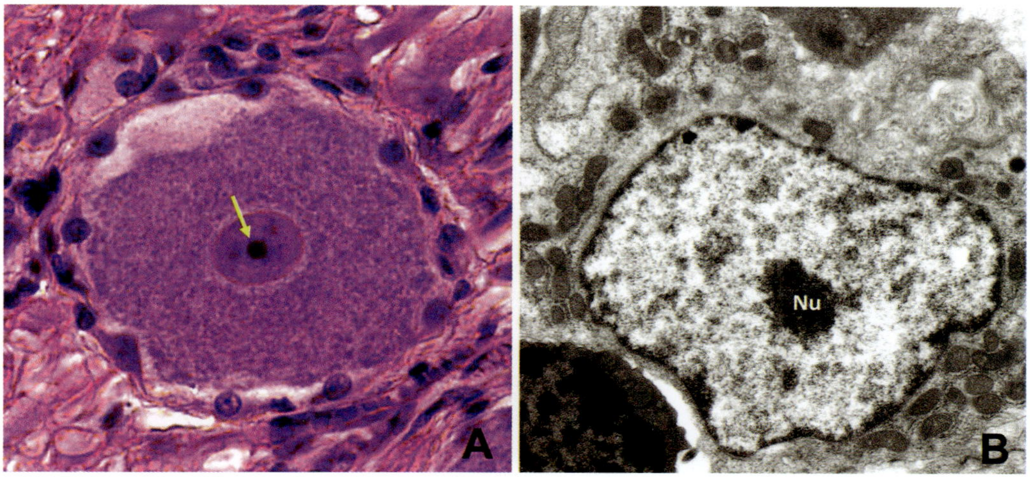

Figure 1-8 **A.** A sensory neuron from a mammal dorsal root ganglion as observed under a light microscope. The nucleus contains a distinct spherical nucleolus (arrow). Its cytoplasm is filled with Nissl substances (representing the abundant rER) as the basophilic, granulated masses. Hematoxylin and eosin (H&E) (×800). **B.** Under the electron microscope, a nucleolus (Nu) is observed as a nonmembranous structure suspended in the nucleus from a reticular cell (×6000).

Cytosol

The **cytosol** makes up approximately half of the cell volume and contains water, ions, sugars, amino acids, nucleotides, and hundreds of soluble enzymes (e.g., of the glycolytic pathway). Additionally, it houses subunits for cytoskeletal components, messenger RNA, tRNA, and myriad other molecules. Actin polymerization is critical in regulating the viscosity of the cytosol. Transition of the cytosol from a gel state to a more soluble (gel-to-sol) state facilitates the formation of extensions (pseudopodia) involved in cell motility.

Organelles

Rough and Smooth Endoplasmic Reticulum and Ribosomes

The endoplasmic reticulum (ER) forms an anastomosing (interconnected) network of membrane-delimited sacs (cisternae) and tubules. The **rough ER** (rER) is densely studded with ribosomes and is involved in protein synthesis (Fig. 1-9), while the **smooth ER** (sER) lacks ribosomes and participates in lipid synthesis, calcium sequestration, steroid hormone synthesis, and detoxification of harmful agents. Both forms of ER are interconnected, with the rER connecting to the outer nuclear membrane. The ribosomes and ER membranes are below the resolution of the light microscope. However, the cytoplasm of cells that synthesize large amounts of proteins is rich in ribosomes and mRNA, making it strongly basophilic. Accumulations of basophilic, well-developed rER are sometimes referred to as **ergastoplasm** in pancreatic cells or **Nissl substance** in neurons (Fig. 1-8).

The sER lacks attached ribosomes and thus is not involved in protein synthesis. Instead, it synthesizes lipids for cellular membranes and steroid hormones. Endocrine cells in the gonads and adrenal cortex have a well-developed system of tubular sER (Fig. 1-10). In addition, several drug-metabolizing enzymes that participate in detoxification of noxious and carcinogenic materials are present in the sER. Finally, the sER performs calcium-sequestering functions in many cells. The release of calcium from the sER can be triggered by various external stimuli, leading to a range of cellular responses. Skeletal and cardiac muscle cells contain an elaborate system of sER, referred to as the sarcoplasmic reticulum, which sequesters calcium ions released during stimulation of muscle contraction.

Ribosomes are either bound to the membranes of rER or present in the cytosol as free ribosomes. Each individual ribosome is formed from two spherical subunits of different sizes. The subunits contain several different proteins, all of which are synthesized in the cytosol, along with rRNA. A variety of cytosolic proteins enter the nucleus through the nuclear pores and are assembled with rRNA in the nucleolus. The immature ribosomal subunits then exit back to the cytoplasm through nuclear pores. Additional ribosomal proteins are incorporated into the ribosomal complex in the cytosol.

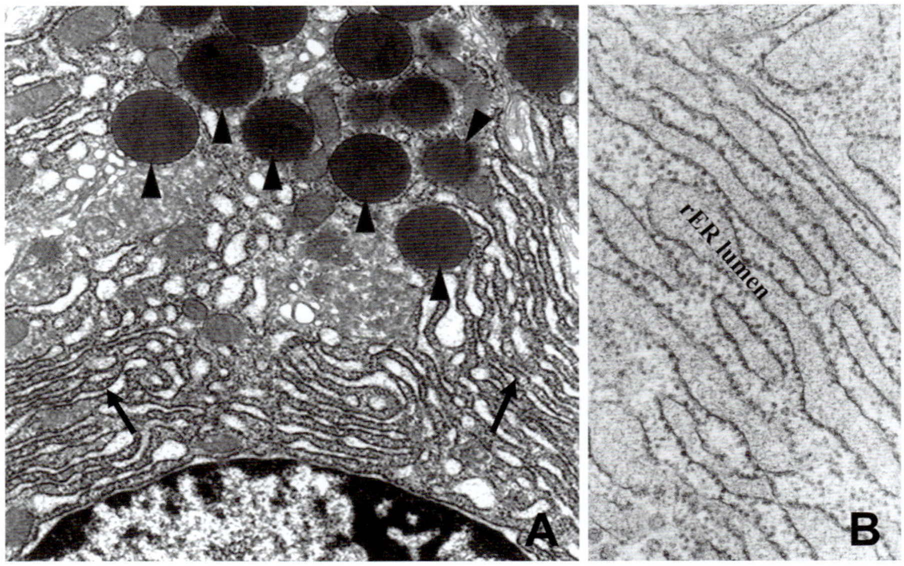

Figure 1-9 **A.** Electron micrograph showing a portion of a pancreatic zymogen cell containing abundant rough endoplasmic reticulum (rER) (arrows) and several secretory granules (arrowheads) (×6600). **B.** The outer surface of rER is densely studded with ribosomes, and its lumen is often dilated in cells undergoing active secretion, indicating protein synthesis (×24,000).

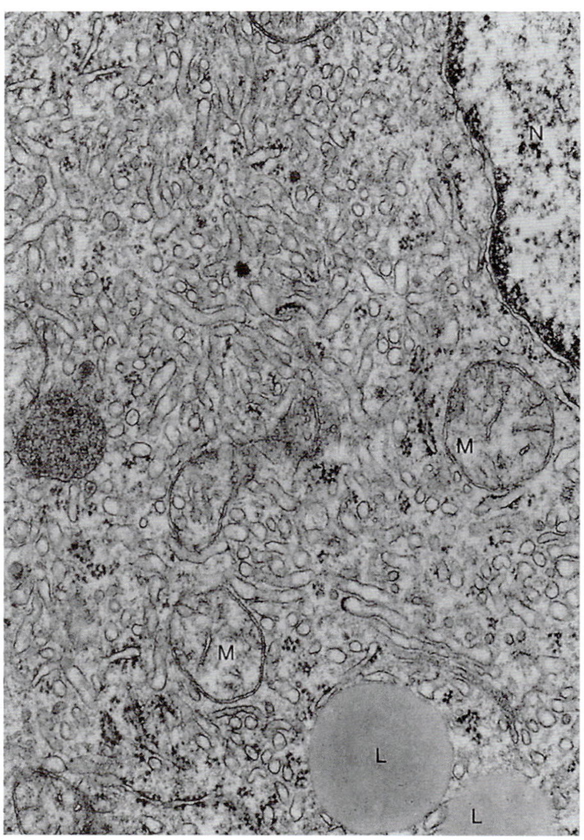

Figure 1-10 Electron micrograph of an adrenal cortical cell containing abundant smooth endoplasmic reticulum, mitochondria (M), and lipid droplets (L) clustered in the vicinity of the nucleus (N) (×27,000).

Proteins are synthesized through the transcription of genes in the nucleus, which results in the formation of **messenger RNAs** (mRNAs). These mRNAs are then exported to the cytosol, where they associate with ribosomal subunits. An mRNA may be simultaneously translated by multiple ribosomes, thus forming a polyribosome (polysome). Multiple **polyribosomes** are often dispersed throughout the cytoplasm of cells.

The nucleotide sequence of mRNA depends upon the sequence of the gene from which it was transcribed and subsequently encodes different proteins. All mRNAs bind to ribosomes at their initiator codon (AUG), which encodes the amino acid methionine and consists of adenine, uracil, and guanine. For every amino acid encoded in the mRNA sequence, there exists a corresponding **tRNA** that transports an amino acid to the mRNA–ribosome complex. The first tRNA carries methionine to the complex. Subsequently, the ribosome moves along the mRNA to the next codon and recruits the next corresponding tRNA. The amino acids released from the tRNAs are joined together by peptide bonds, forming a growing peptide chain that emerges from the mRNA–ribosome complex.

If a protein is predestined for incorporation into lysosomes, membrane insertion, or export from the cell, it will typically start with a short hydrophobic **signal peptide** sequence. This signal peptide binds to a **signal recognition particle** (SRP) present in the cytosol. The resulting complex then attaches to an **SRP receptor** on the cytosolic face of the rER, facilitating the threading of the protein into the cisternae of the ER. Once inside the rER, the protein undergoes several post-translational modifications, including the cleavage of the signal peptide as well as folding and glycosylation.

Cytosolic proteins that are destined to remain within the cell lack signal peptides and are synthesized by free ribosomes (not attached to the rER) in the cytosol.

Golgi Complex and Vesicular Transport

The **Golgi complex** consists of a series (usually 3 to 10) of flattened cisternae with a convex or ***cis*** side that is usually oriented toward the nucleus and a concave or ***trans*** side that generally faces the cell periphery (Fig. 1-11). At the *trans* side, anastomosing tubules and cisternae form the ***trans*-Golgi network** (TGN) (Fig. 1-12). In addition, small vesicles are present at the periphery of the cisternae, while larger vesicles or vacuoles are often detected at the trans side (Fig. 1-10). Although the Golgi complex can be visualized by silver impregnation in light microscopic preparations, electron microscopy is necessary to fully delineate its structure.

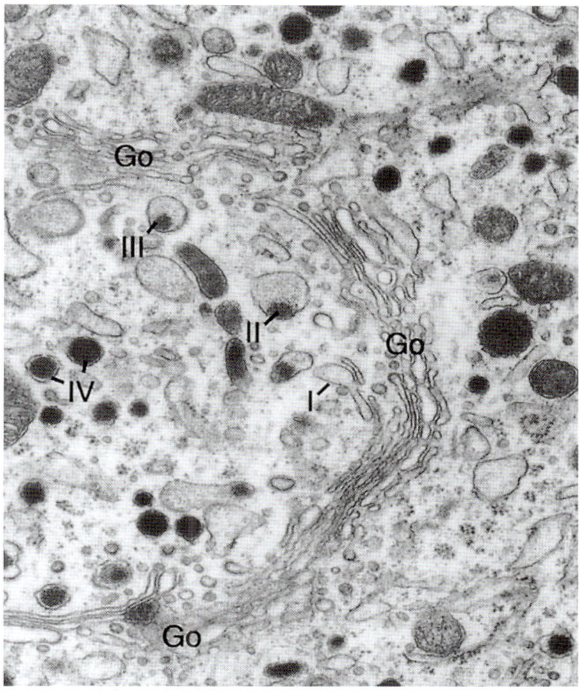

Figure 1-11 Electron micrograph of the Golgi complex (Go) and surrounding cytoplasm of an adenohypophysial cell. As the secretory granules mature, they move away from the concave (*trans*) side of the Golgi complex, and their contents become more electron dense. In the sequence of secretory vesicle maturation, vesicle I is the newest, while vesicle IV is the most mature (×23,700).

Transmembrane, secretory, and lysosomal proteins are transferred from the rER to the Golgi complex. Small transport vesicles filled with newly synthesized proteins bud off from the cisternae of the rER and fuse with the cisternae on the *cis* side of the Golgi complex (Fig. 1-12). Subsequently, the proteins from these vesicles are transported through the Golgi complex in a *cis*-to-*trans* direction. During this transport, the proteins become concentrated and undergo post-translational modifications, including glycosylation. At the *trans* side, appropriately modified proteins are sorted in the TGN and packaged in vesicles. Mannose-6-phosphate-containing lysosomal enzymes bind to specific mannose-6-phosphate receptors in the TGN and are packaged into vesicles destined to become primary lysosomes. Upon budding off from the TGN, these vesicles are coated with the protein **clathrin**.

In specialized digestive glands and hormone-producing cells, secretory products are packaged in condensing vacuoles that mature into **secretory granules** (Figs. 1-12 and 1-13). These granules remain in the cytoplasm until the cell receives a signal to secrete their contents, a process referred to as **regulated secretion**. When a signal is received, the membranes of the secretory vesicles fuse with the cell membrane, leading to the opening of an orifice through which the vesicle contents are expelled (secreted) through **exocytosis**. It is, of course, important that the vesicles fuse with the correct membrane in the cell. To achieve this, both vesicles and target membranes are equipped with complementary "address tags" referred to as **SNAREs** (*S*oluble *N*-ethylmaleimide-sensitive fusion protein *A*ttachment protein *RE*ceptors). The correct combination of vesicle SNAREs and target membrane SNAREs helps to ensure that the appropriate components will fuse.

While regulated secretion is primarily carried out by specialized secretory cells, all cells are capable of **constitutive secretion**, which is the continuous delivery of growth factors and components of membranes and the extracellular matrix to the cell surface. This delivery needs no specific stimulus and is exerted by small vesicles that continuously bud off from the trans region of the Golgi complex. These vesicles then fuse with the cell membrane, releasing their contents through exocytosis.

Both regulated and constitutive secretion result in the delivery of significant amounts of membrane material to the plasmalemma. This accumulation of membranes is balanced by a reverse process referred to as **endocytosis** (Fig. 1-12). Endocytosis involves the plasmalemma invaginating to form small vesicles that bud off into the cytoplasm. Different types of endocytosis occur depending upon the material ingested, and endocytosis serves many functions beyond membrane exchange. Ingestion of solid particulate material by endocytosis is referred to as **phagocytosis**. This process is characteristic of neutrophils and macrophages but can be executed by many different cell types. Phagocytosis serves as a defense mechanism against infectious organisms and aids in removing particles and cell debris. **Pinocytosis**, on the other hand, involves the uptake of fluid, while receptor-mediated endocytosis refers to the uptake of receptor-bound material. An example of **receptor-mediated**

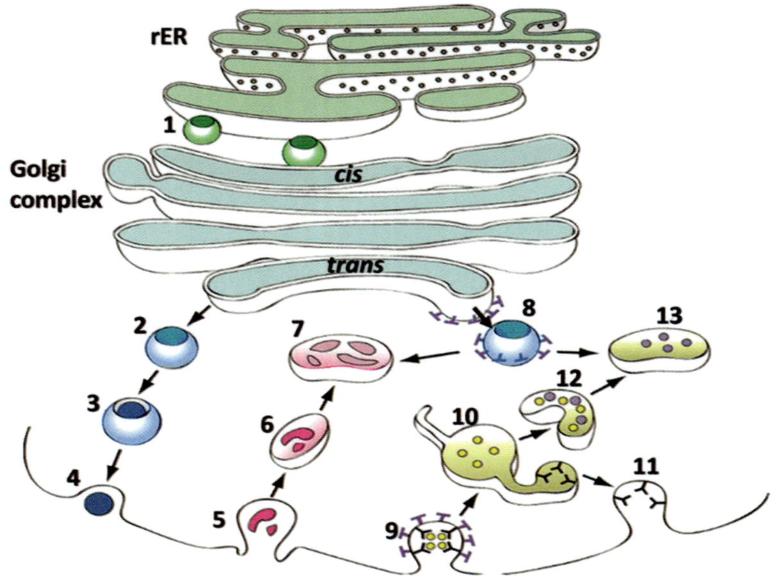

Figure 1-12 Schematic drawing illustrating transport of vesicles in the cell. Small transfer vesicles (1) bud off from the rER and fuse with the *cis* side of the Golgi complex. Secretory granules (2) form from vesicles budding from the *trans*-Golgi network (TGN). Mature secretory granules (3) release their contents through exocytosis (4). Particulate material is taken into the cell by phagocytosis (5), forming a phagosome (6). A secondary lysosome (7) is formed as the phagosome fuses with primary lysosomes (8), derived from clathrin (T)-coated vesicles budding from the TGN. During receptor-mediated endocytosis (9), receptors (Y) and their bound ligands are transferred to early endosomes (10). Dissociated receptors recycle back to the cell membrane through exocytosis (11), while ligands are transported by multivesicular bodies (12) to late endosomes (13). Late endosomes also fuse with primary lysosomes and mature into secondary lysosomes. Secondary lysosomes that contain undigested material may remain in the cell as residual bodies (not shown).

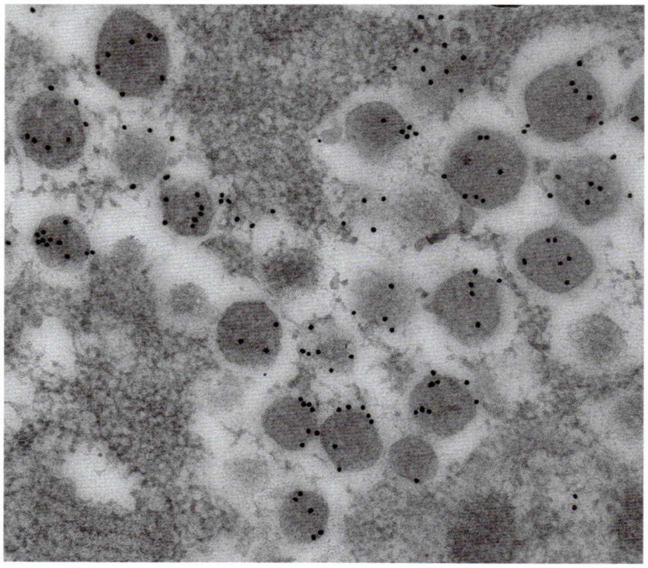

Figure 1-13 Electron micrograph depicting a portion of a pancreatic islet β cell, immunohistochemically stained with insulin antibodies conjugated to 18-nm gold particles. These gold particles appear as electron-dense black dots atop secretory granules storing insulin. Cells engaged in regulated secretion store numerous secretory granules within their cytoplasm. The different sizes and morphologies of these granules facilitate cell identification (×80,000).

endocytosis is the cellular uptake of low-density lipoproteins (LDLs). LDL particles bind to cell-surface receptors and accumulate in **coated pits**, which are clathrin-coated membrane invaginations (Fig. 1-12). These pits then invaginate further to form endocytotic vesicles with the receptor-bound LDL facing the inside. The vesicles transfer their contents to **early endosomes**, which consist of a system of membrane-delimited tubules and vesicles. The internal pH of endosomes is acidic, causing the LDL to dissociate from the receptors. Subsequently, free receptors become enriched in the tubular region of the endosome, which eventually pinches off to form shuttle vesicles that returns the receptors to the cell surface. Meanwhile, the free ligands are sorted to **multivesicular bodies** and further transferred to **late endosomes**. Late endosomes eventually fuse with primary lysosomes, transforming into **secondary lysosomes**. Controversy exists as to whether the different components of the endosomal system (endocytotic vesicles, early and late endosomes, and lysosomes) represent a maturing system or are separate structures shuttling components between themselves.

Transcytosis is the process used for transporting material through cells. Endocytosed material on one surface of a cell is transported through the cytoplasm and exocytosed on the opposite surface (Fig. 1-14). An example of transcytosis is the transport of material from the blood to nearby tissue fluid.

Lysosomal enzymes eventually degrade most extracellular material taken up by phagocytosis, pinocytosis, or receptor-mediated endocytosis, but they do not break down material undergoing transcytosis. These enzymes are sorted to primary lysosomes in the Golgi complex. **Primary lysosomes** are typically very small (down to 50 nm) and inconspicuous in most cells, but they can be larger (up to 500 nm) in specialized phagocytic cells such as neutrophils and macrophages. Material undergoing receptor-mediated endocytosis or pinocytosis passes from early endosomes to late endosomes. The late endosomes receive enzymes from primary lysosomes and then mature into **secondary lysosomes** (Fig. 1-12). Phagocytosed material in phagosomes does not pass through the endosomal structure; instead, it fuses directly with primary lysosomes. These fused structures are also referred to as **secondary lysosomes** or **phagolysosomes**. In addition, constituents of the cell itself can become engulfed into an **autophagosome.** This mechanism represents a way for the cell to digest aged or little-used organelles into useful metabolites. In secondary lysosomes, lysosomal hydrolytic enzymes digest the enclosed material. These enzymes can digest most cellular material and include acid phosphatase, ribonuclease, deoxyribonuclease, proteases, lipases, sulfatases, and β-glucuronidase. All these enzymes have an acidic pH, and a proton pump of the lysosomal membrane ensures that the lysosomal interior is optimally acidic. Despite the multitude of enzymes, some indigestible material remains and is retained within the secondary lysosome, forming a **residual body**. In long-lived cells such as neurons, cardiac myocytes, and liver cells, the gradual accumulation of residual bodies results in the formation of a yellowish-brown age pigment, **lipofuscin** (Fig. 1-15).

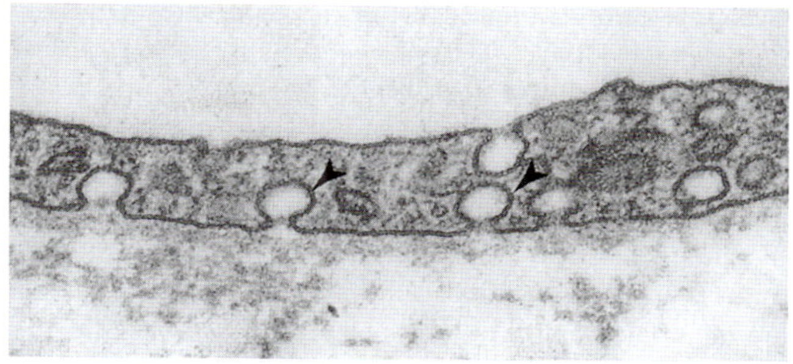

Figure 1-14 Transcytotic vesicles (arrowheads) form at the cell membrane and are present in the cytoplasm of a capillary endothelial cell. The Ω shape of the vesicles indicates that they are in the process of forming or fusing with the plasma membrane (×76,000).

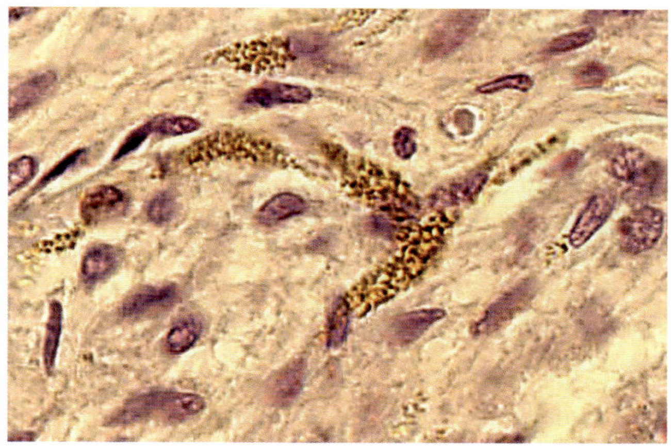

Figure 1-15 Lipofuscin granules, shown as yellowish-brown pigments, are observed in several pituicytes of an aged neurohypophysis. H&E (×800).

Mitochondria

Mitochondria are spherical to oblong membrane-delimited organelles that typically range from 0.3 to 1 μm in diameter and can extend up to 20 μm in length. They become visible under the light microscope when stained with cytochemical methods or vital dyes. Ultrastructurally, mitochondria are bounded by **outer** and **inner membranes** that are separated by an **intermembrane space**. In the classical interpretation of mitochondrial ultrastructure, the inner membrane is folded into **cristae** (Fig. 1-16), which limit a finely granular **matrix** in the intercristal space. Modern microscopic techniques have shown that the cristae also connect to the inner membrane via fine tubules. While most cells contain mitochondria with shelf-like cristae, steroid-producing cells have tubular cristae. While the outer mitochondrial membrane is permeable to many molecules, transport across the inner membrane requires specific channels or carriers.

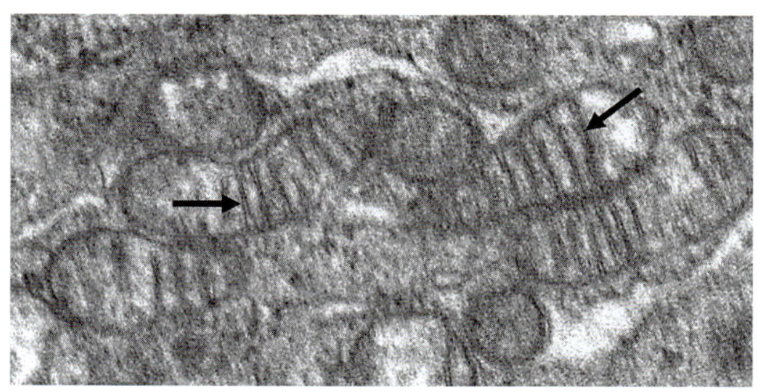

Figure 1-16 Electron micrograph showing mitochondria with cristae (arrows) in a skeletal muscle cell (×60,000).

The mitochondrial matrix contains the majority of the enzymes involved in the citric acid cycle and fatty acid oxidation. Additionally, the inside of each crista is studded with 8.5 nm particles involved in the synthesis of **adenosine triphosphate** (ATP). The energy stored in ATP can easily be utilized by the many energy-demanding reactions in the cell. Thus, the primary function of mitochondria is to convert the inaccessible energy stored in fuels such as glucose and fatty acids into the easily accessible form of ATP.

A process known as **oxidative phosphorylation**, which consumes about 80% of inhaled O_2 and produces CO_2, facilitates this transformation. Glucose metabolism (glycolysis) in the cytoplasm leads to the formation of pyruvate, which is subsequently converted into acetyl-coenzyme A (acetyl-CoA) within the mitochondria. Additionally, mitochondrial fatty acid oxidation yields acetyl-CoA. Acetyl-CoA enters the **citric acid cycle**, which produces nicotinamide adenine dinucleotide (NADH) and flavin adenine dinucleotide ($FADH_2$). Electrons from these molecules traverse carriers in the inner mitochondrial membrane to O_2, and this movement is coupled to the pumping of H^+ ions into the intermembrane space. This process establishes an electrochemical gradient, driving the flow of H^+ through a proton channel that is coupled to the 8.5-nm ATP synthase particles. The narrow tubular connections between the inner membrane and the cristae may compartmentalize the proton gradient and minimize proton leakage through the outer mitochondrial membrane. The flow of protons drives ATP synthesis, with an abundance of cristae increasing the area available to harbor ATP synthase particles. Cells with high-energy demands, such as cardiac muscle cells and flight muscle cells, contain mitochondria with numerous cristae. A protein, **thermogenin**, creates a proton pore in the inner mitochondrial membrane, bypassing the transport of protons through the ATP synthase particles. This uncoupling of oxidative phosphorylation produces heat instead of ATP and is used by hibernating animals, those adapted to cold climates, and newborns to maintain body temperature. Thermoregulation of this type mainly occurs in brown adipose tissue, which has mitochondria rich in thermogenin.

The mitochondrial matrix also contains electron-dense bodies that are rich in calcium in some cell types, although the function of these **dense bodies** remains unknown. Also, the matrix contains the circular DNA of mitochondria, which resembles bacterial DNA, as well as rRNA, mRNA, and tRNA. Some mitochondrial proteins are encoded by mitochondrial DNA and synthesized within the mitochondria, while others are synthesized in the cytosol. The mitochondrial ribosomes are distinct from eukaryotic ribosomes and resemble bacterial ribosomes. Mitochondria are present only in eukaryotes, and it is believed that mitochondria are antecedents of aerobic bacteria that have entered a symbiotic relationship with primitive anaerobic eukaryotic cells. During cell division, mitochondria duplicate their own DNA and divide through a process akin to bacterial fission. Additionally, mitochondria undergo division in response to specific demands, such as following exercise. Under special circumstances, changes in mitochondrial permeability can lead to leakage of an electron carrier, cytochrome C, from the intermembrane space, triggering programmed cell death (apoptosis).

Peroxisomes

Peroxisomes (microbodies) are spherical, membrane-delimited organelles ranging from 0.2 to 1.2 μm in diameter. In some species, they contain a paracrystalloid inclusion. Their name is derived from their ability to metabolize hydrogen peroxide. Peroxisomes contain catalase, which converts hydrogen peroxide into water and oxygen, as well as enzymes involved in the oxidation of fatty acids. Like fatty acid oxidation in mitochondria, peroxisomal fatty acid oxidation also produces acetyl-CoA. However, peroxisomal acetyl-CoA is not used for ATP synthesis but rather is transported to the cytosol, where it participates in different synthetic pathways. Peroxisomes also contain enzymes that oxidize substrates such as L- and D-amino acids while reducing oxygen and hydrogen peroxide. Peroxisomal proteins are synthesized in the cytosol and contain a short amino acid sequence recognized by a receptor in the peroxisomal membrane, facilitating their import into the organelle. Peroxisomes increase in number by division.

Cytoskeleton

The term cytoskeleton is misleading in that it covers structures that function to maintain not only cell shape but also the motility and intracellular transport functions of the cell. There are three main components of the cytoskeleton: microtubules, microfilaments, and intermediate filaments.

Microtubules

Microtubules (Fig. 1-17) play crucial roles in the transport of vesicles and other organelles within the cytoplasm, chromosome separation during cell division, and the motility of cilia and flagella. Each microtubule consists of 13 parallel rows of protofilaments, forming hollow tubes that are 25 nm in diameter. These protofilaments are composed of subunits formed from two proteins, **α**- and **β-tubulin** (Fig. 1-18). Microtubules grow outward from the **microtubule organizing center**, or **centrosome**, situated near the nucleus (Fig. 1-17). Inside the centrosome, two **centrioles** are present, composed of microtubules arranged as nine peripheral triplets and positioned perpendicular to each other (Fig. 1-1). The centrioles are

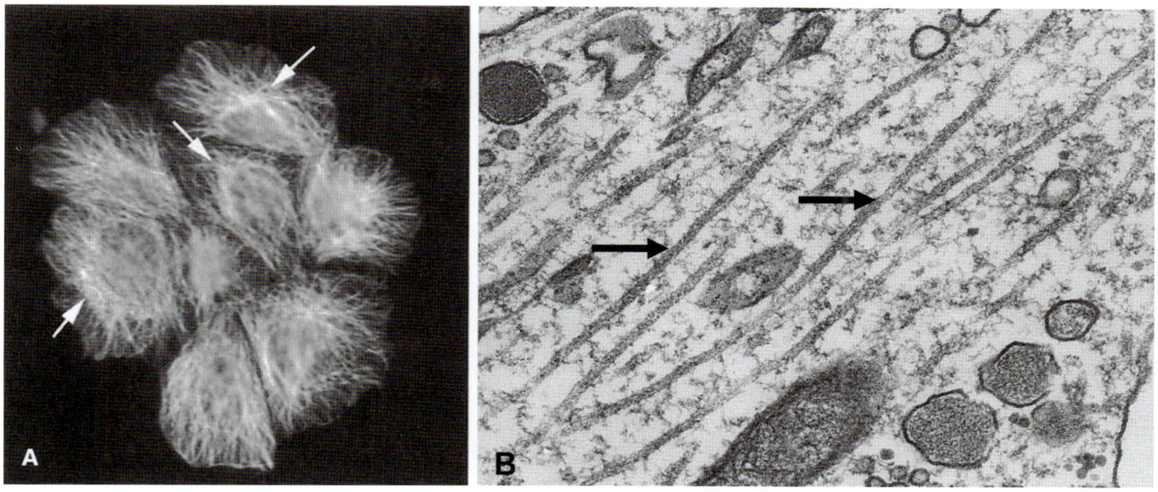

Figure 1-17 **A.** Immunohistochemical staining for tubulin in cultured mammary epithelial cells. Antitubulin antibodies labeled with a fluorescent dye have been used, and microtubules appear in the fluorescence microscope as white structures on a dark background. Note that microtubules converge at microtubule organizing centers close to the nuclei (arrow). **B.** Microtubules (arrows) in axons of neurosecretory neurons (×63,000).

believed to attract centrosome proteins important for tubulin polymerization. Unlike the microtubules of centrioles, cytoplasmic microtubules do not extend directly. Instead, they polymerize on rings of γ-tubulin located near the centrioles. These cytoplasmic microtubules are polarized and exhibit rapid growth at their plus (β-subunit) end. The minus end of the microtubule may either remain attached to the centrosome (e.g., during mitosis) or detach from it, with detached microtubules maintaining their orientation, with their minus end closest to the centrosome. Cytoplasmic microtubules are in equilibrium with free microtubular subunits in the cytosol, and they constantly grow and shrink by a process dependent upon the hydrolysis of guanosine triphosphate. In contrast, microtubules present in cilia and flagella remain stable and do not change in size.

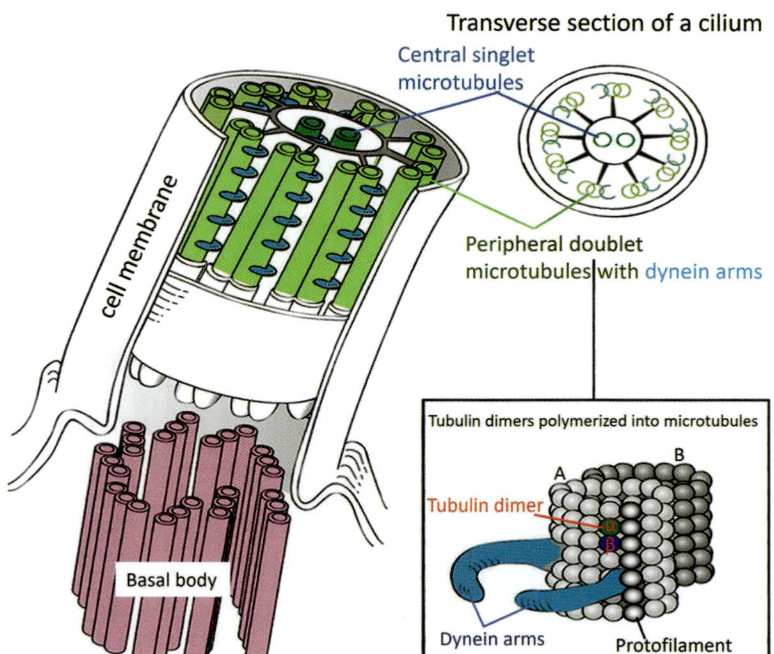

Figure 1-18 Diagram of the structure of a cilium. Nine doublet microtubules are found in the peripheral region of the cilium while two singlets occupy the center, α- and β-tubulin subunits are indicated in the paired microtubules (lower right drawing). Dynein arms extend from the A microtubule to contact the B microtubule of an adjacent doublet. A basal body with nine sets of triplet microtubules is shown at the base of the cilium.

Two **motor proteins**, kinesin and dynein, are important for microtubule function. Kinesin transports vesicles and other materials from the minus end of the microtubules toward the cell periphery (anterograde), while dynein transports vesicles and other materials in the opposite direction (retrograde). Both motor proteins bind to their cargo and "walk" along the microtubule in either the plus (kinesin) or minus (dynein) direction, deriving energy from the hydrolysis of ATP during the process. In developing cells, kinesins pull the ER outward toward the cell periphery, while dyneins pull the Golgi complex in the opposite direction. Retrograde transport up axon microtubules within peripheral nerves can carry viruses (rabies and encephalitis) into the central nervous system.

Microfilaments

Microfilaments (7 nm) are comprised of the protein **actin**. Together with thicker filaments (15 nm) composed of the protein **myosin**, actin constitutes the main protein involved in muscle contraction. In skeletal muscle, actin makes up 10% of all proteins. However, actin is also an abundant protein (1 to 5%) in nonmuscle cells. Actin occurs as a monomer (G-actin), which can polymerize to form 7-nm thick microfilaments (also referred to as actin filaments or F-actin) (Fig. 1-19). Like microtubules, actin filaments are polarized with a plus end and a minus end, enabling the directional movement of motor proteins (in this case, myosin). Microfilaments are also numerous in the cell cortex underlying the plasmalemma. Here, actin filaments associate with transmembrane proteins and stabilize cell shape while simultaneously restricting protein mobility. Receptor-bound hormones and growth factors also interact with cortical actin filaments. At the end of mitosis, actin and myosin filaments form a band that eventually separates the daughter cells from each other. Exposure of cells to agents that stimulate cell migration results in reorganization of the actin cytoskeleton and overlying plasmalemma into finger- or leaf-like projections known as **filopodia** and **lamellipodia**, respectively. These projections probe the cell surroundings prior to the formation of specialized matrix receptors (integrins), which bind to ECM proteins and form focal adhesions. Integrins connect intracellularly to sturdy stress fibers consisting of multiple strands of actin filaments that anchor the cell to its site of attachment. Actin filaments also participate in cell-to-cell adhesion phenomena at zonulae adherens junctions and in supporting microvilli (Fig. 1-21B).

Intermediate Filaments

The diameter of **intermediate filaments** (10 nm) lies between that of thin microfilaments (actin, 7 nm) and thick microfilaments (myosin, 15 nm). Intermediate filaments are not polarized and therefore are not engaged in intracellular transport; instead, they perform anchoring and structural functions. Several different families of intermediate filaments exist, including **keratins** (cytokeratins), **vimentin**, **desmin**, **glial fibrillar acidic protein**, and **neurofilaments**. In addition, filaments that associate with the nuclear lamina (lamins) belong to this group. Keratins are associated with most epithelial cells (Fig. 1-20). Vimentin is expressed by most cells of mesenchymal origin, while desmin is typical in smooth, cardiac, and skeletal muscle cells. Glial fibrillar acidic protein is found in glial cells, while neurofilaments are present in neurons. Certain tumor cells can continue to express the original form of intermediate filaments, allowing immunohistochemistry of the filaments to be used to determine the cell type of origin of the tumor.

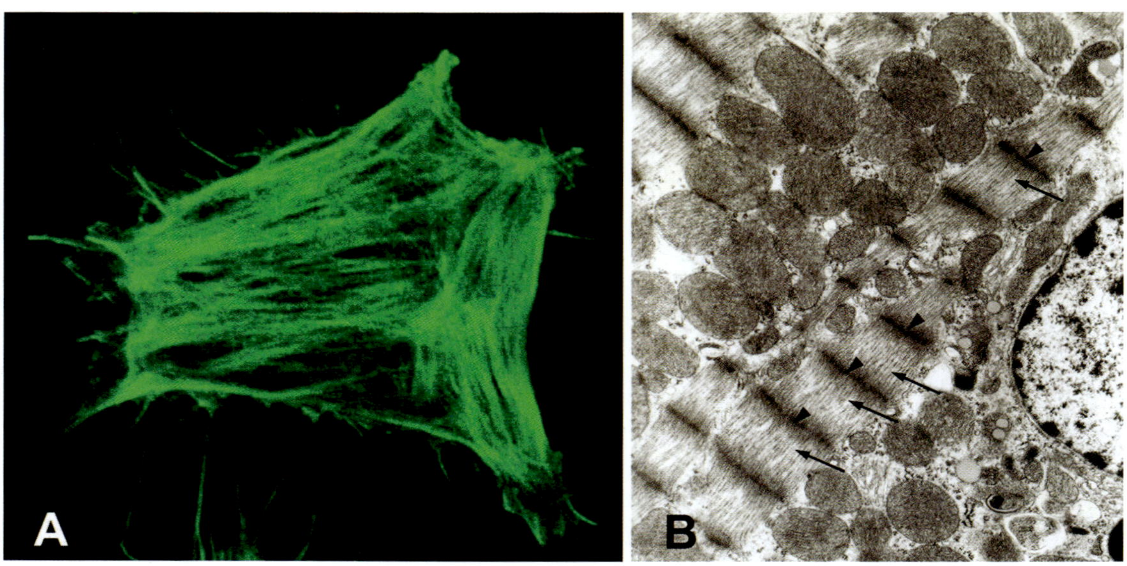

Figure 1-19 **A.** Epithelial cells in culture are stained with phalloidin conjugated with fluorescein isothiocyanate (FITC) to visualize actin filaments (F-actin). Note that F-actin is present in the cell cortex as straight stress fibers underlying the plasmalemma, as well as in hair-like filopodia (×800). **B.** Under the electron microscope, the actin filaments (arrows) in muscle cells are anchored to the electron-dense Z lines (arrowheads) and are well organized in a regularly banded pattern (×20,000).

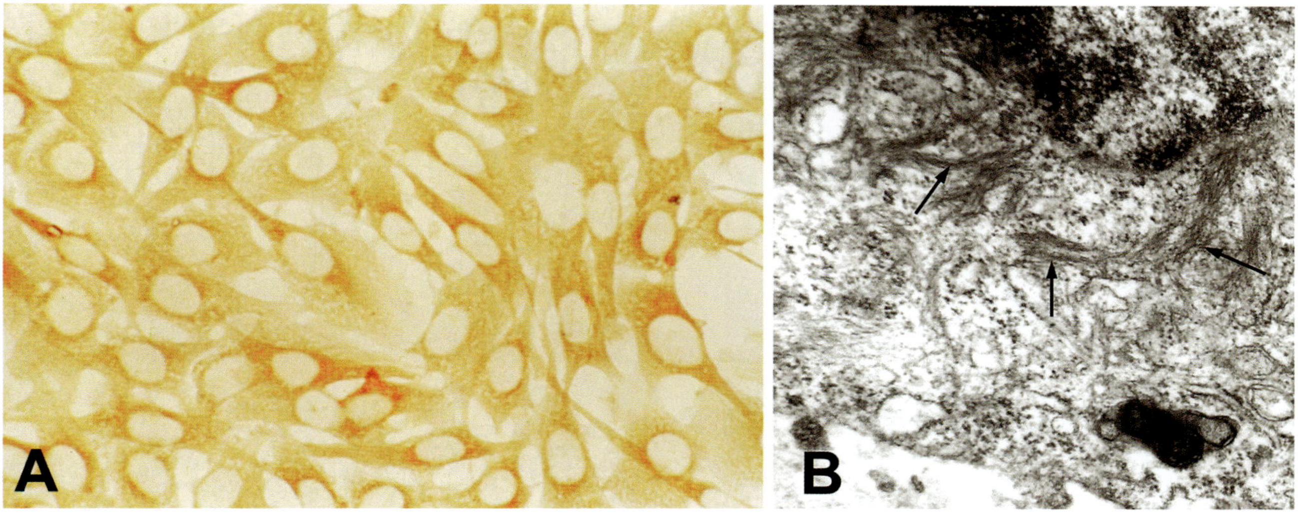

Figure 1-20 **A.** Immunocytochemistry staining shows that thymic epithelial cells in culture contain abundant cytokeratin (brown), a prominent protein component of intermediate filaments in cells with epithelial origin (×400). **B.** Under the electron microscope, the intermediate filaments are organized in bundles (arrows) within the cytoplasm (×20,000).

Inclusions

The cytosol contains several deposits of materials that do not participate in specific chemical reactions and are therefore not classified as organelles. Such inclusions encompass the following substances: (a) **Lipid droplets** (Fig. 1-10), which occur in adipocytes, adrenal cortical cells, and liver cells. In ordinary light microscopic preparations, lipids are dissolved, leaving unstained areas in the cytoplasm. In frozen sections, lipids are retained and can be detected by special dyes such as osmic acid, which imparts a dark coloration of lipids in light and electron micrographs. (b) **Glycogen** deposits, which are frequent in liver and muscle cells. Glycogen is normally not discernible in the light microscope but can be detected by special stains such as PAS or Best's carmine. In the electron microscope, glycogen is seen as fine electron-dense granules and aggregates. (c) **Pigments** such as **lipofuscin** in aging cells, melanin in pigmented cells, and **hemosiderin** derived from the breakdown of hemoglobin. Lipofuscin inclusions (residual bodies) appear light brown in the light microscope and are often seen close to the nucleus in aging cells (Fig. 1-15). Their formation has been described in conjunction with lysosomes, which accumulate the pigment. Melanin inclusions are detectable as minute dark granules present in pigmented epidermal cells, melanocytes, and certain types of neurons, while hemosiderin is a golden-brown pigment detected in macrophages that have phagocytosed red blood cells.

Cell-Surface Modifications

Microvilli are fingerlike projections of the cell membrane that increase the surface area of absorptive cells. Each individual microvillus is so small that can only be resolved using electron microscopes. Under a light microscope, the tightly packed microvilli are collectively identified as the **brush border**, a fuzzy fringe at the surface of the absorptive epithelium (Fig. 1-21A). Microfilaments constitute the core structure of the microvilli (Fig. 1-21B). **Stereocilia** represent a longer variant of microvilli. Both microvilli and stereocilia are nonmotile.

Ciliated cells have numerous, 2- to 10-µm long motile **cilia** on their cell surface that beat in a synchronous manner to produce unidirectional transport of material (Fig. 1-21C). Thus, in the respiratory tract, cilia transport mucus and particles in an oral direction. Flagellated cells, like spermatozoa, normally have a single **flagellum**. The structure of cilia and flagella is very similar (Figs. 1-18 and 1-21D). Both cilia and flagella are delimited by the cell membrane and contain a central region (**axoneme**) characterized by nine peripheral pairs (doublets) plus two central singlets of microtubules. The central singlets of microtubules are separated from the peripheral pairs by a central sheath. A peripheral doublet consists of one

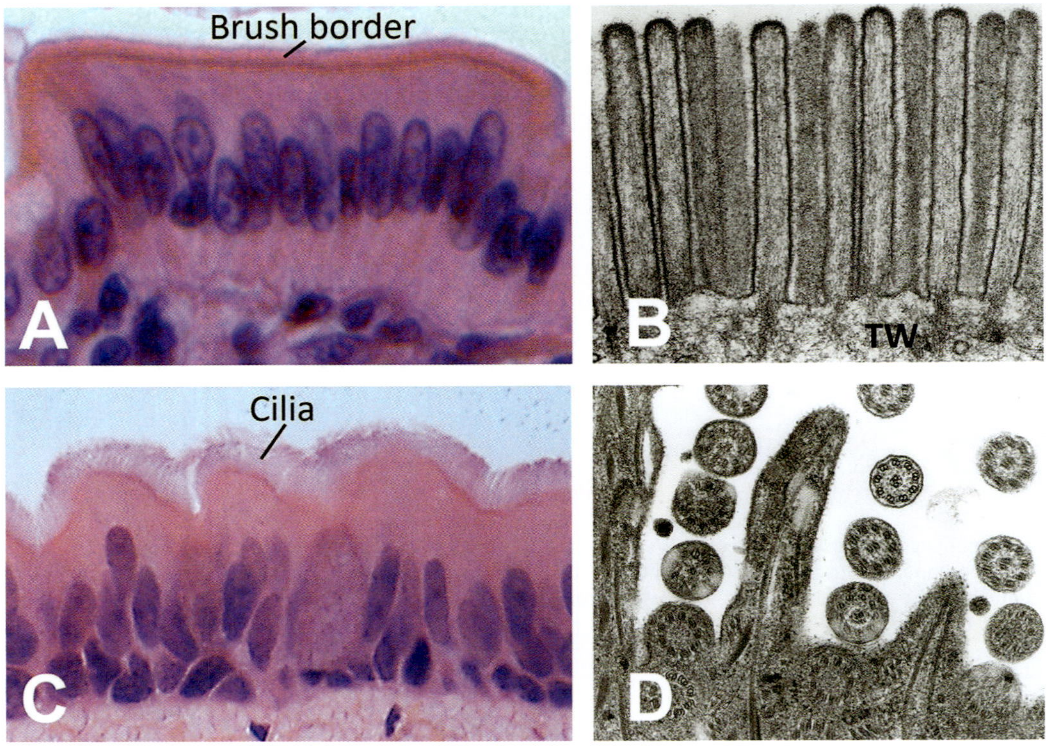

Figure 1-21 **A.** Microvilli in small intestine absorptive epithelial cells are identified as a fuzzy brush border at the apical surface under a light microscope. H&E (×800). **B.** Electron micrograph shows that the brush border is made of tightly packed microvilli containing numerous microfilaments that project into the terminal web (TW) (×51,000). **C.** Cilia on the apical surface of bronchus respiratory epithelial cells under a light microscope. H&E (×800). **D.** Electron micrograph shows that the axonemes of cilia are characterized by nine peripheral doublets plus two central singlets of microtubules (×51,000).

complete A microtubule (composed of 13 protofilaments) and one incomplete B microtubule that shares part of its wall with the A microtubule. The nine peripheral A plus B doublets are connected to each other by protein (nexin) bridges and to the central sheath by radial spokes. Arms of the motor protein **dynein** extend from the A microtubules. During ciliary movement, the dynein arms attach to B microtubules of the adjacent doublet. Because nexin protein bridges connect the microtubules, they cannot slide past each other. Instead, the movement of dynein in the minus direction is translated into a bending motion, which forms the basis for the motility of flagella of spermatozoa and for the ciliary stroke of respiratory epithelium. At the base of each cilium or flagellum, a basal body is present. Like centrioles, basal bodies have nine peripheral triplets of microtubules and no central microtubules. The A and B microtubules of the cilium or flagellum continue directly into the corresponding microtubules of the basal bodies. The central microtubules of the axoneme terminate before the centriole, and the third microtubule of the **basal body** triplets does not extend into the axoneme. Certain plants contain colchicine, which prevents the formation of microtubules. This substance inhibits cell division and vesicle transport and may cause death in cattle feeding on such plants.

Cell Cycle, Cell Division, and Apoptosis

Somatic cells multiply by mitosis, while gametes increase in number through a more complex process referred to as meiosis (see Chapter 13). Before a cell undergoes mitosis, it must duplicate its content of genetic information so that the resulting two daughter cells will contain the same amount of DNA as the parental cell. In addition, since the cytoplasm and organelles are divided between the daughter cells during cytoplasmic division, it is also necessary for the parental cell to increase its size through growth before division. The cell therefore goes through a series of definable steps referred to as the **cell**

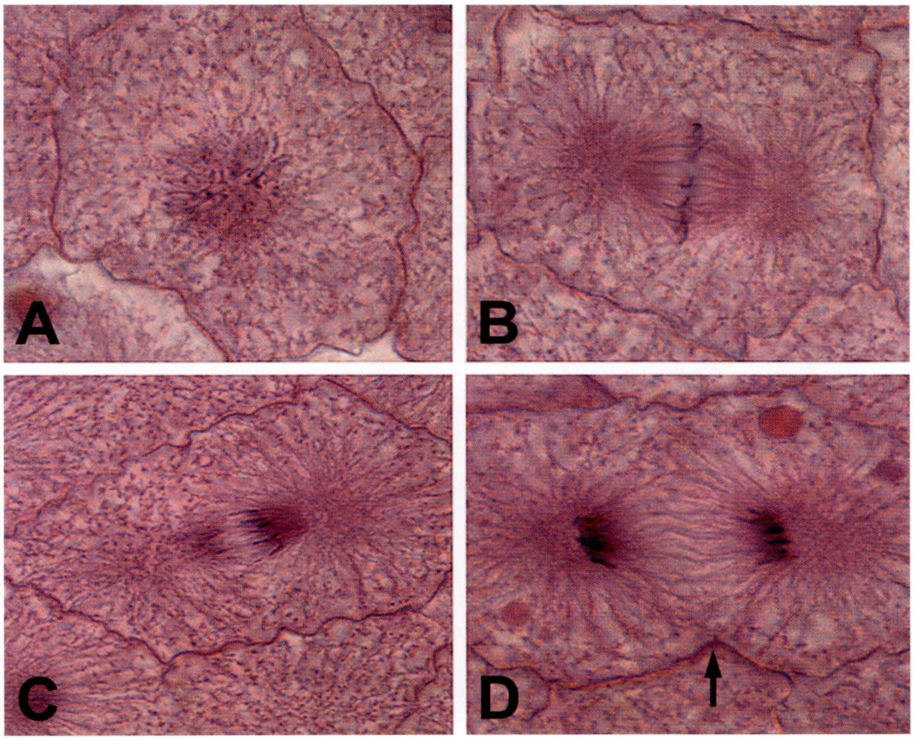

Figure 1-22 **A.** Prophase. **B.** Metaphase. **C.** Anaphase. **D.** Telophase in fetal oral epithelium, stained with iron–hematoxylin (×1000). Note the centrosome and part of the microtubules of the spindle apparatus in **B** and **C** and observe the cleavage furrow (arrow) in **D**.

cycle. These steps are **G1** (gap l), **S** (synthesis of DNA), **G2** (gap 2), and M (mitosis). During **G1**, the cell grows and receives signals (growth factors) from its surroundings that order it to commence preparations for mitosis. While in the **S** phase, the cell doubles its DNA. During **G2**, the cell grows further, checks the quality of the DNA it replicated during the **S** phase, and synthesizes proteins (such as tubulin subunits) needed for the **M** phase. After mitosis, the daughter cells may enter either a new cell cycle or a resting stage (**G0**). Ordered transition through each of these steps is required. At critical checkpoints, the cell will determine if it is of the correct size and if DNA has been correctly replicated. Before proceeding to the next step of the cell cycle, appropriate signals must be received from neighboring cells. Progression is controlled by special proteins called **cyclins.** Different cyclins are needed at different checkpoints and will activate enzymes (**cyclin-dependent kinases** or CDKs) that make it possible for a cell to continue to the next step. Thus, the cell cycle is tightly controlled. Failure of the cell to produce the right cyclin at the right time will stop cell cycle progression and may even result in the demise of the cell through apoptosis. If the cell cycle progresses, the cell will enter mitosis.

Mitosis is characterized by the following morphologically distinguishable phases: prophase, metaphase, anaphase, and telophase (Fig. 1-22). During **prophase** (Fig. 1-22A), chromatin gradually becomes more condensed, resulting in the formation of individual, discernible chromosomes, which stain intensely with hematoxylin or other basic dyes. In addition, nucleoli disappear, and the centrosome divides into two centrosomes that migrate to opposite poles of the cell and begin to organize microtubules into the mitotic spindle. At a later stage of prophase (often termed prometaphase), the nuclear envelope disappears. This is brought about by phosphorylation of the nuclear lamins through an M-phase-promoting CDK, leading to electrostatic repulsion between lamin subunits and ensuing breakdown of the nuclear lamina.

During **metaphase** (Fig. 1-22B), the chromosomes become oriented in the equatorial plane perpendicular to the centrosomes. In metaphase spread preparations (Fig. 1-23), the chromosomes are easily seen to be composed of two closely apposed, identical halves (**chromatids** or **sister chromatids**). The sister chromatids, formed earlier by DNA replication during the S phase, become visible due to increased coiling of the DNA. Chromatids are connected to each other at the **centromere**, which is a constricted, pale-staining structure that contains a protein complex, the **kinetochore**.

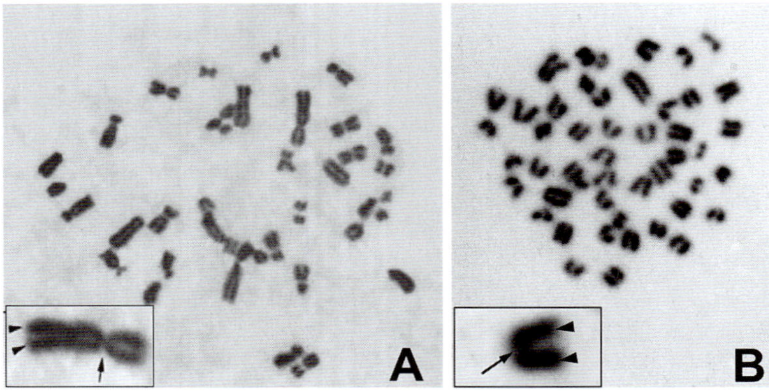

Figure 1-23 **A.** Metaphase chromosomes from a boar. **B.** Metaphase chromosomes from a murine cell line. Note sister chromatids (arrowheads) and centromeres (arrows) in the insets. Mouse chromosomes have centromeres close to one end and have no short arm.

The kinetochore is an attachment point for microtubules emanating from opposite centrosomes. Colchicine prevents polymerization of microtubules and arrests mitosis in metaphase. Techniques using colchicine are sometimes employed to obtain metaphase chromosomes for cytogenetic investigation (Fig. 1-23).

During **anaphase** (Fig. 1-22C), the two sister chromatids separate from each other and are drawn toward opposite centrosomes by the kinetochore microtubules. Anaphase ends when the sister chromatids (now called daughter chromosomes) have completely separated toward opposite sides of the cell.

During **telophase** (Fig. 1-22D), the nuclear envelope reappears, assisted by dephosphorylation of lamins. Chromosomes decondense, and nucleoli reappear. **Cytokinesis** takes place concomitantly with telophase, resulting in a **cleavage furrow** around the equatorial plane of the cell (Fig. 1-22D). This furrow is created by the contraction of actin and myosin filaments and will divide the cytoplasm into two halves surrounding each newly formed nucleus.

The frequency with which cells pass through the cell cycle and divide varies considerably. Certain cells in the adult animal are constantly renewed, such as intestinal absorptive cells, which are replaced every 3 to 5 days. Most cells are either in a permanent or a temporary resting (G0) phase. Some cells, such as neurons, lose their ability to divide in the adult animal and enter a permanent G0 state. Cells in a temporary G0 phase normally do not replicate but are able to do so if the need arises.

Induction of a cell to proliferate involves stimulation by growth factors that are important for activating the cell cycle in Gl. In tumor cells, mutations may result in autonomous activation of growth factor signaling mechanisms. This activation makes tumor cells oblivious to the controlled signaling mechanisms in the body, resulting in continuous proliferation of cells that pay no heed of their surroundings. Since every round of cell division carries the risk of inducing mutations, it is likely that these uncontrolled cells will eventually acquire further mutations that result in invasive, malignant behavior.

Safeguards to avoid mutation exist in the form of a cellular mechanism called **apoptosis** (also referred to as programmed cell death). Apoptosis is defined by a series of morphologic changes leading to the destruction of the cell. In tissue sections, apoptotic cells are recognized by the presence of condensed (**pyknotic**) nuclei due to the abnormal aggregation of heterochromatin, which can be observed under an electron microscope (Fig. 1-24, upper panel). At the late stage of apoptosis, the pyknotic nucleus eventually breaks down into fragments (**karyorrhexis**). The nuclear fragments are encased by corresponding fragments of cytoplasm to form **apoptotic bodies** that are later phagocytosed by surrounding cells. Upon activation of the apoptotic program, a series of biochemical reactions will ultimately destroy the cell's DNA by fragmentation. This can be detected *in situ* by the TUNEL (terminal deoxynucleotidyl transferase biotin-dUTP nick end labeling) method (Fig. 1-24, lower panel). Apoptosis plays a major role in the developmental sculpting of the organism and in the replacement of aged or infected cells.

From Cells to Tissues

In multicellular organisms, cells integrate themselves in a social context with other cells and assume specialized roles with functions that benefit the entire organism. The process of assuming specific functions is called cellular **differentiation**. Social interaction requires that cells make contact with other cells and with the ECM, resulting in the formation of tissues and organs. Moreover, the cells need to continue to communicate with each other by both local and global means.

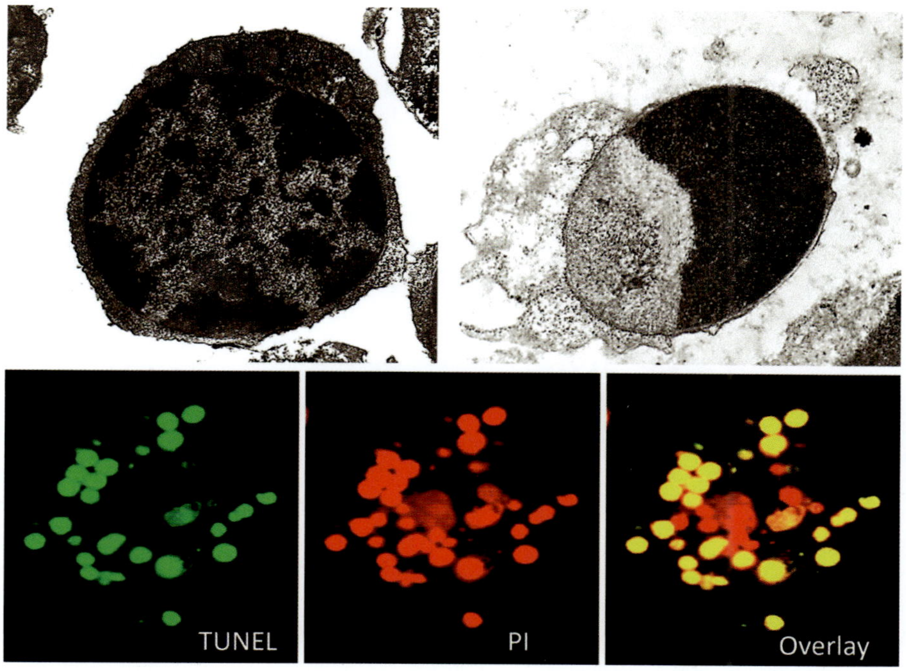

Figure 1-24 Electron micrograph of a normal thymocyte (upper left) and a thymocyte undergoing apoptosis (upper right) (×6600). Note the compromised nuclear structure of the apoptotic thymocyte, which has a large, crescent-shaped condensed heterochromatin aggregation. The confocal fluorescence microscope images at the lower panel show a cluster of apoptotic thymocytes with DNA fragmentation (green) detected by the TUNEL method being phagocytosed by a macrophage in culture. Propidium iodide (PI) counterstains the DNA after fixation (×800).

Intercellular Junctions

Several types of cell junctions (occluding, anchoring, and communicating) occur between cells (Fig. 1-25). Anchoring contacts are present between adjacent cells as well as between cells and the ECM. Occluding and communicating contacts only occur between cells. Intercellular contacts can be ring-shaped (zonulae) or spot-like (maculae).

The presence of occluding contacts between cells is characteristic of epithelial cells. In many epithelia, such as the lining of the gastrointestinal tract, the **zonula occludens** (tight junction) seals off the upper part of the epithelium. This mechanism prevents leakage of material from the lumen into the subepithelial space and vice versa. Additionally, the zonula occludens prevents free mobility of transmembrane proteins in the cell membrane. An individual zonula occludens joins two neighboring cells by a belt-like structure consisting of anastomosing ridges. The junction consists of transmembrane proteins, **occludin** and **claudin**, which join the two cell membranes together. Peripheral cytoplasmic proteins, ZO-1 and ZO-2, link claudin and occludin to spectrin, a structural protein within the cell.

Zonulae adherens and maculae adherens (desmosomes) form cell-to-cell anchoring contacts, while focal adhesions and hemidesmosomes form cell-to-ECM or cell-to-basement membrane contacts. **Zonulae adherens** are comprised of multiple anchoring transmembrane proteins known as **cadherins**. The extracellular region of a cadherin molecule engages in homophilic binding with a cadherin molecule extending from an adjacent cell, thus forming a protein bridge between the cells. Cadherin binding requires Ca^{2+}. Therefore, cell dispersal can often be achieved by restricting Ca^{2+} from cells. On the inside of the cell membrane, cadherins attach to linker proteins, which, in turn, connect to microfilaments. In zonulae adherens junctions, cadherins join microfilaments of neighboring cells into a network. The microfilaments connect with the **terminal web**, which represents a collection of actin, myosin, and keratin filaments (Fig. 1-21B). This connection effectively anchors cells to each other. Moreover, by interacting with myosin, the actin filaments can contract and alter the shape of the epithelium. It is believed that the contraction of actin–myosin filaments connected to zonulae adherens plays a role in the folding of the neuroectodermal epithelium that results in the formation of the neural tube. In tall columnar epithelium, zonulae adherens are present just below the zonulae occludens. Together,

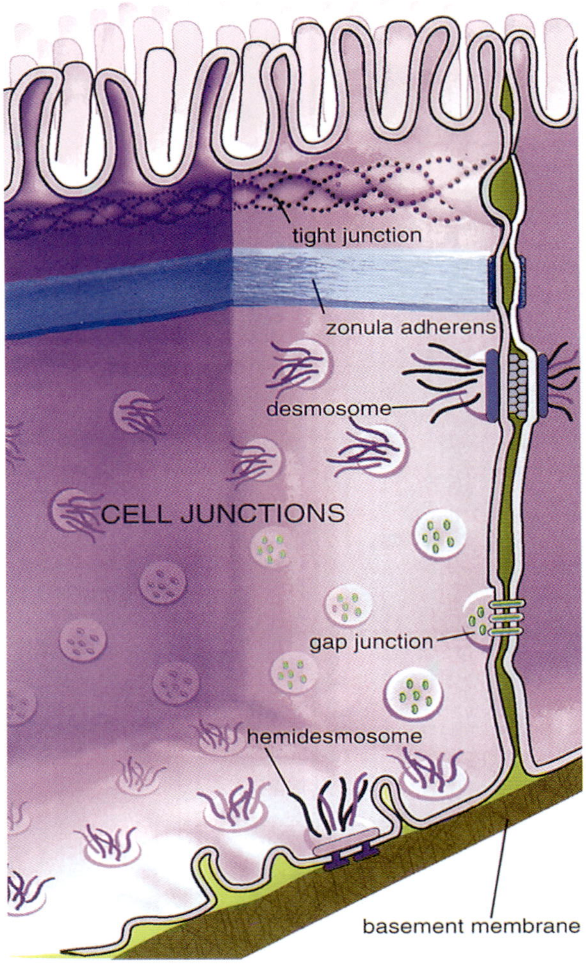

Figure 1-25 Diagrams of intercellular junctions: tight junction, zonula adherens, macula adherens (desmosome), hemidesmosome, and gap junction. (From: Eurell J. *Veterinary histology*. Jackson, WY: Teton NewMedia, 2004.)

these structures form the **terminal bar**, which appears as a dense condensation of the cell membrane when viewed with light microscopy.

Maculae adherens, or desmosomes, are 200- to 400-nm disk-like, cell-to-cell contacts that are particularly well developed in the epidermis of the skin. Like zonulae adherens junctions, maculae adherens have cadherins that function as junctional proteins. The cadherins attach to intracellular adaptor protein complexes that connect to intermediate filaments in neighboring cells, producing a very strong, point-like cell adhesion (Figs. 1-25). Ultrastructurally, maculae adherens are characterized by two prominent, dark-staining plaques located on the inside of the two adjacent cell membranes. These plaques correspond to the adaptor protein complexes. Intermediate filaments extend from the plaques into the cytoplasm. The adjacent cell membranes in the macula adherens are separated by a gap of about 30 nm, which often contains an electron-dense line (Fig. 1-26).

Hemidesmosomes connect cells to the basement membrane complex by way of specific cell-surface matrix receptor proteins called **integrins**. Like maculae adherens, hemidesmosomes connect intracellularly via adaptor proteins to intermediate filaments. Ultrastructurally, hemidesmosomes resemble half desmosomes with a plaque on the inside of the cell membrane from which **intermediate filaments** radiate into the cytoplasm. In the epidermis of the skin, maculae adherens anchor epidermal cells to each other along the lateral margins, while hemidesmosomes anchor cells to the basement membrane above the dermis. Mutations in keratin genes, integrins, or ECM proteins can produce painful diseases such as epidermolysis bullosa, characterized by blister formation due to defective anchoring of epidermal cells.

Focal adhesions also connect cells to the underlying matrix via integrins. The intracellular connection in focal adhesions is via microfilaments, similar to that of zonulae adherens junctions. Focal adhesions are not only involved in anchoring of cells but also have been implicated in cell motility and signaling.

Gap junctions (nexus) are communicating junctions that allow the passage of electrical signals, ions, and small water-soluble molecules (up to 1000 Da) between cells. At these junctions, neighboring cell membranes are separated by a 2- to 4-nm gap. Protein complexes known as **connexons** span the gap and form narrow channels through which small molecules may pass from one cell to another. Gap junctions occur in many cell types. For example, these communicating junctions are important for conducting electrical signals through intercalated disks of cardiac muscle cells, thereby contributing to a coordinated contraction wave throughout the heart muscle.

Cell Communication

Signals from other cells and from the ECM direct cellular functions and processes. Cell communication can be further described as endocrine, neurocrine, and paracrine. **Endocrine** signaling through hormones secreted into the blood and **neurocrine** signaling through neurotransmitters represent distant signaling pathways. **Paracrine** secretion is local transmission of signals to cells within diffusion distance. **Autocrine** signaling refers to a mechanism by which a cell signals to itself. This phenomenon is best known in cancer cells, which use autocrine secretion of growth factors to circumvent normal intercellular control, leading to increased tumor size. Signaling by endocrine, neurocrine, and paracrine mechanisms represents control mechanisms of the body that ensure that all differentiated cells function properly.

Proliferation is only stimulated when need arises and is controlled by **growth factors** that have cell and tissue selectivity. Examples of growth factors include erythropoietin, epidermal growth factor, and platelet-derived growth factor.

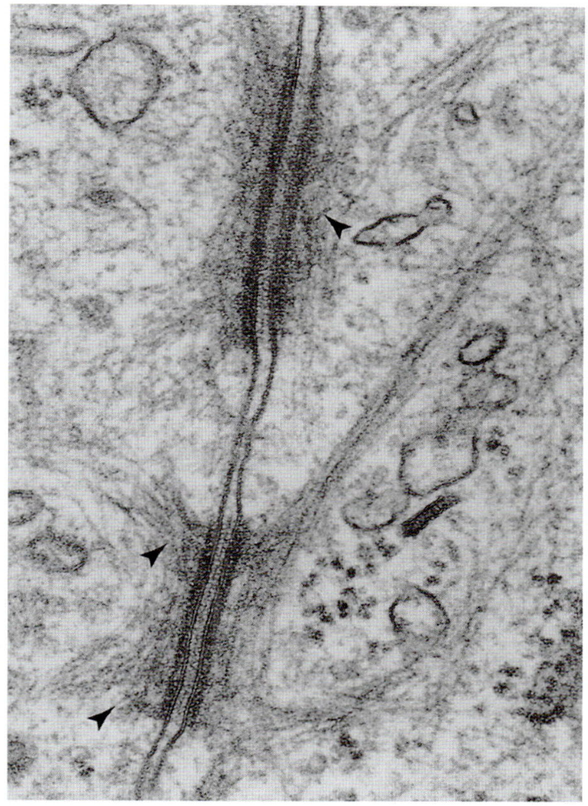

Figure 1-26 Maculae adherens between two neurohypophysial glial cells. Note the distinct central electron-dense lines and the intermediate filaments (arrowheads) that insert into the dense plaques and then make a hairpin turn back into the cytoplasm (×87,500).

Clinical Correlations

Tight (occluding) junctions in the central nervous system (CNS) contribute to the blood–brain barrier. Genetic defects in the connexin 40 gene in gap junctions result in cardiac conduction defects in dogs. Loss of dynein arms on cilia results in ciliary dyskinesia (Kartagener's syndrome), leading to poor respiratory clearance and reproductive sterility in dogs. Retrograde microtubule transport up nerve axons allows for viruses (e.g., rabies and encephalitis) to access the CNS.

Essentials

Interpretation of images relies, in part, on understanding what can or cannot be seen with different basic microscopes. Most of the initial study and/or diagnosis on histology and pathology relies upon H&E-stained sections. Further examinations require cyto/histochemistry and immunocyto/immunohisto-chemistry staining. Nucleus and nucleolus are the most detectable cell structures in H&E-stained sections, while organelles and cytoskeleton in general are not observable in such routine staining but require the transmission electron microscope. However, in some occasions, the accumulation of rER is detectable as the **basophilia** in H&E-stained sections due to its association with abundant mRNA, and Golgi apparatus is observed as a clear zone (lack of staining). **Inclusions:** Not all cell structures are due to organelles, and some structures are considered inclusions (pigments, lipid, crystalline material, storage-secretory granules, and glycogen).

Suggested Readings

Bystricky K. Chromosome dynamics and folding in eukaryotes: Insights from live cell microscopy. *FEBS letters*. 2015;589(20):3014–22.

Di Fiore PP, von Zastrow M. Endocytosis, signaling, and beyond. *Cold Spring Harbor perspectives in biology*. 2014;6(8):a016865.

Eurell J. Veterinary histology. Jackson, WY: Teton NewMedia, 2004.

Falahati H, Pelham-Webb B, Blythe S, Wieschaus E. Nucleation by rRNA dictates the precision of nucleolus assembly. *Current Biology*. 2016;26(3):277–85.

Lodish HF, Berk A, Kaiser CA, Krieger M. Molecular cell biology. 8th Ed. New York: W. H. Freeman & Co., 2016.

Munn EA. The structure of mitochondria. Academic Press; 2014 Jun 28.

Okumoto K, Tamura S, Honsho M, Fujiki Y. Peroxisome: metabolic functions and biogenesis. *Peroxisome Biology: Experimental Models, Peroxisomal Disorders and Neurological Diseases*. 2020:3–17.

Paz J, Lüders J. Microtubule-organizing centers: towards a minimal parts list. *Trends in cell biology*. 2018;28(3):176–87.

Perkins GA, Frey TG. Recent structural insight into mitochondria gained by microscopy. *Micron* 2002;31:97–111.

Pol A, Morales-Paytuví F, Bosch M, Parton RG. Non-caveolar caveolins–duties outside the caves. *Journal of cell science*. 2020;133(9):jcs241562.

2

Epithelium

John J. Turek and Marxa L. Figueiredo

CHAPTER MENU

Introduction

Cells, Tissues, and Organs

The animal body is composed of cells organized into tissues which then make up the various organs (Fig. 2-1). There are four basic types of tissue: **epithelium, connective tissue, muscle**, and **nervous tissue**.

Dellmann's Textbook of Veterinary Histology, Seventh Edition. Edited by Marxa L. Figueiredo and John J. Turek.

Companion website: www.wiley.com/go/figueiredo/vethistology7e

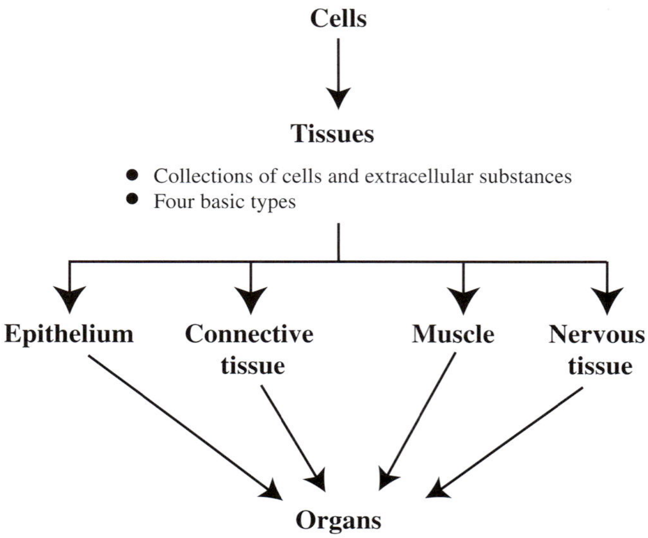

Figure 2-1 Structural organization of the animal body.

Table 2-1 Characteristics of Epithelium

Covers body surfaces (surface epithelium)
Forms secretory cells of glands (glandular epithelium)
Cells are functionally diverse
Cells contain cytoplasmic cytokeratin filaments
Cells are capable of mitosis (regeneration)
Contacts a basement membrane
Devoid of blood vessels (avascular)
Derived from each of the three embryonic germ layers

Characteristics of Epithelium

Epithelium exists in two major forms: surface epithelium and glandular epithelium. **Surface epithelium** consists of sheets of cells of similar type, which cover all of the external surfaces and line all of the internal surfaces of the body. **Glandular epithelium**, the secretory cells of endocrine and exocrine glands, results from the proliferation of surface epithelial cells into underlying connective tissue (CT). Table 2-1 summarizes the main characteristics of epithelium as a tissue.

Epithelial tissues are specialized for protection, absorption, secretion, and excretion, and form barriers for selective permeability. In mammals, all epithelial cells contain cytoplasmic filaments composed of the protein **cytokeratin**, an exception being endothelial cells. Cells not of epithelial origin (e.g., mesenchymal cells) lack cytokeratin. This characteristic is used in diagnostic pathology to identify the cell of origin of malignant neoplasms (cancers), which consist of cells that are unrecognizable by routine histologic methods.

At the basal surface of all epithelial cells there is an extracellular matrix material that is the **basement membrane**. In some organs, such as the trachea, the basement membrane is thick and can be observed with hematoxylin and eosin (H&E) staining. In most other organs, the basement membrane is not visible with H&E staining but can be demonstrated with the periodic acid-Schiff (PAS) technique or silver stains. In transmission electron microscopic images, the basement membrane beneath an epithelial cell is observed to consist of a basal lamina and a reticular lamina. The basal lamina has an electron-lucent region containing laminin and fibronectin (lamina lucida) and a denser region containing collagen IV (lamina densa) (Fig. 16-9). The basal lamina is linked via type VII collagen to an underlying reticular lamina (sublamina densa), composed of type III collagen and proteoglycans. These two laminae are synthesized by the epithelial cells. The reticular lamina is composed principally of reticular fibers (type III collagen) and connects the lamina densa to the subepithelial CT. In addition to providing attachment for the epithelium, this layer permits stretching and recoil of the epithelium in distensible organs. The basement membrane is described in greater detail in Chapter 16.

In addition to underlying all epithelia that contact CT, a basement membrane is found between two epithelial layers in both the renal corpuscle of the kidney and the pulmonary alveolus. In these locations, the reticular lamina is absent, and the structure is referred to simply as the **basal lamina**. A basal lamina also surrounds many individual cells, including smooth, skeletal, and cardiac muscle cells, as well as adipocytes and Schwann cells.

The basement membrane serves in a variety of purposes. In the renal corpuscle, it is an ultrafilter in capillaries and acts as a selective barrier to the exchange of macromolecules. Epithelia are avascular, and all epithelial cells receive their nutritional support by diffusion through the basement membrane from capillaries in the underlying connective tissue.

All three embryonic germ layers contribute to the formation of epithelium. **Ectoderm** gives rise to the epithelium of the external body surfaces, such as the epidermis of the skin. Most of the lining epithelium (i.e., that lining the luminal surfaces of the digestive and respiratory systems) originates from **endoderm**, while **mesoderm** gives rise to the lining of the vascular system, the lining of the serous membrane body cavities, and certain parts of the urinary and reproductive systems.

Surface Epithelium

Classification

Epithelial types are classified by the number of layers and the shape of the epithelial cells. A **simple epithelium** consists of a single layer of cells resting on a basement membrane. In contrast, a **stratified epithelium** has two or more cell layers, with only the basal layer attached to the basement membrane. The stratified epithelia are categorized based on the shape of the surface cells. A surface epithelium is considered **pseudostratified** if all of its cells contact the basement membrane but not all extend to the free surface. As a result, nuclei are located at different levels within a pseudostratified epithelium, giving the impression of stratification. Fig. 2-2 depicts the classification of epithelial tissue.

Microscopic Structure

Simple Squamous Epithelium

Simple squamous epithelium consists of a single layer of thin, flat, scale-like cells. On surface view (Figs. 2-3A and 2-4), the cells exhibit an irregular shape with a slightly serrated border and fit together to form a continuous sheet. The nucleus, typically spherical to oval in shape, is centrally located within the cell. In cross section, the cell appears thicker in the region of the nucleus and exhibits thin, attenuated strands of cytoplasm on either side (Fig. 2-4).

Simple squamous epithelium lines the internal serous membranes of body cavities and the internal surface of the circulatory system (heart, blood, and lymph vessels). The simple squamous epithelium lining the serous membrane body cavities (pleural, pericardial, and peritoneal cavities) is referred to as **mesothelium**, while the lining of the circulatory system is referred to as **endothelium**. Simple squamous epithelium is also found lining the pulmonary alveoli, the anterior chamber of the eye, the internal surface of the tympanic membrane, the membranous labyrinth of the internal ear, the glomerular capsule, and a portion of the loop of the nephron.

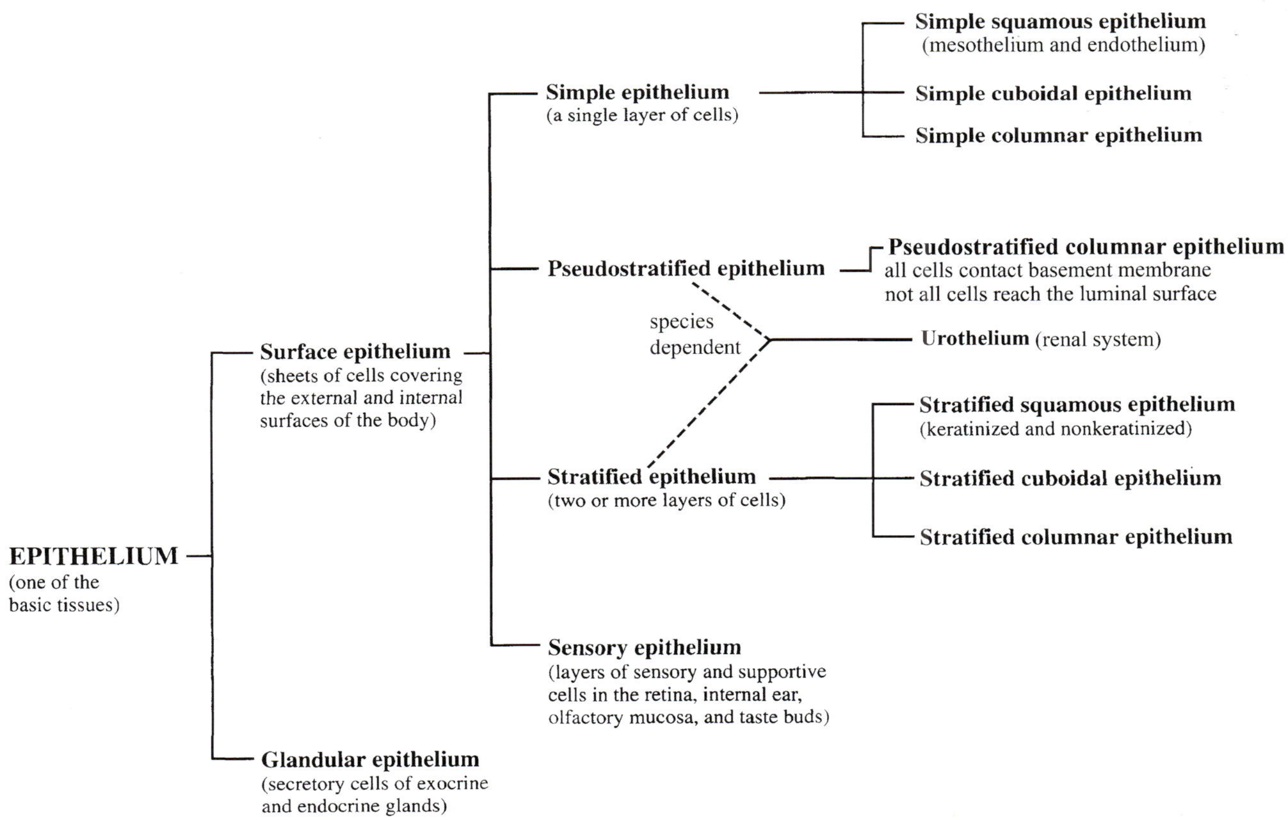

Figure 2-2 Classification of the various forms of epithelial tissue.

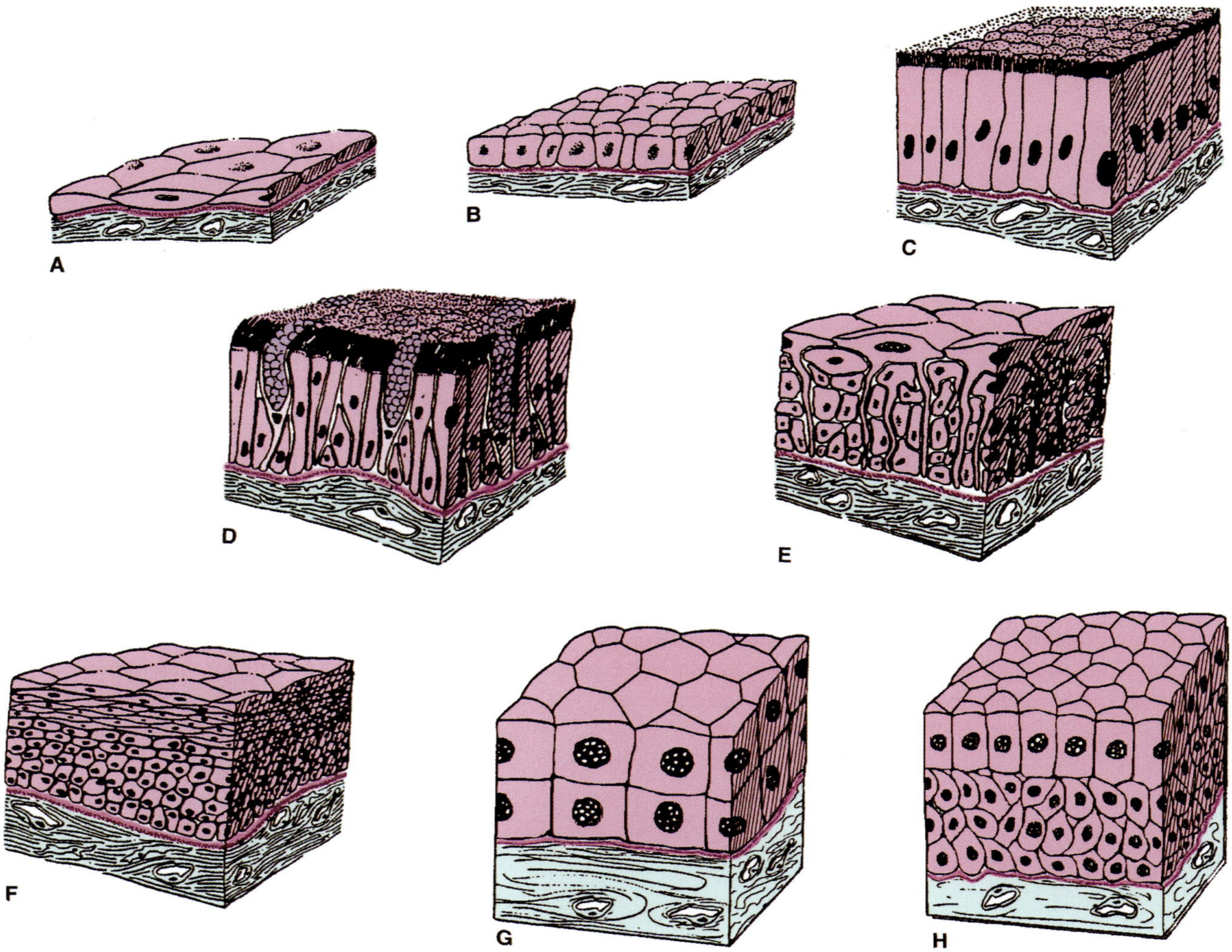

Figure 2-3 Schematic drawings illustrating the major types of surface epithelia. **A.** Simple squamous epithelium. **B.** Simple cuboidal epithelium. **C.** Simple columnar epithelium bearing microvilli. **D.** Pseudostratified columnar epithelium with cilia and goblet cells. **E.** Transitional epithelium (urothelium). **F.** Stratified squamous epithelium, nonkeratinized. **G.** Stratified cuboidal epithelium. **H.** Stratified columnar epithelium.

Simple Cuboidal Epithelium

Simple cuboidal epithelium consists of a single layer of cells that have similar width and height. The height of the cell can vary between a low cuboidal (height is slightly less than the cell width) or a tall cuboidal (height is slightly greater than the width). These cells appear as squares in cross sections but are more hexagonal when viewed from the surface (Figs. 2-3B and 2-5).

Simple cuboidal epithelium lines the ducts of many exocrine glands and the collecting ducts of the kidney. It is also found in the choroid plexus in the brain and ciliary body of the eye, and lining the follicles of the thyroid gland. The epithelium of the lens of the eye and the retinal pigment epithelium are also examples of simple cuboidal epithelium.

Simple Columnar Epithelium

Simple columnar epithelium consists of tall, narrow cells with greater height than width (Figs. 2-3C and 2-6). The nuclei are oval and are located near the base of the cell. Simple columnar epithelium lines the surface of organs involved in absorptive or secretory functions. Examples include the glandular stomach, the small and large intestines, and the gallbladder in the digestive system, the bulbourethral gland in the male reproductive system, and the uterus and uterine tube in the female reproductive system.

Pseudostratified Epithelium

In pseudostratified epithelium, all of the cells contact the underlying basement membrane, but not all of them reach the free surface.

Pseudostratified Columnar Epithelium **Pseudostratified columnar epithelium** is a single layer of cells. However, the irregular size and shape results in their nuclei being located at various levels, giving the appearance of multiple layers (Figs. 2-3D and 2-7). All cells in this epithelia type are in contact with the basement membrane, though not all reach the surface. Those cells that reach the surface extend a process from the basement membrane to the surface. This process can be a cilium (a hair-like structure), a microvillus (a small protrusion involved in absorption), or another type of specialized cellular extension. Pseudostratified columnar epithelia can consist of **ciliated** or **nonciliated epithelial cells** and **goblet cells** (unicellular mucous glands). **Basal cells** are attached to the basement membrane but do not reach the surface of the epithelium. By division and differentiation, basal cells replace other epithelial cell types lost by attrition.

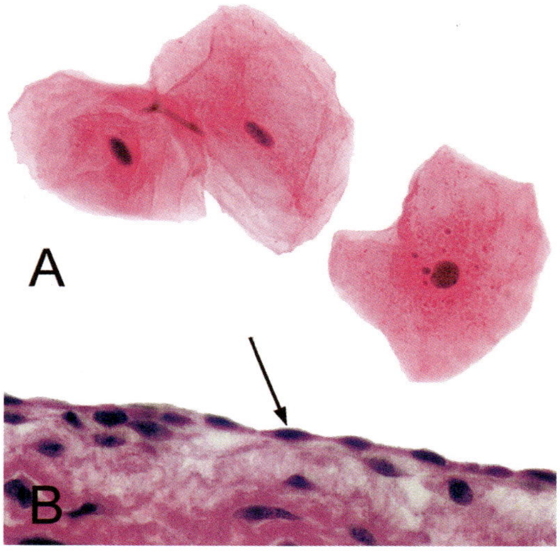

Figure 2-4 **A.** Squamous epithelial cells spread on a glass slide. Note the irregular shape of the cells. The basophilic nucleus is located in the center of the acidophilic cytoplasm. Oral cavity, H&E (×400). **B.** Simple squamous epithelium (arrow) lining the thoracic aorta of the pig. H&E (×600). (Images by W.E. Haensly.)

Ciliated, pseudostratified columnar epithelium with goblet cells lines the greater part of the nasal cavity, paranasal sinuses, and nasopharynx, as well as the auditory tubes, the trachea, and the larger bronchi. In the respiratory system, goblet cells contribute to a thin mucous film over the epithelium. Dust particles in the inhaled air become trapped in this mucus, and the current created by the ciliated cells moves the dust-laden mucus to the body openings. A pseudostratified columnar epithelium with stereocilia but lacking goblet cells is found lining the duct of the epididymis and the ductus deferens.

Urothelium (Transitional Epithelium) **Transitional** is a term that has been applied to several different types of epithelium. The epithelium in the renal system (renal pelvis and calices, ureter, urinary bladder, and urethra) is often referred to as transitional epithelium. However, this is a unique epithelium that is now more properly referred to as **urothelium**. Urothelium has a one cell thick basal cell layer, followed by an intermediate cell layer of several layers (species-dependent), and finally, an outer single layer of umbrella cells. Evidence in the literature supports classifying urothelium as either stratified or pseudostratified, with recent findings indicating that this classification is species-dependent (Figs. 2-3E and 2-8). When the epithelium is stretched, the cells become flattened and elongated, and the total height of the epithelium decreases.

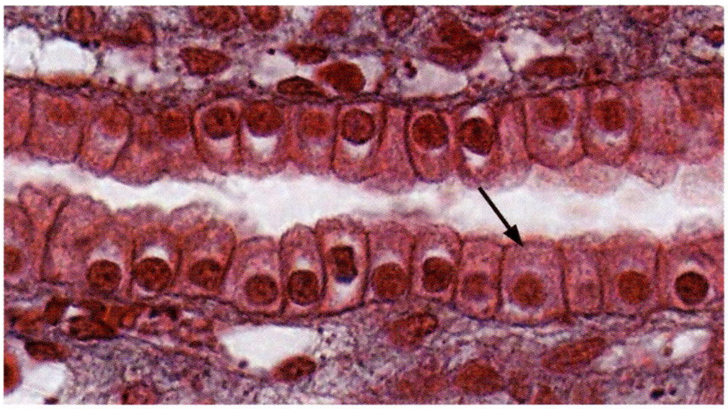

Figure 2-5 Simple cuboidal epithelium, collecting duct, kidney. Modified Masson trichrome (×500). (With permission of Purdue University.)

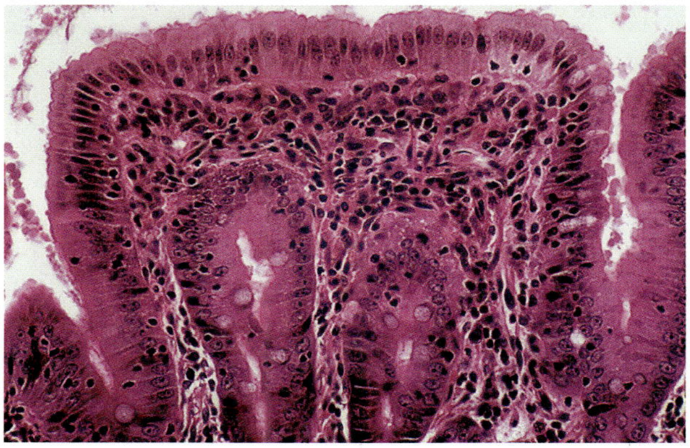

Figure 2-6 Simple columnar epithelium, duodenum, pig. Hematoxylin and eosin (H&E) (×400). (Image by W.E. Haensly.)

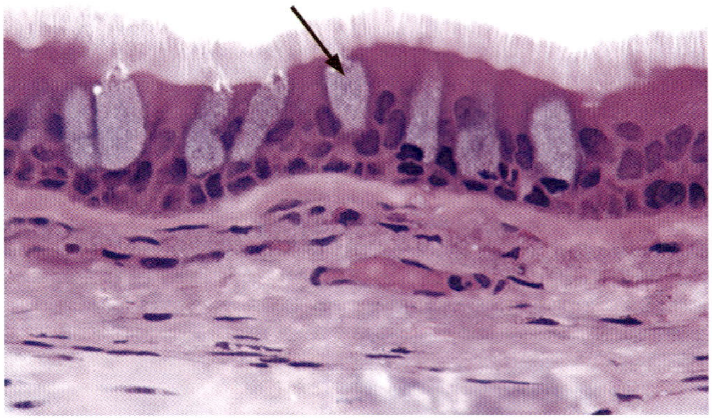

Figure 2-7 Pseudostratified columnar epithelium with cilia and goblet cells (arrow), trachea. H&E (×1000). (Image by J. Eurell.)

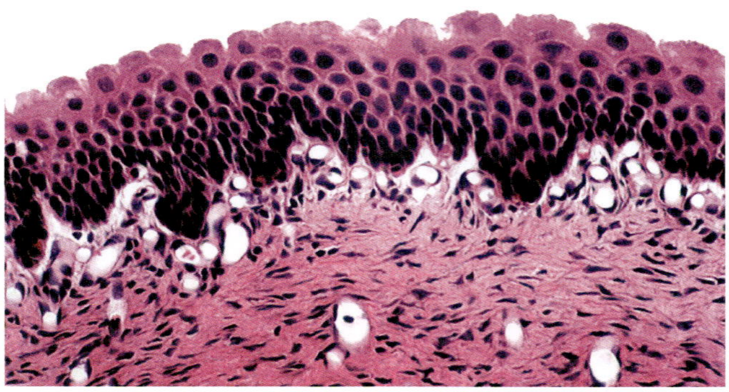

Figure 2-8 The cells of urothelium (transitional epithelium) increase in size from the basal layer to the surface. The surface cells have a scalloped umbrella shape that flattens and elongates as the epithelium is stretched. Urinary bladder, cat, H&E (×400). (Image by W.E. Haensly.)

The luminal surface of transitional epithelial cells appears relatively smooth with the light microscope. In electron micrographs, however, areas of thickened plasmalemma (*plaques*) anchored by numerous cytoplasmic filaments are seen on the luminal surface of the cell. The region between the membrane plaques is a normal cell membrane, and when the bladder contracts, the plaques fold together much like a hinge. Upon distention of the bladder, the plaques unfold, allowing expansion of the luminal surface.

Epithelium termed "transitional" is also found in the larynx, nasopharynx, and the palpebral conjunctiva, but this is different than what is found in the urinary system. In the respiratory system, there are at least four different types of epithelia. In between squamous epithelium and more classical respiratory epithelium, ciliated or nonciliated cuboidal to columnar epithelium can be found, which has been referred to as transitional. Similarly, in the turbinates, cuboidal and ciliated or nonciliated epithelium has been called transitional.

The surface epithelium of the urinary bladder forms a barrier to the diffusion of water from the subepithelial tissue to the hypertonic urine stored in the lumen. Morphologic evidence of this diffusion barrier includes (a) the increased thickness of the outer lamina of the trilaminar cell membrane, compared to the inner lamina; (b) a concentration of tonofilaments, which are cytoskeletal filaments, immediately beneath the luminal surface; and (c) junctional complexes, such as tight junctions, located between the adjacent surface cells that prevent intercellular diffusion.

Detailed studies of transitional epithelium indicate that when the epithelium is relaxed, the cells elongate and overlap each other, giving the appearance of a multilayered epithelium. All of the transitional epithelial cells remain attached to the basement membrane by slender cytoplasmic processes, much like the attachment seen in pseudostratified columnar epithelium (Fig. 2-3E). This attachment allows the cells to align parallel to each other when the urinary bladder is distended, resulting in the observation of fewer cell layers.

Stratified Squamous Epithelium

Stratified squamous epithelium has several layers of cells, where the superficial cells have a squamous shape (Fig. 2-3F). There are two types of stratified squamous epithelia (Fig. 2-9). In **keratinized stratified squamous epithelium**, the surface layer cells have lost their nuclei and are filled with keratin. In **nonkeratinized or parakeratinized stratified squamous epithelium**, the cells contain keratin, but the flattened superficial cells retain their nuclei.

Typically, three to five distinct cell layers are present in stratified squamous epithelium (see also Chapter 16). The deepest layer of cells next to the basement membrane is the **stratum basale** (Figs. 2-3F and 2-9), which is a single layer of cuboidal to columnar cells. The cells of the stratum basale are mitotically active and continually divide, giving rise to new cells that move into the upper layers of the epithelium through a process of cell turnover or renewal.

The next layer is the **stratum spinosum** (Fig. 2-9), composed of a varying number of layers of polyhedral cells tightly adhered to each other by numerous **desmosomes (maculae adherens)**. In ordinary histologic preparations, the cytoplasm between the desmosomal attachments shrinks, and wherever the cells remain attached, small spiny processes

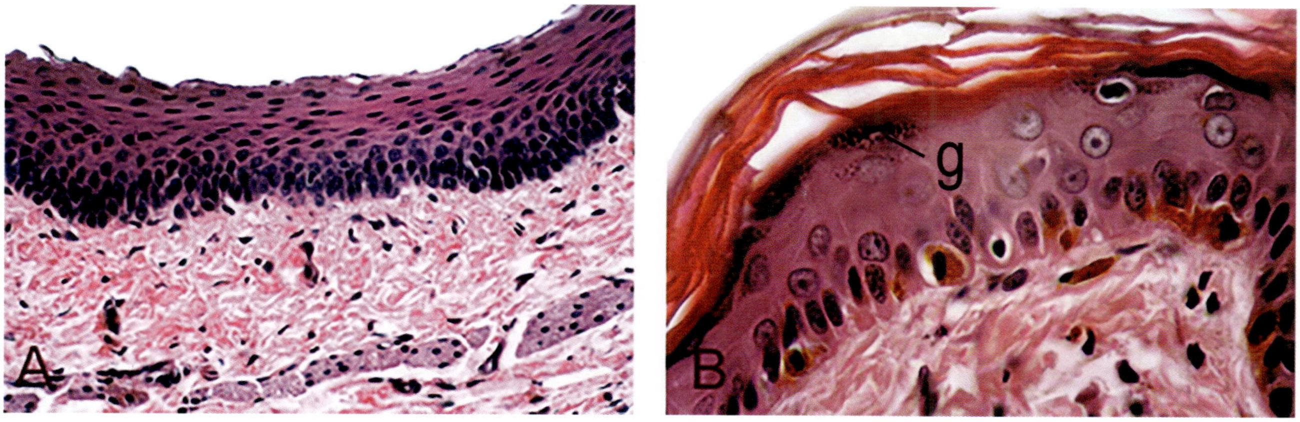

Figure 2-9 **A.** Nonkeratinized stratified squamous epithelium. The upper cell layer is flattened and retains the nucleus. Esophagus, cat (×400). **B.** Keratinized stratified squamous epithelium. Several cells containing brown pigment are present in the deepest layer of this stratified squamous epithelium. As the epithelial cells migrate from the basal layer to the surface, they flatten, acquire dark-staining granules (g, stratum granulosum), and eventually lose their nuclei. Cell remnants in the upper layers of the epithelium form the keratinized layer. Pinna, cat (×1000). (Images by W.E. Haensly.)

radiate from the surface of the cells. This appearance gives rise to the name of the layer, stratum spinosum or "spiny layer." These spiny processes contain **cytokeratin filaments**, termed **tonofilaments**, which are condensed at the site of the desmosomes (Fig. 16-6).

As the cells of the stratum spinosum move toward the surface, they become more flattened and accumulate **keratohyalin granules**, which contribute to the formation of keratin, and **lamellar granules**, which contain lipids important for skin barrier function, in their cytoplasm. This layer of cells, known as the **stratum granulosum**, is absent from nonkeratinized stratified squamous epithelium. It is also absent from keratinized forms that produce hard keratin, such as those found in the wall of the hoof and in the horn of ruminants, where keratinization proceeds to form a tough, durable structure.

The **stratum lucidum** occurs only in nonhairy skin regions (Fig. 16-2C). This layer of flattened keratinized cells, situated between the stratum granulosum and the stratum corneum, has a translucent appearance because it contains **eleidin**, a protein similar to keratin but with a different affinity for histologic stains.

The outermost layer of keratinized stratified squamous epithelium is the **stratum corneum**, composed of dead, keratinized cells. To reach the keratinized state, epithelial cells undergo a series of transformations as they move from the stratum basale to the stratum corneum. The process of **keratinization** involves the gradual disappearance of the nuclei, Golgi complexes, and mitochondria, along with decreased lysosomal activity and a concurrent accumulation of **tonofilaments**. Germinative cells in the stratum basale, rich in polyribosomes, synthesize cytokeratin. As these cells move up into the stratum spinosum, tonofilaments condense into bundles visible with the light microscope (**tonofibrils**) and become attached to desmosomes. In the stratum granulosum, flat cells contain numerous **keratohyalin granules** and lamellar granules, which are readily visible with the light microscope. With the electron microscope, the tonofilaments are observed to extend into the periphery of the cell, intermingling with the granules. The cells of the stratum granulosum also contain unique, oval, membrane-bounded granules (100 to 500 nm) composed of alternating light and dark lamellae. These Golgi-derived **lamellar granules** (**membrane-coating granules**) are located at the cell periphery. By the time the cells reach the stratum lucidum, they become elongated and flattened, with all organelles gone. The stratum corneum cells, visible only as outlines under light microscopy, exhibit densely packed tonofilaments embedded in a dense matrix, likely derived from keratohyalin granules. In the stratum corneum, the contents of lamellar granules are secreted by exocytosis, contributing to the intercellular substance between cells, crucial for epithelial barrier properties. Groups of cells in the outermost layer of the stratum corneum eventually become loose and separate. This process gives rise to the descriptive term **stratum disjunctum**.

A stratum corneum is absent in nonkeratinized stratified squamous epithelium found on moist surfaces (Fig. 2-9). Instead, the layer of keratin-containing cells that fail to lose their nuclei as they migrate to the surface of the epithelium is termed the **stratum superficiale**.

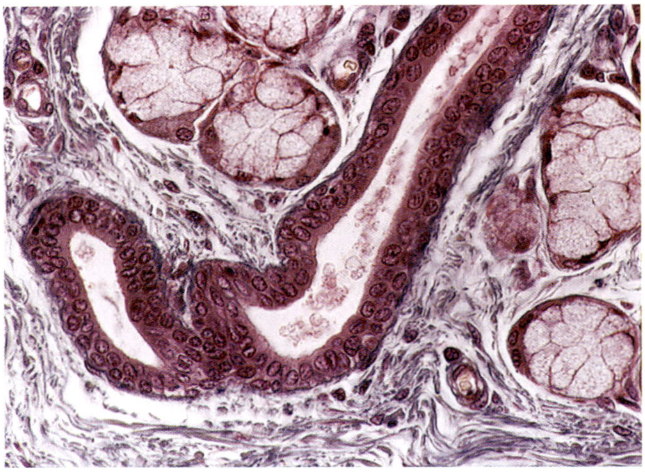

Figure 2-10 Stratified cuboidal epithelium, duct of carpal gland (pig). H&E (×1400).

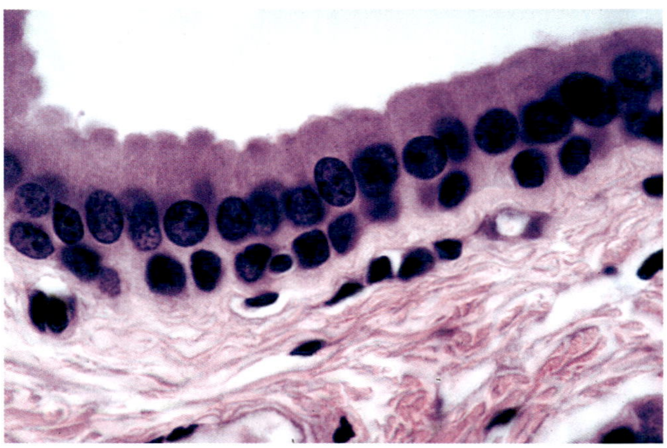

Figure 2-11 Stratified columnar epithelium, penile urethra (horse). H&E (×620). Note that the surface cells are columnar, and the nuclei form a fairly regular row.

Stratified Cuboidal Epithelium

Stratified cuboidal epithelium consists of two or more layers of cells with a surface layer of typical cuboidal cells. It is found as a distinct two-layered epithelium lining the excretory ducts of glands (Figs. 2-3G and 2-10).

Stratified Columnar Epithelium

Stratified columnar epithelium consists of several layers of cells. The superficial layer is composed of tall cells that do not extend to the basement membrane (Figs. 2-3H and 2-11). The deeper layers are composed of smaller polyhedral cells that do not reach the surface. This type of epithelium may be found lining the distal portion of the urethra, in circumscribed areas within transitional epithelium, as well as in the parotid and mandibular ducts, and in the lacrimal sac and duct.

Sensory Epithelium

Epithelia containing supportive (sustentacular) cells and specialized receptor cells are found in the retina of the eye, the internal ear, the olfactory mucosa, and the taste buds. These highly specialized **sensory epithelia** mediate the senses of vision, hearing, equilibrium, smell, and taste. These epithelia are described in detail in Chapters 9, 10, and 17.

Glandular Epithelium and Glands

The secretory cells of endocrine and exocrine glands constitute **glandular epithelium**. These cells derive from the proliferation of surface epithelial cells into underlying CT. A **gland** is a structure that may consist exclusively of glandular epithelium or may include a complex duct system, lined by surface epithelium, and a supportive framework of CT, known as the **stroma.** Glands are found, in one form or another, in most organs of the body.

Classification of Glands

Glands are classified based on **morphologic characteristics**, the **nature of the secretory product**, and the **mode of release of the secretory product** (Table 2-2).

Morphologic Characteristics

Unicellular glands consist of a single secretory cell embedded within a nonsecretory surface epithelium. An example of this type of gland is the **goblet cell**, a specialized epithelial cell that produces **mucinogen**. Upon synthesis, the mucinogen is released onto the epithelial surface as **mucin**, a key component of **mucus**. As this secretory material is synthesized, it accumulates in the apical portion of the cell, causing it to expand and push the nucleus into the slender basal portion, resulting in the characteristic goblet shape (Fig. 2-7). Unicellular endocrine glands are found throughout the epithelial linings of the tubular organs of the gastrointestinal, respiratory, urinary, and reproductive systems, as well as in the adrenal and thyroid glands, and the heart and kidney. These cells are part of the diffuse neuroendocrine system and are referred to

Table 2-2 Classifications of Glands

Based on Morphologic Characteristics	Based on the Nature of the Secretory Product
Unicellular glands	Serous
Multicellular glands	Mucous
Intraepithelial	Seromucous (mixed)
Extraepithelial	
Endocrine	**Based on the Mode of Release of the Secretory Product**
Exocrine	Merocrine (eccrine)
Simple	Apocrine
Tubular—straight, coiled, branched	Holocrine
Acinar/Alveolar—single, branched	Cytocrine
Tubuloacinar/tubuloalveolar	
Compound	
Tubular	
Acinar/alveolar	
Tubuloacinar/tubuloalveolar	

as **APUD cells** (*a*mine *p*recursor *u*ptake and *d*ecarboxylation cells) due to their ability to uptake amine precursors and produce amine or peptide hormones via decarboxylation. APUD cells are described in detail in Chapter 12.

Multicellular glands are composed of more than one cell, and most glands fall into this classification. They may occur as a cluster of only a few secretory cells within a surface epithelium, forming **intraepithelial glands**, or as large accumulations of cells that have proliferated into the underlying CT, forming **extraepithelial glands**.

Endocrine glands are multicellular glands that do not have a system of ducts and secrete their products (hormones) directly into the intercellular fluid. These hormones are then picked up by fenestrated capillaries and lymph vessels, through which they are transported systemically to the site of action.

Exocrine glands are multicellular glands with a system of ducts through which their secretory products are transported to the sites of utilization. Exocrine glands can be either **simple** or **compound. Simple glands** consist of one to several secretory units connected to the surface through an unbranched duct, while **compound glands** have many secretory units emptying into a highly branched duct system.

Simple Glands **Simple exocrine glands** have secretory units of various shapes and dispositions. **Simple straight tubular glands**, such as those in the large intestine, follow a straight, unbranched course in the surrounding tissue and open directly onto the surface (Figs. 2-12A and 2-13). **Simple coiled tubular glands** have a coiled or convoluted terminal portion. In histologic sections, the secretory unit appears as a cluster of cross-sectional profiles (Figs. 2-12B and 2-14). Sweat glands of the skin serve as good examples of this type. **Simple branched tubular glands** feature a branched terminal portion (Figs. 2-12C and 2-15). The branches converge into a single duct near the opening onto the surface, and both portions are lined with secretory cells. The glands of the stomach represent typical simple branched tubular glands.

Simple acinar and **simple alveolar glands** share similarities as they both have enlarged, spherical secretory units connected to the surface by short ducts (Figs. 2-12D, 2-12E, and 2-16). The **acinus** has a small and narrow lumen, whereas the **alveolus** has a large and distended one (Fig. 2-17). These types of glands are rare; some sebaceous glands are of the simple acinar type, whereas simple alveolar glands are found in the respiratory system of the chicken. **Simple branched acinar** and **simple branched alveolar glands** are more common than their unbranched counterparts. In these branched types, two or more acini or alveoli occur together, and their secretory product empties through a common duct (Fig. 2-12D and E). Many of the larger sebaceous glands of the skin are of the simple branched acinar type, while simple branched alveolar glands are found in the respiratory system of the chicken.

Simple tubuloacinar and **simple tubuloalveolar glands** have secretory units composed of a tubular portion with a terminal acinus or alveolus, and they occur only in the branched form. The minor salivary glands that empty into the oral cavity are classified as this type.

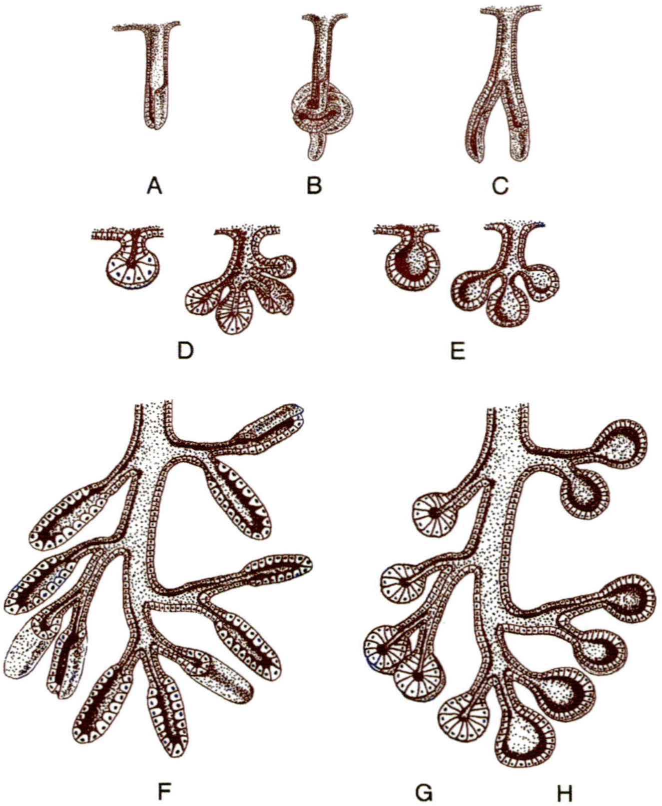

Figure 2-12 Schematic drawings illustrating the types of exocrine glands. **A.** Simple tubular gland. **B.** Simple coiled tubular gland. **C.** Simple branched tubular gland. **D.** Simple acinar gland and simple branched acinar gland. **E.** Simple alveolar gland and simple branched alveolar gland. **F.** Compound tubular gland. **G.** Compound acinar gland. **H.** Compound alveolar gland. Compound tubuloacinar/tubuloalveolar glands consist of either a mixture of tubular and acinar/alveolar secretory units or tubular secretory units "capped" by acini or alveoli.

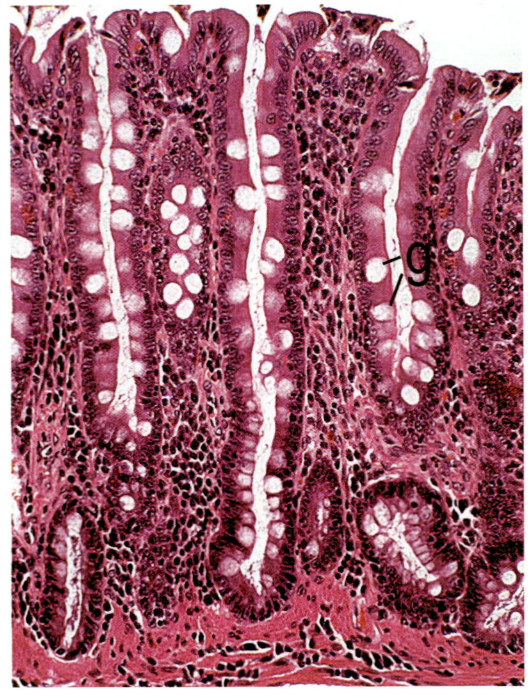

Figure 2-13 Simple straight tubular gland follows a straight, unbranched course from the surface of the epithelium and is lined by simple columnar epithelium with goblet cells (g). Rectum, cat, H&E (×250). (Image by W.E. Haensly.)

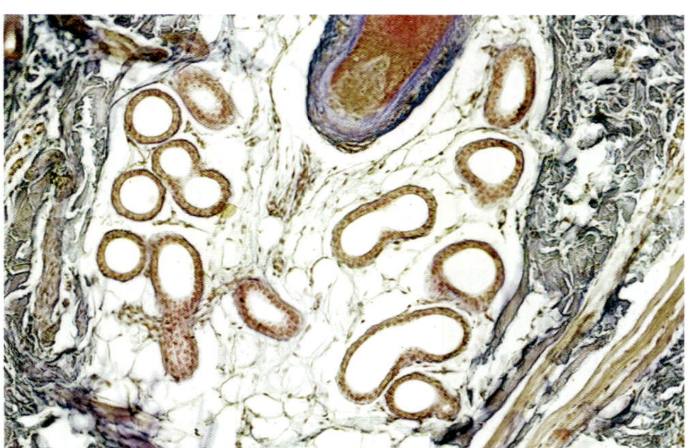

Figure 2-14 Simple coiled tubular gland. Ceruminous gland, ear canal. Masson's trichrome (×120). (Image by John J. Turek.)

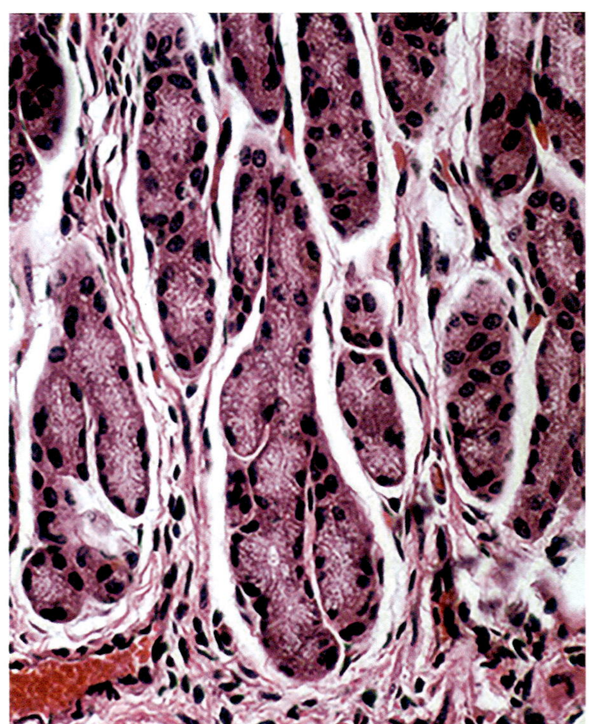

Figure 2-15 The duct system of a simple branched tubular gland branches repeatedly. Stomach, pyloric gland, horse, H&E (×400). (Image by W.E. Haensly.)

Compound Glands **Compound glands** contain the same types of secretory units as those of the simple glands but have *elaborate duct systems that branch repeatedly*. Compound glands are classified as tubular, acinar, alveolar, tubuloacinar, or tubuloalveolar types. For example, a gland with a highly branched duct system whose secretory units consist of tubules of glandular epithelium would be classified as a **compound tubular** gland, whereas a **compound tubuloacinar gland** contains either a mixture of acinar and tubular secretory units or tubular secretory units with terminal acini. Fig. 2-12F, G, and H and Fig. 2-18 illustrate the various types of secretory units and ducts found in compound glands.

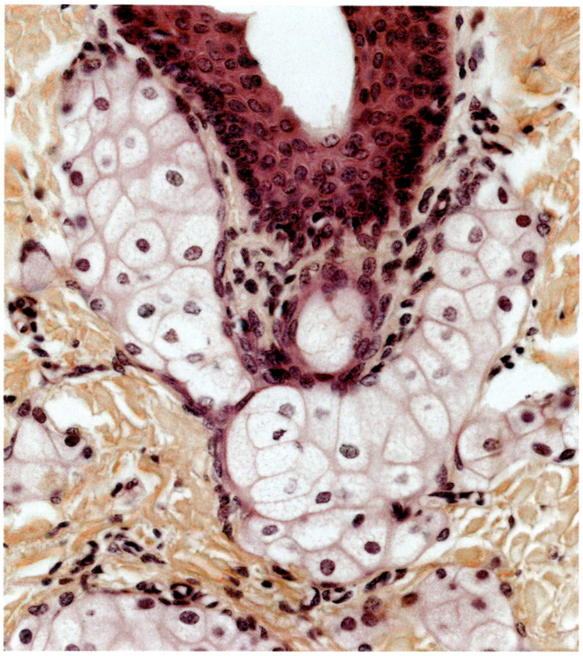

Figure 2-16 Simple acinar gland. Sebaceous gland, ear. Masson's plus elastin stain (×300).

Parenchyma Compound glands are composed of secretory units and ducts, collectively termed **parenchyma**, while the supportive or CT elements comprise the **stroma**. Large glands are partly or completely divided into **lobes**, which are large, easily recognized structural units. The lobes are further subdivided by CT into **lobules**, each composed of numerous **secretory units** (Fig. 2-18). Some of the smaller compound glands have only lobules and secretory units. The various segments of the duct system of compound glands are identified by their location within the gland.

Secretory product produced in tubules, acini, or alveoli of a compound gland first flows into an **intralobular duct**, usually located in the center of the lobule. Intralobular ducts continue as **interlobular ducts** when they emerge from the lobule to enter the interlobular CT. Interlobular ducts converge to form large **lobar ducts**, which drain individual lobes of the gland. The **main duct** is formed by the convergence of the lobar ducts (Fig. 2-18).

In some glands, such as the parotid salivary gland, portions of the intralobular ducts also contribute to the secretory product and thus are called **secretory ducts**. These ducts also are known as **striated ducts** because their cells contain many mitochondria oriented perpendicularly to the long axis of the cell and located between folds of the basal

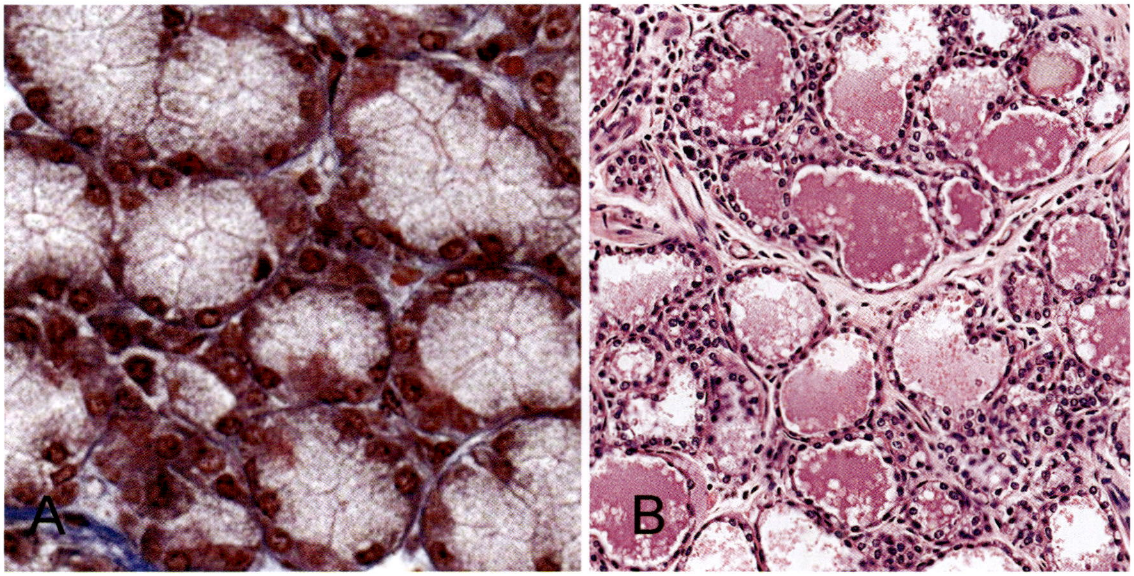

Figure 2-17 Types of secretory units. **A.** Acini, characterized by a small lumen, parotid salivary gland (dog). Masson's trichrome (×400). **B.** Alveoli, mammary gland (sow). Note the large lumen. H&E (×300). (Image by John J. Turek.)

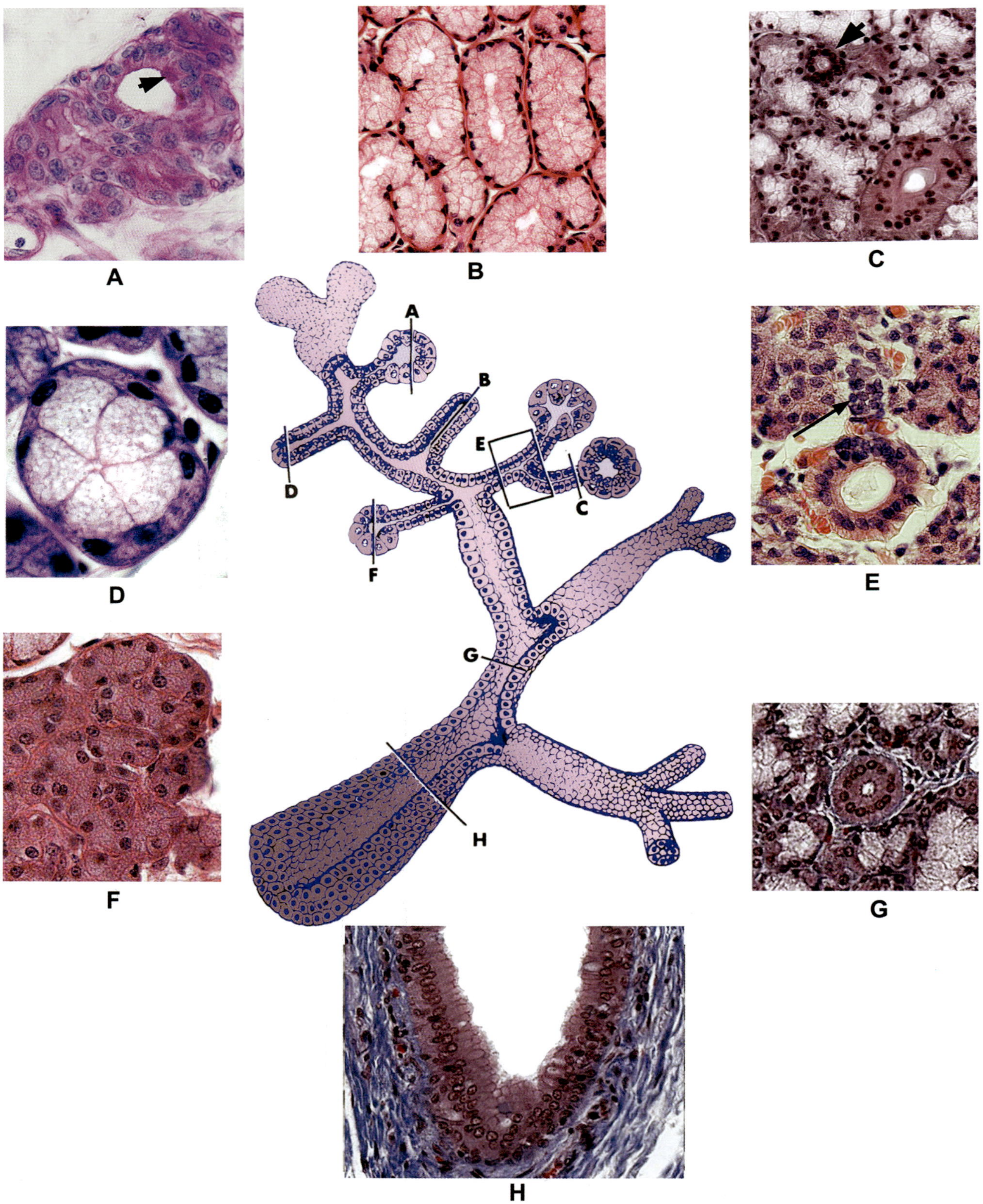

Figure 2-18 Schematic composite drawing and photomicrographs of the duct system and secretory units of a compound gland. The photomicrographs correspond to the areas labeled A through H. **A.** Seromucous alveolus, Mucous cell (arrow). Trachea (pig). PAS (×400). **B.** Mucous tubular secretory unit, bulbourethral gland (bull). H&E (×400). **C.** Cross section of intercalated duct, salivary gland (dog). Masson's trichrome (×400). **D.** Mucous acinus with serous demilunes, seromucous salivary gland (horse). H&E (×1000). **E.** Longitudinal section through intercalated duct (arrow), parotid salivary gland (dog). H&E (×480). **F.** Serous acinus, parotid salivary gland (dog). H&E (×400). **G.** Striated intralobular duct, salivary gland (dog). Masson's trichrome (×400). **H.** Interlobular duct, parotid salivary gland (dog). Masson's trichrome (×300). (Drawing from Stinson AW, Brown EM. Veterinary Histology Slide Sets. East Lansing, MI: Michigan State University, Instructional Media Center, 1970.). (With permission of Purdue University.)

plasmalemma, giving the cells a striated appearance (Fig. 2-18G). **Intercalated ducts** are small, nonsecretory intralobular ducts that connect the secretory units with the secretory (striated) duct (Fig. 2-18C and E). Intercalated ducts are prominent in the parotid salivary gland and are present also in the mandibular and sublingual salivary glands, as well as the pancreas.

The general term **excretory duct** describes any of the previously mentioned ducts that function only to transport the secretory product to the site of utilization. Unlike secretory ducts, excretory ducts do not contribute to the secretory product.

Stroma The **stroma** of compound glands includes the capsule and the internal supportive framework. The **capsule**, composed of collagen, elastic, and reticular fibers, completely surrounds the gland and gives rise to CT sheets (**septa**) or strands (**trabeculae**) that extend deep into the parenchyma. Septa distinctly delineate the lobes and lobules while providing support for the various lobar and interlobular ducts. Fine **reticular fibers** encircle the individual secretory units.

Nature of the Secretory Product

Both simple and compound glands can be classified as mucous, serous, or seromucous (mixed), depending on the nature of their secretory product. **Serous glands** produce a thin, watery product. The cells of the secretory units usually have spherical nuclei near the center of the cells, and the apical cytoplasm is filled with small secretory granules (Fig. 2-18F). These granules are precursors of enzymes produced by many of the serous glands and are called **zymogen granules**. The parotid salivary gland and the exocrine part of the pancreas are typical serous glands.

Mucous glands produce a thick, viscous secretion, called **mucin**, which contributes to a protective coating over the lining of hollow organs that communicate with the outside of the body (Fig. 2-18B). This protective coating is termed **mucus** and contains cast-off epithelial cells and leukocytes, in addition to mucin. The cells of the mucus-secreting units are filled with **mucinogen**, the precursor of **mucin**, which stains lightly with H&E. The nuclei are displaced toward the basal part of the cell and usually are flattened against the cell membrane.

Glands that contain both mucous and serous cells are described as **seromucous, mucoserous,** or simply "**mixed**." The combinations of these two types of cells vary considerably from one gland to another. Some secretory units contain intermixed serous and mucous cells (Fig. 2-18A). Other seromucous glands are composed of a mixture of all-mucous acini and all-serous acini rather than each acinus containing some serous and some mucous cells. Most commonly, the serous cells are located at the periphery of the mucous secretory unit and are half-moon- or crescent-shaped cells called **serous demilunes** (Fig. 2-18D). They empty their serous secretory product into the lumen of the secretory unit by way of small channels between the mucous cells called intercellular canaliculi. Some seromucous tubuloacinar glands have a mucous tubular unit with a terminal serous acinus.

Mode of Release of the Secretory Product

The mechanism by which the secretory product is released from the cell forms the basis for a third classification of glands. Four different modes of release are recognized: merocrine or eccrine, apocrine, holocrine, and cytocrine.

During the **merocrine** (sometimes called **eccrine**) mode of secretion, the contents of small secretory granules are released as the secretory product (Fig. 2-19A). The secretory granules are usually enclosed within a membrane. When the secretory granule reaches the cell surface, its membrane fuses with the plasmalemma, thereby discharging the secretory product via **exocytosis**.

In the **apocrine** mode of secretion, a large, single secretory granule migrates within the cytoplasm to the cell apex. The plasmalemma (plasma membrane) and a portion of the neighboring cytoplasm surround the granule. Eventually, the plasmalemma constricts beneath the granule, causing the projection containing the granule to bulge into the gland lumen (Fig. 2-19B). Constriction of the plasmalemma proceeds until the membrane-bounded granule and its accompanying cytoplasm and plasmalemma are separated from the cell, leaving the rest of the cell plasmalemma intact.

Apocrine glands in the secretory state are easily recognized; however, when they are in a resting phase with no secretory "droplets," their differentiation from merocrine glands is difficult. Examples of apocrine glands include the mammary glands and the sweat glands found throughout the body.

In the **holocrine** mode of secretion, entire cells are released as the secretory product (Fig. 2-19C). The sebaceous glands of the skin are typical holocrine glands. As the cells fill with lipid granules, they migrate toward the gland's duct. Eventually, the cells disintegrate, releasing their contents into the duct.

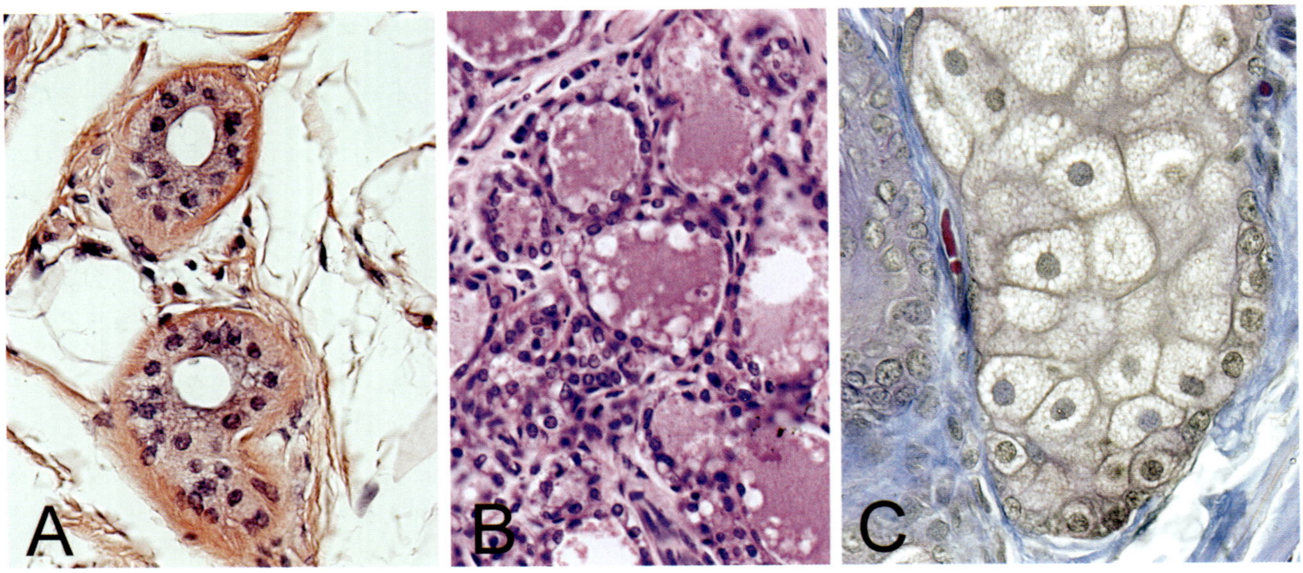

Figure 2-19 Secretory units illustrating the various modes of release of the secretory product. **A.** Merocrine sweat gland, skin (dog). H&E (×400). **B.** Apocrine lactating mammary gland (pig). H&E (×400). **C.** Holocrine gland, sebaceous gland (dog). Masson's trichrome (×400). (Image by John J. Turek.)

In the **cytocrine** mode of secretion, secretory material is transferred from one cell to the cytoplasm of another cell. This mode is exemplified in the epidermis, where melanocytes transfer the brown pigment melanin into the cytoplasm of the keratinocytes.

Myoepithelial Cells

In some glands, **myoepithelial cells** are located between the base of the secretory cells and the basement membrane. As implied by their name, myoepithelial cells possess characteristics of both muscle cells (actin and myosin filaments) and epithelial cells (cytokeratin). When stimulated, these cells contract and force the secretory product of the epithelial cells into the duct system. Myoepithelial cells are particularly well developed in sweat glands and mammary glands (Fig. 2-19B). In the mammary gland, myoepithelial cells are stimulated by oxytocin.

Clinical Correlations

Epithelial hyperplasia of the mammary gland is a common occurrence in intact female dogs, involving an increase in epithelial cell numbers, especially during estrus and pregnancy, as well as in response to hormonal therapies or certain medications. This abnormal proliferation leads to enlargement of the gland and the formation of palpable masses. While epithelial hyperplasia is not inherently malignant, it may increase the susceptibility to mammary tumors, such as adenomas and carcinomas. Regular palpation and monitoring of mammary glands are critical for early detection. Spaying before the first heat cycle mitigates the risk of mammary hyperplasia and associated neoplasia. The surgical removal of palpable masses, coupled with histopathological examination, is recommended to determine whether there is any malignant transformation and to help guide subsequent therapy. Histological evaluation informs the extent and severity of hyperplastic changes, contributing to treatment planning and prognosis determination.

In addition, cancers of epithelial origin (**carcinomas**) may develop from an organ or gland (adenocarcinoma), or from squamous epithelium (squamous cell carcinoma). Loss of dynein arms on cilia microtubules causes **Kartagener's syndrome**, which manifests as poor respiratory clearance of mucus and infertility. Defects in collagen VII can cause a canine dystrophic epidermolysis bullosa.

Essentials

1) Epithelium covers surfaces, and the cells have polarity. Top (apical) portions may have specializations for absorption (microvilli or stereocilia with actin cytoskeleton) or motility (cilia with microtubules). Exocrine and endocrine glands are derived from epithelial tissues.
2) Tight junctions (zonula occludens) separate the apical from the lateral surface. The lateral surface contains (1) belt desmosomes or zonula adherens, which connect to the actin cytoskeleton; (2) spot desmosomes or macula adherens, which are connected to intermediate filaments; and (3) gap junctions for chemo-electrical connection.
3) The base of the cell is attached to a basement membrane, composed of the basal lamina and reticular lamina. The major components of the basal lamina include type IV collagen and laminin. The amorphous basal lamina attaches to the reticular lamina (primarily type III collagen) through type VII collagen fibrils that link type IV collagen to type III collagen. Cells also attach via hemidesmosomes, which connect the internal intermediate filament cytoskeleton to the extracellular matrix and basal lamina via transmembrane integral proteins (integrins).
4) Exocrine glands secrete through ducts and can produce mucus, serous, or mixed secretions. Many exocrine glands have a duct structure (small to large), beginning with intercalated ducts, progressing to intralobular ducts, and finally to interlobular ducts. Exocrine glands will secrete via merocrine, apocrine, or holocrine mechanisms.
5) Endocrine glands secrete into CT spaces, where hormones are picked up by fenestrated capillaries, or they may secrete hormones directly into the bloodstream.

Suggested Readings

Dalghi MG, Montalbetti N, Carattino MD, et al. The urothelium: life in a liquid environment. *Physiol. Rev.* 2020;100:1621–1705.

Franke WW, Jahn L, Knapp AC. Cytokeratins and desmosomal proteins in certain epithelioid and nonepithelial cells. In: Osborn M, Weber K, eds. Cytoskeletal Proteins in Tumor Diagnosis. Cold Spring Harbor, NY: Cold Spring Harbor Laboratory, 1989.

Halfter W, Oertle P, Monnier CA, et al. New concepts in basement membrane biology. *FEBS J.* 2015;282(23):4466–4479. doi: 10.1111/febs.13495.

Harkema JR, Carey SA, Wagner JG. The nose revisited: a brief review of the comparative structure, function, and toxicologic pathology of the nasal epithelium. *Toxicol Pathol* 2006;34(3):252–269. doi: 10.1080/01926230600713475.

Hashimoto K. The eccrine and apocrine glands and their function. In: Jarret A, ed. The Physiology and Pathophysiology of the Skin. New York: Academic Press, 1978: 5.

Krstić RV. General Histology of the Mammal. New York: Springer-Verlag, 1985.

Krstić RV. Ultrastructure of the Mammalian Cell. New York: Springer-Verlag, 1979.

Rousselle P, Laigle C, Rousselet G. The basement membrane in epidermal polarity, stemness, and regeneration. *Am J Physiol Cell Physiol.* 2022;323(6):C1807–C1822. doi: 10.1152/ajpcell.00069.2022.

3

Connective and Supportive Tissues

Marxa L. Figueiredo and John J. Turek

CHAPTER MENU

Dellmann's Textbook of Veterinary Histology, Seventh Edition. Edited by Marxa L. Figueiredo and John J. Turek.

Companion website: www.wiley.com/go/figueiredo/vethistology7e

Connective and supportive tissues connect other tissues, provide a framework, and support the entire body by means of cartilage and bones. These tissues also play an important role in thermoregulation and in defense and repair mechanisms. Connective tissues are also a reservoir for various hormones and cytokines that play an important role in growth and development.

Most connective and supportive tissues are derived from mesoderm, which arises from the somites and lateral layers of the somatic and splanchnic mesoderm. In addition, neural crest cells from surface ectoderm form the head mesenchyme, which subsequently develops into the connective tissue of the rostral head. Connective and supportive tissues are composed of **cells**, **fibers**, and amorphous **ground substance** in varying proportions. Embryonic mesenchyme is a unique connective tissue because it lacks fibers during early development. Based on occurrence, connective and supportive tissues are classified as embryonic or adult with several subgroups.

Connective Tissue Cells

The cells of connective tissue (CT) proper are diverse and have varied functions, ranging from production of CT components to phagocytosis and antibody formation. Many cells of CT, such as fibrocytes, remain as resident cells in a fixed location within the tissue. Other CT cells, such as macrophages, are capable of moving through the tissue as mobile or wandering cells.

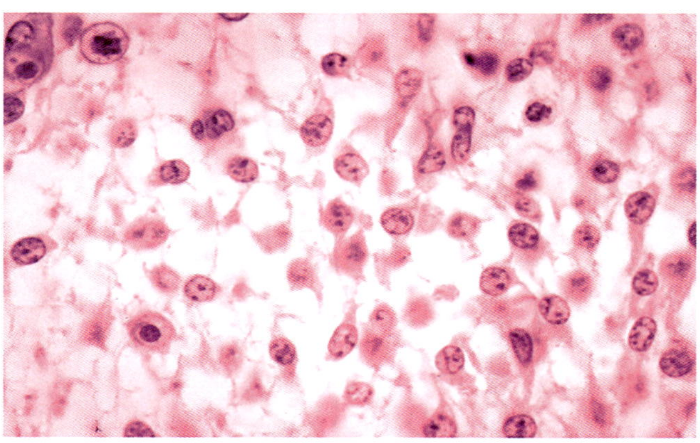

Figure 3-1 Mesenchyme (rat embryo). Note the stellate mesenchymal cells in an amorphous ground substance. Hematoxylin and eosin (H&E) (×800).

Mesenchymal Cells

Mesenchymal (or stromal) cells are irregularly shaped with multiple processes (Fig. 3-1). They are smaller than fibroblasts and have fewer cytoplasmic organelles. The large, oval nucleus has a prominent nucleolus and fine chromatin. The mesenchymal cell population serves as a reservoir of pluripotent cells that can differentiate into other types of CT cells as needed.

Fibrocytes and Fibroblasts

The most common CT cell is the **fibrocyte** (Fig. 3-2B). Fibrocytes are elongated and spindle-shaped and may have processes that contact adjacent cells and fibers. Their sparse, pale cytoplasm contains a nucleus with abundant heterochromatin. Secretory vesicles in the

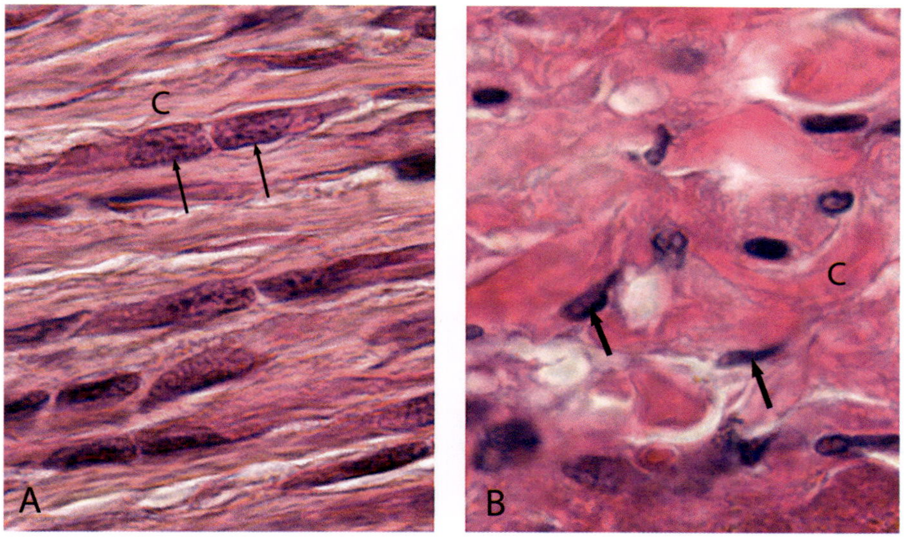

Figure 3-2 **A.** Fibroblasts (arrows) have larger, more euchromatic nuclei than fibrocytes in image **B** (arrows). The fibroblasts are more active in the production of fibers and ground substance of connective tissue (CT) than the fibrocyte. Collagen fibers (C) are present between the cells that produced them. Left: Tendon, puppy. H&E (×1200). Right: Liver, CT, dog. H&E (×1200). (Image by J. Eurell)

cytoplasm discharge their contents (e.g., procollagen, proteoglycans, and proelastin) into the surrounding microenvironment. At the transmission electron microscopic level, the cytoplasm has sparse rough endoplasmic reticulum (rER) and a small Golgi complex. Free ribosomes, mitochondria, lysosomes, and vesicles are also present. Actin filaments occur as bundles in the cell processes. Fibrocytes maintain the CT matrix by forming the fibers and constantly renewing the ground substance.

The **fibroblast** has a larger, more euchromatic nucleus and more abundant, basophilic cytoplasm than the fibrocyte (Fig. 3-2A). At the electron microscopy (EM) level, the cytoplasm shows abundant rER and a prominent Golgi complex. These structural characteristics suggest that fibroblasts are more actively involved in CT matrix production compared to fibrocytes. Fibroblasts may arise directly from undifferentiated (stem) mesenchymal stromal cells or are transformed from fibrocytes in response to microenvironmental factors (e.g., cytokines). In certain situations, fibroblasts may differentiate into adipose cells, chondroblasts, or osteoblasts.

Myofibroblasts are a type of fibroblast that contain actin filaments associated with dense bodies (smooth muscle α-actin); hence, they resemble smooth muscle cells. It is believed that myofibroblasts play a role in the contraction of the wound during healing.

Reticular Cells

Reticular cells are similar in appearance to the fibrocyte (Fig. 3-3A). They are stellate-shaped cells with a spherical nucleus and basophilic cytoplasm. Reticular cells produce **reticular fibers**, which form the fine-structural supportive network of organs such as the lymph nodes, spleen, and bone marrow (Fig. 3-3B). These cells are fixed in the tissue and are capable of phagocytosis. Reticular cells should not be confused with the reticulocyte, an immature erythrocyte.

Adipocytes

Adipocytes are also referred to as fat cells or adipose cells (Fig. 3-4). Individual adipocytes or clusters containing multiple cells are normal components of loose CT, but when the fat cells outnumber other cell types, the tissue is

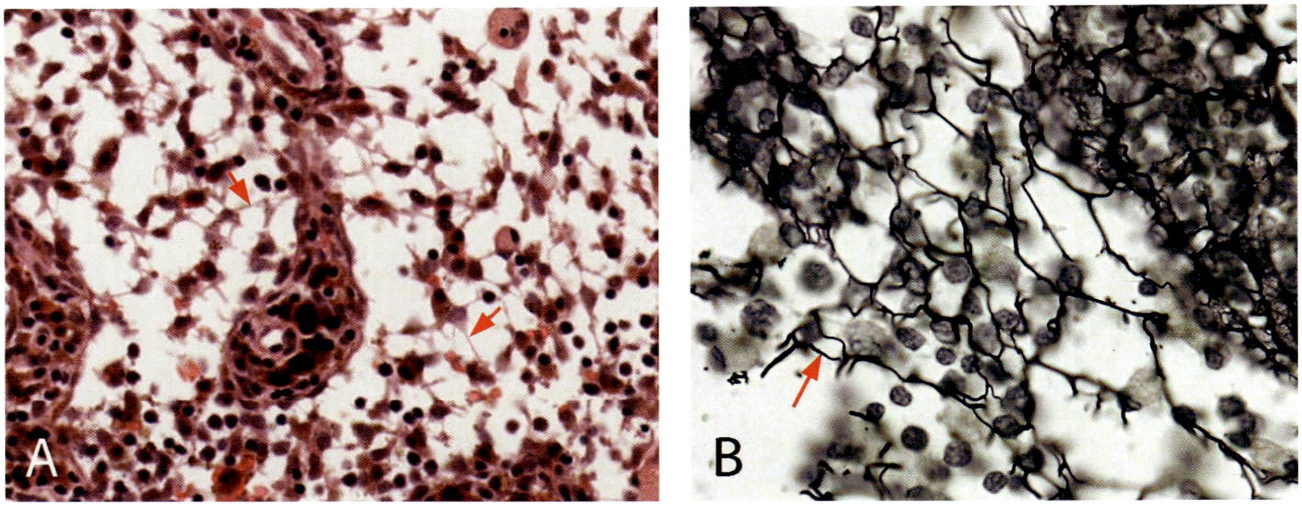

Figure 3-3 **A.** Reticular CT in medullary sinus of a lymph node (pig). Arrows indicate the interconnected reticular cells, which form a three-dimensional network. H&E (×600). **B.** Silver-stained lymph node with reticular fibers (arrow) (×800). (Image by John J. Turek.)

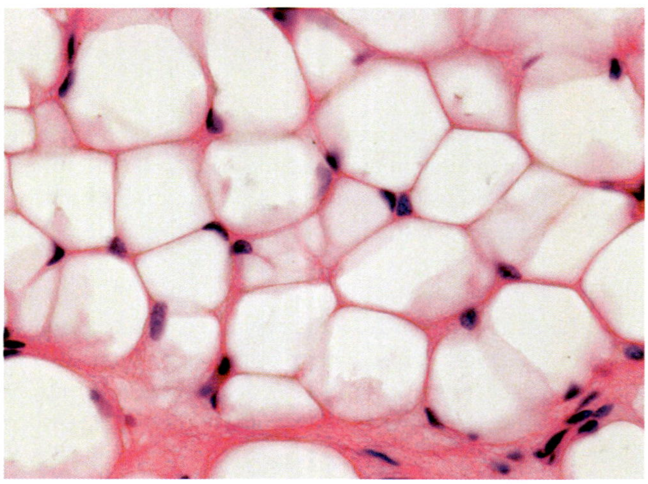

Figure 3-4 White adipose tissue in the hypodermis of pig skin. H&E (×400). (Image by John J. Turek.)

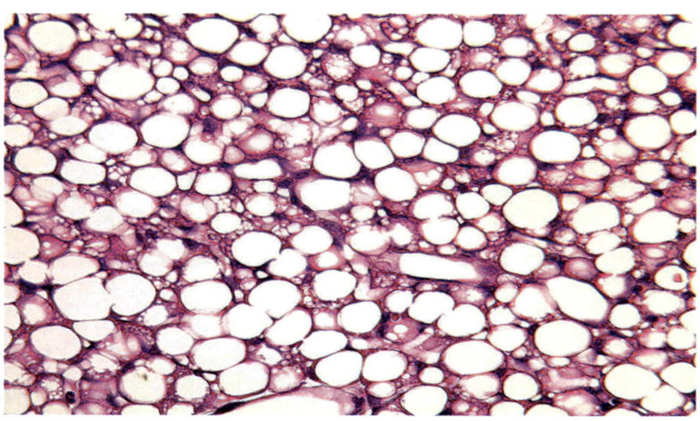

Figure 3-5 The cells of brown adipose tissue contain multiple lipid vacuoles of varying size. This tissue is found in neonates and hibernating animals and may play a role in thermoregulation. Adipose tissue ventral to vertebral column, dog. H&E (×400). (Image by J. Eurell.)

called **adipose tissue** (see more on this in the section "Adipose Tissue"). Mature **unilocular adipocytes** are spherical or polyhedral cells that measure up to 120 µm in diameter. Most of the cell is occupied by a single, large nonmembrane-bounded lipid droplet surrounded by a thin layer of cytoplasm. The cell nucleus is displaced to the periphery by the lipid droplet, which is surrounded by cytoplasm that contains a small Golgi complex, mitochondria, rER, and microfilaments.

In contrast, mature **multilocular adipocytes** contain a more centrally located nucleus with multiple lipid droplets in the cytoplasm (Fig. 3-5). Both the Golgi complex and rER are rather inconspicuous, but many mitochondria are present. The high concentration of cytochromes in the mitochondria is primarily responsible for the brown color of aggregates of multilocular adipocytes, which are referred to as brown fat (described below).

Unilocular adipocytes produce chemical energy, whereas multilocular adipocytes metabolize lipid to produce heat. Leptin, a protein produced by unilocular fat cells, regulates the amount of adipose tissue in the body. Thermogenin, a transmembrane protein in the mitochondria of brown fat, channels protons away from adenosine 5'-triphosphate (ATP) synthesis and into heat production instead.

Because fat is rapidly dissolved by most of the dehydration and/or clearing agents commonly used for the preparation of histologic sections, the lipid droplets appear as clear spaces surrounded by cytoplasm (Fig. 3-4). When rapidly processed, the lipid can be preserved and stained with certain agents, such as osmium tetroxide or Sudan III stain.

Pericytes

Pericytes or periendothelial cells are elongated cells that are located adjacent to the endothelium lining capillaries and postcapillary venules. The cells share a common basement membrane (BM) with endothelial cells, and both produce BM factors. Pericytes make frequent contact with the underlying endothelial cells by extending processes through the lamina. Pericytes resemble fibrocytes in appearance but have contractile filaments similar to smooth muscle. Proposed functions of pericytes include regulating capillary blood flow, serving as multipotent mesenchymal stromal cells with specific ability to form vascular smooth muscle cells, phagocytosing, and regulating new capillary growth. Pericytes also have the ability to differentiate into adipocytes, osteoblasts, and phagocytes.

Mast Cells

Mast cells are common in loose CT, especially around nerve endings and microcirculation. The cells are found in the dermis of the skin and CT of the respiratory tract and gastrointestinal system. Mast cells are bone marrow-derived and tissue-homing secretory cells.

Mast cells are large, polymorphic, spherical, or ovoid cells that contain a prominent, centrally located nucleus. Numerous secretory granules are present in the cytoplasm (Fig. 3-6). These cells can be identified with immunocytochemistry or a **metachromatic stain**, which has the capacity to stain elements of a cell or matrix a different color from that of the dye solution (e.g., toluidine blue, a blue dye that shifts the staining color of heparin-containing granules towards purple). At the EM level, the mast cell granules are membrane bounded and have crystalline, lamellar, or fine granular characteristics. The remaining cytoplasm is occupied by an extensive Golgi complex, cisternae of rER, free ribosomes, and mitochondria (Fig. 3-7).

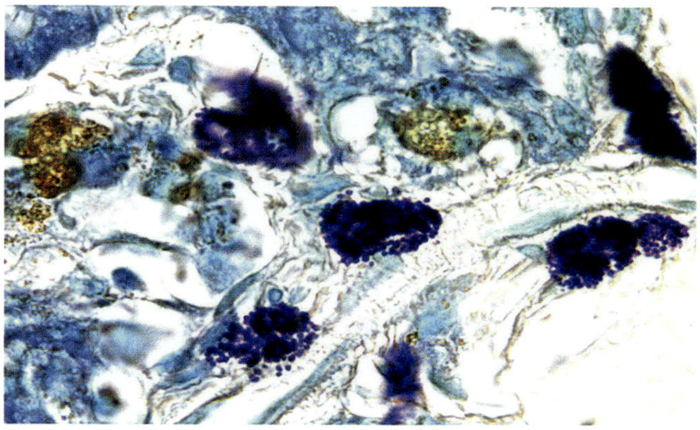

Figure 3-6 Mast cells scattered between pale blue CT fibers and cells. The mast cell granules stain dark purple to blue and often obscure the nucleus. Macrophages in this tissue sample have phagocytized gold-colored material. Skin, rat, toluidine blue (×1000). (Image by J. Eurell)

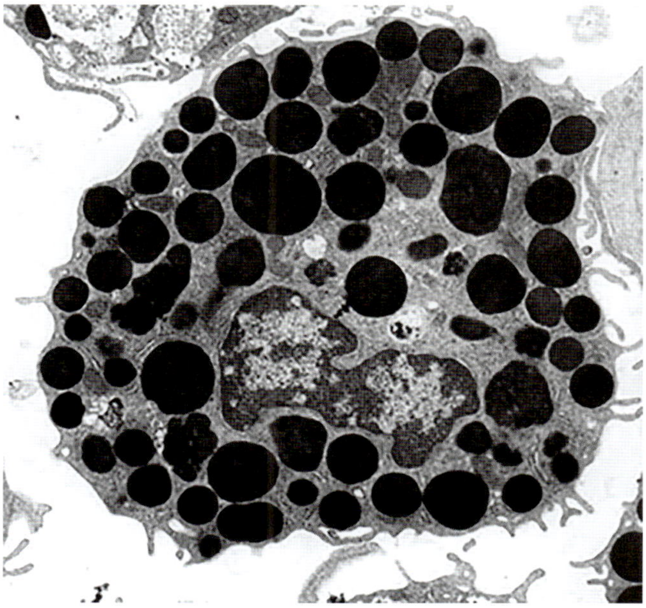

Figure 3-7 A rat mast cell featuring prominent granules. Electron micrograph by Dr. Constance Oliver and Dr. Celia Jamur. (Reproduced with permission from R.P Siraganian (1998) / ELSEVIER).

Mast cell granules contain histamine, heparin, and various proteases. **Histamine**, a biogenic amine, is a vasoconstrictor that causes increased permeability of small venules, thereby permitting leakage of plasma, resulting in tissue edema. This localized inflammatory reaction is designed to dispose of foreign antigens rapidly. Histamine also stimulates smooth muscle contraction in small airways. **Heparin**, a glycosaminoglycan, acts as an anticoagulant and is believed to stimulate angiogenesis. Mast cells can be activated to release their contents (degranulate) by physical stimuli such as trauma or sunlight; immunogenic stimuli including immunoglobulin (Ig) E, complement, or cytokines; and neurogenic stimuli such as neuropeptides.

Three populations of mast cells based on protease content have been identified. The mucosal mast cell (MC_T) contains tryptase only, while the connective tissue mast cell (MC_{TC}) contains tryptase, chymase, carboxypeptidase, and cathepsin. A third mast cell type (MC_C) has chymase and carboxypeptidase. The dog and cat have about 70% MC_{TC} cells. Proteases can destroy nearby cells and tissue matrix and activate complement components. Arachidonic acid products (leukotrienes) and cytokines (e.g., various interleukins, stem cell factor, and tumor necrosis factor alpha [TNF-α]) are also produced by the mast cell and immediately released without storage in the cytoplasmic granules. In the past, the mast cell has been described as a "tissue basophil," but despite some similarities, the mast cell and the basophil are different cells. Both cells develop from the same pluripotent stem cell (CD34+), and both have basophilic cytoplasmic granules that contain similar inflammatory products. However, basophils are terminally differentiated before they enter the blood circulation, while mast cells leave the bone marrow, pass through the circulation, and differentiate in tissues outside the bone marrow. The mast cell can undergo mitotic division while the basophil cannot. Also, basophils have a short lifespan of days while most mast cells can survive for weeks to months.

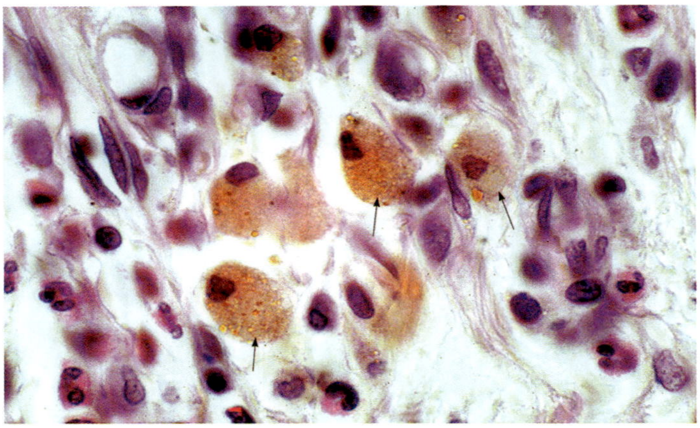

Figure 3-8 Macrophages (arrows) are large, ovoid, or spherical cells. They are phagocytic and contain numerous cytoplasmic vacuoles and phagolysosomes. Liver, rat. H&E (×1000). (Image by W.E. Haensly)

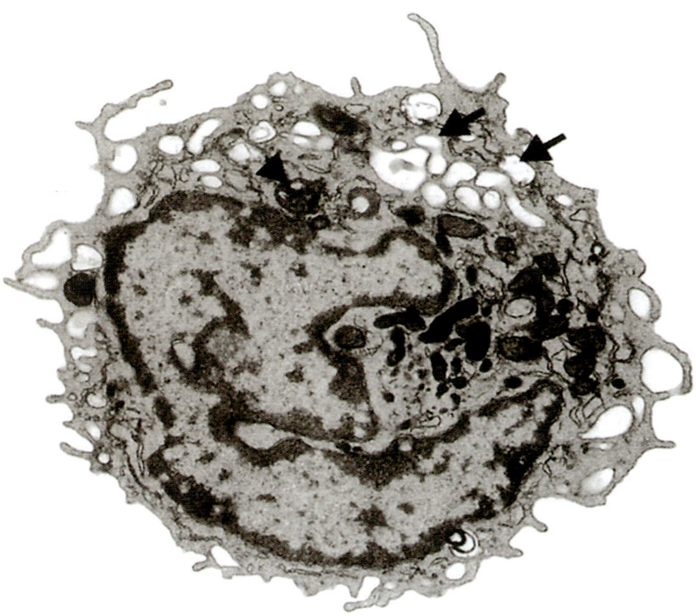

Figure 3-9 Macrophage containing abundant pinocytotic vacuoles (arrows) and phagolysosomes (arrowhead) (×8000).

Macrophages

Macrophages are phagocytic cells that are scattered throughout the body and form the **mononuclear phagocyte system**. They are derived from a bone marrow precursor cell (CFU-GM) that divides and produces monocytes that circulate in the blood. The monocytes then migrate across blood vessel walls into CT or organs and differentiate into macrophages. Mobile (free) macrophages wander through the tissues performing their phagocytic function, while fixed macrophages remain in one location. The fixed macrophage of CT is also known as the **histiocyte**. Other macrophages located in specific tissues include the stellate macrophage of the liver (Kupffer cell), the intraepidermal macrophage (Langerhans cell), and preosteoclasts.

Macrophages are large, ovoid, or spherical cells that contain cytoplasmic vacuoles and are readily distinguishable with the light microscope (Fig. 3-8). At the EM level, they are characterized by numerous lysosomes, phagosomes, phagolysosomes, and pseudopodia (footlike extensions of the cell membrane) (Fig. 3-9). Abundant ribosomes, rER, smooth ER (sER), mitochondria, and a Golgi complex are also present. Histochemical stains for lysosomal enzymes, such as acid phosphatase, facilitate the identification of macrophages. Once activated, the macrophage changes morphology with increased microvilli and lamellipodia, which are sheet-like extensions of cytoplasm. The lamellipodia form transient adhesions with the surrounding substrate, enabling the cell to move.

The number of tissue macrophages is sustained by monocyte influx from blood, local monocyte proliferation, and macrophage turnover through apoptotic cell death (lifespan in tissue <3 weeks). A variety of chemotactic stimuli (e.g., infectious agents and cytokines) cause macrophages to migrate to locations in the body where foreign material must be removed. Macrophages engulf material such as cell debris, abnormal matrix components, neoplastic cells, bacteria, and inert substances by pinocytosis and phagocytosis. Phagocytosis may be indiscriminate (e.g., dust particles in the lung) or may involve specific interaction with receptors on the macrophage surface (e.g., Fc receptors, IgG, and IgM). Macrophages also act as antigen-presenting cells, which process and display foreign substances so that lymphocytes can recognize and respond more effectively to the challenge.

Inflammation can be characterized as acute or chronic based on the relative proportions of neutrophils and macrophages. Acute inflammation has a higher number of neutrophils compared to macrophages, whereas chronic inflammation has a predominance of macrophages over neutrophils. When stimulated, macrophages may form clusters of epithelioid cells, which resemble epithelial cells in morphology. Multinucleated giant cells or foreign-body cells (Fig. 3-10) arise during chronic inflammation and are a result of the fusion of several macrophages in response to the presence of foreign material.

Macrophages synthesize and secrete many substances that reflect their multiple functions. These substances include enzymes such as lysozyme, which lyses the wall of many bacteria; cytokines (interferons and interleukin); complement components (C2, C3, C4, and C5); coagulation factors; and reactive chemical species (hydrogen peroxide, hydroxyl radicals, and nitric oxide), which are important components of the bactericidal and cytocidal (e.g., tumor cells) activities of macrophages. Recent research has expanded our understanding of macrophage functions, revealing a broader cytokine repertoire production beyond interferons, including TNF-α, IL-1, and IL-6. Additionally, while macrophages produce reactive species, these molecules also play roles in signaling and inflammation. Macrophages exhibit different polarization states that influence their functional roles in various physiological and pathological contexts. M1 macrophages, or "classically activated", are induced by pro-inflammatory stimuli such as IFN-γ and LPS, leading to high production of pro-inflammatory cytokines such as TNF-α, IL-1β, and IL-6, which enhance their role in defending against pathogens and tumors but can also contribute to tissue damage if excessively activated. In contrast, M2 macrophages, or "alternatively activated," are stimulated by anti-inflammatory cytokines such as IL-4 and IL-13, and are important in tissue repair, inflammation resolution, and immune regulation, via the production of anti-inflammatory cytokine IL-10, for example. This polarization indicates that macrophages have high functional plasticity and can participate in diverse functions beyond traditional immune responses.

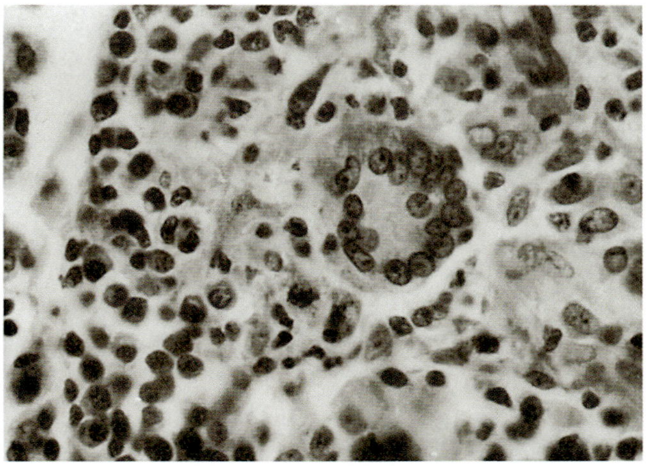

Figure 3-10 Multinucleated giant cell, lymph node (sheep). Crossman's trichrome (×435).

Plasma Cells

Plasma cells are spherical, ovoid, or pear-shaped cells with a spherical, eccentric nucleus. The chromatin is often arranged in peripherally located clumps or in centrally converging strands that give the nucleus a "cartwheel" appearance (Fig. 3-11). The cytoplasm is intensely basophilic, and a negatively stained Golgi region is usually present. At the fine-structural level, in addition to an extensive Golgi complex, the cytoplasm has an abundant rER with dilated cisternae containing slightly granular and moderately electron-dense material as well as spherical inclusions referred to as *Russell bodies*, which contain immunoglobulins (Fig. 3-12). Free ribosomes and mitochondria are also present in the cytoplasm.

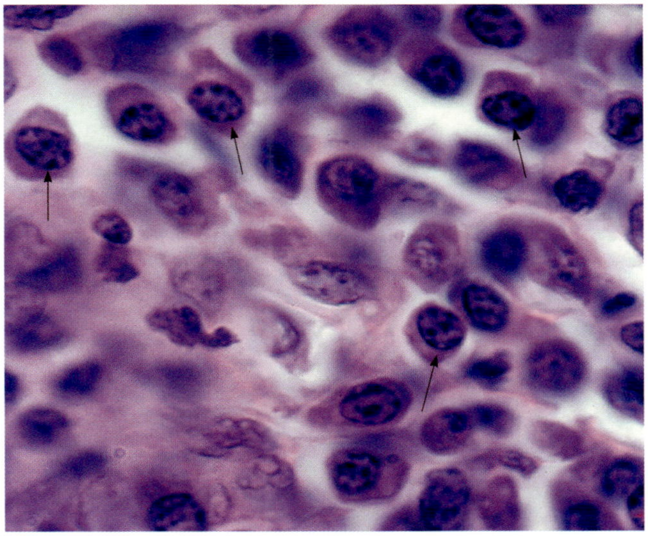

Figure 3-11 Plasma cells (arrows) are spherical or ovoid-shaped and have an eccentric nucleus. The nuclear chromatin is often arranged in peripheral clumps. A light-staining area in the cytoplasm adjacent to the nucleus is the site of the Golgi complex. Soft palate, cat. H&E (×1000). (Image by W.E. Haensly).

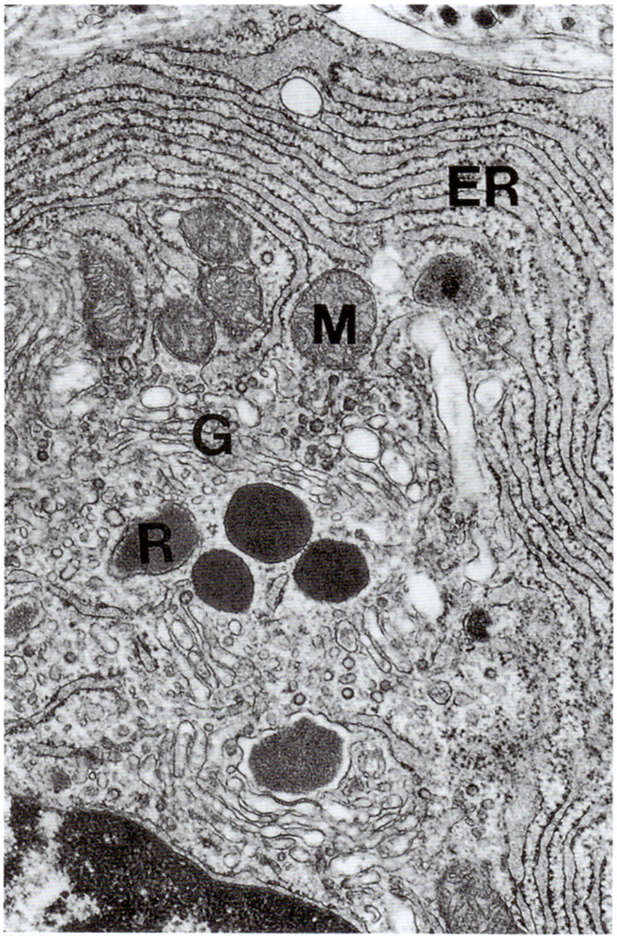

Figure 3-12 Part of a plasma cell with abundant rough endoplasmic reticulum (ER), mitochondria (M), extensive Golgi complex (G), and Russell bodies (R) (×19,500).

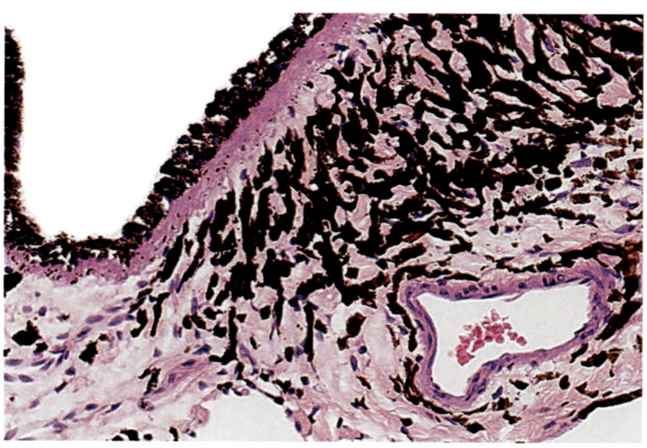

Figure 3-13 CT of the iris of the eye with pigment-containing cells. Eye, dog. H&E (×400). (Image by John J. Turek.)

Plasma cells are most numerous in lymphatic tissue, especially in the center of medullary cords of lymph nodes. They are also particularly abundant in bone marrow, the loose CT underlying the epithelium of the gastrointestinal tract, the respiratory system, and the female reproductive system. This distribution reflects their role in immune surveillance and antibody production in various locations of the body.

Plasma cells do not originate in loose CT but develop from B lymphocytes that immigrate into CT from the blood; they produce circulating or humoral antibodies (see Chapter 8).

Pigment Cells

Other cells in CT may contain pigments, including melanin in domestic animals or pteridines and purines in fish and amphibians (Fig. 3-13). When present in large numbers, the cells impart color to the CT. They occur in various locations such as the dermis, uterine caruncles of sheep, meninges, choroid, and iris. Their significance is context dependent and described in connection with the specific organs in which they are located.

Other Cells of Loose Connective Tissue

Depending on its location and various other factors (infestation by parasites, presence of bacteria, and the like), loose CT may contain a varying number of lymphocytes, monocytes, and granulocytes (especially eosinophils and neutrophils). The structure and function of these infiltrating cells are described in the section on blood (see Chapter 6).

Globule leukocytes are mononuclear cells with acidophilic and metachromatic cytoplasmic granules. These cells are found in epithelium and CT of the respiratory, digestive, reproductive, and urinary systems. Globule leukocytes were traditionally considered mucosal mast cells, but there is emerging evidence proposing their origin as a subpopulation of T lymphocytes.

Connective Tissue Fibers

Structural CT fibers include collagen, reticular, and elastic fibers. In addition, **fibrous adhesive proteins** such as fibronectin and laminin bind structural fibers together or help cells attach to the CT matrix.

Collagen Fibers

Collagen is the principal fiber type in mature CT. The turnover rate of collagen is tissue-specific and can vary even within the same tissue. Most collagen digestion occurs through the action of metalloproteinases (e.g., collagenase) and serine proteases.

Collagen polypeptide chains are synthesized in the rER as pro-α chains that contain extension peptides (propeptides) at both ends (Fig. 3-14). Multiple α chains have been recognized. Within the rER cisternae, these pro-α chains assemble into triple helices to form **procollagen** molecules. The molecules are then transferred to the Golgi complex, packaged into secretory vesicles, and released by exocytosis. At this point in synthesis, collagen can be classed as fibril-forming, FACIT (*f*ibril-*a*ssociated *c*ollagens with *i*nterrupted *t*riple helices), sheet-forming, multiplexin, connecting and anchoring, or transmembrane collagen. Twenty-eight collagen types are currently recognized.

Fibril-forming collagen then undergoes extracellular enzymatic cleavage of the propeptides to yield collagen molecules. These molecules in turn assemble in the extracellular matrix (ECM) to form **collagen fibrils**. The fibrils are only visible with the electron microscope, are up to several micrometers in length, and vary in diameter (10 to 300 nm), with characteristic cross-striations repeated at 67 nm intervals (Figs. 3-14 and 3-15). Bundles of these fibrils form **collagen fibers** that are visible by light microscopy (Fig. 3-2A). Fibril-forming collagen includes

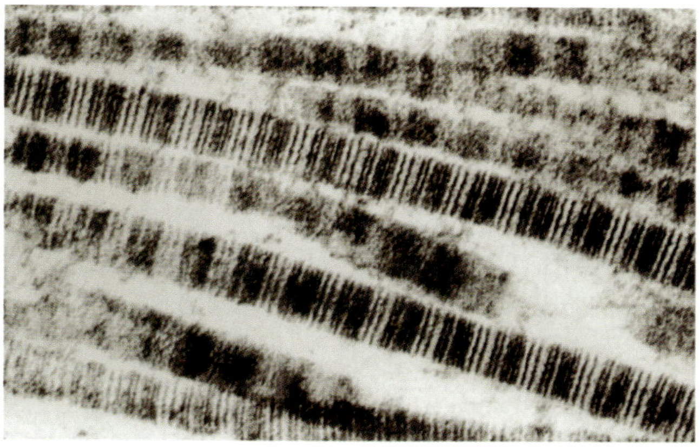

Figure 3-15 Electron micrograph of collagen fibrils with characteristic cross-striations (×88,000).

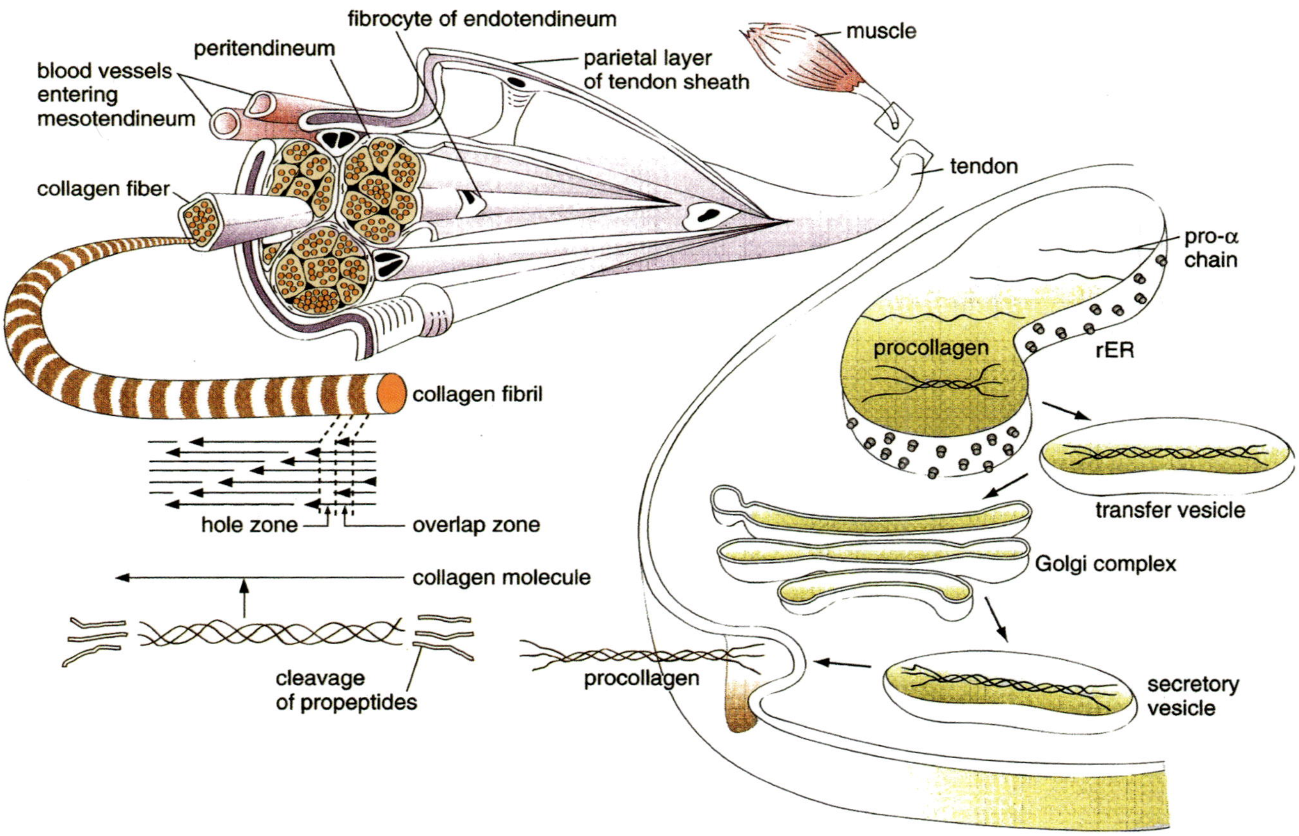

Figure 3-14 Collagen polypeptide chains are synthesized within the cell and released into the extracellular space as procollagen. In fibril-forming collagen, peptides are then cleaved from the procollagen, resulting in a collagen molecule. The collagen molecules are assembled in such a way that hole zones are created, which stain dark, in contrast to overlap zones, which exclude stain. Bundles of light- and dark-banded fibrils form collagen fibers. In a tendon, individual collagen fibers are surrounded by endotendineum and bundles of fibers are bound by peritendineum. In this drawing, the sheath surrounding the tendon is reflected to show the collagen fiber bundles (fascicles) inside. Blood vessels pass through the mesotendineum to supply the tendon.

types I, II, III, V, XI, XXIV, and XXVII. Fibers composed of type I collagen account for 90% of the body collagen. Type I collagen is found in skin, tendon, bone, and dentin, while type II collagen is specific for cartilage and vitreous humor. Frequently colocalized with type I collagen, type III collagen is essential for normal collagen I fibrillogenesis. Type V collagen is necessary for ECM assembly in CT; it is present in fetal tissues and the placenta. Type XI collagen is found in hyaline cartilage and type XXIV collagen is distributed in developing cornea and bone.

Fresh collagen fibers are white, and in histologic preparations, they stain with acid dyes. Thus, they are red to pink in hematoxylin and eosin (H&E)-stained sections, red with van Gieson's method, and blue in Mallory's and Masson's triple stains (green when light green stain is used). The fibers are flexible and can adapt to the movements and changes in size of the organs with which they are associated. Collagen fibers are characterized by a high tensile strength and a poor shear strength, and stretch is limited to approximately 5% of their initial length. Consequently, they are found wherever high tensile strength is required, such as in tendons, ligaments, and organ capsules.

The **FACIT collagens** include types IX, XII, XIV, XX, XXI, and XXII. These collagens serve as molecular bridges that are important in the organization and stability of extracellular matrices. Glycosaminoglycans (GAGs) are linked to type II collagen of hyaline cartilage by collagen IX. Type XX collagen is prevalent in corneal epithelium. The ECM of blood vessel walls contains type XXI collagen, while the ECM at tissue junctions contains type XXII collagens. Some FACIT collagens (types XVI and XIX) are unable to bind fibers and are referred to as FACIT-like collagens.

Sheet-forming collagen forms a flexible framework of sheets rather than fibrils. Collagen IV forms the basal lamina of epithelia. In the eye, the posterior limiting lamina (Descemet's membrane) of the cornea is formed from type VIII collagen. Type X collagen is found in the hypertrophic zone of the physis.

Multiplexins (*multiple* triple-heli*x* domains and *in*terruptions) are collagens that are associated with BMs. This subgroup includes types XV and XVIII.

Connecting and anchoring collagen binds to the surface of fibril-forming collagen and may mediate the interactions of fibrils with one another and with other matrix components. Collagen types VI and VII are believed to perform this function. Type VI collagen forms unique beaded filaments, while collagen VII forms **anchoring fibrils** that link collagen IV of the basal lamina of the epidermis to the collagen of underlying CT.

Transmembrane collagens include XIII, XVII, XXIII, and XXV. Collagen XVII, a transmembrane collagen of the skin, is associated with hemidesmosomes and mutates in diseases that cause blisters (epidermolysis bullosa). Type XXIII collagen is associated with metastatic tumor cells, while type XXV collagen is a neuronal collagen.

Collagen XXVI is unclassified and is found in the testes and ovary.

Reticular Fibers

In routine histologic preparations, reticular fibers cannot be distinguished from other small collagen fibers. These fibers can be identified only with certain silver impregnations due to their affinity for silver salts (thus the term **argyrophilic** or **argentaffin fibers**) (see Fig. 3-3B) or with the periodic acid-Schiff (PAS) reagent. These fibers are actually individual collagen fibrils (type III collagen) coated by proteoglycans and glycoproteins. This coating increases the affinity of the fibers for silver salts. When individual reticular fibers are bundled to form collagen fibers, the coating is supposedly displaced and the argyrophilia decreases.

Reticular fibers form delicate, flexible networks around capillaries, muscle fibers, nerves, adipose cells, and hepatocytes and serve as a scaffolding to support cells or cell groups of endocrine, lymphatic, and blood-forming organs. They are an integral part of BMs.

Elastic Fibers

Elastic fibers and/or sheets (laminae) are present in organs in which normal function requires elasticity in addition to tensile strength. Elastic fibers can be stretched as much as two and one-half times their original length to which they return when released. Elastic fibers are found in organs requiring elasticity in addition to tensile strength, such as the pinna of the ear, vocal cords, and lungs. Found also in the epiglottis ligamentum nuchae, dermis, aorta, and muscular arteries, elastic fibers are one of the most resilient CT fibers, withstanding chemical maceration and autoclaving.

Elastic fibers usually occur as individual, branching, and anastomosing fibers. Their diameters vary within a wide range, from 0.2 to 5.0 μm in loose CT to as large as 12 μm in elastic ligaments, such as the ligamentum nuchae in the neck. In H&E-stained histologic sections, the larger elastic fibers in elastic ligaments are readily distinguished as highly refractile, amorphous, light pink strands; they are stainable by certain selective dyes, such as orcein and resorcin-fuchsin (Fig. 3-16).

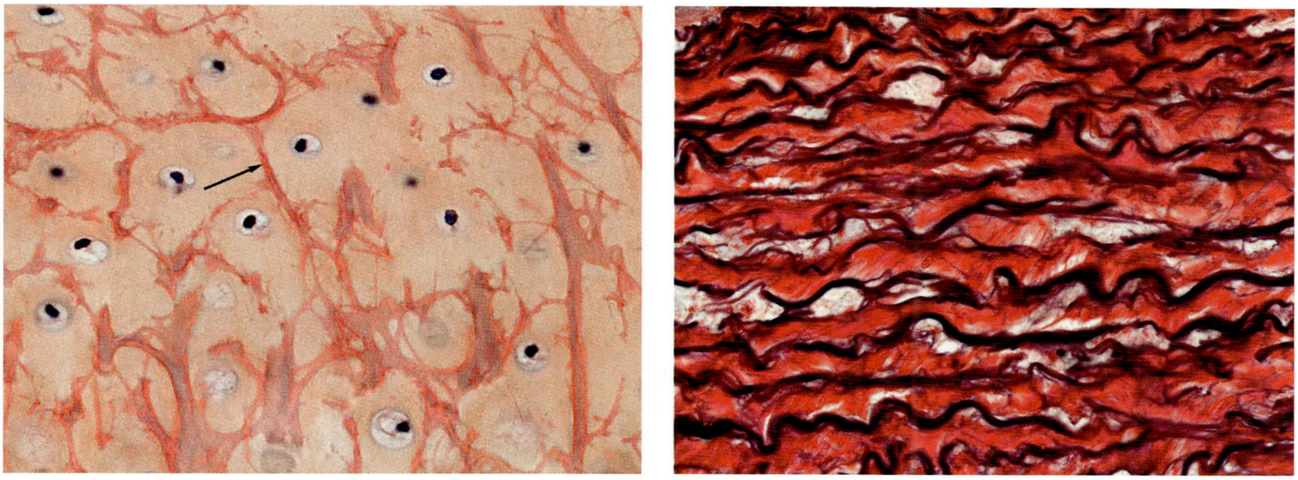

Figure 3-16 Left: Elastic fibers (arrow) within elastic cartilage of ear pinna of a dog (×400). Right: Elastic fibers within the aorta (pig) (×400). Elastin stains. (Image by John J. Turek.)

The main component of elastic fibers is **elastin**, which contains a network of **fibrillin** microfibrils providing a scaffold. Elastin, rich in proline and glycine, undergoes stretch and recoil due to its randomly coiled structure, stabilized by cross-links containing desmosine. The coils of elastin can stretch and then recoil as needed. Elastin is synthesized by fibroblasts and smooth muscle cells.

The secondary component of elastic fibers is 10 nm microfibrils that surround and are embedded within the elastic core of the fiber, contributing to its integrity (Fig. 3-17). The microfibrillar material is composed of a glycoprotein, **fibrillin**, which is necessary for elastic fiber integrity.

During the development of the elastic fiber, fibrillin microfibrils are secreted before elastin and provide a scaffold onto which elastin is deposited. This initial stage of fiber development is referred to as **oxytalan**. In the subsequent stage, elastin is deposited between the microfibrils, forming **elaunin**. As elastin continues to accumulate, mature **elastic fibers** are formed. Developmentally, the elastic fiber is the last fiber to appear in organs (e.g., lung) or CT.

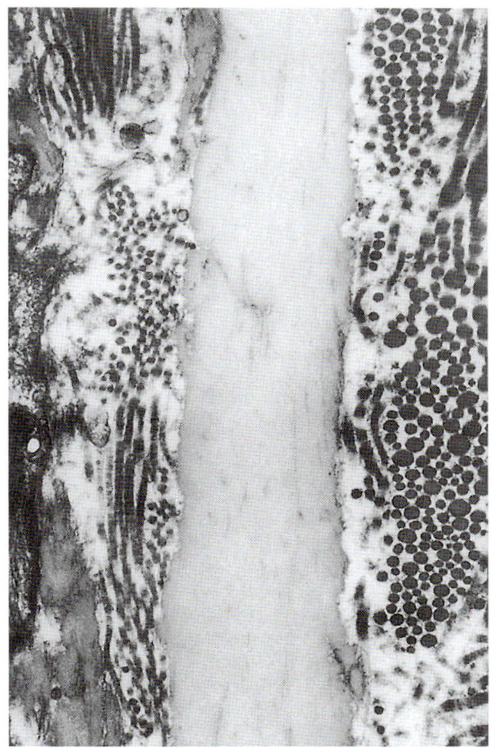

Figure 3-17 Electron micrograph of an elastic lamina between collagen fibrils (longitudinal and cross sections). The electron-dense thin lines in the elastic lamina are microfibrils (×21,000).

Fibrous Adhesive Proteins

The ECM contains noncollagenous fibrous proteins crucial for matrix organization and cell adhesion. **Fibronectin**, a major product of mesenchymal cells, is a fibril-forming protein that binds to various structures, including the cell membrane, collagen, elastin, and proteoglycans, and mediates the connection between the cytoskeleton and the ECM. Fibronectin plays a role in a variety of processes, such as cell adhesion, cell differentiation, cell growth, and phagocytosis.

Laminins, on the other hand, are large glycoproteins that are a major constituent of the BM. They are synthesized by cells in contact with the BM, such as epithelial cells, smooth muscle cells, and Schwann cells (Fig. 4-12). Laminins are present in both the lamina lucida (lamina rara) and the lamina densa of the BM. They are connected to type IV collagen by the adhesive glycoprotein nidogen (entactin). Laminins form a structural network in the BM to which other glycoproteins and proteoglycans attach. Additionally, laminins act as signaling molecules that stabilize cell-surface receptors.

Ground Substance

The cells and fibers of CT are embedded in an amorphous ground substance composed of GAGs, proteoglycans, plasma constituents, metabolites, water, and ions. The ground substance forms a hydrated gel that, by virtue of its high water content, has unique properties of resiliency.

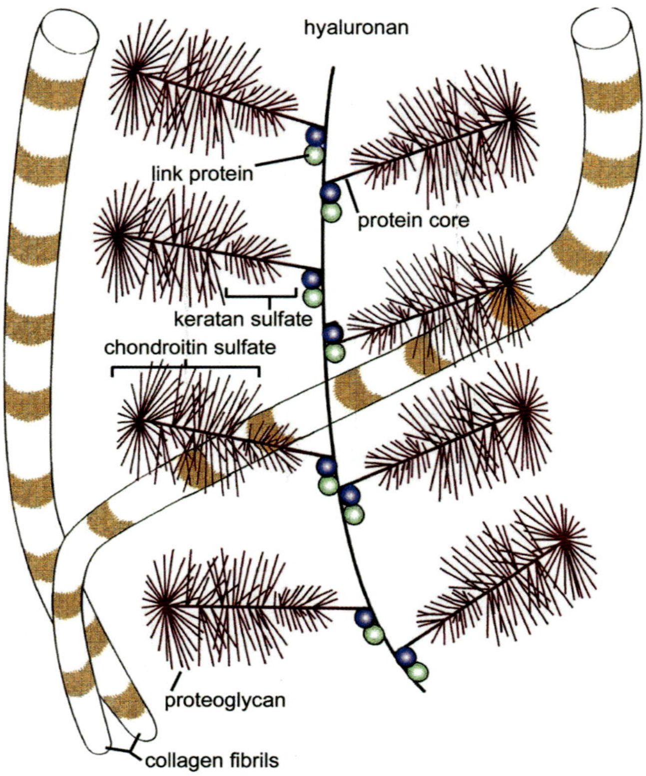

Figure 3-18 The matrix of cartilage contains aggrecans, which are composed of proteoglycans bound to a hyaluronic acid chain by link proteins. The proteoglycans are composed of glycosaminoglycans, such as chondroitin and keratan sulfate, bound to a protein core.

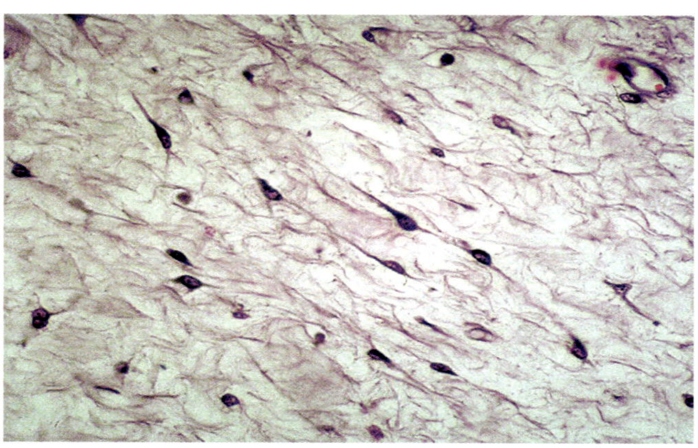

Figure 3-19 Stellate fibroblasts form the matrix of mucous CT. The matrix consists of collagen fibers and a ground substance of glycosaminoglycans or proteoglycans. Umbilical cord. H&E (×400). (Image by W.E. Haensly.)

Glycosaminoglycans are comprised of unbranched polysaccharides of alternating uronic acid and hexosamine residues. Seven major types of GAGs can be distinguished. **Hyaluronan** (hyaluronic acid) is a nonsulfated GAG. It is a large, long molecule that forms networks with spaces that are filled with tissue fluid. The resulting gel is particularly abundant in the vitreous humor of the eye and in synovial fluid; it is also found in the umbilical cord, loose CT skin, and cartilage. Hyaluronan binds proteoglycans into a larger molecule called an **aggrecan** (Fig. 3-18). **Chondroitin-4-sulfate** and **chondroitin-6-sulfate** are abundant in cartilage, arteries, skin, and cornea. A smaller amount is found in bone. **Dermatan sulfate** is found in skin, tendon, ligamentum nuchae, sclera, and lung. **Keratan sulfate** is present in cartilage, bone, and cornea. **Heparan sulfate** is found in arteries and the lung, whereas **heparin** is found in mast cells, the lung, the liver, and skin. The latter six GAGs are of the sulfated variety.

Proteoglycans are formed by covalently linking GAGs to a protein core and range in size from small molecules (decorin, M_W 40,000) to large aggregates (aggrecan, M_W 210,000) (Fig. 3-18). Proteoglycans play essential roles in filling space in the CT matrix and contribute to its unique biomechanical properties. Also, they are involved in regulating the passage of molecules and cells in the intercellular space and are believed to play a significant role in chemical signaling between cells.

Proteoglycans are typically not detected in low concentrations in routine H&E-stained sections, but when present in higher concentrations, as in hyaline cartilage, they stain with basophilic dyes. When stained with toluidine blue or crystal violet, a metachromatic change occurs that promotes a color shift to pink or magenta.

Embryonic Connective Tissues

Mesenchyme

Mesenchyme, the CT of the developing embryo, is composed of irregularly shaped undifferentiated mesenchymal cells and amorphous ground substance (Fig. 3-19). The cell processes contact adjacent cells and thus form a three-dimensional network. Mesenchymal cells undergo numerous mitotic cell divisions and continuously change their shape and location to adapt to the transformations that occur during embryonic growth. During early development, mesenchyme lacks fibers, and the intercellular spaces are filled with abundant ground substance. Importantly, mesenchyme serves as a precursor to various types of adult CT, as well as blood and blood vessels.

Mucous Connective Tissue

Mucous or gelatinous CT is primarily found in the embryonic hypodermis and umbilical cord (Fig. 3-19). It is characterized by stellate fibroblasts that form a network. The large intercellular spaces are occupied by a viscous, gel-like amorphous ground substance that has a positive reaction for GAGs or proteoglycans. Collagen fibers (types I and III) are also present. In the adult organism, gelatinous CT occurs in the papillae of omasal laminae and reticular crests, the bovine glans penis, and the core of the rooster comb.

Adult Connective Tissues

Adult connective tissues are classified based on the quantity and arrangement of fibers within the matrix. The properties of cell structure and the biochemical composition of fibers and ground substance are generally similar across different types of CT.

Loose Connective Tissue

Loose CT, also known as areolar CT, is the most widely distributed type in the adult animal (Fig. 3-20A). The cells and fibers of loose CT are widely separated by spaces filled with ground substance. Compared to other types of CT, the cells in loose CT are more abundant and include both fixed and mobile populations. All three fiber types (reticular, collagen, and elastic) are present. The relative abundance and orientation of fibers can vary widely depending on the location-specific function of the tissue. In cases of injury, the stage of healing can also influence the arrangement of fibers, with early CT being highly cellular with fine reticular fibers and later CT having predominantly thick collagen fibers.

The amorphous ground substance of loose CT is composed of proteoglycans that bind a significant quantity of tissue fluid. This ground substance allows substances dissolved in the tissue fluid to diffuse through it, providing ready access to CT cells. Circulating tissue fluid is formed at the arterial end of capillaries and absorbed by either venous or lymphatic capillaries.

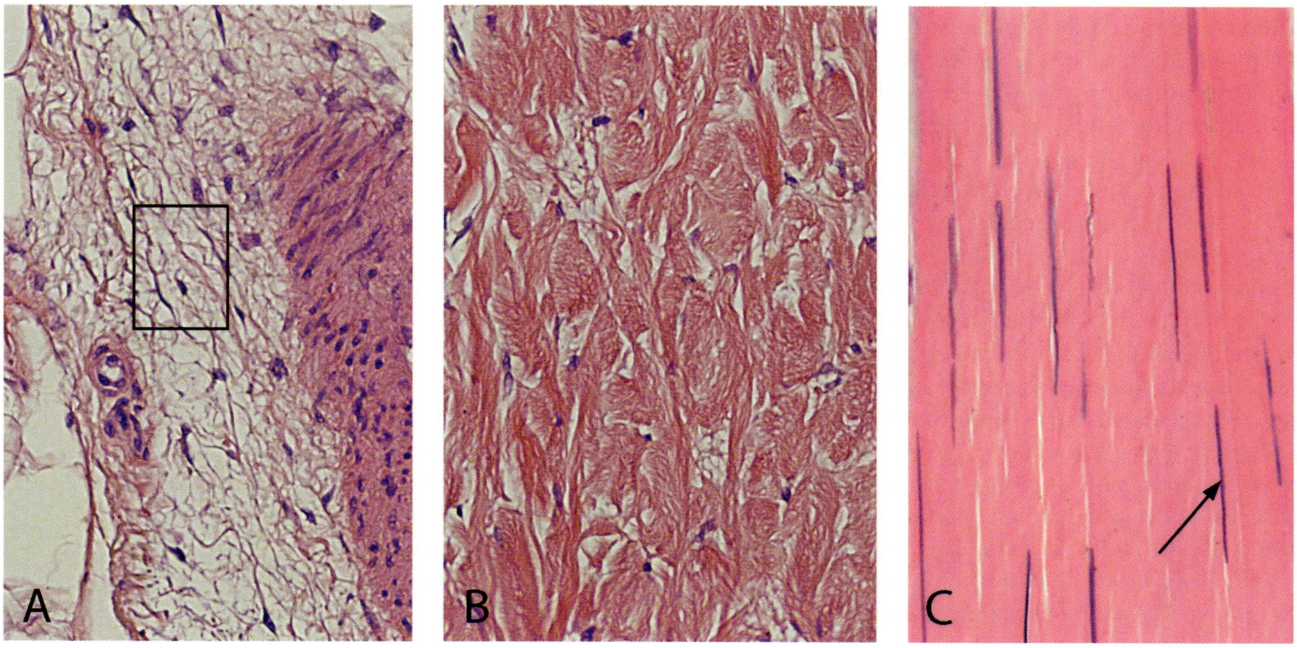

Figure 3-20 **A.** Loose CT adjacent to an artery (skin, pig) (box), liver (dog). **B.** Dense irregular CT (dermis, pig). **C.** Dense regular CT with fibrocytes a nucleus at the (arrow), tendon. H&E (×500). (Image by John J. Turek.)

Loose CT is present beneath many epithelia, providing support and a vascular supply. This tissue also forms the interstitial tissue in most organs, allowing for easy movements and shifting of organs. Loose CT surrounds nerve and skeletal muscle bundles as named tissue layers (e.g., epineurium) and is present between the layers of smooth musculature of hollow organs. The pia mater and arachnoid of the brain and spinal cord are also composed of loose CT.

The functions of loose CT are diverse, ranging from mechanical support and dampening biomechanical effects in various locations, such as the hypodermis, to more sophisticated roles in tissue repair and defense activities, including inflammation.

Dense Connective Tissue

Dense CT is characterized by a higher abundance of fibers relative to cells and amorphous ground substance. This CT type is commonly classified as either **dense irregular CT**, with a random (mesh-like) orientation of the fiber bundles, or **dense regular CT**, in which fibers are oriented in a regular (parallel) pattern.

Dense Irregular Connective Tissue

Fibrocytes are the predominant cell population in **dense irregular CT** (Fig. 3-20B). Collagen fibers are generally arranged in bundles that cross each other at varying angles. In thin aponeuroses or muscle fasciae, these bundles are located in a single layer. In heavier aponeuroses, organ capsules, or dermis, the bundles are superimposed in several layers and interlace with one another in multiple planes. This irregular configuration allows adaptation to changes in the size of an organ or the diameter of a muscle, and stretching forces can be withstood in any direction. Continuation of surface CT into the organ or muscle enhances strength. Elastic networks within the tissue contribute to its ability to rapidly return to resting conditions.

Dense irregular CT is found in a variety of locations, such as the lamina propria of the initial portions of the digestive system, the capsule of the lung (visceral pleura) and other organs (spleen, liver, kidney, and testis), fasciae, aponeuroses, joint capsules, pericardium, and dermis. Special functional and morphologic features are described with the various organ systems.

Dense Regular Connective Tissue

Dense regular CT occurs as collagenous tendons and ligaments or as elastic ligaments (Fig. 3-20C). In both types, all fibers are arranged in the same direction according to specific functional requirements.

Collagenous Tendons and Ligaments The great tensile strength of collagenous tendons is reflected in their structure. They consist of fascicles of parallel collagen fibers (Fig. 3-14). Individual collagen fibers are surrounded by fibrocytes, which form the **endotendineum**. These fascicles are bound together by sparse, loose CT (the **peritendineum**) that forms a protective sheath around the blood vessels and nerves of the tendon. The peritendineum is continuous with the **epitendineum**, the dense irregular CT around the entire tendon. The fibrocytes between the collagen fibers of the tendon are long, flat cells of varying shape. Wing-like cytoplasmic processes extend between adjacent collagen fibers and give the fibrocytes a stellate appearance in cross sections of tendon. Following injury, the fibroblasts of surrounding CT sheaths proliferate and contribute to the repair process.

The typical tendon structure may be altered at points of insertion into bone or cartilage or where the tendon courses around bones. Wherever tendons or ligaments insert on bone or cartilage, the dense regular collagenous tissue of the tendon gradually changes to fibrocartilage and then to mineralized fibrocartilage before the point of osseous penetration. Collagen fibers from the tendon or ligament are embedded in the bone matrix as **perforating fibers** (Sharpey's fibers). The function of this arrangement is to gradually transmit biomechanical forces from a flexible fibrous unit to a stiffer osseous unit. In areas where tendons wrap around bones, they are subject not only to tension but also to compression, which causes the cells to enlarge and to become encapsulated, resembling fibrocartilage.

The mobility of the tendon is ensured either by the surrounding epitendineum or the **tendon sheath**, which consists of a visceral and a parietal portion (Fig. 3-14). The visceral portion is tightly anchored to the epitendineum of the tendon and is separated from the parietal portion by a fluid-filled synovial cavity. Both the parietal and the visceral portions of the tendon sheath comprise dense irregular CT and a synovial layer, the structure of which is similar to that of synovial membranes (see *synovial joints* below). Blood vessels supplying the tendon pass through a gap between the opposing edges of the synovial sheath known as the **mesotendineum**. This arrangement permits smooth movement of the tendon within its sheath while providing vascular supply to the tendon.

Collagenous ligaments contain a lower percentage of ground substance relative to tendons, which makes them less compliant and more resistant to deformation. Also, the collagen fibers are organized more randomly relative to the parallel arrangement seen in tendons. Unlike tendons, ligaments typically do not have named CT sheaths associated with them. Ligaments are instead either surrounded by loose CT or are partially integrated into joint capsules or other surrounding structures.

Elastic Ligaments Large elastic fibers that branch and interconnect predominate in **elastic ligaments**, providing the ligament with elasticity and resilience. The fibers are surrounded by loose CT. The ligamentum nuchae and some dorsal ligaments (ligamenta flava) of the vertebral column are examples of elastic ligaments.

Reticular Connective Tissue

The stroma of all lymphatic organs (spleen, lymph node, hemal node, and tonsils), diffuse lymphatic tissue, solitary lymphatic nodules, and bone marrow is made of reticular CT. This tissue is composed of stellate reticular cells and a complex three-dimensional network of reticular fibers (Fig. 3-3B) (see Chapter 8), which provide a framework for the cells and other components within these tissues.

Adipose Tissue

Adipose tissue, or fat, is a specialized type of CT that, in addition to performing insulating and mechanical functions, plays an important role in the metabolism of the organism. One of the most important functions of adipose tissue is its participation in fat metabolism. The turnover of intracellular fat is rapid, with a continuous cycle of withdrawal and deposit, even if the organism has to draw on its fat reserves to supplement food intake.

Intracellular lipids are synthesized primarily from fatty acids but also from carbohydrates and proteins. The fatty acids necessary for lipid synthesis are derived from the enzymatic breakdown, by lipoprotein lipase, of the triglycerides contained in blood chylomicrons or lipoproteins; after their uptake by the adipocytes, the fatty acids are reassembled into triglycerides for storage.

Under hormonal (insulin) or nervous (norepinephrine) control, intracellular enzymatic hydrolysis of triglycerides takes place, and fatty acids and glycerol are released into the blood and catabolized in energy-yielding reactions. In brown adipocytes, a unique feature is that mitochondrial respiration is uncoupled from ATP synthesis; thus, the oxidation of stored fat generates heat rather than ATP, causing a rise in body temperature in arousing hibernating mammals or in response to cold exposure.

In mammalian subcutaneous CT, the adipose-tissue component serves as a thermal and mechanical insulator. In the foot pads and digital cushions, adipose tissue is associated with bundles of collagen and elastic fibers. This combination of fibers and fat cells allows the adipose tissue to act as a dampening cushion, and at the same time, the cells are protected by the great tensile strength of the collagen fibers. After deformation, the elastic fibers allow the adipose cells to return to normal shape.

Two types of adipose tissue, white and brown, are distinguished in most mammals by differences in color, vascularity, structure, and function.

White Adipose Tissue

The cells of **white adipose tissue** are separated by septa of loose CT into clusters of adipose cells, or adipocytes, referred to as lobules. Each adipocyte is surrounded by a delicate network of collagen and reticular fibers that supports a dense capillary plexus and nerve fibers (Fig. 3-4). In addition, the narrow intercellular spaces contain a few fibrocytes, mast cells, and sparse amorphous ground substance.

Brown Adipose Tissue

Brown adipose tissue (brown fat or BAT) is composed of aggregates of multilocular adipocytes (Fig. 3-5). The intercellular CT consists of fibrocytes, collagen, and reticular fibers. Capillaries form a dense plexus, and the adipocytes are directly innervated by adrenergic axons.

BAT is particularly common and abundant in rodents and hibernating mammals. It is located primarily in the axillary and neck regions (interscapular fat body), along the thoracic aorta and in the mediastinum, in the mesenteries, and around the abdominal aorta and vena cava near the kidney. BAT may also be found in the same locations in other domestic mammals. The high abundance of BAT in these regions reflects its importance in thermoregulation.

Adult Supportive Tissues

Cartilage

Cartilage is specialized for a supportive role in the body. It possesses considerable tensile strength because the intercellular substance has a supportive framework of collagen and/or elastic fibers. The ground substance of cartilage is firm but pliable, enhancing its weight-bearing ability. In general, this tissue is avascular, alymphatic, and aneural in mature forms. However, during development and growth, blood vessels can penetrate certain cartilagenous structures, particularly in areas such as the epiphyses of developing bones.

Cartilage Cells

Two cell types are recognized in cartilage: the **chondroblast** and the **chondrocyte**.

Chondroblast The **chondroblast** is found in growing cartilage (Fig. 3-21). The cell is oval shaped with a spherical nucleus and a prominent Golgi apparatus. The cytoplasm is basophilic due to abundant rER. The chondroblast actively forms the matrix of cartilage that surrounds the perimeter of the cell.

Chondrocyte After cartilage matrix formation is complete, the chondroblast differentiates into a less active cell, the **chondrocyte** (Fig. 3-21). The chondrocyte's shape varies from elongated to spherical, depending on the location within the cartilage. Each chondrocyte is located within a **lacuna**, a cavity within the semirigid cartilage matrix. In living cartilage or at the fine-structural level, the cell fills the lacuna. Short cytoplasmic processes extend into the intercellular substance. In most light microscopic preparations, the cell surface appears separated from the lacunar walls because of shrinkage. The chondrocyte has a spherical nucleus with one or more nucleoli and abundant rER and prominent Golgi complex. As chondrocytes age, they may accumulate glycogen and lipids, leading to vacuolation seen in routine preparations. Although considered a less active cell than the chondroblast, the chondrocyte is responsible for continual ongoing maintenance of the surrounding matrix.

Cartilage Matrix

The matrix of cartilage is composed of fibers and ground substance as found in other connective tissues, but the **cartilage matrix** has unique biomechanical properties. Collagen forms the framework of the matrix. The major cartilage collagen is type II, but type I predominates in fibrocartilage. Various other collagen types are present in cartilage, though in smaller amounts.

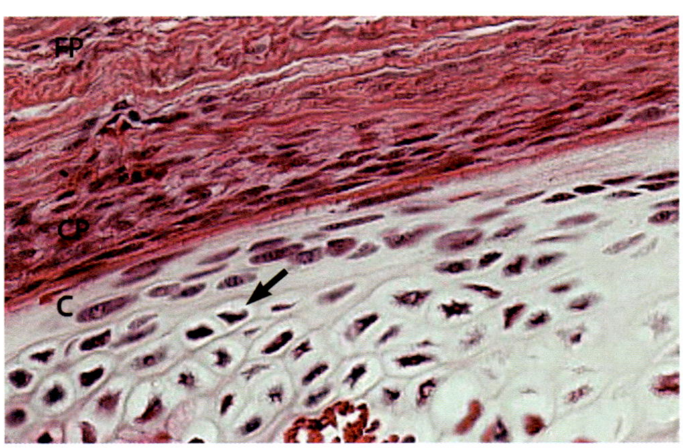

Figure 3-21 Immature hyaline cartilage (dog). The fibrous layer (FP) and cellular layer (CP) of the *perichondrium* border the cartilage (C) containing chondroblasts (arrow). H&E (×300). (Image by John J. Turek.)

The ground substance contains the GAGs chondroitin sulfate, keratan sulfate, and hyaluronic acid, all of which play an important role in transporting water and electrolytes as well as in binding water to give hyaline cartilage its resiliency, i.e., an ability to withstand compressive forces. GAGs complex with a protein backbone to form proteoglycans (Fig. 3-18). Numerous proteoglycans join to a hyaluronan core with the help of **link proteins**, thus forming a large **aggrecan**. The proteoglycans of the aggrecan are also bound to adjacent collagen fibrils, thereby forming a loose network that functions as a molecular sieve. The sieve-like structure serves to limit the movement of larger molecules through the cartilage matrix, contributing to its selective permeability and function in nutrient transport and waste removal.

Additional components of the cartilage matrix include the adhesive molecules, **chondronectin**, **anchorin CII**, and **fibronectin**, which contribute to cell–matrix and cell–cell interactions between collagen and chondrocytes. The matrix is mineralized by calcium phosphate, present in the form of **hydroxyapatite** crystals, in the deep regions of articular cartilage and zones of hypertrophy, resorption, and ossification of the growth plate (physis).

Overall, the matrix is slightly basophilic when stained with H&E, reacts positively with PAS due to the presence of GAGs and proteoglycans, and exhibits a marked metachromasia (color shift) with metachromatic stains such as toluidine blue or alcian blue. Staining intensity can vary across the matrix due to variations in its biochemical composition related to biomechanical stresses.

Classification of Cartilage

On the basis of different structural characteristics of the matrix, three types of cartilage are distinguishable: **hyaline cartilage**, **elastic cartilage**, and **fibrocartilage**.

Hyaline Cartilage **Hyaline cartilage** is found on the articulating surfaces of bones in synovial joints and provides support in the nose, larynx, trachea, and bronchi. It forms most of the entire appendicular and axial skeleton in the embryo.

The chondrocytes in mature hyaline cartilage vary in size (Fig. 3-22A). Chondrocytes near the surface of cartilage are small and have elliptical lacunae with their long axes oriented parallel to the surface. Deep within the cartilage, the cells are larger and more polyhedral. Some lacunae contain only one cell; others contain two, four, or sometimes six cells. These multicellular lacunae are called **cell nests or isogenous cell groups**.

The amorphous ground substance of hyaline cartilage is a firm gel containing a network of type II collagen fibrils. Since the fibrils have the same refractive index as the amorphous ground substance, they cannot be seen in standard preparations. Surrounding each chondrocyte is a thin layer of **pericellular matrix** that has proteoglycans but lacks collagen. This region plays a role in regulating cellular activities and providing a microenvironment for chondrocyte function. The **territorial matrix** surrounds the pericellular matrix and is composed of a network of fine collagen fibrils and ground substance. The **interterritorial matrix** lies outside the territorial matrix and fills the remaining matrix space. This region contains large collagen fibrils and abundant proteoglycans. Differences in collagen and proteoglycan content account for the staining differences between regions as observed with the light microscope.

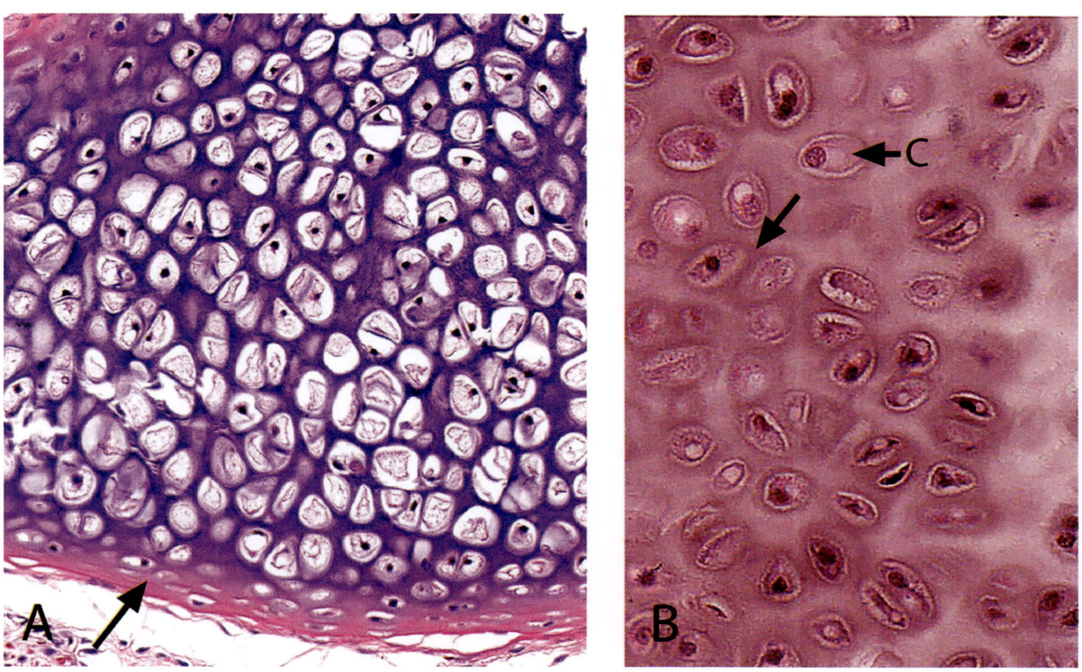

Figure 3-22 **A.** Mature hyaline cartilage (larynx, rat). The fibrous perichondrium (arrow) surrounds the cartilage mass (×300). **B.** The chondrocytes (C) lie in lacunae. The territorial matrix (arrow) is darker than the interterritorial matrix (D). H&E (×400). (Image by John J. Turek.)

At the ultrastructural level, **matrix granules** are adjacent to the chondrocytes. These granules contain proteoglycans secreted by the chondrocytes and represent the early stages of matrix production. The granules later contribute to the formation of aggrecans within the surrounding matrix. This process is important for the synthesis and organization of the cartilage matrix.

Except on articular surfaces, hyaline cartilage is surrounded by a vascular CT called the **perichondrium**, which is composed of two distinct layers (Fig. 3-21). The layer immediately adjacent to the cartilage is composed of chondroblasts and a network of small blood vessels; it is called the **cellular** or **chondrogenic layer**. The cellular layer contributes to cartilage growth and maintenance. The outer **fibrous layer** of the perichondrium consists of irregularly arranged collagen fibers and fibroblasts, providing mechanical support and anchorage for the cartilage.

Elastic Cartilage **Elastic cartilage** is found in areas where elasticity, as well as some rigidity, is required, such as in the epiglottis and external auditory canal. It is also part of the corniculate and cuneiform processes of the larynx.

In addition to all of the structural components of hyaline cartilage, elastic cartilage possesses a dense network of elastic fibers that are visible in ordinary H&E preparations. The density of elastic fibers is low near the perichondrium, but they form a dense network within the cartilaginous mass (Fig. 3-23). Chondrocytes located away from the surface of elastic cartilage contain many fat vacuoles. Later in adults, these fat-containing cells can often become adipose tissue.

Fibrocartilage Of the three cartilage types, **fibrocartilage** occurs least frequently. It is often interposed between other tissues and hyaline cartilage, tendons, or ligaments. Fibrocartilage is found in the intervertebral disks and forms the menisci of the stifle joint. In intervertebral disks, it provides cushioning and stability to the vertebral column, whereas in menisci, it contributes to joint stability and load distribution. In dogs, fibrocartilage is found also in the cardiac skeleton, which joins the atrial and ventricular heart muscles.

The most striking characteristic of fibrocartilage is the presence of prominent type I collagen fibers in the matrix (Fig. 3-24). The microscopic appearance of fibrocartilage may vary with location. Fibrocartilage that attaches ligaments and tendons to bone has large collagen fiber bundles oriented parallel to the direction of pulling forces. These collagen bundles are interspersed with rows of small lacunae containing chondrocytes (Fig. 3-24). In the fibrocartilaginous cardiac skeleton (fibrous trigone) of the dog, the chondrocytes and collagen fibers are distributed more randomly, reflecting the tissue's adaptation to its specific biomechanical requirements. The amorphous ground substance is most abundant in the vicinity of the cells, whereas the remainder of the matrix contains primarily collagen fiber bundles. Fibrocartilage lacks a distinct perichondrium; the cartilage is surrounded by collagen fibers in some locations, but a cellular layer is absent.

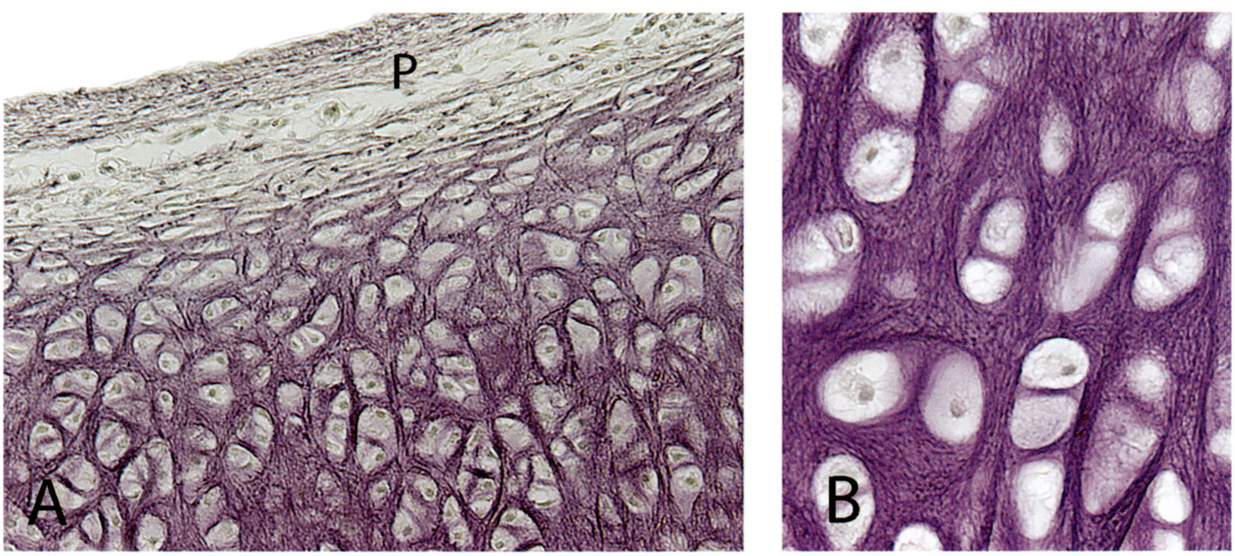

Figure 3-23 Elastic cartilage, epiglottis (dog). **A.** A perichondrium (P) covers elastic cartilage similar to hyaline cartilage (×200). **B.** Higher magnification illustrates elastic fibers coursing through the matrix surrounding the chondrocytes. H&E (×400). (Image by John J. Turek.)

Development of Cartilage

The initial step in cartilage formation within the embryo involves a clustering of mesenchymal cells. These cells enlarge, withdraw their processes, and synthesize and secrete amorphous ground substance and procollagen (type II). They are then referred to as chondroblasts, and the cell clusters are called **centers of chondrification**. As the intercellular matrix increases, the cells become spherical and isolated from each other in lacunae; at this point, they are mature cartilage cells called **chondrocytes**.

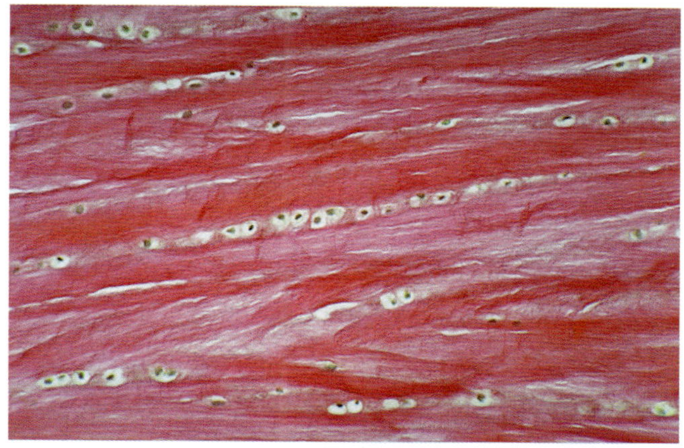

Figure 3-24 Fibrocartilage at ligament insertion on bone (dog). The lacunae (arrows) are oriented in the plane of pulling forces. H&E (×300). (Image by W.E. Haensly).

Chondroblasts undergo several mitotic divisions, and after each division, a new intercellular matrix separates the two resulting daughter cells. This process leads to substantial expansion of the cartilage from within and is referred to as **interstitial growth**. Concurrently, the mesenchyme surrounding the cartilage primordium differentiates into the perichondrium. Chondroblasts from the cellular layer of the perichondrium undergo division and deposit additional matrix onto the surface of the existing cartilage. This process, known as **appositional growth**, contributes to the expansion of cartilage. In the adult, although the chondrogenic layer retains the capacity to produce cartilage, this ability is dormant until the demand for new cartilage arises.

During the development of elastic cartilage, fibroblasts initially produce undifferentiated fibrils. Some of these fibroblasts later transform into chondroblasts, which then produce mature elastic fibers hat become incorporated into the matrix of elastic cartilage.

Nutrition of Cartilage

Unlike other connective tissues, most cartilage is avascular. Therefore, the chondrocytes must depend on the diffusion of nutrients through the gelled matrix. These nutrients diffuse from nearby capillaries within the perichondrium or from synovial fluid bathing the cartilage surface. When the intercellular matrix becomes calcified, diffusion is no longer possible, and the chondrocytes die. This phenomenon occurs in aging and is natural in endochondral bone development.

When cartilage surpasses a 3 mm^3 volume, then vessels may penetrate the matrix. An example of vascularized cartilage is the hyaline cartilage of developing epiphyses of long bones, which contain blood vessels and nerves surrounded by CT structures called **cartilage canals**.

Bone

Bone is a CT with cells and fibers embedded in a hard, mineralized substance that is well suited for supportive and protective functions. Functioning as an organ, bone provides internal support for the entire body as well as attachment sites for the muscles and tendons necessary for movement. It protects the brain and organs in the thoracic cavity and contains the bone marrow within its medullary space. Bone functions metabolically by providing a source of calcium to maintain proper blood calcium levels and various growth factors (e.g., transforming growth factor beta [TGF-β]) that play a role in remodeling.

Bone is a dynamic tissue that is renewed and remodeled throughout the life of all mammals. Its construction is unique because it provides the greatest tensile strength with the least amount of weight of any tissue.

Bone Cells

Osteoblast The **osteoblast** is the cell responsible for active formation and mineralization of bone matrix. The cells range from columnar to squamous in shape and are located on surfaces of bone where new bone is being deposited (Figs. 3-25 and 3-26). The nucleus is located in the basal region of the intensely basophilic cytoplasm. The Golgi apparatus and rER are prominent between the nucleus and the secretory surface of the osteoblast. The cell deposits **osteoid** (collagen I and proteoglycans), the unmineralized matrix of bone. In addition, the osteoblast produces various growth factors and signaling mediators including fibroblast growth factors, insulin growth factor, platelet-derived growth factor, bone morphogenetic proteins, prostaglandins, and TGF-β.

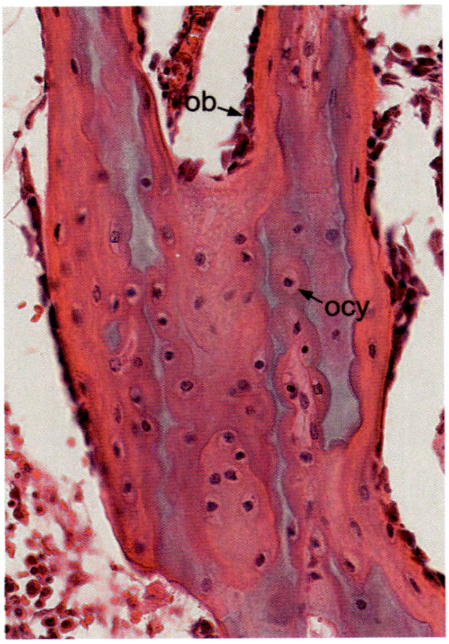

Figure 3-25 Trabecular bone of endochondral osteogenesis has osteoblasts (ob) and osteocytes (ocy) within lacunae. Basophilic cartilage still remains. H&E (×200). (Image by John J. Turek.)

Osteoblasts originate from pluripotent mesenchymal stem cells that also give rise to chondroblasts, fibroblasts, and other cell types. The **osteoprogenitor cell**, which ultimately develops into a differentiated osteoblast, does not have a typical morphologic appearance, but specific cell-surface molecules expressed during differentiation help identify the cell line. Bone morphogenetic proteins (BMPs), proteins from the bone matrix, play an important role in the differentiation of stem cells into osteoblasts.

Flattened, quiescent (resting) osteoblasts are known as **bone lining cells**. These cells are found on the surfaces of adult trabeculae and cortical (compact) bone. They are capable of becoming active osteoblasts when appropriately stimulated.

Osteoblasts have receptors for parathyroid hormone (PTH) on their surface. When PTH binds to the osteoblast, the cell releases factors that stimulate osteoclastic activity indirectly. Osteoblasts primarily regulate osteoclastic activity by secreting RANKL (receptor activator of nuclear factor kappa-β ligand) and OPG (osteoprotegerin).

Osteocyte As matrix secretion approaches completion, approximately 10% of the osteoblasts surround themselves with osteoid and modulate into osteocytes. The **osteocyte** is the principal cell in mature bone and resides in a **lacuna** surrounded by calcified interstitial matrix (Fig. 3-25). Numerous long, slender processes extend from the cell body into **canaliculi** within the matrix to connect with adjacent osteocytes. Gap junctions are present at the contact points and provide communication between osteocytes. Further, the long cellular processes of the osteocyte are able to shorten and lengthen. This activity may serve as a "pump" to move fluid through lacunae and canaliculi to transfer metabolites from the surface of the bone. The organelles of young osteocytes resemble osteoblasts, but as they mature, the Golgi complex and rER are less prominent and lysosomes increase in number. This reflects the shift in cellular function from active matrix production by the *osteoblast* toward maintenance and regulation within mature bone by the *osteocyte*.

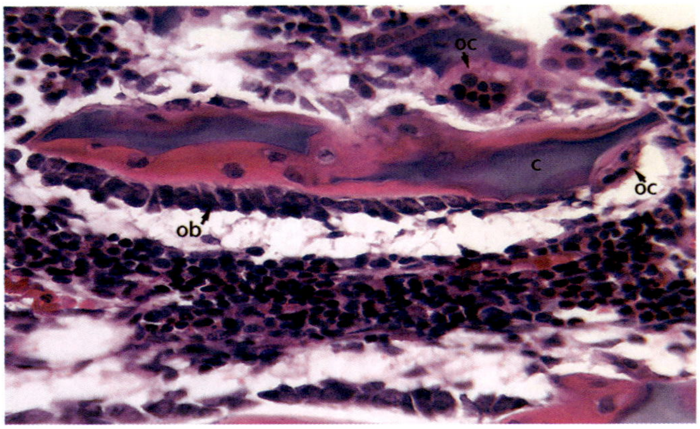

Figure 3-26 Multinucleated osteoclasts (oc) resorb bone on the surface of trabeculae. Nearby osteoblasts (ob) form new bone. Within the bone of the trabeculae, osteocytes are responsible for maintenance of the tissue. Purple calcified cartilage matrix (c) is still present in this primary spongiosa. Digit, dog. H&E (×400). (Image by J. Eurell).

The exact way in which osteocytes preserve the integrity of bone matrix is not completely understood. Osteocytes are essential in preserving bone structure because, upon their death, signals including RANKL and other factors attract osteoclasts immediately to the area, where they begin to resorb the bone. Therefore, signals from apoptotic osteocytes may be part of a signaling pathway to initiate bone remodeling. Other signals that osteocytes may utilize to regulate bone formation include sclerostin, for regulating osteoblast activity.

Osteocytes may also play a role in calcium homeostasis, although the osteoclast is primarily responsible for calcium release through bone resorption. Osteocytes remove and replace perilacunar bone, which refers to a 1 μm layer of bone immediately surrounding the lacunae where osteocytes reside. Perilacunar bone removal is called **osteocytic osteolysis**. The extent to which this process normally occurs is unclear.

The ECM surrounding osteocytes within the lacunae and canaliculi contains various proteins and proteoglycans, including GAGs. The maintenance of this matrix by osteocytes is important to maintain the integrity of this tissue.

Osteoclast The **osteoclast** is a large, multinucleated cell located on the surface of bone (15 to 30 nuclei per cell, and ranging from 40 to 100 μm in diameter) (Fig. 3-26). Occasional mononuclear osteoclasts are much less common, but can be present during early stages of osteoclast formation. The cytoplasm is acidophilic and contains a small amount of rER, ribosomes, numerous smooth vesicles, and mitochondria. These organelles are involved in the metabolic activities of the osteoclast, including enzyme secretion and bone resorption.

The activated osteoclast has a ruffled border created by extensive in foldings of the cell membrane that sweep across the bony surface. The cell secretes acid and lysosomal enzymes into this region. The cell membrane immediately adjacent to the ruffled border adheres tightly to the bony surface, thereby sealing the area of active bone resorption. As the osseous matrix is enzymatically digested, an **erosion lacuna** (Howship's lacuna) is formed. The lacuna persists after the osteoclast is no longer present, thus indicating prior areas of bone resorption. Osteoclasts may also be found in bone remodeling units as part of a cellular complex that remodels cortical bone in the adult (described later in this chapter). In addition to the release of mineral and protein components of bone, osteoclasts are also responsible for the release and activation of TGF-β from the matrix. TGF-β is a multifunctional cytokine involved in various aspects of bone metabolism and remodeling. Osteoclasts are stimulated by PTH, interleukins, and RANKL; they are inhibited by calcitonin, OPG (a decoy receptor for RANKL), and gonadal steroids.

Osteoclasts are derived from pluripotent stem cells (CFU-GM) of the bone marrow that also give rise to monocytes and macrophages. Final differentiation to an osteoclast from a circulating monocyte occurs after the cells are recruited to bone resorption sites. Once at these sites, under the influence of various factors such as macrophage colony-stimulating factor (M-CSF) and RANKL, monocytes are promoted to fuse and form multinucleated osteoclasts. At the end of their cell lifespan, osteoclasts undergo apoptosis, a process that helps regulate bone remodeling and turnover.

Bone Matrix

The matrix of bone is composed of osteoid produced by the osteoblasts. Mineralization of the osteoid occurs as hydroxyapatite crystals are deposited in the osteoid framework.

The organic intercellular substance of bone contains sulfated GAGs, glycoproteins, and collagen. Glycoproteins of bone include alkaline phosphatase, osteonectin, osteopontin, and sialoprotein. These glycoproteins are thought to play various roles in bone mineralization, cell signaling, and matrix organization. Osteocalcin, a noncollagenous protein produced by osteoblasts, indirectly regulates the activity of osteoclasts. While the primary function is in bone mineralization and turnover, osteocalcin also modulates the production of factors involved in bone remodeling, such as OPG and RANKL. These factors affect osteoclast formation, function, and survival. Type I collagen predominates in bone matrix with traces of types III, V, and X. The collagen fibrils in each osteonal lamella course in a spiral direction with respect to the long axis of the central canal. In addition to their spiral orientation, the collagen fibrils in each cylindrical osteon alternate at right angles to those in each adjacent lamella. This alternating arrangement, known as a "crossed lamellar" structure, imparts considerable resilience to each osteon by distributing forces in multiple directions.

The inorganic component of bone consists of submicroscopic hydroxyapatite crystals deposited as slender needles within the collagen fibril network. Such an efficient arrangement enhances the tensile strength that is characteristic of bone. The principal ions in bone salt are Ca^{2+}, CO_3^{2-}, PO_4^{3-}, and OH^-. Smaller amounts of Na^+, Mg^{2+}, and Fe also are present. Bone, then, is a major storehouse for calcium and phosphorus, which are vital for various physiological processes including bone mineralization, muscle contraction, and nerve function. These minerals can be mobilized from bone whenever they are needed, such as during periods of low dietary intake or increased demand.

Structural and Functional Characteristics

Adult bone is distinguished from cartilage by the presence of both a canalicular system and a direct vascular supply. The growth process of bone also differs from that of cartilage.

Adult cartilage depends entirely on diffusion for nourishment, as it lacks blood vessels. In contrast, bone has a unique lacunar–canalicular system for supplying the bone cells with metabolites in a mineralized matrix in which diffusion is not an option (Figs. 3-27 and 3-28). Canaliculi extend from one lacuna to another and to the bone surface, where they open into the CT surrounding the capillaries. The canalicular system provides a conduit system for nourishment of the mature osteocytes located deep in the bone, and the extensive capillary supply of bone further enhances the efficiency of the canalicular system.

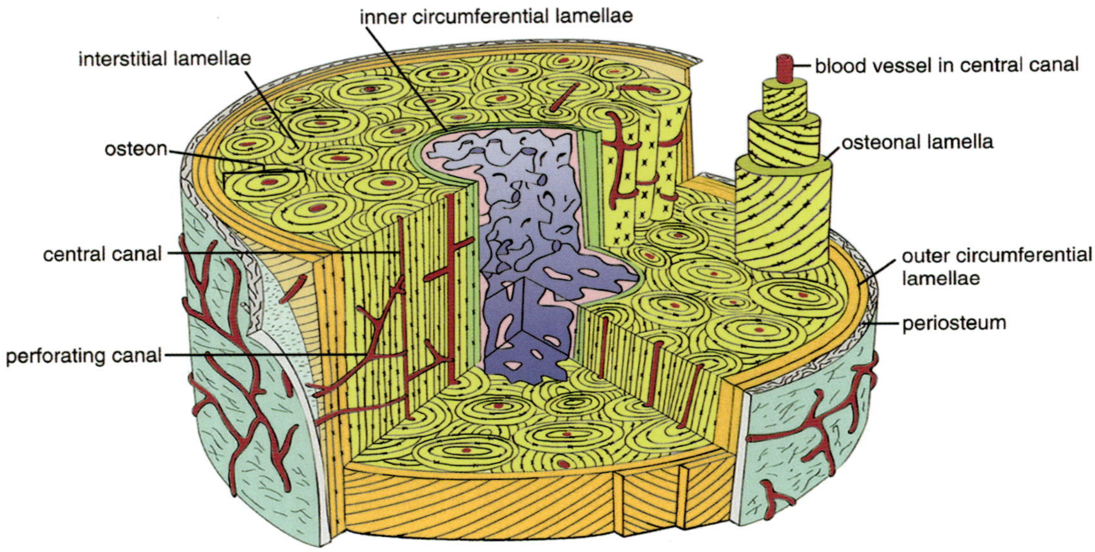

Figure 3-27 The structural unit of compact bone is the cylindrical osteon. In this drawing, an osteon is telescoped to show the concentric osteonal lamellae that surround the central canal. Blood vessels reach the central canal through perforating canals from either the periosteal or endosteal surface. The space between adjacent osteons is filled by interstitial lamellae. Inner and outer circumferential lamellae form the surfaces of compact bone.

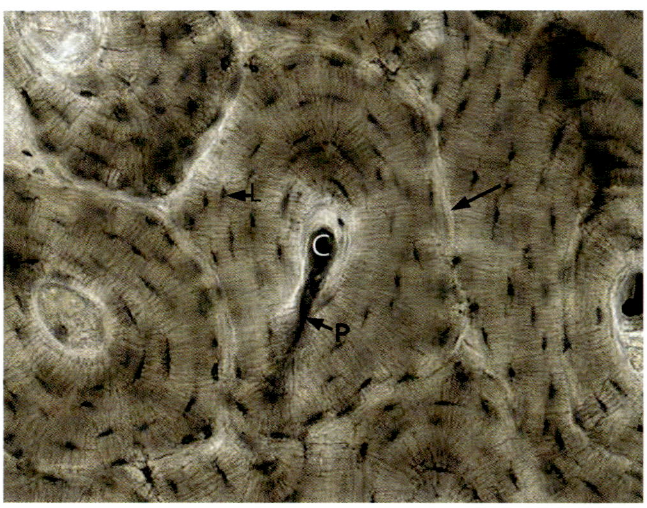

Figure 3-28 Osteon of ground bone surrounded by a light cement line (arrow). The central canal (C) carries blood vessels, lymphatics, and nerves, and branches into a transverse perforating canal (P). Lacunae (L) are located between lamellae of compact bone that surround the central canal. Fine canaliculi extend from each lacuna. Unstained (×250).

Unlike cartilage, bone grows by apposition only. Because the intercellular substance mineralizes so rapidly, interstitial growth of bone is not possible. Therefore, bone changes shape and increases or decreases in size by adding layers to or removing layers from one or more of its existing surfaces over time in response to mechanical stresses or physiological needs.

Macroscopic Structure An adult long bone (e.g., humerus) comprises enlarged ends (**epiphyses**) connected by a hollow cylindrical shaft (**diaphysis**) (Fig. 3-29). The ends of the epiphyses are covered by a thin layer of hyaline cartilage called **articular cartilage**, whereas the remainder of the external bone surface is covered by a vascular fibrous membrane, the **periosteum** (Figs. 3-27 and 3-30). Each region of the bone is composed of lamellar bone, arranged to optimize its biomechanical function. The epiphyses have a thin shell of dense bone (subchondral bone) beneath the articular cartilage. **Spongy bone**, comprised of a network of **trabeculae**, extends from the subchondral bone, forming the central part of the bone. The wall of the diaphysis is composed of **compact bone**, containing osteons. The inner (medullary) cavity of bone is lined by the **endosteum** and contains adipose tissue or red (hematopoietic) or yellow (adipose) bone marrow, depending on the age of the animal or the region of the bone.

In the growing animal, the diaphysis and epiphysis are separated by the **physeal–metaphyseal** region (Fig. 3-31). This region consists of a specialized hyaline cartilage plate called the physis and the metaphysis, a region of trabecular bone located beneath the physis. The physis, also known as the cartilaginous growth plate, drives the longitudinal growth of the animal's bones. During the growth process, temporary trabeculae with cartilaginous cores form in the metaphysis and are later remodeled into permanent bony trabeculae (Figs. 3-29 and 3-32). When growth ceases, the cartilage cells in the

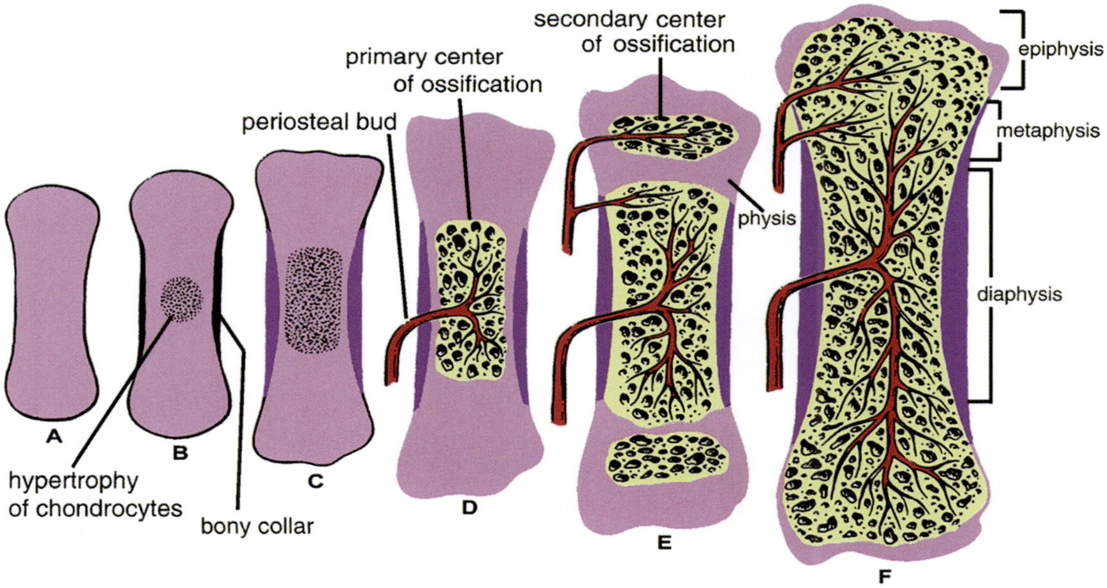

Figure 3-29 The stages of endochondral ossification of a long bone. **A.** A hyaline cartilage model forms initially. **B.** The chondrocytes in the center of the model hypertrophy. **C.** A bony collar begins to form around the cartilage model. **D.** Blood vessels from the periosteum (periosteal bud) invade the cartilage model, bringing bone-forming cells to initiate the primary center of ossification. **E.** The physis (growth plate) and secondary centers of ossification are established. **F.** The physis closes in the mature bone, and a confluent marrow cavity from the epiphysis to the diaphysis is formed.

physis stop proliferating, but bone formation continues on the metaphyseal side of the physis. Eventually, a transverse, perforated plate of bone (epiphyseal scar) replaces the physis in the skeletally mature animal. The epiphyseal scar may appear as the epiphyseal line on radiographs.

Histologic Preparation Because of its dense mineral deposits, bone is difficult to section and process for histologic procedures. Decalcification before histologic processing removes the mineral from the bone, leaving behind the organic matrix and the bone cells for study (Fig. 3-30). If examination of osseous mineral content is required, undecalcified sections can be prepared using special techniques (Fig. 3-28).

Microscopic Structure The outermost layers of the shaft of a long bone consist of compact bone arranged as **outer circumferential lamellae** (2 to 8 µm thick). Deep to the outer circumferential lamellae are osteons (Haversian systems) formed by concentric lamellae surrounding longitudinally oriented vascular channels (**central canals**) (Fig. 3-27). Internal surfaces of compact bone from adult animals are composed of **inner circumferential lamellae** encircling the medullary cavity.

Lacunae are located between each lamella of the compact bone (Fig. 3-28). Radiating from the lacunae are the branching **canaliculi** that penetrate and join canaliculi of adjacent lamellae. Thus, the lacunae and canaliculi form an extensive system of interconnecting passageways for the transport of nutrients.

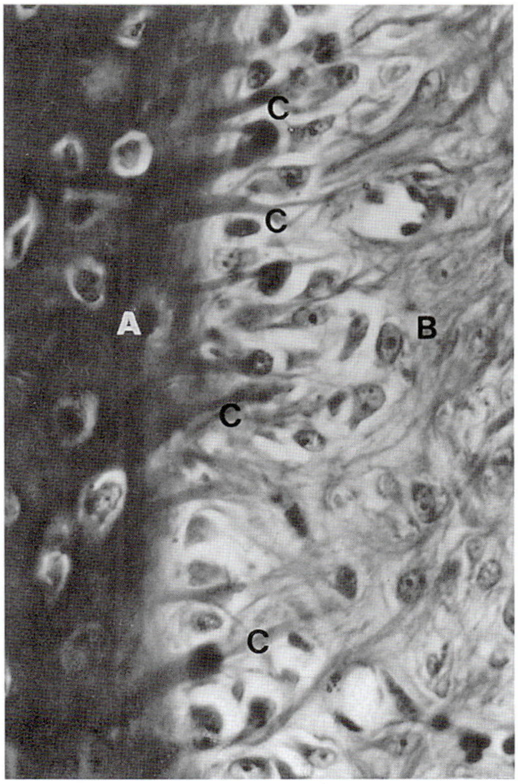

Figure 3-30 Decalcified bone (cat). Bone (A) with periosteum (B) attached by perforating fibers (C). H&E (×500). (Courtesy of A. Hansen).

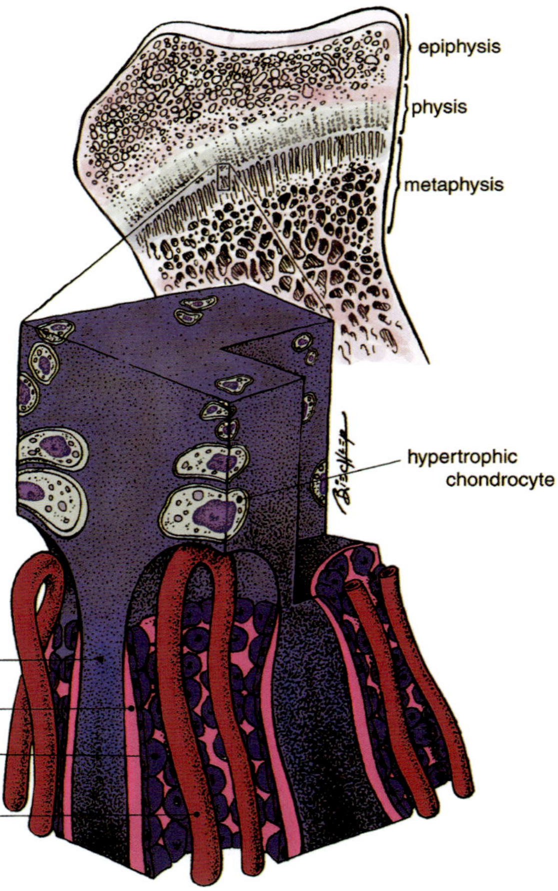

Figure 3-31 Metaphyseal blood vessels make a sharp bend in the zone of resorption. Capillary loops invade the lacunae of the degenerating hypertrophic chondrocytes. Osteoblasts form bone on the remnants of the calcified physeal cartilage.

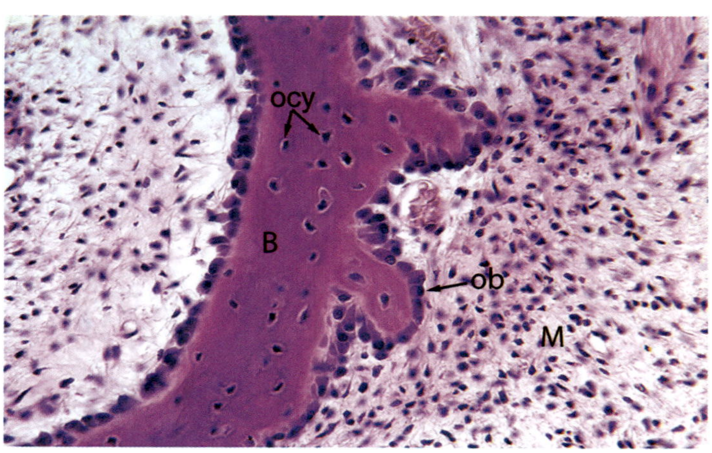

Figure 3-32 Intramembranous bone development. Bone (B) develops directly from mesenchyme (M). Osteoblasts (ob) differentiate from mesenchymal cells and deposit bone matrix. As development progresses, some osteoblasts are surrounded by matrix and become osteocytes (ocy) within the bone. Head, fetal pig. H&E (×250). (Image by J. Eurell).

The **central canal** (Haversian canal) of each osteon contains capillaries, lymphatic vessels, and nonmyelinated nerve fibers, all supported by reticular CT. Central canals are connected with each other and with the free surface by transverse or horizontal channels called **perforating canals** (Volkmann's canals) (Figs. 3-27 and 3-28).

Most bones are invested with a tough CT layer, the **periosteum** (Figs. 3-27 and 3-30). It has two layers: an inner **osteogenic layer** that provides cells necessary to form bone and an outer **fibrous layer** made of irregularly arranged collagen fibers and blood vessels. The vessels branch and enter the perforating canals and ultimately reach the central canal of the osteons. The cellular layer is more evident in young animals than in adults. The periosteum is attached firmly to the bone by bundles of coarse collagen fibers that have been incorporated into the outer circumferential lamellae of the bone. These fibers are called **perforating (Sharpey's) fibers** (Fig. 3-30). A periosteum is absent over the surface of hyaline articular cartilage and at sites where tendons and ligaments insert on bones.

The marrow cavity, central, and perforating canals are lined with a layer of bone-lining cells, including osteoprogenitor cells, osteoblasts, and osteoclasts known as the **endosteum**. Some endosteal cells send processes into canaliculi to connect with nearby osteocytes. Recently, it has been suggested that these cells form an ion barrier, separating the fluid within the lacunae and canaliculi from the interstitial fluid. In addition, endosteal cells may regulate mineral homeostasis by controlling the flow of calcium and phosphate into and out of bone fluids, thus maintaining an optimal microenvironment for the growth of bone crystals.

Osteogenesis

Bone formation occurs through a two-step process. First, osteoid is deposited by osteoblasts, followed by mineralization of the osteoid several days later. Two theories exist regarding the initiation of bone mineralization. The **nucleation theory** proposes that the hole regions of type I collagen fibrils serve as the major site for calcium phosphate crystal deposition. A second theory involves **matrix vesicles**, membrane-bounded structures that form along the osteoblast membrane. These vesicles contain lipids, accumulated calcium ions, and alkaline phosphatase, all essential for initiating and sustaining the process of mineralization.

Bone is classified based on the arrangement of collagen fibrils in the matrix (woven versus lamellar bone) or by the type of precursor CT (intramembranous versus endochondral ossification).

Woven bone exhibits collagen fibrils arranged in an irregular anastomosing fashion (Fig. 3-32), whereas **lamellar bone** features a more organized matrix deposited in layers (Fig. 3-28). Woven bone forms rapidly and is considered an immature form of bone; it is usually replaced by lamellar bone. Woven bone is commonly found in developing bone, fracture repair sites, and certain bone tumors. Calcified cartilage and woven bone appear to mineralize in association with matrix vesicles, whereas the mineralization of lamellar bone appears to follow the nucleation theory.

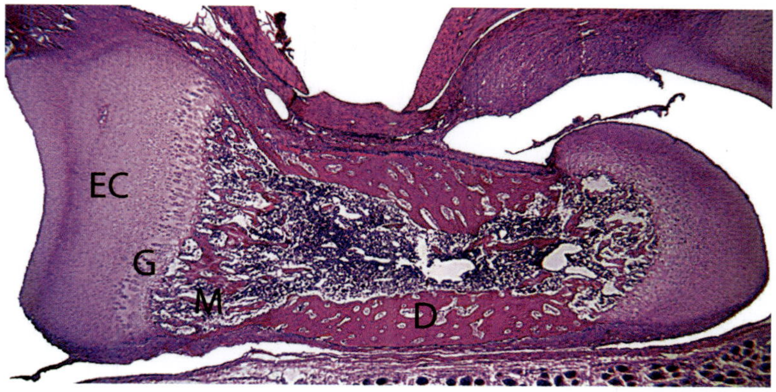

Figure 3-33 Endochondral bone formation. The primary center of ossification expands within the model to form the diaphyseal (D) and metaphyseal regions (M). The epiphyseal cartilage (EC) is a remnant of the original cartilage model. The growth plate (G) is responsible for growth in length of the developing bone until skeletal maturity is reached. Phalanx, dog. H&E (×25). (Image by J. Eurell).

Regardless of the site, bone develops through a process of transformation from existing CT. The two types of bone development depend on specific cells differentiating within distinct microenvironments. When bone forms directly from CT, the process is termed **intramembranous ossification** (Fig. 3-32). This term originates from the arrangement of soft tissue located where bone will form, which is membranous. The process of bone formation in pre-existing cartilage models is termed **endochondral** or **intracartilaginous ossification** (Fig. 3-33). During this process, calcified cartilage is replaced by bone. The terms intramembranous and endochondral indicate the type of microenvironment in which the bone forms, rather than the type of adult bone. For example, both intramembranous and endochondral bone formation can give rise to spongy bone in the adult.

Intramembranous Ossification

The process of intramembranous ossification occurs within well-vascularized CT, such as that found in the diploe of the developing calvaria of the skull. Osteoprogenitor cells differentiate into osteoblasts, which begin synthesizing and secreting osteoid. The first secreted component of osteoid is collagen, followed by the production of other ground substance constituents. During early intramembranous osteogenesis, osteoblasts become surrounded by a partially mineralized matrix containing visible collagen fibrils (Fig. 3-32). Gradually, more osteoid is produced, followed by complete mineralization. As a result, some osteoblasts become trapped within their lacunae and mature into osteocytes. These small, isolated pieces of developing bone within the CT are called the **centers of ossification**, which ultimately radiate in several directions to form trabeculae (Fig. 3-25). This type of bone is referred to as **trabecular**, **spongy**, or **cancellous** bone.

The bony trabeculae expand in width and length through the addition of new lamellae, resulting in the formation of a primary spongiosa of trabecular bone. In regions where compact bone develops within the spongiosa, the mesenchymal space between trabeculae is filled with osseous tissue, leaving a central canal housing the vasculature of the new osteon. Conversely, in regions where spongy bone persists, the mesenchymal soft tissue located between trabeculae becomes bone marrow.

Endochondral Ossification

Bones of the extremities, vertebral column, pelvis, and base of the skull are formed initially as hyaline cartilage models that are replaced by bone in the developing embryo.

Primary center of ossification. As the cartilage model grows both in width and in length, it reaches a stage when most of the remaining growth concentrates at its ends. Chondrocytes in the midsection mature and enlarge, leading to thinning of the matrix between hypertrophied cells (Fig. 3-35). At the same time, these chondrocytes release matrix vesicles, similar to those of osteoblasts, that promote calcification of the surrounding cartilage matrix. This calcification impedes adequate nutrition to the hypertrophied chondrocytes, resulting in their degeneration and eventual death.

In the meantime, the perichondrium is invaded by numerous capillaries. This event changes the microenvironment of the chondrogenic layer to one that favors osteogenesis on the cartilage model's surface. The osteoprogenitor cells within

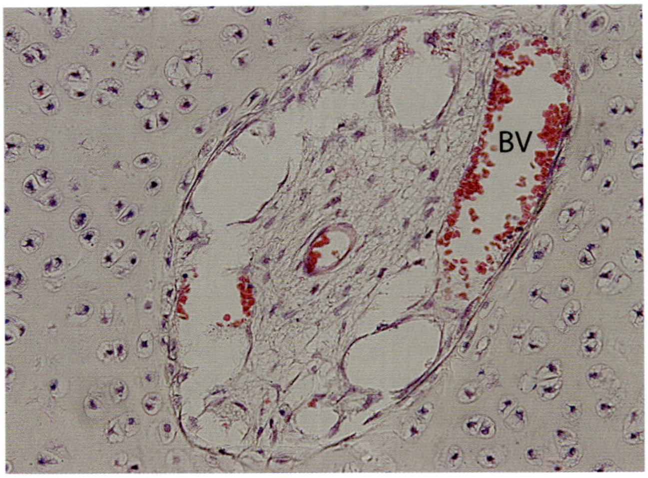

Figure 3-34 During endochondral bone development, cartilage canals containing blood vessels (BV) penetrate the epiphyseal cartilage. The cartilage then mineralizes to begin formation of the secondary ossification center. Humerus, dog. H&E (×200). (Image by John J. Turek.)

this layer differentiate into osteoblasts, encasing the midsection of the cartilage model with a thin bone shell. This **periosteal band** or **bony collar** forms by intramembranous ossification, with the perichondrium becoming the periosteum. Blood vessels are essential in activating the osteogenic potential of the inner layer of the perichondrium, whose cells retain the capacity to differentiate into either chondroblasts or osteoblasts throughout their lifespan. This ability holds particular significance in fracture healing, during which cartilage forms in areas that are relatively devoid of capillaries, but endochondral ossification occurs as soon as capillaries grow into the area.

After the formation of the bony collar around the model's midsection, blood vessels from the periosteum invade the area where hypertrophied chondrocytes are degenerating, thereby increasing the oxygen level (Figs. 3-29 and 3-34). Osteoprogenitor cells from the periosteum, pericytes, and undifferentiated mesenchymal cells all accompany the invading capillaries. These blood vessels and their associated cells constitute the **periosteal bud**. When the periosteal bud reaches the interior of the midsection of the cartilage model, the **primary center of ossification** is established. Simulated by inductive bone-forming factors in the blood plasma, osteoprogenitor cells accompanying the capillaries differentiate into osteoblasts. These cells cluster around fragments of the calcified cartilage to synthesize and secrete osteoid, eventually contributing to the mineralization process. This osteoblastic activity persists until bone trabeculae containing cores of calcified cartilage are formed.

While the primary center of ossification is forming, the cartilage at each end of the model continues to proliferate by interstitial growth, lengthening the model. Simultaneously, the bony collar surrounding the diaphysis continues to increase in thickness and length, rendering the primitive bone in the primary center of ossification unnecessary for support. Therefore, most of the bone in the primary center is resorbed by osteoclasts, creating the marrow cavity, which becomes filled with hemopoietic tissue developed from the undifferentiated mesenchymal cells introduced with the periosteal bud.

Secondary centers of ossification. The cartilaginous epiphyses of larger long bones develop additional centers of ossification referred to as **secondary centers** (Fig. 3-29). The epiphyseal cartilage of newborn animals is well supplied with **cartilage canals** containing arterioles, venules, and nonmyelinated nerve fibers, all surrounded by CT (Fig. 3-34). These canals arise from the perichondrium and are evenly spaced throughout the epiphysis, providing nutrients to a given area. The blood vessels do not enter the physis or penetrate the future articular cartilage. The arterioles of these canals end in a capillary glomerulus, and the initial sites of ossification occur as multiple foci adjacent to the glomeruli. When ossification begins, the chondrocytes next to the glomerulus of the cartilage canal hypertrophy and degenerate, and the surrounding matrix calcifies. This process is followed by the appearance of circularly oriented layers of hypertrophic and dividing chondrocytes, resembling the cellular arrangement of growth zones in the physis. Because the CT in the cartilage canals is continuous with the perichondrium, these cells have the same osteogenic potential for bone formation. Ultimately, these foci fuse into a single secondary center of ossification, forming spongy bone in the epiphysis.

Ossification does not replace all of the epiphyseal cartilage. Sufficient cartilage remains, allowing the epiphyseal portion to serve as a template for enlarging the end of the bone, while the surface portion functions as the articular cartilage. A transverse plate of cartilage is left between the diaphysis and each epiphysis. In domestic animals, this physis persists until puberty, after which it also is replaced by bone.

Growth in Length

Growth in length occurs through the function of the physis and metaphysis, which is a scaffolding for constructing metaphyseal cancellous bone. The continued interstitial growth of the cartilage in the physis, involving chondrocytic hyperplasia, synthesis of proteoglycans, and chondrocyte hypertrophy, serves to lengthen the long bones.

A longitudinal section through the physis reveals five distinct zones from the epiphysis to the metaphysis (Fig. 3-34):

1) The **reserve zone** (resting zone) is adjacent to the bone and marrow cavity of the epiphysis (Fig. 3-35). Here, the small chondrocytes are dispersed irregularly and nourished by epiphyseal blood vessels, arranged in glomeruli (Fig. 3-36). Chondrocytes in this zone form matrix vesicles, membrane-bounded structures similar to those produced by osteoblasts, but matrix mineralization does not occur until deeper in the physis.
2) In the **zone of proliferation**, chondrocytes are larger and form rows or columns parallel to the long axis of the developing bone (Figs. 3-35 and 3-36). New cells are produced through cell division at the top of the columns. Each cell in the columns possesses all the organelles necessary for the synthesis of matrix and is separated from the cell in an adjacent lacuna by a layer of matrix.
3) As maturation progresses in the **zone of hypertrophy**, cells enlarge and accumulate calcium, which is released into the matrix of the deep hypertrophic zone (Fig. 3-37). Matrix vesicles absorb calcium, and enzymes such as alkaline phosphatase increase local phosphate levels. This rise in calcium and phosphate causes matrix mineralization. The last few hypertrophied cells in each column are surrounded by calcified matrix, while transverse septa remain uncalcified. Some of these hypertrophied cells become shrunken, and their pyknotic nucleus appears to attach to the transverse septum.
4) The metaphyseal capillaries make a sharp U-shaped bend in the **zone of resorption** and return to the medullary circulation (Figs. 3-31 and 3-38). Individual capillary loops and perivascular CT invade the lacunae of the degenerating hypertrophic chondrocytes located at the base of the cell columns.
5) In the **zone of ossification**, osteoblasts differentiate from cells accompanying the invading capillaries and deposit bone on the remnants of the calcified cartilage, forming the **primary spongiosa** (Figs. 3-31 and 3-38).

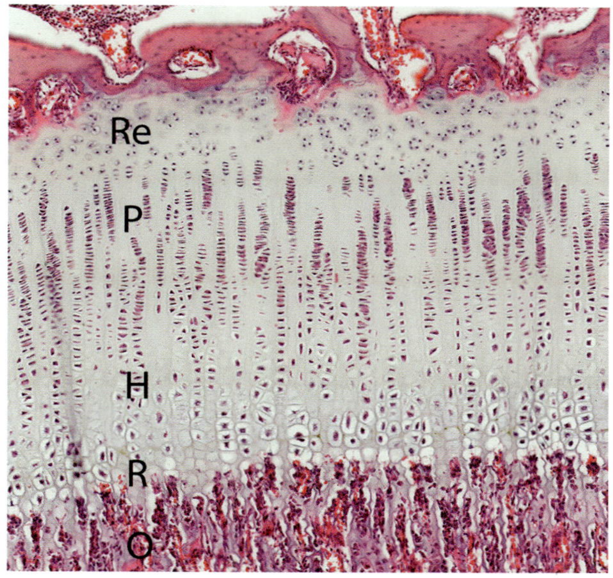

Figure 3-35 Canine growth plate. Chondrocytes in the reserve zone (Re) are scattered in the matrix. In the zone of proliferation (P), chondrocytes are arranged in columns. The cells increase in size in the zone of hypertrophy (H). Metaphyseal capillaries enter the zone of resorption (R), and bone is formed on the cartilage remnants of the physis in the zone of ossification (O). H&E (×200). (Image by John J. Turek.)

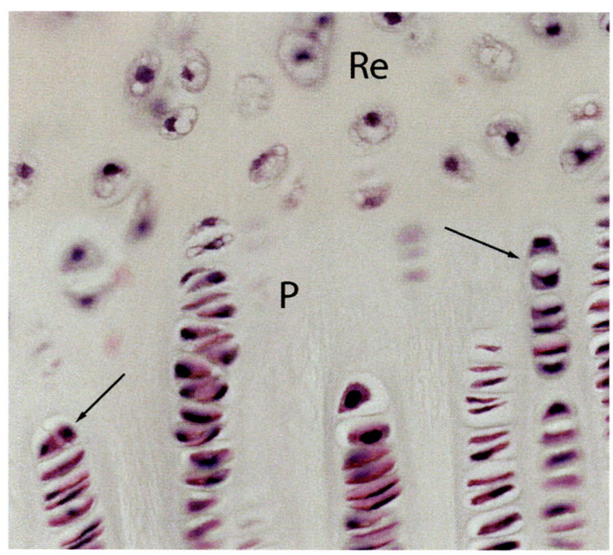

Figure 3-36 Chondrocytes of the reserve zone (Re) are scattered and spherical. New cells are produced at the top of the columns (arrows) in the zone of proliferation (P). H&E (×400). (Image by John J. Turek.)

Many trabeculae in the primary spongiosa are covered by osteoclasts extending a short distance into the metaphysis. Osteoclast precursors arrive with the invading metaphyseal vessels and differentiate into functional osteoclasts within the bone. These osteoclasts resorb bone from the trabecular surface, reducing the number of trabeculae.

Because the cartilage cores of the trabeculae are continuous with the cartilaginous matrix of the physis, the new bony trabeculae are anchored firmly to the physis. In longitudinal sections through the growth plate, the bony trabeculae and their cartilage cores resemble separate stalks attached to the growth plate. In a cross-section taken through the metaphyseal side of the physis, however, each trabecula is actually a wall between adjacent tubes filled with osteogenic cells and capillaries (Fig. 3-31).

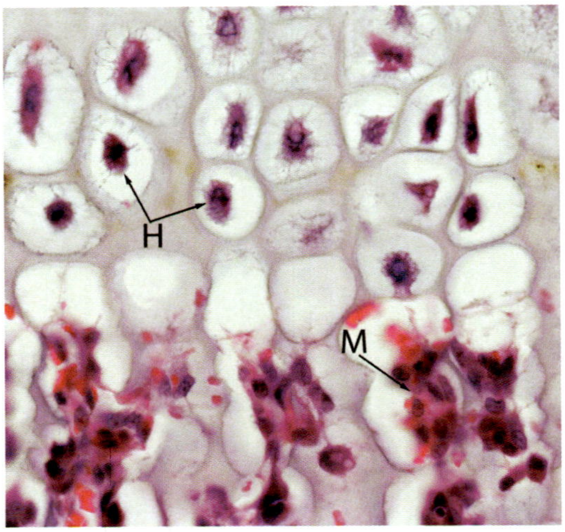

Figure 3-37 Hypertrophic chondrocytes (at arrow tips) degenerate within the zone of hypertrophy (H) just above the zone of resorption. In the zone of resorption, metaphyseal blood vessels (M) invade the lacunae of the degenerating chondrocytes. H&E (×400).

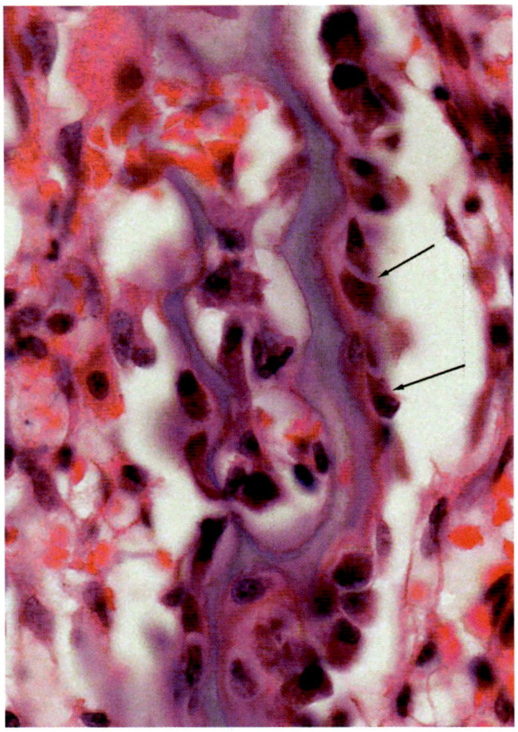

Figure 3-38 Osteoblasts (arrows) form bone on basophilic staining cartilage in the zone of ossification. H&E (×400). (Image by John J. Turek.)

Deeper into the metaphysis, trabeculae of the primary spongiosa decrease, and trabeculae composed of lamellar bone predominate. Trabecular bone without cartilage cores is known as the secondary spongiosa.

Growth in Width and Circumference

The trabecular bone that formed in the original bony collar is converted to compact bone composed of primary osteons. Concurrent periosteal bone formation and endosteal bone resorption enlarge the marrow cavity and increase the width of the diaphysis. Because endosteal resorption lags behind periosteal production, the thickness of the shaft wall slowly enlarges as the circumference increases.

The outer surface of an actively growing bone is uneven, owing to numerous longitudinal ridges and grooves. Within these grooves, osteoblasts from the adherent periosteum deposit bone around the periosteal vessels. Eventually, the edges of the groove meet, forming a tube lined with osteogenic cells and enclosing the blood vessel derived from the periosteum. The osteogenic cells produce concentric layers of bone around the blood vessel within the new central canal. In this way, new **primary osteons** are added to the periphery of an actively growing young bone. Primary osteons comprising the cortical bone are gradually replaced with more orderly **secondary osteons**.

Primary osteons are smaller than secondary osteons, lack cement lines, and often have two or more blood vessels in their central canal. Secondary osteons are surrounded by cement lines, which are basophilic (in H&E) or lighter (in ground bone, Fig. 3-28), composed of mineralized matrix deficient in collagen. Between the secondary osteons are many irregularly shaped groups of lamellae called **interstitial lamellae**.

Finally, the bone growth slows, and appositional growth in the subperiosteal and endosteal regions adds more layers, which smooth the surface. These layers are the inner and outer circumferential lamellae.

The important principle to note is that growth in length is the result of endochondral ossification, whereas growth in width is the result of intramembranous ossification. Each type of growth responds to different rules, and each can be affected separately without necessarily influencing the other.

Bone Modeling

The changes in size and shape of bones during the growth process are called **modeling**. The concurrent action of bone resorption and formation on different surfaces of a bone alters the overall shape. The process of modeling continues over most of the skeleton until the adult shape of the bones is reached. Modeling is rapid and results in a net gain of bone in the body. Examples of modeling include the drifting of the diaphysis during growth, shaping of the metaphyseal funnel, and enlargement of the cranial vault.

In the diaphysis, bone formation occurs on the periosteal surface while bone is resorbed on the endosteal surface, resulting in a wider diaphysis and larger marrow cavity (Fig. 3-39). If the modeling process occurs in an eccentric fashion, the entire diaphysis may drift in a specific direction.

In contrast, the shaping of the metaphyseal region is accomplished by periosteal resorption on the external surface to narrow the funnel shape in the direction of the diaphysis. Concurrent endosteal bone formation creates a thickened metaphyseal cortex.

Bone Remodeling Throughout life, bone is constantly being turned over. Early woven bone is of poorer quality than mature lamellar bone. In addition, as bone ages, the quality also diminishes. **Bone remodeling** is the process by which bone is constantly replaced.

In contrast to modeling, bone remodeling occurs in a cyclical fashion at a slower rate. The process generally does not alter the shape or size of the bone. Remodeling is coupled; it initiates and proceeds in only one way. First, activation of remodeling occurs, perhaps caused by a change in biomechanics. Osteoclastic bone resorption is then followed by osteoblastic bone formation. Balance between bone resorption and formation is important for healthy bone; however, bone resorption is often greater than bone formation, leading to net bone loss (e.g., osteoporosis related to aging).

Cortical bone is remodeled by **cortical remodeling units**. The unit, when viewed longitudinally, consists of a leading **cutting cone** composed of osteoclasts, which resorb compact bone without respect to osteonal barriers (Fig. 3-40). The cutting cone is followed by a **reversal zone**, in which resorption switches to osteoblastic bone formation. The structure terminates as a **closing cone**, in which osteoblasts close the newly excavated osteon by adding centripetal layers of lamellar bone inward from the cement line boundary. The osteoclasts of the cutting cone are supported metabolically by a glomerulus, whereas the osteoblasts of the closing cone are within close diffusion distance from the blood vessel of the new central canal.

In spongy bone, remodeling is accomplished on the endosteal surface of the trabecula. Osteoclasts resorb bone from the surface of the trabecula. Osteoblasts then form new bone in either the same location where the resorption occurred or on the opposing surface of the trabecula. If bone is formed on the opposing surface, the alignment of the trabecula is changed in the direction of the bone formation.

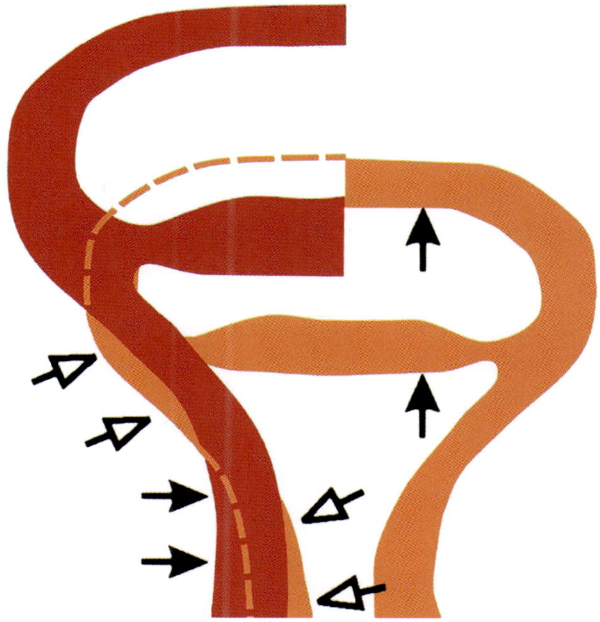

Figure 3-39 During growth, modeling occurs as new bone is added on the outer periosteal surface of the diaphysis and within the metaphysis and epiphysis (solid arrows). Bone is concurrently resorbed on both the endosteal and periosteal surfaces to shape the adult bone (open arrows).

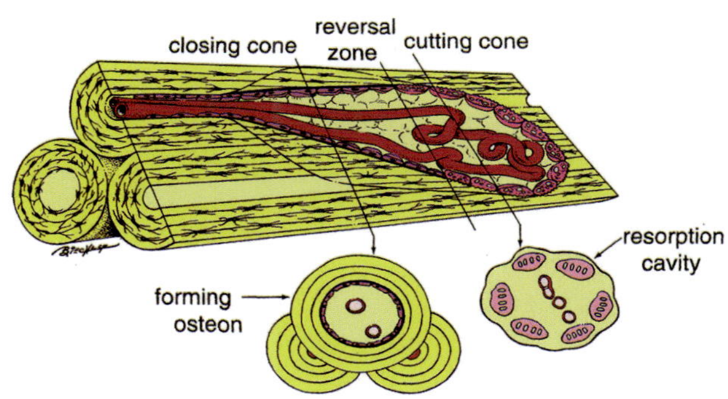

Figure 3-40 The remodeling unit of cortical bone is composed of a cutting cone of osteoclasts, which resorbs bone. Osteoclasts are followed by osteoblasts at the reversal zone and the osteoblasts of the closing cone fill in the resorption cavity to create a new osteon.

Fracture Repair After a midshaft fracture of a bone, a certain sequence of events occurs during the healing process. Fracture repair involves changes in blood supply that affect cellular proliferation and differentiation as well as bone resorption.

The trauma that causes the bone to break also tears the adjacent soft tissues and blood vessels. The blood clot that forms at the fracture site stops circulation and results in necrosis or death of the surrounding tissue. Likewise, the interruption of the blood vessels within the osteons causes cessation of blood supply and death of the osteocytes on each side of the fracture site.

New tissue developing at the fracture site forms a bridge between the fragments. This formation is termed a **callus** and is composed of two parts. The **internal callus** develops between the opposing ends of the bone, and the **external callus** surrounds the outermost surface of the broken bone.

The cells involved in callus formation are the osteogenic cells of the periosteum and endosteum. Early in the healing process, the cells of the periosteum proliferate to such an extent that the fibrous layer of the periosteum is lifted away from the bone. In addition, the endosteal cells proliferate, resulting in a thickened endosteum. The undifferentiated marrow cells increase in number in the same area. Differentiation of these cells takes place in one of two ways and depends on the vascular supply available. Those nearest to the bone fragments differentiate in the presence of blood vessels; consequently, they become osteoblasts and form bony trabeculae. Those farther away from the bone proliferate in an area relatively devoid of capillaries; consequently, they form chondroblasts, which produce cartilage in the external callus. The cartilage is a temporary splint that eventually is replaced by bone, following the same sequence of events that occurs in endochondral ossification. Gradually, the callus is remodeled by resorption of the trabeculae at the periphery, until the original outline of the bone is restored.

No external callus develops when a bone fracture has smooth, even, opposing surfaces that are perfectly aligned without any space between the fragments, and the fragments are held rigidly throughout the healing period. In this situation, dead bone extends for some distance on both sides of the fracture line. Osteogenic cells and capillaries in the living bone proliferate and grow into the adjacent dead bone. Simultaneously, osteoclasts invade the area and form cortical remodeling units that cross the fracture line. Resulting new osteons extend into the cortical bone on the other side of the fracture (primary osteosynthesis).

Fractures that are realigned in direct apposition but have a small space between the two fragments heal similarly, as long as rigid fixation is maintained. The only difference is that the two bone ends are joined initially by woven bone rather than by new osteons. Remodeling occurs as a secondary event.

Joints

Joints connect two or more bones. The various types of joints are classified according to the type of tissue that makes up the structure and the degree of movement permitted. As the result of aging, certain fibrous and cartilaginous joints may become **synostoses**, as the respective connective tissues are eventually replaced by bone.

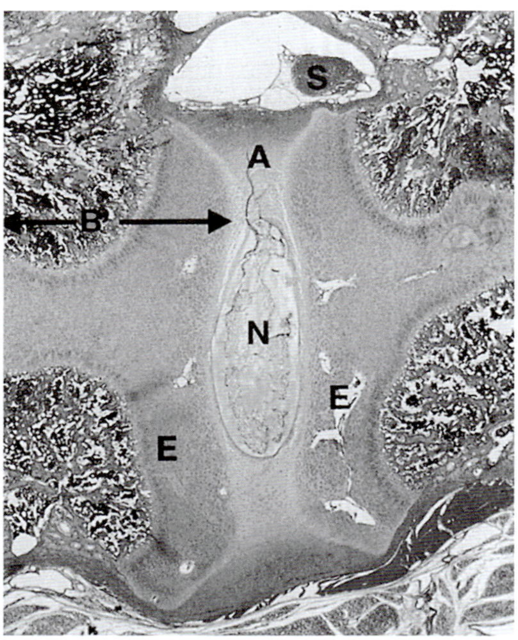

Figure 3-41 Vertebral column, longitudinal section (puppy). The central nucleus pulposus (N) of the intervertebral disk is surrounded by the annulus fibrosus (A). The disk attaches to the cartilaginous end plates (E) of the vertebral bodies (B). A spinal nerve (S) exits from the spinal cord through the intervertebral foramen above the disk. H&E (×8).

Fibrous Joints

Bones held together by collagenous or elastic dense CT are called **syndesmoses** or **sutures**. An example of a syndesmosis is the fibrous articulation between the radius and ulna. Sutures are typical of the skull.

Cartilaginous Joints

Joints in which the two bones are connected by cartilage are called **synchondroses**, such as the physis. In the **symphysis** joint, the hyaline cartilage caps of adjacent bones are joined by thick fibrous bands. Between the hyaline cartilage and the collagen fibers is a transition zone of fibrocartilage. The pelvic symphysis is an example of this type of joint.

The intervertebral disk is a symphysis that consists of an outer lamellated **annulus fibrosus** and an inner dorsally eccentric cavity, which is filled with a gelatinous **nucleus pulposus** in young animals (Fig. 3-41). The nucleus becomes more rigid with age and may calcify in some breeds of dogs at approximately 5 years of age. The annulus is thicker ventrally than dorsally, and its fibers insert into a thin layer of hyaline cartilage covering the ends of adjacent vertebrae. The cells in the peripheral laminae of the annulus resemble fibrocytes, whereas the cells of the deeper lamellae are more representative of chondrocytes. The annulus is avascular and hence is sustained by diffusion from the vessels in the medullary cavity and periosteum of the vertebrae.

Synovial Joints

Synovial (diarthrodial) joints are characterized by the presence of articular cartilage on the opposing bony surfaces, a lubricating synovial fluid within the closed joint cavity, and a joint capsule enclosing the entire joint (Fig. 3-42).

The articulating surfaces of synovial joints are covered by a specialized complex, the **articular cartilage**, which consists of hyaline cartilage, tidemark, and calcified cartilage (Fig. 3-43). The hyaline cartilage segment is devoid of perichondrium and can be divided into three zones based on the morphology of the chondrocytes and the arrangement of the type II collagen fibrils in the matrix: (a) the **superficial zone** has flat cells that lie among layers of collagen fibrils oriented parallel to the surface; (b) the **middle zone** has larger, more spherical cells, displays a random arrangement of collagen fibrils, and stains the most intensely of all zones for GAGs; and (c) the **deep zone** has cells that are arranged perpendicular to the articular surface between columns of collagen fibrils. These fibrils are anchored into the calcified cartilage, which forms the deepest layer of articular cartilage. The calcified cartilage is joined to underlying subchondral bone by simple adherence without traversing collagen fibrils. Although uncalcified articular cartilage (superficial, middle, and upper deep zone) may vary in thickness during life, the thickness of the calcified cartilage layer remains constant.

The **tidemark** is a thin layer of clusters of mineral, glycoproteins, and lipids located between the calcified and uncalcified layers of the deep zone. In decalcified sections, the tidemark stains with hematoxylin. Multiple tidemarks may be present in older animals and indicate that mineralization of the cartilage was interrupted and then resumed several times. This contrasting interface between calcified and uncalcified tissues is prone to fracture.

The highly anionic GAGs (e.g., chondroitin sulfate and keratan sulfate to a lesser degree) of articular cartilage normally bind water, which is released upon compression of the cartilage. Conversely, when the compression is released, the water is absorbed into the matrix and rebinds with the GAGs. This process provides a "weeping" lubrication of the articular surfaces, as well as a circulation of nutrients to and waste products from the articular chondrocytes. This fluid circulation is important since the articular cartilage is avascular and alymphatic.

The joint capsule encloses the entire joint and comprises an inner **synovial membrane** and outer **fibrous layer** (Fig. 3-42). The synovial membrane, in turn, is composed of synovial cells (synoviocytes) and subcellular CT, which may be loose, fibrous, or adipose. The predominating CT type in the synovial membrane varies with the location in the joint and classifies the type of synovial membrane. The outer fibrous layer is composed of dense irregular CT and is continuous with the periosteum of adjacent bones.

Synoviocytes, the specialized cells residing in the synovial membrane, are classified into two main types. Type A synoviocytes are macrophage-like or phagocytic and function to engulf

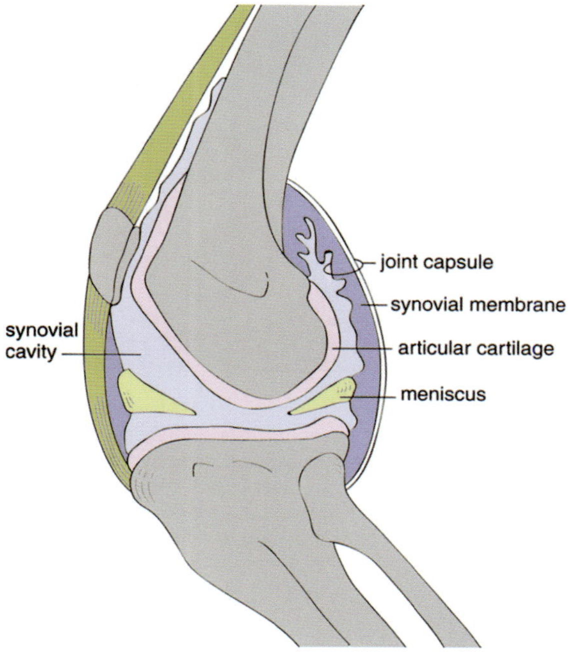

Figure 3-42 Articular cartilage covers the opposing bony surfaces of a synovial joint as shown in this diagram of a stifle. The joint space is filled with synovial fluid produced by the synovial membrane of the surrounding joint capsule. A meniscus composed of fibrocartilage extends into the joint cavity.

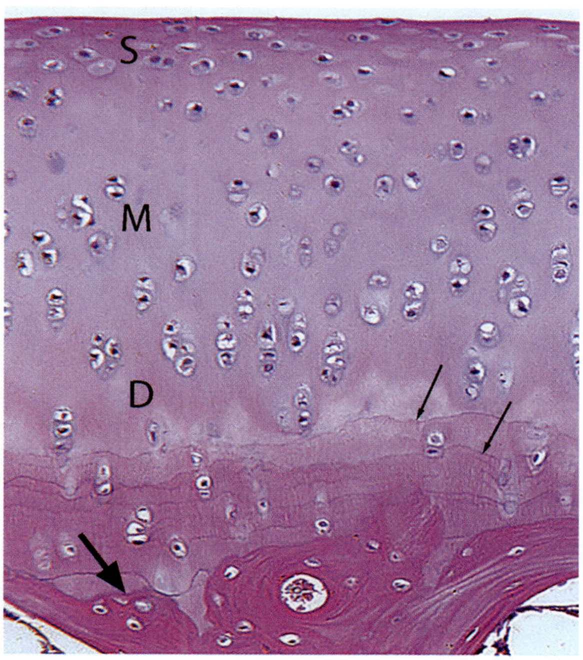

Figure 3-43 Articular cartilage zones: superficial (S), middle (M), and deep (D). Multiple tidemarks (small arrows) are present in the calcified cartilage region. The junction of the articular cartilage with the subchondral bone is indicated by the large arrow. H&E (×290).

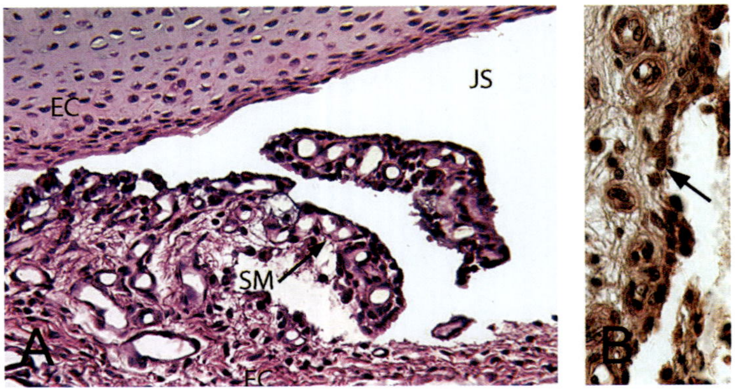

Figure 3-44 **A.** Synovial membrane (SM) lines the joint capsule of synovial joints. Type A synoviocytes are phagocytic, whereas the fibroblast-like Type B synoviocytes secrete synovial fluid into the joint space (JS). The outer fibrous layer (FC) of the joint capsule is composed of dense irregular CT. Humerus, puppy. H&E (×250) (Image by J. Eurell). **B.** Synoviocyte (arrow) on the surface of a bovine synovial membrane (×400).

and remove cellular debris, pathogens, and foreign particles in the joint. They also participate in antigen presentation and immune surveillance. In contrast, type B synoviocytes are fibroblast-like and are responsible for synthesizing and maintaining the synovial fluid and extracellular matrix. They secrete key components including hyaluronic acid and lubricin, contributing to the lubrication and viscosity of the synovial fluid, while also producing structural proteins to support the integrity of the synovial membrane. The two synoviocyte types play crucial roles in maintaining joint health and function (Fig. 3-44).

The synovial cavity is filled with **synovial fluid**, which has a composition similar to plasma. This fluid is derived as an ultrafiltrate of the blood with the addition of a substantial amount of polymerized hyaluronic acid from synovial cells. Synovial fluid provides the lubrication for the articulating surfaces of joints.

Some synovial joints (stifle) have intraarticular **menisci** composed of fibrocartilage (Fig. 3-42). Usually, menisci are anchored on one side to the fibrous layer of the joint capsule. If the cartilages are removed after traumatic injury, a new structure can develop from the fibrous layer of the capsule; however, it is composed of dense collagen rather than fibrocartilage. These structures are important to the biomechanics of the joint, and the ends (horns) are heavily innervated with proprioceptive nerves.

Clinical Correlations

Mast cell tumor (**mastocytoma**) is a common canine skin tumor.

Inheritable genetic disease is the most common cause of CT disorders in animals. Defects in various collagens are the cause. **Type V** collagen is involved in type I collagen fibrillogenesis, and a defect is a cause of Ehlers-Danlos syndrome in dogs. Similarly, hyperelastosis cutis (HC) or hereditary equine regional dermal asthenia (HERDA), occurs in Quarter Horses. HC is caused by a missense mutation in cyclophilin B that is necessary for triple helix folding of collagen. **Type VII** collagen anchors the epithelial basal lamina to the reticular lamina, and a defect in this protein causes dystrophic epidermolysis bullosa in dogs.

Essentials

1) CT is characterized by the types of **cells**, **fibers**, and the **ground substance**. The fibroblast/fibrocyte is the primary cell for collagenous tissues. Type I collagen is the predominant fiber in collagenous tissues (loose and dense). Type III collagen is a major fiber in reticular CT. The ECM **ground substance** consists primarily of proteins linked to GAGs, linkage to hyaluronic acid (aggrecan), and various glycoproteins (fibronectin and laminin are most important).
2) *Cells*: Other than the fibroblast, CT can contain a variety of other cells: **mast cell** (type I hypersensitivity, related to blood basophil); **eosinophil** (parasite immune response); **neutrophil** (first cell in inflammatory reaction); **lymphocytes** (regulators of immune function); **plasma cell** (antibody production); **pericytes** (stem cell around some capillaries/postcapillary venules important in wound healing); and **macrophages** (phagocytes and immune regulators).
3) *CT types*: 1. **Embryonic** (mucus and mesenchyme). 2. **Loose** (below epithelium, around blood vessels, and nerves); **dense irregular** (dermis, organ capsules; type I collagen); **dense regular** (ligaments, tendons only; type I collagen); **adipose tissue** (white fat for energy storage, endocrine function with receptors for insulin, growth hormone, and glucocorticoids, brown fat for heat generation); **reticular** (framework for lymphoid organs; type III collagen); and **dense regular elastic** (elastic arteries).

4) *Fibers*: **Type I** collagen is most common, secreted as procollagen, cleaved to tropocollagen, and assembled into **fibrils**. Individual fibrils cluster together to form **fibers**. **Type III** reticular fibers react with silver stain and are found in lymphoid tissue and the reticular portion of basement membranes. **Elastic fibers** are amorphous fibers of elastin and fibrillin found in multiple locations where elasticity and strength are needed.

Suggested Readings

Alberts B, et al. Molecular Biology of the Cell. 6th ed. New York: Garland Science; 2014.

Athanasiou KA, Darling EM, Hu JC, et al. Articular cartilage. CRC Press; 2017 Oct 19.

Bartl R, Bartl C. Bone disorders: biology, diagnosis, prevention, therapy. Springer; 2016 Sep 20.

Birbrair A. Pericyte biology: development, homeostasis, and disease. *Pericyte Biology-Novel Concepts*. 2018:1–3.

Bronner F, Farach-Carson MC, Roach HI, editors. Bone-Metabolic functions and modulators. Springer Science & Business Media; 2012 Jun 12.

Cheville NF. Cell Pathology. 2nd ed. Ames, IA: Iowa State University Press; 1983.

Florencio-Silva R, Sasso GR, Sasso-Cerri E, et al. Biology of bone tissue: structure, function, and factors that influence bone cells. *BioMed Research International*. 2015;2015:421746.

Keene DR, Tufa SF. Transmission electron microscopy of cartilage and bone. *Methods in Cell Biology*. 2010;96:443–73.

Novack DV, Mbalaviele G. Osteoclasts—key players in skeletal health and disease. *Myeloid Cells in Health and Disease: A Synthesis*. 2017;2017:235–55.

Shapiro IM, Risbud MV. Intervertebral Disc. Springer Verlag Gmbh; 2016.

Sprangers S, Everts V. Molecular pathways of cell-mediated degradation of fibrillar collagen. Matrix Biology. 2019;75:190–200.

4

Nervous Tissue

Olalekan M. Ogundele

CHAPTER MENU

Dellmann's Textbook of Veterinary Histology, Seventh Edition. Edited by Marxa L. Figueiredo and John J. Turek.

Companion website: www.wiley.com/go/figueiredo/vethistology7e

Nervous tissue parenchyma consists of **neurons** and supportive cells called **neuroglia**. This tissue forms the nervous system, which may be divided into the central nervous system (CNS) and the peripheral nervous system (PNS). The **CNS** includes the brain and spinal cord. The **PNS** consists of cranial nerves, spinal nerves, nerve roots, and ganglia. Motor (visceral efferent) nerves and the associated ganglia that innervate viscera constitute the **autonomic nervous system**.

Neurons

Neurons are the structural and functional units of the nervous system. They are also trophic units because they often transform and sustain the structures they innervate. Generally, neurons must last a lifetime because, with some exceptions (e.g., olfactory neurons and neuronal stem cells), mature neurons are incapable of mitosis. However, recent evidence of new neuron formation in several regions of the brain has been discovered. This concept is described as adult neurogenesis and has been mapped to the hippocampus and olfactory bulb brain regions.

Morphologically, neurons feature elongated processes termed axons and dendrites, which extend variable distances from the cell body (perikaryon) (Fig. 4-1). Metabolically, neurons are actively involved in maintaining their structural integrity and in synthesizing, packaging, transporting, and releasing secretory products, including neurotransmitters, neuromodulators, and (neurotransmitter) hormones.

Neurons communicate by releasing chemical agents (neurotransmitters, neuromodulators, or neurohormones) that act as ligands for various receptors and ion channels located in other neurons and cells. These ligands are packaged in vesicles, trafficked by cytoskeleton/motor proteins, and delivered through exocytosis to the vicinity of the target neuron/cell.

Neurons are excitable cells. In this context, excitation involves a change in the electrochemical gradient across the hydrophobic barrier formed by the neuronal plasma membrane. Protein receptors and ion channels embedded in the neuronal membrane facilitate ion movement, leading to depolarization of the neuronal membrane and triggering "firing events" called action potentials. Depending on the type of neurotransmitter released and the receptors expressed by target neurons or cells, an action potential event may lead to excitation or inhibition of the target cell.

Neuronal Structure

Neurons assume a variety of shapes and sizes, related to their functional roles. Neuronal processes are configured according to the connections that must be made. Neurons with processes that extend over long distances tend to be larger than those with shorter connections. Because larger processes conduct electrical signals more rapidly than smaller ones, neurons that convey urgent information are large. Also, neurons that are highly branched are more readily excitable.

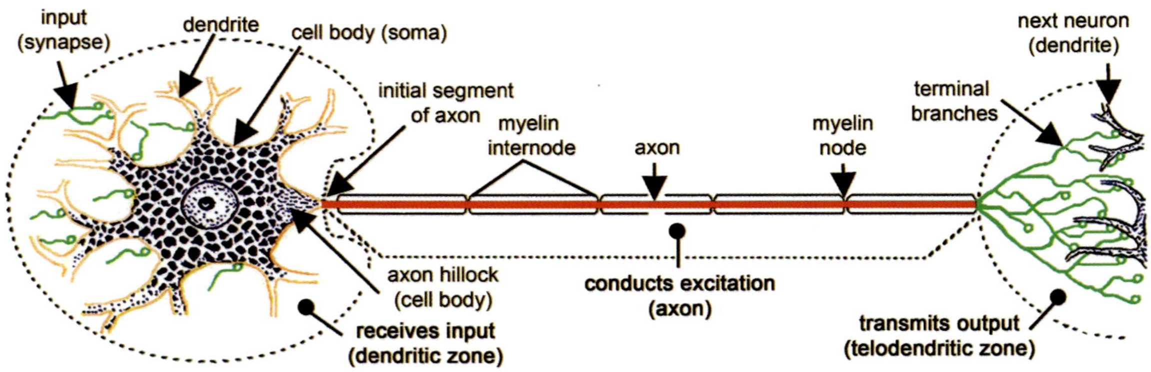

Figure 4-1 Schematic illustration of a typical (multipolar) neuron, showing multiple dendrites and one axon emanating from the cell body. Functional regions include the dendritic zone (cell body and dendrites), which receives synaptic input; the telodendritic zone (axon terminals), which makes synaptic contact with other neurons; and the axon, which conducts excitation between the two zones. This axon is drawn myelinated. The myelin insulation is interrupted by nodes (gaps). The myelin of each internode is formed by individual glial cells (not shown).

Cell Body

The **cell body** (perikaryon; soma) of a neuron consists of the nucleus plus the surrounding cytoplasm and a plasma membrane (Fig. 4-1). In routinely stained histologic sections, the cell body is the most identifiable feature of a neuron. Cellular constituents are synthesized within the cell body and then transported distally into neuronal processes (axon and dendrites).

Cell bodies can range in diameter from less than 10 μm to over 100 μm. The size of the cell body is proportional to the total volume of the neuron, although it represents a minor portion of the total volume and an even smaller fraction of the total surface area. In multipolar neurons, where the plasma membrane of the cell body integrates synaptic input, smaller cell bodies are more easily excited to reach the threshold for triggering action potentials compared to larger ones. This is because smaller neurons have higher input impedance, by virtue of their size.

Nucleus

Typically, the nucleus of a neuron is centrally positioned, spherical or ovoid, and relatively euchromatic, reflecting its high synthetic activity. Small neurons have rather heterochromatic nuclei. Neurons in the autonomic ganglia often have eccentrically positioned nuclei. Nuclear size is proportional to neuron size. The nucleus appears relatively large within a neuron because the surrounding cell body cytoplasm represents only a minor fraction of the total cell volume.

A prominent nucleolus is evident within the nucleus. In females of some species, **sex chromatin** (Barr body) may be evident in the vicinity of the nucleolus (cats and rodents) or the nuclear membrane (primates).

Cell Body Cytoplasm

Many proteins are synthesized in the cell body cytoplasm of the neuron, including cytoskeletal proteins (e.g., for neurofilaments and microtubules), membrane proteins (e.g., ion channels and receptors), enzymatic proteins (e.g., for glucose metabolism and neurotransmitter synthesis), and secretory peptides (e.g., neuromodulators and neurohormones).

The cell body cytoplasm of large neurons stained with aniline dyes and examined under light microscopy features clumps of **chromatophilic substance** (Nissl substance). This substance represents aggregations of rough endoplasmic reticulum (rER), free ribosomes, and polyribosomes. Chromatophilic substance extends into the trunks of dendrites, but it is absent from the axon and **axon hillock**—a pale-staining region of the cell body where the axon originates. Instead, the hillock contains neurofilaments and grouped microtubules. In small neurons, cytoplasmic chromatophilia appears relatively pale and diffuse.

When a neuron is injured (e.g., by transection of its axon), several changes occur: the cell body swells, the nucleus shifts to an eccentric position, and ribosomes disperse, leading to the disappearance of chromatophilic substance from the center of the cell body (**chromatolysis**). This response to injury is called the **axonal reaction** (Fig. 4-2) and typically begins within days of the injury and may persist for several weeks. The reaction is considered pathologic evidence of nervous tissue damage in the CNS. Depending on the proximity of the damage to the cell body, axonal and neuronal degeneration may occur. In severe cases, axonal degeneration progresses toward the cell body (retrograde degeneration), ultimately leading to cell death. On the other hand, if degeneration occurs distal to the injury site (anterograde degeneration), axonal regeneration and guidance to target sites are more likely.

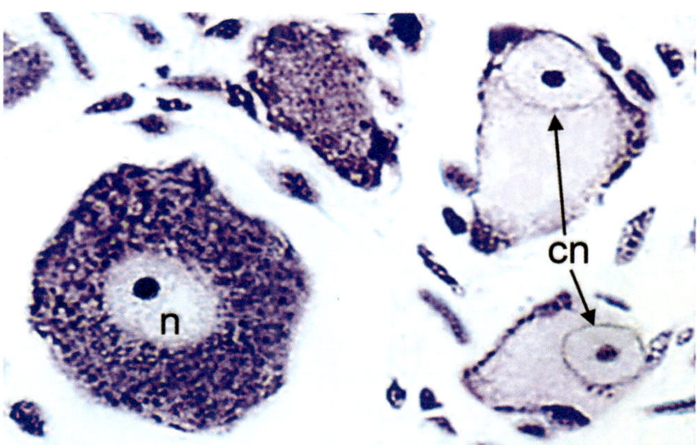

Figure 4-2 The cell body of a multipolar neuron at the lower left (n) appears normal. The two cell bodies on the right are undergoing chromatolysis in response to axonal transection. The chromatolytic cell bodies are swollen, their nuclei (cn) have eccentric positions, and chromatophilic substance is lost except at the margin. Spinal cord, dog, Nissl stain (×200). (Image by A.J. Beitz and T.F. Fletcher.)

Organelles in the cell body cytoplasm of the neuron include numerous mitochondria, which support the aerobic energy needs of the cell. **Mitochondria** in neurons are particularly enriched at synapses, providing energy for high ion exchange activity with a concentration of ion channels and receptors. Neurons also contain a prominent network of Golgi complexes that underscores their high rate of protein synthesis and vesicle trafficking. **Secretory vesicles** originate from these Golgi complexes and are transported along the axon to synaptic boutons, which are expansions of the axon terminal. These vesicles commonly contain neuroactive peptides that influence the excitability or growth of target cells. In certain hypothalamic neurons, secretory vesicles carry neurohormones that are released in proximity to blood vessels and ultimately enter the bloodstream.

Synaptic vesicles containing neurotransmitters are concentrated in axon terminals, where they fuse with the plasma membrane and release neurotransmitters into the synaptic cleft. Long-lived neurons may accumulate **lipofuscin granules** in the cytoplasm as a residue of lysosomal activity.

Microtubules (25 nm in diameter) and **neurofilaments** (10 nm in diameter) are numerous in the cell body. Microtubules are involved in the rapid transport of membrane-bounded organelles within the neuron. This transport is facilitated by the interaction between building blocks of microtubule assembly ($\alpha\beta$ tubulin dimers) and motor proteins (kinesin and dynein) that drag vesicles away or toward the cell body. Groups of neurofilaments, referred to as neurofibrils, provide structural stability and maintain the shape of connective neurons and associated projections. These can be visualized with light microscopy.

Neuron Processes

A typical neuron has a single axon and multiple dendrites originating as processes from its cell body (Fig. 4-1). The axon ends in terminal branches that synapse with dendrites and cell bodies of other neurons, or it innervates muscle or glandular epithelium. Each type of neuronal process has a distinct functional role within the neuron, characterized by different populations of plasma membrane proteins such as channels, receptors, transporters, and pumps.

A synapse is formed between two neurons or between a neuron and an excitable cell (e.g., muscle cell). The neuron that contributes the terminal branches (telodendrion) is presynaptic, whereas the neuron that contributes the target dendritic membrane or density is the postsynaptic neuron or cell. The space between the pre- and postsynaptic membrane is the synaptic cleft (typically ~35 nm). When a presynaptic neuron is excited, ion currents (mostly Ca^{++}) associated with the action potential trigger vesicle activity, releasing neurotransmitters into the synaptic cleft. These neurotransmitters bind to receptors expressed on the postsynaptic membrane, either to drive an action potential or to suppress neuronal activity in the postsynaptic neuron or cell.

Synapses are classified into structural, chemical, and functional categories. Structural classifications include axodendritic (axon to dendrite), axoaxonal (axon to axon), and axosomatic (axon to cell body), among others. Chemical classification is based on the types of neurotransmitters (ligands) and receptors present at the synapse (e.g., glutamate, gamma-aminobutyric acid (GABA), dopamine, etc.). Functional classification depends on the effect of neurotransmitters across the synapse. For example, excitatory synapses lead to the firing of the postsynaptic neuron when the presynaptic neuron fires (e.g., glutamate and acetylcholine). Conversely, inhibitory synapses suppress the activity of the postsynaptic neuron when the presynaptic neuron fires (e.g., GABA and glycine).

Dendrites **Dendrites** are highly branched processes specialized to receive numerous synaptic contacts from other neurons. Resembling a tree, each dendrite emerges as a main trunk that divides repeatedly into smaller and smaller branches. The trunk has an organelle content similar to that of the cell body. Small dendritic branches feature predominantly microtubules, augmented by neurofilaments, mitochondria, and smooth endoplasmic reticulum (sER). Dendrites are further organized into dendritic spines that can be visualized by silver staining methods and light microscopy. In typical electron microscopic preparations, dendritic spines contain postsynaptic densities with large mitochondria bodies.

Synaptic sites on dendrites are distinguished by a band of electron-dense cytoplasm of variable thickness along the **postsynaptic membrane**, which faces a **presynaptic element** across a **synaptic cleft** (Fig. 4-3). This dense material represents proteins (receptors, channels, enzymes, etc.) responsible for postsynaptic activity.

Many neurons display numerous **dendritic spines** (gemmules), which serve as the postsynaptic partner in excitatory synapses. A spine is a short, expanded process attached to a dendritic branch by a narrow stalk, like a bud on a twig (Fig. 4-4). A **spine apparatus consisting of alternating membrane sacs and dense plates** may be found within the spine. Spines increase dendritic surface area and act to restrict the spread of postsynaptic excitation. For over a century, dendritic spines were considered as largely static structures. However, recent research has shown that the structure of the spine is very dynamic. Time-lapse imaging has shown that adult spines can change shape up to 30% of their length or width within a few seconds to minutes. Furthermore, high-frequency stimulation induces protrusion of new dendritic processes and even spine bifurcation within minutes. These findings suggest that changes in spine number or shape may contribute to synaptic plasticity, potentially serving as a lasting structural substrate for newly encoded memories. The loss of dendritic spines in various brain regions also underlies several neurological, neurodevelopmental, and neurogenerative disorders.

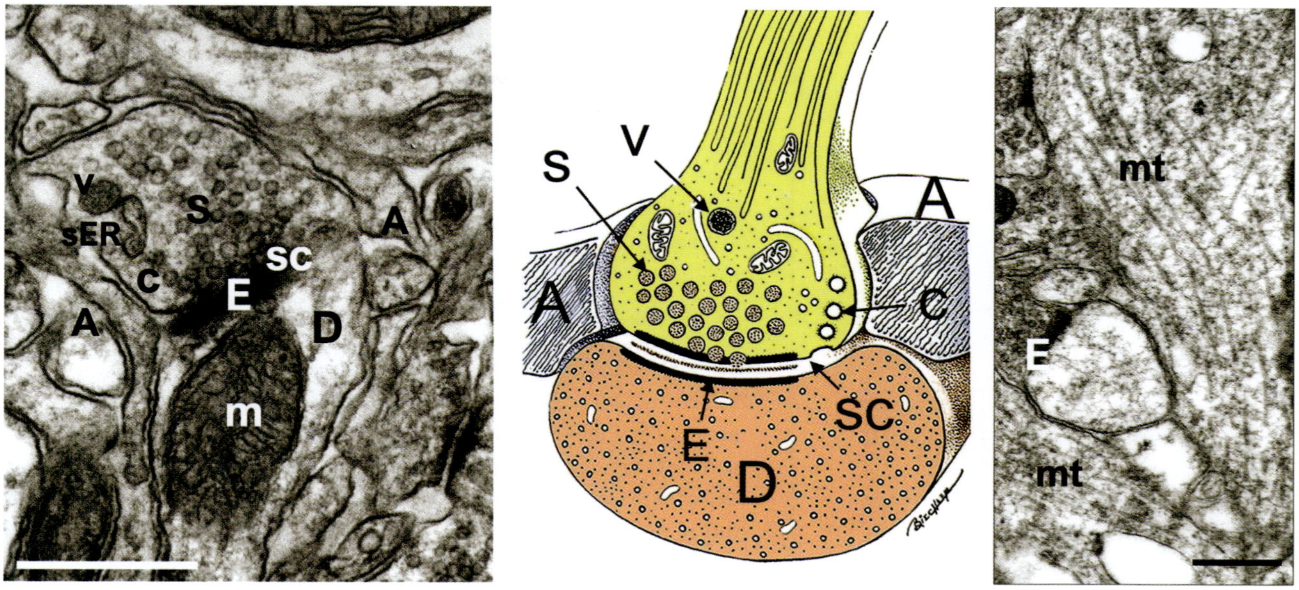

Figure 4-3 Schematic illustration and transmission electron photomicrographs (mouse brain; scale: 500 nm) of an axodendritic synapse. The axon terminal bulb and dendrite (D) are separated by a synaptic cleft (SC) containing glycoprotein material, bordered bilaterally by astrocyte processes (A). Within the terminal bulb, synaptic vesicles (S) are clustered around an active zone with an electron-dense band lining the plasma membrane. Ca^{++} influx triggers synaptic vesicles to dock with the plasma membrane and release neurotransmitters by exocytosis. Vesicle membranes, as coated vesicles (C), are recycled via smooth endoplasmic reticulum (sER). A solitary, large, dense-core secretory vesicle (possibly containing a peptide or monoamine neuroactive substance) is also shown (V), along with mitochondria, microtubules, and neurofilaments. The transverse section of the dendrite features an electron-dense band (E) along the postsynaptic membrane, a large mitochondrion (m), numerous microtubules (mt), neurofilaments, and a few sER profiles.

Axon The **axon** is a relatively long, cylindrical process that extends from the axon hillock of the cell body and ends in terminal branches and synaptic boutons, as described below. While the axon typically emerges directly from the cell body, in some neurons such as those found in parasympathetic ganglia or in the brain, the axon may originate as a branch of a dendrite. Apart from its terminal ends, axonal branches are sparse. When branches are present along the course of the axon, they emerge at right angles (from nodes in the case of myelinated axons) and are called **collateral branches**. The **axoplasm**, which is the cytoplasm of the axon, contains microtubules, neurofilaments, mitochondria, and sER. Devoid of rER, the axoplasm is not well stained by hematoxylin and eosin (H&E) or other routine histologic stains.

The **initial segment** of the axon is located just distal to the axon hillock, where action potentials normally originate. It is narrower than the rest of the axon. Ultrastructurally, bundled microtubules are present, and electron-dense material is evident along the inner surface of the plasma membrane of the initial segment. This density corresponds to protein accumulation associated with ion channels and pumps. Similar accumulations of electron-dense proteins are also found at the nodes of myelinated axons.

A slow flow of cytoplasm (1 mm/day) and a slow transport of cytoskeletal elements (10 mm/day) progress along the axon from the axon hillock to terminal branches (anterograde transport). In addition, axons have a fast transport capability (up to 400 mm/day) involving microtubule-linked movement of mitochondria and vesicles containing various constituents. There is also a retrograde transport mechanism that rapidly returns organelle remnants from terminal branches back to lysosomes within the cell body. This pathway can also transport viruses (e.g., rabies) and neurotoxins (e.g., tetanus toxin) to the cell body. To study connections between parts of the nervous system, researchers use anterograde and retrograde axonal transport of vesicles to deliver contrast and fluorescence molecules. Anterograde tracing labels cell bodies within a nucleus or ganglion, followed by the axons of these neurons, thereby mapping their axon terminals in target regions of the nervous system. On the other hand, retrograde tracers are picked up at axon terminals and label the cell bodies at their origin.

Axons are capable of regenerative conduction, that is, they convey an excitation signal to the end of the axon with the same magnitude as it originated from the initial segment. Large axons conduct signals more rapidly than smaller ones. However, to further increase conduction velocity, large axons are myelinated, which involves a myelin sheath formed by

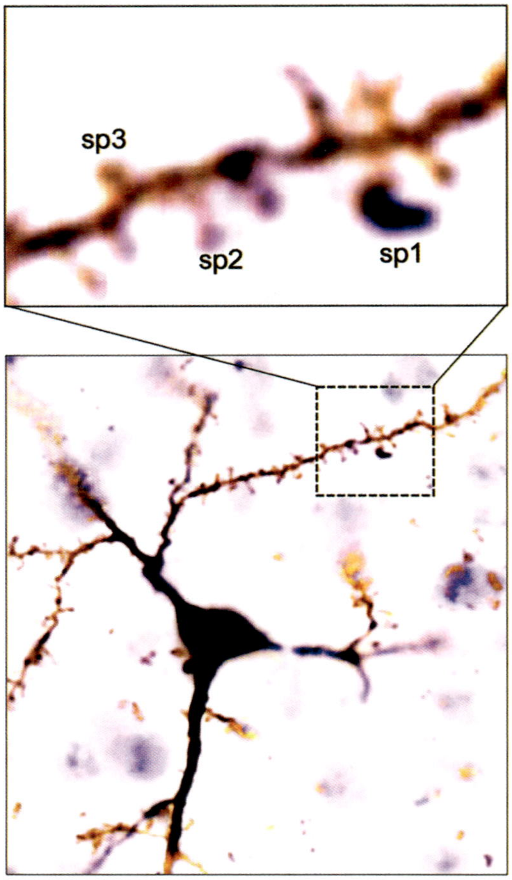

Figure 4-4 A pyramidal neuron from the cerebral cortex is shown using Golgi silver impregnation, counterstained with hematoxylin. This multipolar neuron has a pyramidal cell body from which apical and basal dendrites extend. A single axon (not visible) emerges from the lower surface of the cell body. Dendritic spines (sp) can be observed along the dendrites. *Inset*: A magnified view of the apical dendrite, highlighting dendritic spines of various sizes and shapes (*sp1* > *sp2* > *sp3*).

glial cells. In peripheral nerves, small axons that are nonmyelinated are still ensheathed by glial cells. However, in the CNS, small axons may not be ensheathed at all.

Axon degeneration may be linked causally to the physiologic and behavioral deficits observed in aged animals. Traditionally, the decline in memory function and behavioral dysfunction that accompany normal aging in animals have been attributed to loss of neurons in certain areas of the brain. However, recent data suggest that aging does not induce prominent cell loss in the brain but rather leads to the degeneration of axons that innervate certain forebrain structures.

Terminal branches (telodendrites) Axons terminate by successively branching (Fig. 4-1). The collective terminal branches form the axon terminal (telodendritic) zone of a neuron. Each terminal branch ends in an enlargement called a **terminal synaptic bulb** (synaptic bouton). Along the nonmyelinated terminal branches, synapses occur at multiple focal swellings called axonal varicosities (preterminal boutons). The number of axonal varicosities is substantial; for instance, a single hippocampal cell axon makes 50,000 synapses over a distance of only 200 mm. Both axonal varicosities and terminal synaptic boutons are sites where neurotransmitter molecules are packaged and stored within synaptic vesicles.

The most common **synaptic vesicle** is spherical (40 to 50 nm in diameter) with an electron-lucent (agranular) core (Figs. 4-3 and 4-5). Such vesicles may contain any one of a number of neurotransmitters. Inhibitory synapses are associated with electron-lucent synaptic vesicles that appear flattened when exposed to solutions of high osmolarity. Additionally, some neurons have spherical vesicles (40 to 60 nm in diameter) with an electron-dense (granular) core. These electron-dense synaptic vesicles usually contain dopamine or norepinephrine molecules.

Synaptic vesicle proteins are synthesized in the cell body and transported rapidly to axon terminal sER, where they supplement local production of synaptic vesicles from recycled vesicular membranes. Transporter proteins embedded in the vesicle membrane then load these newly formed synaptic vesicles with recycled neurotransmitter molecules. Linked together by cytoskeletal actin filaments, synaptic vesicles are clustered together in ready reserve for plasma membrane docking and exocytosis during synaptic activity (Fig. 4-3). In addition to synaptic vesicles, terminal branches may contain **secretory vesicles** that store neuroactive peptides (several dozen have been identified). These peptides are encapsulated within spherical, electron-dense vesicles that of relatively large size (100 to 200 nm in diameter). The secretory vesicles are synthesized in the cell body and transported to preterminal and terminal synaptic boutons for storage and release. The peptides generally act as neuromodulators (agents that augment neurotransmitter effects). Secretory vesicles of certain hypothalamic neurons contain peptide hormones (e.g., vasopressin and oxytocin), which are stored and released in the neurohypophysis.

The sprouting of new terminal branches and the degeneration of existing branches in response to environmental change are major mechanisms of neural plasticity, enabling neural development and, subsequently, behavioral modification and learning.

Classification

Neurons are anatomically classified as unipolar, bipolar, or multipolar according to the number of processes that emanate from the cell body (Fig. 4-6).

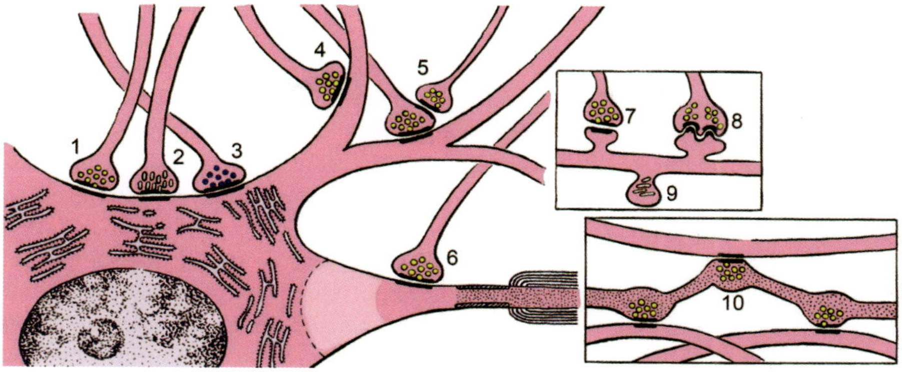

FIGURE 4-5 Schematic illustrations of various types of CNS synapses. **1.** Axosomatic synapse with electron-lucent, spherical, synaptic vesicles. **2.** Axosomatic synapse with synaptic vesicles that appear flattened (an artifact associated with inhibitory synapses). **3.** Axosomatic synapse with electron-dense synaptic vesicles. **4.** Axodendritic synapse. **5.** Axoaxonic synapse in which one terminal bulb synapses on another (associated with presynaptic inhibition). **6.** Synapse on an axon hillock, close to the initial segment of the axon. **7.** Axodendritic synapse on a dendritic spine. **8.** Relatively elaborate synapse on a dendritic spine. **9.** Dendritic spine exhibiting a spine apparatus (sER plus electron-dense material). **10.** Three axonal varicosities making synapses in passing (en passant).

In a **unipolar** neuron, the cell body gives off a single axon that quickly bifurcates into central and peripheral branches. The peripheral branch terminates in receptors sensitive to environmental stimuli, while the central branch conveys these stimuli-induced excitations into the CNS. Unipolar cell bodies are found in sensory ganglia located within roots of the cranial and spinal nerves. Mammalian unipolar neurons are often referred to as pseudo-unipolar because they originate as bipolar cells during development and only adopt a unipolar morphology later. The unique geometry of pseudo-unipolar sensory neurons can lead to spontaneous discharge in their cell bodies, potentially disrupting the accurate transmission of afferent signaling in normal animals. More importantly, following nerve injury, this ectopically generated discharge from spinal ganglion cells significantly increases, contributing to neuropathic dysesthesias and chronic pain. Pseudo-unipolar neurons primarily transmit general somatic (afferent) sensations (e.g., skin corpuscles). Their cell bodies are located in the dorsal root ganglion.

In a **bipolar** neuron, two processes emanate from the cell body, which is located either within the axon itself (as seen in vestibulocochlear afferent neurons and bipolar cells of the retina) or at the juncture of the axon and a single dendrite (as observed in olfactory afferent neurons). Like unipolar neurons, bipolar neurons are afferent neurons that convey sensory information to the CNS. The cell bodies of bipolar neurons are typically found in laminated structures within the organs they innervate. Their dendrites are specialized into receptive end organs, while their axons coalesce to form nerves traveling to the CNS.

In a **multipolar** neuron, the cell body gives rise to multiple branches, including several dendrites and typically a single axon. Nearly all of the billions of neurons comprising the CNS are multipolar, as well as those found in the autonomic ganglia of the peripheral nervous system (PNS).

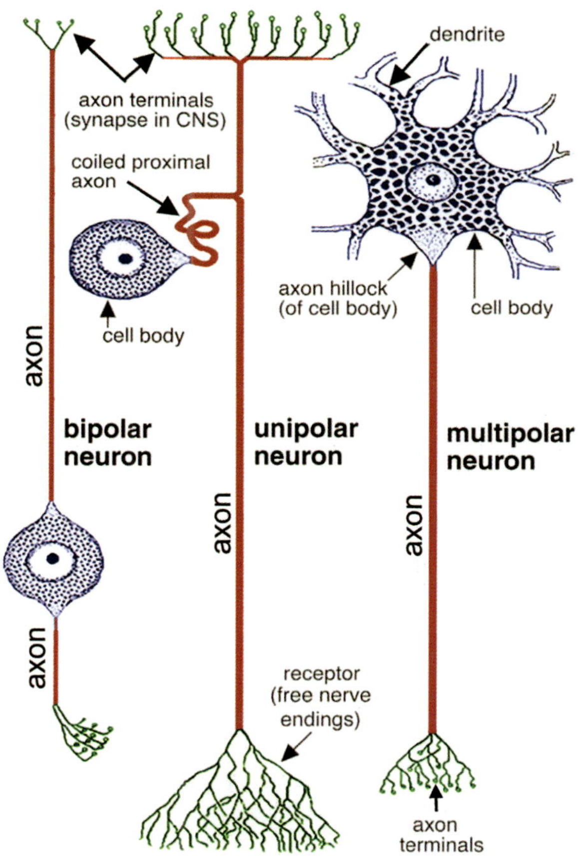

Figure 4-6 Schematic illustration of a bipolar neuron (left), a unipolar neuron (center), and a multipolar neuron (right). Neurons are anatomically classified according to the number of processes emanating from the cell body. Unipolar and bipolar neurons are primarily sensory. While most neurons are multipolar, their shapes can vary considerably. The cytoplasm of the cell bodies features clumps of chromatophilic substance (Nissl substance).

Regions of a Neuron

Neurons are bounded by a lipid bilayer membrane rich in ion channels and receptors. These proteins maintain a stringent electrochemical gradient across the membrane such that the resting membrane potential is approximately −70 mV. A typical neuron becomes excited by depolarization of its membrane, which increases electropositivity above a certain threshold to generate an action potential at its input region. Subsequently, the axon conducts excitation to its output region and transmits it via chemical secretion at synapses (Fig. 4-1). The processes of reception, conduction, and transmission of excitation require functionally distinct ion channels and cellular components. Thus, each neuron has several distinct regions: (a) an input region or **dendritic zone**, where initial excitation is received; (b) an output region or **telodendritic (axon terminal) zone**, where excitation is transmitted to other cells; (c) an **axon**, which conducts excitation between the dendritic and axon terminal zones; and (d) a **cell body**, which provides nourishment and supports the neuron.

In a typical multipolar neuron (Fig. 4-1), the receptive dendritic zone features a large surface area encompassing the cell body and highly branched dendrites. A long, cylindrical axon originates from the cell body. At the distal end of the **axon** lies the axon **terminal zone**, which is **highly branched**. Within this terminal zone, there are **localized expansions (boutons or bulbs)** where neurotransmitter molecules are stored and released at synapses. In contrast, a unipolar afferent neuron has its cell body situated along the axon. Its dendritic zone consists of receptors that convert environmental energy into neural excitation. In bipolar afferent neurons, the dendritic zones may involve receptors (such as those for olfaction) or synaptic contacts with receptor cells (as found in the retina and inner ear). From dendritic zones, excitation is conveyed along the axon to terminal branches within the CNS.

The protein composition of the plasma membrane varies significantly across the functional regions of a neuron. For example, in the dendritic zone, the membrane has ligand-reactive protein receptors that activate ion channels, either directly or through second messengers. Here, the term "receptor" refers to membrane proteins interacting with extracellular physiologic signals and translating them into intracellular effects. Conversely, the axon membrane has voltage-gated Na^+ channels that enable membrane polarity reversal and regenerative conduction of action potentials. The membrane of terminal branches and synaptic boutons has voltage-gated Ca^{++} channels responsible for mediating the influx of calcium ions. Ca^{++} play a key role in the release of neurotransmitter molecules. Additionally, this membrane region contains membrane-associated receptors for the reuptake of released neurotransmitters.

Neuronal Communication

Neurons communicate extensively among themselves, with glial cells, and with the muscles and glands they innervate. The alterations in excitation transmitted from one neuron to another constitute the basis of nervous system function.

Among the billions of neurons that comprise the nervous system, the primary means of communication is the localized release of neurotransmitter molecules at interneuronal chemical synapses. Similar chemical synaptic arrangements are encountered between efferent neurons and the muscles and glands they innervate (see the Peripheral Nervous Tissue section). A few neurons communicate through gap junctions (electrotonic synapses), especially in invertebrates and fish. However, in mammals, gap junction communication is more common between neuroblasts during embryonic development and is relatively rare between mature neurons. Additionally, some neurons communicate by producing a gas that freely passes through neuronal membranes. Gases such as nitric oxide and carbon monoxide are increasingly appreciated as major neurotransmitters. NO and CO transmit signals between neurons by binding to a heme moiety at the active site of soluble guanylyl cyclase, leading to an increase in the intracellular second messenger molecule cyclic guanosine 5′-monophosphate.

Interneuronal Chemical Synapses

An **interneuronal chemical synapse** is a specialized site where one neuron influences the excitability of another by releasing neurotransmitter molecules stored in synaptic vesicles. The majority of **neurotransmitters** are biogenic amines (e.g., glutamate, glycine, dopamine, norepinephrine, serotonin, acetylcholine, etc.). Generally, each neurotransmitter can interact with a variety of membrane receptors.

A **receptor** is a binding site on a membrane protein where a neurotransmitter briefly attaches. This receptor protein may function as an ion channel that undergoes conformational changes to allow selective ion passage. Alternatively, the receptor may be coupled to a G-protein cascade that can directly or indirectly open ion channels by activating second messengers (such as cyclic adenosine monophosphate). Second messengers provide a means of amplifying the scope and impact of a neurotransmitter signal, as well as prolonging its duration. Autoreceptors, located on the presynaptic plasma membrane, regulate neurotransmitter synthesis and release via second messenger systems. Neuromodulators, such as peptides released from secretory vesicles, also typically exert their effects through second messengers.

Ionotropic membrane receptors represent one large class of neurotransmitter receptors in which the receptor protein forms part of an ion channel–receptor protein complex. When activated, the complex opens or closes the ion channel, resulting in a change in membrane permeability. In contrast, **metabotropic receptors** represent another major class of neurotransmitter receptors. These receptors do not directly function as ion channels but instead interact with G proteins or other intermediary proteins. Upon activation by neurotransmitter binding, metabotropic receptors initiate signaling cascades that may involve enzyme activation or inhibition and potentially modulate ion channels or other cellular functions. This process leads to broader changes in cell function rather than immediate changes in ion permeability.

Based on the ion channel or G-protein coupling, receptors may be excitatory or inhibitory. Thus, the receptor type, rather than the neurotransmitter itself, determines the function of a synapse (e.g., excitatory or inhibitory, short or long acting, etc.). Nonetheless, certain neurotransmitters (e.g., glutamate) are associated with excitatory synapses, while others (e.g., GABA and glycine) are associated with inhibitory synapses. It is worth noting that glutamate receptors are the most prevalent excitatory neurotransmitter receptors in the brain, and they mediate almost all excitatory communications between CNS neurons. Thus, it is perhaps not surprising that epileptic seizures often result from overactivation of neurons primarily driven by glutamate synapses.

Most synapses between neurons involve terminal synaptic boutons of one neuron contacting the input region of another neuron, forming axodendritic or axosomatic synapses (Fig. 4-5). However, among the trillions of synapses in the nervous system, every possible synaptic combination has been observed, including axoaxonic, dendrodendritic, dendrosomatic, somatodendritic, and somatosomatic synapses.

The input region of a typical multipolar neuron receives thousands of synaptic contacts. Excitatory and inhibitory synaptic effects are collectively summed and integrated at the cell body of the target neuron so that the cell body membrane potential continually registers the net effect of total synaptic input to the neuron. In turn, the cell body influences the membrane potential at the nearby initial segment of the axon. At any moment, the collective synaptic input to a neuron may either trigger an action potential at the initial segment of the axon or be insufficient to do so.

The influence that one neuron has on another depends on the number of synaptic contacts it makes with the target neuron and where the synapses are positioned. Synapses close to the initial segment exert greater influence in triggering action potentials compared to synapses located on distal dendrites.

Synaptic Ultrastructure and Function

Ultrastructurally, an interneuronal chemical synapse may be identified by the juxtaposition of a presynaptic element, a synaptic cleft, and a postsynaptic membrane (Fig. 4-3). The **presynaptic element** contains multiple synaptic vesicles clustered around an active zone marked by electron density (protein accumulation) just inside the plasma membrane. The **synaptic cleft**, approximately 20 to 30 nm wide in the CNS (the same width as the general intercellular space), contains proteins that hold the presynaptic and postsynaptic membranes together. The **postsynaptic somatodendritic membrane** contains many types of protein receptors that aggregate to form functional microdomains opposite the presynaptic terminal boutons releasing neurotransmitters. These domains are associated with postsynaptic densities, visible under the electron microscope as electron-dense material facing the presynaptic active zone. The **postsynaptic density**, composed of adhesive proteins such as cadherin–catenin complexes, receptor proteins, subsynaptic scaffolding proteins, and elements of the cell's cytoskeleton, is involved in the stabilization and trafficking of receptors and in facilitating signal transduction.

When an action potential reaches the end of an axon, it passively depolarizes the presynaptic element (e.g., terminal synaptic bouton). Voltage-sensitive channels in the presynaptic membrane open to allow Ca^{++} influx. Elevated cytoplasmic Ca^{++} activates enzymes that phosphorylate synaptic vesicle proteins responsible for reversibly linking vesicles to cytoskeletal actin filaments and merging vesicles with the plasma membrane. This mobilizes synaptic vesicles, enabling them to dock with the plasma membrane and release several thousand neurotransmitter molecules by exocytosis. These molecules diffuse into the synaptic cleft and bind with various receptors and transporters.

Synapses are highly dynamic structures where receptors constantly move into and out of synaptic membranes. Recent data have shown that rapid turnover of neurotransmitter receptors at synaptic sites involves both endocytosis and exocytosis, as well as lateral diffusion within the plane of the membrane. These processes are interdependent and regulated by neuronal activity and interactions with scaffolding proteins. Thus, it is known that activity-dependent increases in postsynaptic intracellular calcium concentration triggers the rapid receptor immobilization and local accumulation of receptors on the neuronal surface. Neurotransmitter receptor movement into and out of the synaptic membrane is one of the core mechanisms for rapidly changing the number of functional receptors during synaptic plasticity.

Synaptic activity ceases through various mechanisms. First, neurotransmitter molecules are removed from the synaptic cleft through degradation by enzymes such as acetylcholinesterase (acetylcholine), monoamine oxidase, and catechol-O-methyl transferase (serotonin, dopamine, epinephrine, and norepinephrine). The target receptors of neurotransmitters also can be internalized at the postsynaptic membrane and degraded in lysosomes. Neurotransmitter molecules also are actively transported intracellularly by transporters (protein pumps) located in the presynaptic membrane or in membranes of adjacent glial cells. Thus, neurotransmitter molecules are recycled to minimize the need for synthesis within the presynaptic cytoplasm. Furthermore, the synaptic vesicle membrane undergoes recycling. The vesicle membrane is extracted from the presynaptic plasma membrane and transported as coated vesicles to the sER within the presynaptic cytoplasm (Fig. 4-3).

Neuroglia

Neuroglia (gliocytes) comprise over 90% of the cells that make up the nervous system. Recent studies have shown that glia are not simply the support structure in which neurons are embedded. While the biology of glial cells is poorly understood, it is clear that glial–neuronal and glial–glial interactions are essential for many critical functions in the nervous system. Neurons communicate with glial cells by releasing ATP at synapses and from axons during conduction. Glial cells have vital roles in neuronal development, metabolism, activity, plasticity, and recovery from injury.

Neuroglia possess a rich assortment of ionic channels, neurotransmitter receptors, and transport mechanisms that enable the gliocytes to respond to many of the same signals that affect neurons and to modulate neuronal responses. In parallel to the sequential flow of information along chains of neurons, glia communicate with other glial cells through intracellular waves of calcium and via the intercellular diffusion of chemical messengers. By releasing neurotransmitters and other extracellular signaling molecules, glia can affect neuronal excitability and synaptic transmission, perhaps coordinating activity across networks of neurons. Moreover, glia secrete cytokines, growth factors, and other trophic factors that regulate the long- and short-term survival of neurons, as well as the elaboration and retraction of synaptic connections. Some glial cells, specifically astrocytes, also form specialized tripartite synapses where they regulate ion concentrations and clear excess neurotransmitters from synaptic spaces.

From a histologic perspective, neuroglial cells are relatively small. With routine histologic stains, only their nuclei and cell bodies are evident, making them distinguishable primarily by the size and shape of their cell bodies and the chromatin pattern of their nuclei in tissue sections. However, the use of modern immunocytochemical staining for specific cell surface or internal markers allows definitive identification of glial cells in brain sections. It should be noted that unlike mature neurons, glial cells remain capable of mitosis, and thus they can give rise to tumors of the nervous system.

Except for microglial cells, which migrate into the CNS from mesoderm, CNS gliocytes are derived from the ectodermal cells that form the embryonic neural tube. Neurolemnocytes of the PNS are also derived from the embryonic neural crest, similar to neurons with cell bodies located in ganglia.

Central Nervous System Gliocytes

The gliocytes of the CNS include astrocytes, oligodendrocytes, microglia, and ependymal cells.

Astrocytes

With routine stains, **astrocytes** are identified by their pale, ovoid nuclei, which are the largest among glial nuclei. With silver stains, astrocytes exhibit numerous processes that contain glial fibrils. In white matter, these processes are long, slender, and moderately branched, while in gray matter, they appear shorter and highly branched. Thus, white matter is said to contain **fibrous astrocytes**, whereas gray matter contains **protoplasmic astrocytes** (Fig. 4-7).

Under the electron microscope, astrocytes feature packed bundles of intermediate filaments (8 nm in diameter) and pale cytoplasm. The **glial filaments**, which are composed of glial fibrillar acidic protein, are unique to astrocytes and form the **glial fibrils** seen with light microscopy. The density of these filaments is greater in fibrous astrocytes compared to protoplasmic ones.

Adjacent astrocytes are connected by gap junctions. In response to local stimulation, an excitatory wave of elevated cytoplasmic Ca^{++} can propagate outward from cell to cell via the gap junctions. The adjacent astrocytes also are linked by small, button-like adhering junctions (spot desmosomes).

Astrocyte processes terminate in expansions called **end feet**. Collections of end feet form a **glial-limiting membrane** to which the pia mater is attached at the surface of the CNS. End feet are prominent in the subependymal glial layer, and they form septa in the spinal cord. End feet of specialized astrocytes cover vessels within the brain and spinal cord, where they are believed to be responsible for inducing the formation of tight junctions between capillary endothelial cells, contributing to the blood–brain barrier (further described in later chapters).

Astrocytes provide structural support through their glial fibrils, but, in addition, these cells play critical roles in several aspects of brain function. By storing glycogen and releasing glucose, they represent a source of reserve energy. Astrocyte plasma membranes have ionic pumps that regulate K^+ levels within the narrow extracellular space of the CNS. Astrocyte processes insulate synapses and release substances that modulate synaptic sensitivity. Astrocytes also can take up neurotransmitter molecules from the synaptic cleft to stop ongoing synaptic activity.

Recent data have revealed that astrocyte activity is likely influenced by neuronal activity and that astrocytes have the capacity to signal not only to each other but also back to neurons. Furthermore, since astrocytes can detect synaptic activity, it is thought that they are pivotal intermediaries between neurons and the brain microcirculation. In this regard, increased synaptic activity triggers calcium waves in astrocytes, causing their end feet to release substances that promote local vasodilation. Thus, astrocytes can act to synchronize brain activity not only with energy demands but also with blood flow requirements.

Finally, astrocytes also appear to have immune functions; they can present antigens to T lymphocytes and secrete a wide array of chemokines and cytokines. This capability allows them to influence T helper cell responses and monocyte/microglia effector functions. It should be noted that the reaction of astrocytes following brain trauma or in certain pathologic states is characterized by astrocyte proliferation and hypertrophy, elongation of astrocyte processes, and upregulation of various intermediate filaments. In cases of severe trauma or pathology, these reactive astrocytes can form a dense glial scar. This process is referred to as astrogliosis, where the hypertrophied processes of reactive astrocytes fill in the spaces left by the loss of myelin and neurons.

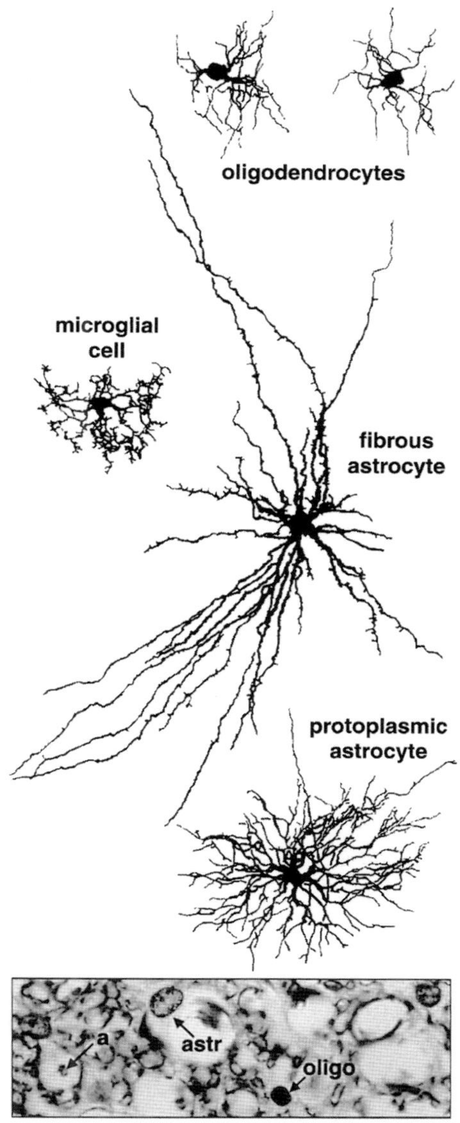

Figure 4-7 Central nervous system (CNS) gliocytes are drawn as they appeared following Golgi silver impregnation of monkey cerebral cortex (×700). The inset at the bottom shows an astrocyte nucleus (astr) and an oligodendrocyte nucleus (oligo) as they appear in white matter stained with Luxol blue and hematoxylin. An axon (a) surrounded by a myelin vacuole and neurokeratin can be seen. (Adapted from Weiss L. Cell and Tissue Biology. A Textbook of Histology. 6th Ed. Baltimore, MD: Urban & Schwarzenberg, Inc., 1988.)

Oligodendrocytes

Oligodendrocytes have relatively few branches (Fig. 4-7). In routine stains, they are recognized by their small, spherical, densely stained nuclei. Ultrastructurally, oligodendrocyte cytoplasm is electron-dense and rich in microtubules and organelles, especially rER and mitochondria. Oligodendrocytes lack gap junctions.

In gray matter, oligodendrocytes serve as perineuronal satellites. Recent studies indicate that oligodendrocytes also serve as providers of growth factors. They synthesize specific growth factors and release trophic signals to nearby neurons. They also appear to be highly responsive to neurotrauma.

In white matter, oligodendrocytes wrap **myelin sheaths** around axons, which enhances the speed of action potential propagation in the CNS. Intracellular trafficking of membrane constituents plays an essential role in the biogenesis and maintenance of myelin. The requisite proteins and lipids are synthesized elsewhere in the cells and transported to the myelin sheath via intracellular carrier vesicles that move along the cytoskeleton.

Microglia

Microglia are cells of mesodermal origin that infiltrate the CNS during its embryological vascularization. They are sparse and difficult to find in normal tissue. In routine stains, microglia are identified by their small, elongated, chromophilic nuclei. With silver impregnation, they are seen as small, elongated cells with polar processes (Fig. 4-7). Under physiologic conditions, microglia synthesize and release trophic factors. However, in response to CNS injury, microglia become activated, proliferate, and express protective or, under certain circumstances, cytotoxic properties. Microglial activation often precedes reactions of other cell types in the brain, and once activated, they transform into macrophages with antigen-presenting and phagocytic capabilities. Reactive microglia also secrete cytokines, including tumor necrosis factor and IL-1β, which can influence synaptic transmission and exert trophic effects on neurons. Microglia have been recognized to play crucial roles in various diseases, including viral infections, autoimmune conditions, and neurodegenerative disorders.

In addition to microglia, other cell types also respond to CNS damage. Hematogenous macrophages can invade the CNS, while pericytes, cells associated with CNS capillaries and believed to have contractile capability, are also considered to be phagocytic. Although the functional role of glial scarring is not completely understood, it has been suggested to be an attempt by the CNS to restore homeostasis by isolating the damaged region.

Ependymal Cells

Ependymal cells form an epithelium that lines the ventricular cavities in the brain and the central canal of the spinal cord. These cells are typically cuboidal or columnar with numerous motile cilia on their apical surfaces (Fig. 4-8). Ependymal cells are interconnected by zonulae adherens and gap junctions near their luminal borders. In the adult brain, mature ependyma is not merely a passive lining but likely regulates the transport of ions, small molecules, and water between the cerebrospinal fluid and neuropil. Ependyma serves as a critical barrier that protects neural tissue from potentially harmful substances. Although the mechanisms are still incompletely understood, this function is believed to involve ion and metabolite secretion. Ependymal cells have only limited regenerative capacity and typically do not undergo mitotic proliferation. Tearing of the epithelium leaves discontinuities that become filled with processes from subventricular astrocytes.

Specific modified ependymal cells, called **choroid plexus epithelium**, cover the surfaces of choroid plexus villi and produce cerebrospinal fluid through active secretion of Na^+. These modified ependymal cells are cuboidal in shape and have microvilli extending into cerebrospinal fluid instead of cilia. Adjacent cells are connected by relatively impermeable junctions (zonulae occludens or tight junctions), establishing a localized ependymal barrier. This barrier is associated with a locally reduced blood–brain barrier due to the presence of fenestrated capillaries.

Tanycytes are modified ependymal cells found in the wall of the third ventricle in the hypothalamus. The luminal border of a tanycyte has microvilli, while their basal border features elongated processes that contact capillaries and neurons. Tanycytes are thought to guide hypothalamic axons and facilitate transport mechanisms between the ventricle and the blood vessels of the hypothalamic–hypophysial portal system. Thus, tanycytes can influence the release of hypothalamic hormones.

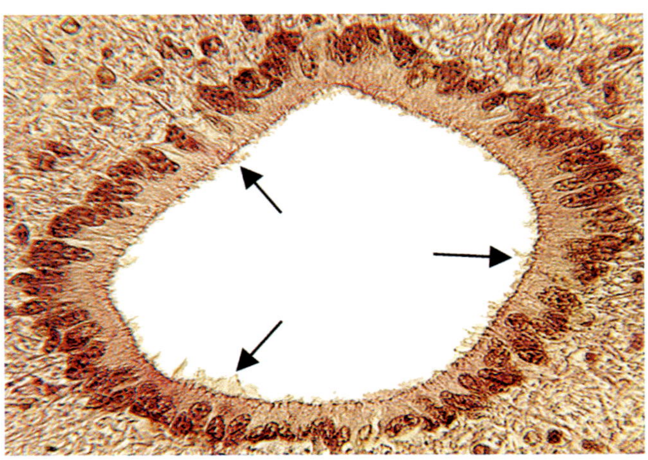

Figure 4-8 Ependymal cells (simple columnar epithelium) line the central canal of a canine spinal cord. Motile cilia projecting into the lumen of the central canal are evident (arrows). H&E.

At certain sites, neuronal processes extend between ependymal cells to make contact with cerebrospinal fluid. These processes end in bulbous structures containing stereocilia, which are presumed to serve a receptive function. Also, neurons containing secretory vesicles can be found among ependymal cells; they are believed to release catecholamines.

Peripheral Nervous System Gliocytes

The gliocytes of the PNS include ganglionic gliocytes and neurolemnocytes (Schwann cells).

Ganglionic Gliocytes

Ganglionic gliocytes (satellite cells) encapsulate neuron cell bodies in the PNS. In cranial nerve and spinal (sensory) ganglia, each neuron cell body is tightly surrounded by a capsule formed by ganglionic gliocytes (Fig. 4-9). In autonomic ganglia (Fig. 4-10), the capsules formed by ganglionic gliocytes are incomplete and may enclose more than one postganglionic cell body. Away from the cell body, ganglionic gliocytes are replaced by neurolemnocytes that sheathe or myelinate axons.

Neurolemnocytes

Neurolemnocytes (Schwann cells) are gliocytes of the PNS that sheathe and myelinate axons. They create a protective environment for PNS neurons, which is crucial for axonal function and survival. Each neurolemnocyte is enclosed by a basal lamina. Neurolemnocytes can proliferate and become phagocytic in the event of nerve damage, aiding in debris removal and facilitating nerve regeneration.

Every axon in the PNS is sheathed or myelinated along its entire length by neurolemnocytes, except for the most terminal branches in some cases. Because an individual neurolemnocyte is less than 1 mm in length, a tandem series of many neurolemnocytes is required to enclose the entire length of a long axon.

For small axons, an individual neurolemnocyte sheathes multiple axons simultaneously, and these axons (nerve fibers) are considered **nonmyelinated** (Fig. 4-11). Each axon resides in a furrow, protected by a pair of neurolemnocyte processes so that the space surrounding the axon communicates with the general interstitial space only through a narrow gap known as the **mesaxon**. In the case of PNS axons larger than 1 µm in diameter, each neurolemnocyte encloses a single axon, and glial processes wrap around the axon to form a **myelin sheath** (Fig. 4-12).

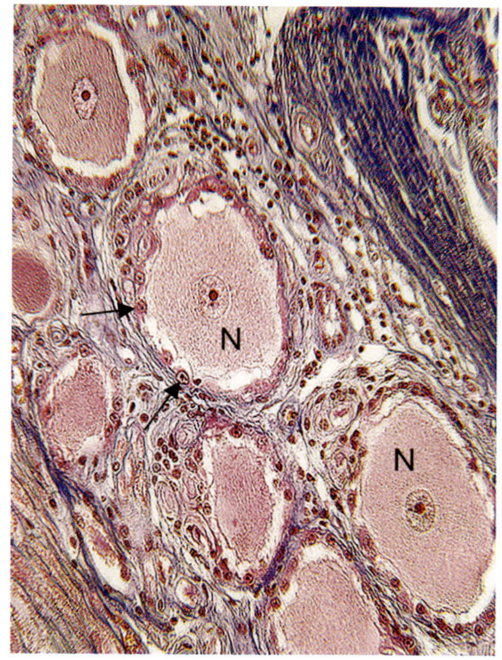

Figure 4-9 Canine spinal ganglion. Unipolar neuron cell bodies (N) are surrounded by ganglionic gliocytes (satellite cells) (arrow) within the ganglion. Triple stain.

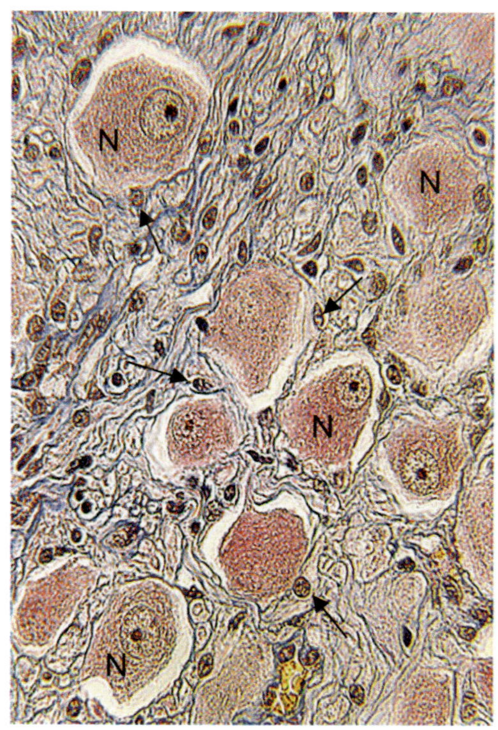

Figure 4-10 Canine autonomic ganglion. The cell bodies (N) of postganglionic neurons are multipolar, with nuclei positioned eccentrically. Ganglionic gliocytes (satellite cells) (arrows) form an incomplete capsule around individual neuron cell bodies. Triple stain.

Myelin Sheath

The term **myelin sheath** (myelin) refers to layers of glial cell plasma membrane that wrap around an axon, providing insulation it to speed up conduction. Myelin is formed by oligodendrocytes in the CNS and by neurolemnocytes in the PNS.

In the PNS, a transverse section of a myelinated fiber viewed by light microscopy reveals an axon enclosed in a myelin sheath surrounded by neurolemnocyte cytoplasm (Fig. 4-13). With electron microscopy, the myelin sheath appears as multiple layers of neurolemnocyte plasma membrane, with the neurolemnocyte itself surrounded by a basal lamina (Fig. 4-12).

Myelin formation in the PNS begins with a neurolemnocyte wrapping around a solitary axon, establishing a simple mesaxon (Fig. 4-14). Stimulated by the axon itself, neurolemnocyte processes elongate, slide past one another, and proceed to form multiple layers of neurolemnocyte wrappings around the axon. During this process, cytoplasm is extruded from the wrappings, leaving behind concentric lamellae of plasma membrane that constitute the myelin sheath.

In transmission electron microscopic images, the myelin sheath exhibits a periodic pattern of concentric **major dense lines** separated

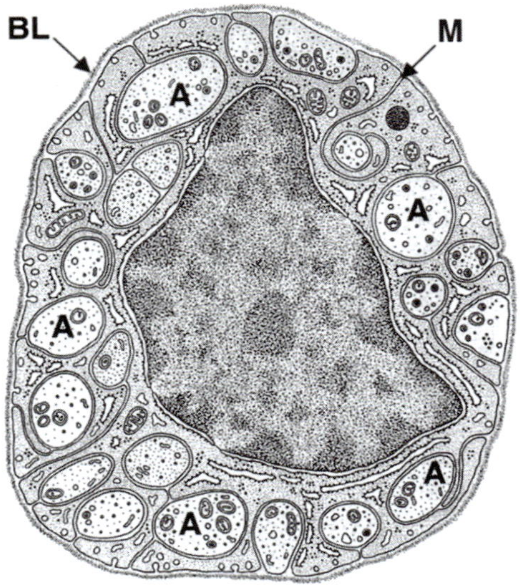

Figure 4-11 Drawing of the ultrastructure of a peripheral nerve neurolemnocyte sheathing 22 nonmyelinated axons (A). Each axon is enveloped by neurolemnocyte processes. Mesoaxons (M) are formed where the processes meet. A basal lamina (BL) surrounds the entire cell. (From Lentz TL. Cell Fine Structure. Philadelphia, PA: WB Saunders, 1971.)

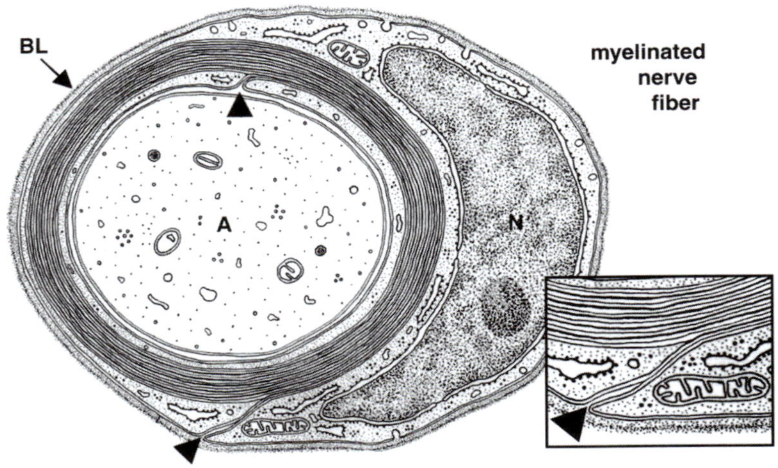

Figure 4-12 Ultrastructural drawing of a transected myelinated nerve fiber from the peripheral nervous system (PNS). A neurolemnocyte has enveloped a single axon (A) with a myelin sheath consisting of multiple layers of neurolemnocyte plasma membrane. Paired neurolemnocyte processes form outer and inner mesaxons (arrowheads at 12 and 6 o'clock, respectively). The nucleus of the neurolemnocyte is labeled (N). A basal lamina (BL) surrounds the neurolemnocyte. The inset (lower right) shows an enlarged view of the outer mesaxon and myelin sheath. Note that stained myelin exhibits major dense lines (formed by fusion along the inner surface of neurolemnocyte plasma membrane), separated by intraperiod lines (formed by apposition of outer surfaces of neurolemnocyte plasma membrane). (From Lentz TL. Cell Fine Structure. Philadelphia, PA: WB Saunders, 1971.)

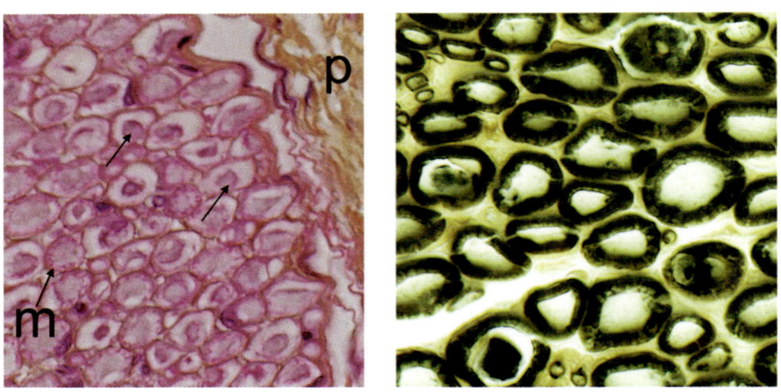

Figure 4-13 **Left panel:** Transverse section through myelinated fibers of a canine peripheral nerve. The myelin sheath surrounding the axon (arrow) is often clear due to solvents used in sample preparation. The myelin sheath (arrow) is observed on a few axons. H&E (×200). **Right panel:** Peripheral nerve preserved with osmium tetroxide fixation. The myelin sheath around the axon is well preserved (×200).

by intraperiod lines. Each major dense line is formed by the fusion of inner surfaces of plasma membrane as cytoplasm is extruded during myelin sheath formation. An **intraperiod line** appears where the outer surfaces of adjacent plasma membranes are separated by a small gap. This gap is continuous with the **inner mesaxon** and the **outer mesaxon**, all of which are derived from the original simple mesaxon during early myelin sheath development. Occasionally, a major dense line may appear to split and contain a pocket of cytoplasm. Adjacent pockets of cytoplasm can extend throughout the thickness of the myelin sheath, thereby establishing a **myelin incisure** in the sheath.

A longitudinal view of a myelinated nerve fiber shows gaps in the myelin sheath where adjacent gliocytes meet (Fig. 4-15). Each gap is referred to as a **node** (of Ranvier), and the myelin sheath between nodes is called an **internode**. The internodal transition region immediately adjacent to a node is referred to as a **paranode** (Fig. 4-16), where major dense lines split and cytoplasm-filled processes overlap, contacting the axon plasma membrane. The outermost cytoplasmic processes of adjacent neurolemnocytes enclose the node in the PNS, surrounded by a continuous basal lamina. At the node, the axon bulges slightly and exhibits subplasmalemmal electron-dense material. In normal axons, sodium channels are present at high density within the nodal gap, facilitating nerve conduction, while voltage-dependent potassium channels

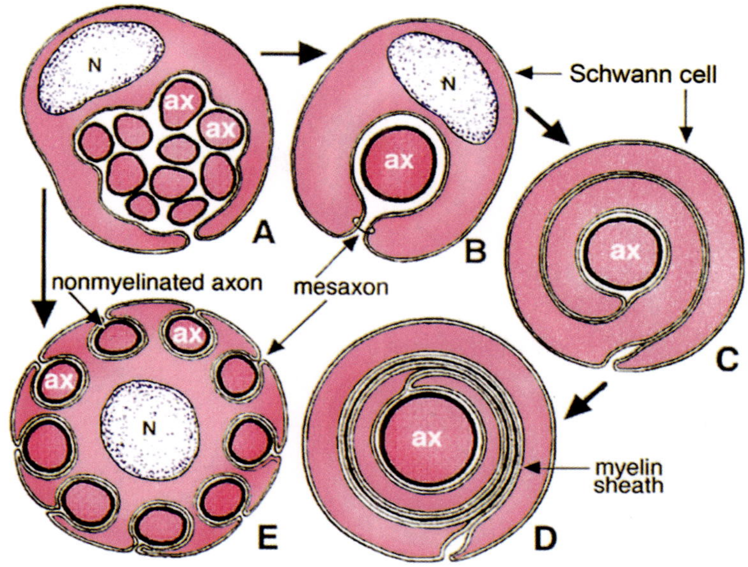

Figure 4-14 Schematic illustration of the developmental relationships between myelinated and nonmyelinated axons (ax) and neurolemnocytes in cross-sectional perspective. **A.** Early in development, several axons are sheathed together by a single neurolemnocyte. **B.** After neurolemnocyte proliferation, a solitary large axon destined to be myelinated is sheathed, forming a mesaxon where neurolemnocyte processes converge. **C.** Neurolemnocyte processes elongate and encircle the axon, thereby lengthening the original mesaxon. **D.** A myelin sheath is formed when cytoplasm is extruded from encircling neurolemnocyte processes, leaving layers of plasmalemma. Cytoplasm is retained internally and externally to the myelin sheath, showing an inner mesaxon and an outer mesaxon. **E.** Nonmyelinated axons feature neurolemnocyte invaginations providing separate compartments and mesaxons for each axon. Neurolemnocyte nucleus (N). (Adapted from Copenhaver WM, Bunge RP, Bunge MB. Bailey's Textbook of Histology. 16th Ed. Baltimore, MD: Williams & Wilkins, 1971.)

are clustered at the internodal side of the paranode, a region known as the juxtaparanode. The juxtaparanode and its associated potassium channels appear to stabilize nerve conduction and help maintain the internodal resting potential.

In the CNS, myelin sheaths are formed by oligodendrocytes, and nodes lack covering cytoplasmic processes, being exposed to the extracellular space (Figs. 4-16 and 4-17). Internodes are shorter and nodes are wider in the CNS compared to the PNS. A single oligodendrocyte can contribute internodes to as many as 50 myelinated fibers. The outer cytoplasm of the internode is restricted to a single ridge connected to the oligodendrocyte perikaryon by a thin process.

It is well established that myelin sheaths provide electrical insulation, enabling action potentials to jump from node to node instead of propagating continually as in nonmyelinated axons. This process, called **saltatory conduction**, is much faster than nonmyelinated conduction. The speed of conduction increases with longer internodes, which are proportional to myelin sheath thickness and axon diameter. Neurolemnocytes develop early associations with axons during development, resulting in longer internodes for axons that grow farther (e.g., in the limbs), compared to axons in closer proximity (e.g., in the head).

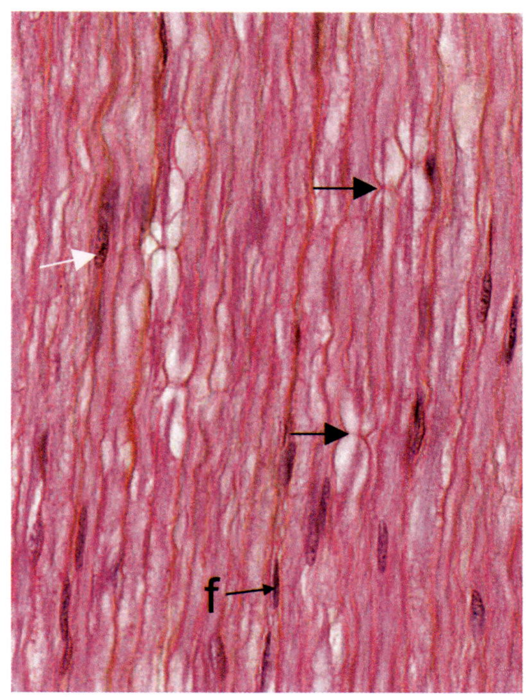

Figure 4-15 Light micrograph of a longitudinal section of a canine peripheral nerve. An axon passing through a myelin node (black arrows) is evident at the center. Nuclei in the section belong to fibrocytes (f) or neurolemnocytes (white arrow). H&E (×400). (With permission of Purdue University.)

The recent discovery of tight junctions and adhering junctions between myelin lamellae may help elucidate other roles played by this compact multilamellar structure. Whereas in epithelial cells these junctions are formed between different cells, in myelinating glia these so-called autotypic junctions are found between membrane lamellae of the same cell. Such junctions were initially proposed to link adjacent membranes for increased mechanical strength. However, tight junctions in other cell types play critical roles in paracellular functions, including signal transduction and fluid movement through aqueous pores and channels. This knowledge, taken together with evidence from studies on normal and pathologic myelin, supports the possibility that in addition to mechanical support, junctional plaques likely regulate perfusion of the periaxonal space.

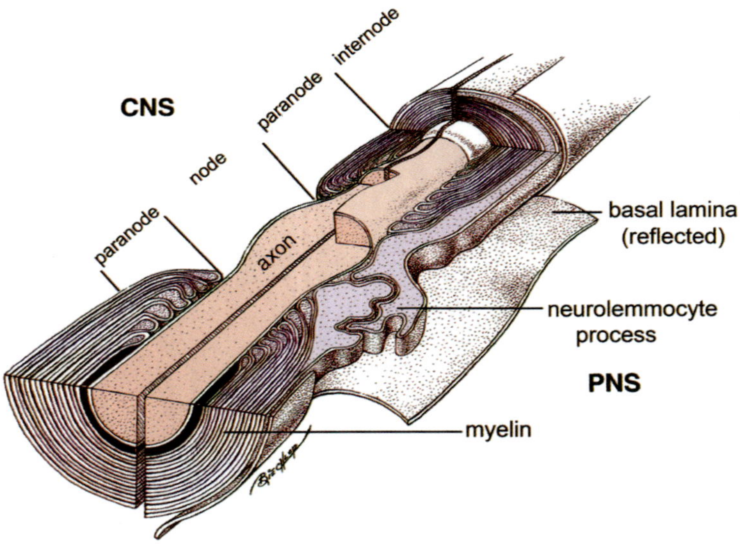

Figure 4-16 Schematic illustration of nodal and paranodal regions of myelinated fibers from the CNS (left) and the PNS (right). In the CNS, myelin is formed by oligodendrocytes and nodes are broadly exposed to the extracellular space. In the PNS, outer cytoplasmic processes of adjacent neurolemnocytes (Schwann cells) overlap to restrict node exposure to the extracellular space. Also, neurolemnocytes are surrounded by a continuous basal lamina. Myelin consists of compressed membranes of glial cells, distinguished by a series of major dense lines separated by intraperiod lines. At each paranode, major dense lines split to contain terminal cytoplasmic loops that contact the axon plasma membrane and impede ionic flow beyond the node.

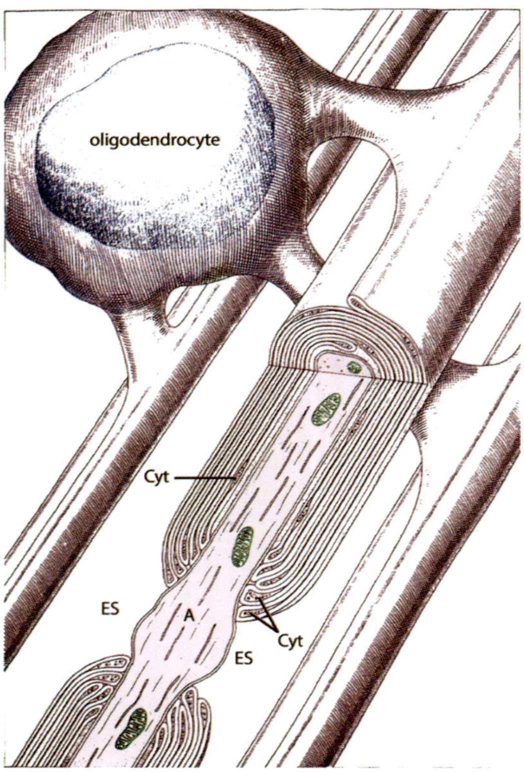

Figure 4-17 Illustration of an oligodendrocyte providing myelin internodes to three axons. A bisected view of a node, adjacent paranode regions, and part of an internode are shown in the foreground. The axon (A) bulges at the node and is exposed to extracellular space (ES). Cytoplasm loops (Cyt) contact the axon at the paranodal regions. Cytoplasm is retained along the ridges associated with inner and outer mesaxons, and small cytoplasmic pockets may be seen interrupting major dense lines. (Adapted from Bunge MB, Bunge RP, Ris H. Ultrastructural study of remyelination in an experimental lesion in adult cat spinal cord. J Biophys Biochem Cytol 1961;10:67–94.)

Peripheral Nervous Tissue

Tissue in the PNS consists of cranial and spinal nerves, including their roots, distal branches, and ganglia. **Cranial nerves** originate from the brain and exit the cranial cavity through various openings called foramina. **Spinal nerves** originate from the spinal cord and exit the vertebral canal through the intervertebral foramen. A **nerve root** is the proximal region of a cranial or spinal nerve enveloped by meninges within the cranial cavity or vertebral canal. The term **nerve fiber** refers to a single axon within a nerve. In the case of a myelinated axon, the term **nerve fiber** (or myelinated nerve fiber) includes the axon, myelin sheath, and surrounding neurolemnocyte.

Individual nerve fibers may be classified as either afferent or efferent. **Afferent fibers** are sensory because they conduct excitation to the CNS. Typical afferent neurons have pseudo-unipolar cell bodies located in cranial nerve and spinal (sensory) ganglia (such as the dorsal root ganglion). The dendritic zone of an afferent neuron consists of receptors or postsynaptic endings, such as sensory epithelial cells in sense organs. **Efferent axons** arise from multipolar cell bodies located in the brain or spinal cord, or in autonomic ganglia. They activate muscles, glands, or neurons in the autonomic ganglia.

Individual nerve fibers are also classified as somatic or visceral. **Somatic fibers** innervate skin, skeletal muscles, and joints, whereas **visceral fibers** innervate cardiac and smooth muscles and glands. Visceral efferent fibers, in particular, and visceral fibers, in general, are components of the **autonomic nervous system (ANS)**. The visceral efferent pathway involves two neurons: the first (preganglionic) neuron has its cell body in the CNS, while the cell body of the second (postganglionic) neuron is located in an autonomic ganglion.

The ANS, a part of the motor (efferent) outflow system, is divided into two parts based on its neurochemical anatomy: the *sympathetic system*, which promotes energy consumption (catabolism), and the *parasympathetic system*, which promotes energy conservation and storage (anabolism). The interaction between preganglionic and postganglionic neurons in the autonomic ganglia is driven by cholinergic neurotransmission. However, beyond the ganglia, these systems differ in their energy modulation requirements and specificity of targeting. The sympathetic system utilizes a rapid and diffuse mode of action, achieved through a direct release of catecholamines (adrenaline/nor-adrenaline) from postganglionic neurons into the bloodstream or target organs. On the other hand, the parasympathetic system utilizes localized effects by releasing acetylcholine from postganglionic neurons to modulate cholinergic receptors in target tissues.

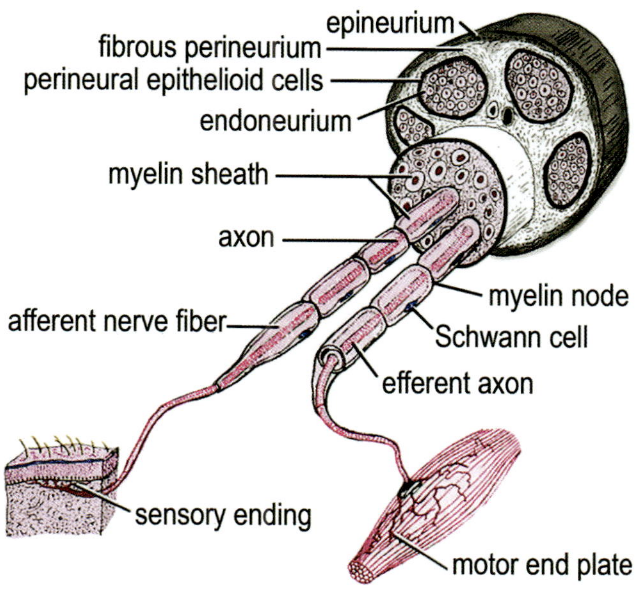

Figure 4-18 Diagram of peripheral nerve constituents: five fascicles surrounded by epineurium connective tissue (CT). Each fascicle is encircled by perineurium, composed of layers of perineural epithelioid cells surrounded by fibrous tissue. Within each fascicle, endoneurium surrounds individual myelinated fibers consisting of axons encased in myelin sheaths formed by neurolemnocytes and interrupted by nodes. Somatic afferent and efferent myelinated fibers are illustrated. (Modified from Jenkins TW. Functional Mammalian Neuroanatomy. 2nd Ed. Philadelphia, PA: Lea & Febiger, 1978).

Nerves

A **nerve** typically consists of thousands of axons, each sheathed or myelinated by neurolemnocytes and all organized into fascicles enveloped by connective tissue (CT) (Fig. 4-18). A **nerve fascicle** is delimited by the **perineurium**, which consists of fibrous tissue surrounding epithelioid cells. The multiple fascicles of a nerve are bound together by CT called **epineurium**. Within each fascicle, fibrocytes and collagen fibers surrounding individual neurolemnocytes constitute the **endoneurium**. Blood vessels supplying a nerve are designated as **vasa nervorum**.

Individual perineural epithelioid cells are interconnected by zonulae occludens and enveloped by basal laminae. Multiple concentric sheets of the squamous cells, along with interposed collagen fibrils, form a continuous tube that encloses nerve fibers and endoneurium within a fascicle. A perineural epithelioid tube may have a dozen concentric layers at its origin, where it meets its meningeal-covered root. The number of layers gradually decreases as a nerve branches. A single layer surrounds terminal branches, although epithelioid cells proliferate to encapsulate certain receptors. A **blood–nerve barrier** exists, constituted by the epithelioid cells and the endothelium of endoneurial microvessels. This barrier serves to protect axons and the internal nerve environment from fluctuations in blood plasma levels of hormones, ions, and toxic substances. However, the enclosed intrafascicular space may also serve as a channel for infectious or toxic agents once they breach the epithelioid cell barrier.

The **perineural epithelioid cells** are squamous and arranged in concentric sheets. The **fibrous perineurium** is collagenous CT. The morphologic distinction between fibrous perineurium, which surrounds individual fascicles, and epineurium, which binds fascicles together, varies by species. In dogs, for example, nerves are composed of a few relatively large fascicles with dense fibrous perineurium and flimsy, fatty epineurium. In contrast, bovine nerves have multiple small fascicles where fibrous perineurium and epineurium tend to blend indistinguishably.

Ganglia

Aggregations of neuronal cell bodies exists in both the CNS and the PNS. Those in the CNS are called nuclei, whereas such cell bodies constitute a ganglion in the PNS. Thus, a ganglion is an aggregation of neuronal cell bodies outside the CNS. Structurally, a **ganglion** is a localized enlargement of a nerve caused by the accumulation of neuron cell bodies. Spinal ganglia located in dorsal spinal roots and ganglia in cranial nerve roots are referred to as **sensory ganglia** because they contain cell bodies of primary afferent neurons (Fig. 4-9). Afferent neurons are pseudo-unipolar, except in certain sense organs (vestibular apparatus, cochlea, retina, and olfactory epithelium), where they are bipolar.

Within a sensory ganglion, unipolar cell bodies are distributed superficially and nerve fibers course through the center of the ganglion. These cell bodies range in size from large (30 to 50 μm in diameter) to small (15 to 25 μm in diameter), and each cell body gives rise to a single axon that may coil initially before bifurcating into central and peripheral branches. Typically, the peripheral branch is thicker than the central branch. Large cell bodies give rise to myelinated axons that bifurcate at a node. Each cell body is tightly encapsulated by ganglionic gliocytes.

Autonomic ganglia are accumulations of multipolar cell bodies within autonomic nerves (Fig. 4-10). These neuron cell bodies, which have eccentric nuclei and marginally distributed chromatophilic substance, are loosely encapsulated by ganglionic gliocytes. Synapses occur within autonomic ganglia, where terminals of cholinergic preganglionic neurons synapse with dendritic zones of postganglionic neurons. Microscopic accumulations of postganglionic cell bodies within nerve plexuses of visceral organs (especially the gut) constitute terminal autonomic ganglia.

Postganglionic neurons are classified as either **cholinergic** if they synthesize and release acetylcholine (parasympathetic) or **adrenergic** if their associated neurotransmitter is noradrenaline (norepinephrine; sympathetic). Adrenergic neurons feature dense-core synaptic vesicles. Some autonomic ganglia contain a few **small intensely fluorescent (SIF) cells**, which have numerous large, dense-core vesicles containing dopamine, released under neural control. The significance of SIF cells is unknown, but they form somatodendritic synapses and thus appear to function as interneurons.

Efferent Neurons

Somatic efferent neurons (α motor neurons) innervate skeletal muscle. Each neuron, along with all the muscle fibers it innervates, constitutes a **motor unit**. When excited, the muscle fibers contract synchronously as a unit. A motor unit may have few or several hundred muscle fibers, depending on muscle size. Typical muscles have a mix of large and small motor units. **Small motor units** have fatigue-resistant muscle fibers innervated by small neurons. These neurons are among the first to begin firing and the last to cease firing during muscular contraction. In contrast, **large motor units** have hundreds of muscle fibers innervated by large neurons. The muscle fibers are readily fatigued and, because large neurons require additional synaptic input to reach activation threshold, they fire only when strong muscle contractions are needed.

A **neuromuscular synapse** consists of a presynaptic neuronal end plate overlaying a postsynaptic muscle sole plate at the midregion of a muscle fiber (Fig. 4-19). A **motor end plate** is formed by very short branches within a circumscribed zone (plate) at the end of one terminal branch of an efferent neuron. Each branch of the end plate lies within a corresponding trough of the **sole plate**. The width of the neuromuscular gap is normally 40 to 50 nm; however, this gap is widened by junctional folds, where the sarcolemma of the trough undergoes transverse enfolding. Neurolemnocytes cover the end plate, and the associated basal lamina extends into the neuromuscular gap and junctional folds (Fig. 4-20).

The end-plate cytoplasm contains numerous mitochondria and agranular synaptic vesicles (40 nm in diameter). These vesicles store acetylcholine, which is released at active sites opposite the junctional folds. Acetylcholine molecules diffuse across the neuromuscular gap and bind to postsynaptic receptor sites that open cation channels, leading to muscle fiber

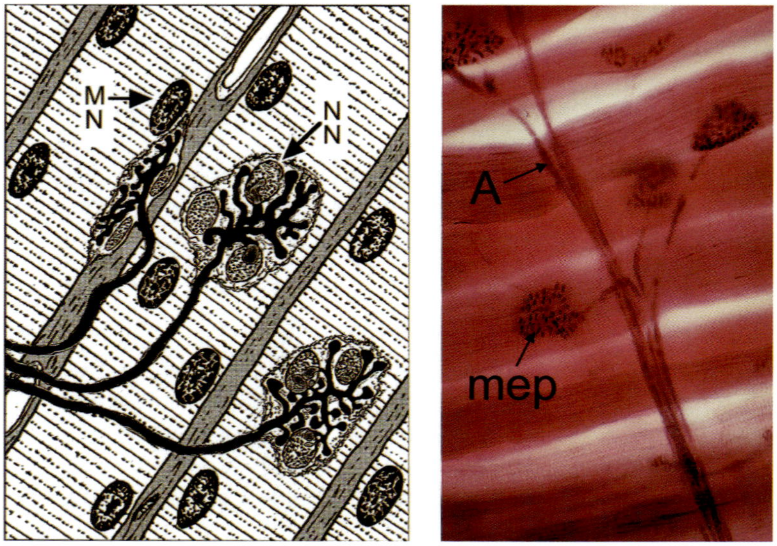

Figure 4-19 Motor end plates synapsing on skeletal muscle fibers. **Left:** Drawing of three motor end plates synapsing on skeletal muscle fibers. Each of the three terminal branches of an axon ends in a perfusion of short branches collectively designated an end plate. The top end plate is viewed from its edge. Neurolemnocytes that ensheathe axon terminal branches proceed to overlay the end plate branches. Neurolemnocyte nucleus (N. nuc.); muscle fiber nucleus (M. nuc.). (Adapted from Krstić RV. General Histology of the Mammal. New York: Springer-Verlag, 1985). **Right:** The axons (A) of a motor neuron branch end as motor end plates (mep) on skeletal muscle fibers. Snake, H&E (×250). (Image by W.E. Haensly).

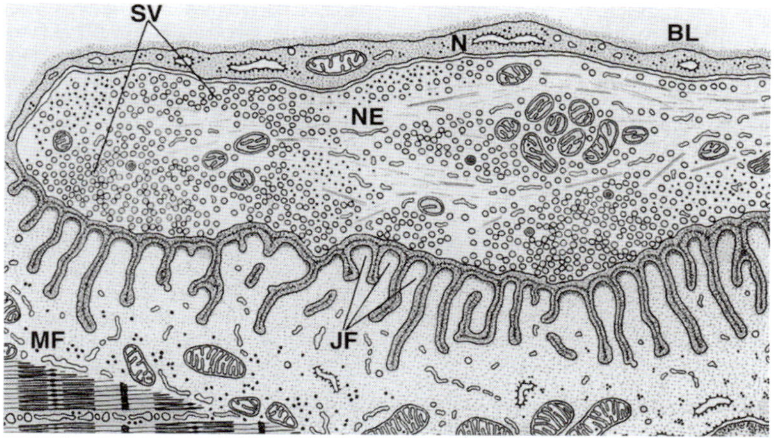

Figure 4-20 Ultrastructural drawing of one nerve ending (NE) of a branched motor end plate synapsing on a muscle fiber (MF). The nerve ending contains numerous synaptic vesicles (SV). The muscle fiber plasma membrane features junctional folds (JF) that greatly expand the synaptic cleft. The cleft contains basal lamina (BL) continuous with that covering the muscle fiber and the neurolemnocyte (N) overlaying the nerve ending. (From Lentz TL. Cell Fine Structure. Philadelphia, PA: WB Saunders, 1971.)

depolarization. Some binding sites are occupied by cholinesterase enzymes, which degrade acetylcholine to cease synaptic activity. Transporter protein molecules are present in the presynaptic membrane to recapture and recycle choline.

The **fusimotor** or **γ motor neuron** is another type of somatic efferent neuron. It innervates intrafusal muscle fibers within muscle spindles. These relatively small neurons have myelinated axons that terminate as end plates or trail endings, forming multiple synaptic contacts along the muscle fiber surface.

Preganglionic autonomic neurons originate in the CNS and synapse on postganglionic neurons in autonomic ganglia, forming typical interneuronal synapses. **Postganglionic autonomic neurons** have nonmyelinated axons that innervate cardiac muscle, smooth muscle, or glands. These axons terminate in branches that individually extend long distances without forming specialized contacts with muscle or gland cells.

Ultrastructurally, terminal autonomic nerves consist of isolated neurolemnocytes sheathing one or more terminal branches. The terminal branches have numerous preterminal synaptic varicosities along their course. Each preterminal varicosity protrudes beyond the neurolemnocyte sheath and contains a concentration of synaptic vesicles. This allows neurotransmitter release from multiple sites, diffusing variable distances to bind with receptors on target cells. Postsynaptic specializations are not evident.

There are several lines of evidence indicating that postganglionic sympathetic axons innervating immune organs, such as the spleen and lymph nodes (see Chapter 8), regulate cytokine production by immune cells. This occurs via the release of noradrenaline from nonsynaptic axonal varicosities, resulting in the suppression of immune responses. Conversely, immune cells can release neurotrophic factors, such as nerve growth factor and brain-derived neurotrophic factor, which act on receptors present on neurons and astrocytes, exerting neuroprotective effects. This highlights the fact that the nervous and immune systems are closely interconnected such that physiologic or pathologic effects on one system may affect the other.

Receptors

Afferent axons convey information to the CNS from receptors or sense organs. Sense organs are organized collections of sensory epithelial cells, neurons, and supporting cells that detect visual, auditory, olfactory, or taste stimuli. In contrast, **receptors** are individual, isolated stimulus detectors that are widely distributed in the body (Fig. 4-21). Generally, the peripheral branch of an afferent axon branches repeatedly, with each branch terminating at a receptor. All receptors of a single neuron have the same structure and function.

Receptors are classified in several ways. By location, **exteroceptors, proprioceptors**, and **enteroceptors** are found on body surfaces, in musculoskeletal structures, and in viscera, respectively. Receptors are also classified according to the type of stimulus they detect, such as **mechanoreceptors, chemoreceptors**, and **thermoreceptors**. Morphologically, receptors may be classified as **encapsulated** and **nonencapsulated**. The following is a list of common receptors.

Nonencapsulated Receptors

Free nerve endings are found throughout the body and detect stimulation described as pain (noxious), warmth, cold, or touch. Simultaneously, the same stimulus information is used for subconscious reflex activity. These receptors are associated with nonmyelinated or thinly myelinated axons that branch extensively to innervate a wide area known as the receptive field. The actual receptors are simply unsheathed terminal branches enveloped by basal lamina (Fig. 4-21).

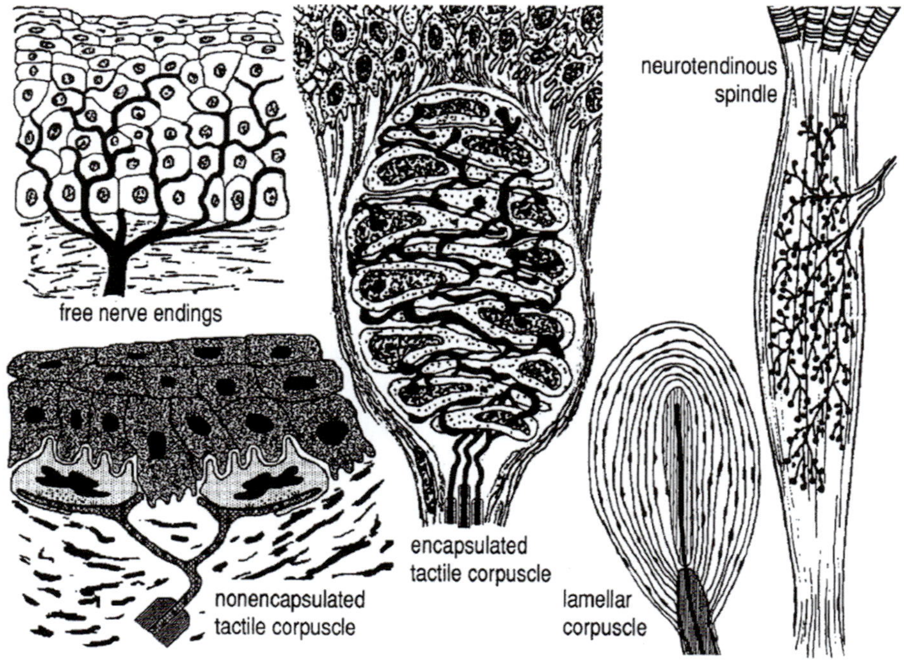

Figure 4-21 Schematic drawings of five receptors at various magnifications. Free nerve endings branch within the epidermis. Two nonencapsulated tactile corpuscles are shown at the base of the epidermis, each consisting of a terminal branch contacting a specialized tactile cell (Merkel's cell). An encapsulated tactile corpuscle (Meissner's corpuscle) is located in the dermis, with dendritic branches from multiple myelinated axons weaving among flattened neurolemnocytes within a perineural epithelioid cell capsule. A lamellar corpuscle (Pacini's corpuscle) features the dendritic branch of a myelinated axon encased in a core of flattened neurolemnocytes within a laminated capsule of perineural epithelioid cells. A neurotendinous spindle splays among the collagen bundles of a small tendon, enclosed in a thin capsule and associated with a myelinated axon (not shown). (Encapsulated tactile corpuscle and neurotendinous spindle from Krstić RV. General Histology of the Mammal. New York: Springer-Verlag, 1985).

Hair follicle terminals, which detect displacement of body hairs, are derived from myelinated axons that branch extensively to innervate hundreds of follicles. Each follicle is encircled by a nonmyelinated plexus that disperses free nerve endings among follicle epithelial cells. A different situation prevails for tactile hair follicles (vibrissae), each of which receives several myelinated axons, giving rise to several types of receptors.

Nonencapsulated tactile corpuscles are often collected at the base of a slight elevation in the skin called a tactile pad (Fig. 4-21). Each tactile corpuscle consists of an expanded axonal terminal branch embraced by processes of an epithelioid tactile cell (Merkel cell). The epithelioid cell, which develops under the trophic influence of the nerve ending, contains large dense-core vesicles. Individual tactile corpuscles are innervated by a myelinated axon that distributes to a restricted receptive field. These corpuscles are capable of persistent firing (tonic receptors).

Encapsulated Receptors

Encapsulated tactile corpuscles (Meissner's corpuscles) are oval, encapsulated phasic mechanoreceptors for touch and superficial pressure found in the dermal papillae of mammalian skin (Fig. 4-21). Several myelinated axons give rise to nonmyelinated branches that penetrate a stack of flattened neurolemnocytes encapsulated by perineural epithelioid cells. Tactile corpuscles and their associated afferent nerve fibers adapt rapidly and provide great sensitivity to minute skin deformations.

Lamellar corpuscles (Vater's and Pacini's corpuscles) are widely distributed throughout the body and are large enough to be seen without magnification (0.5 × 1.0 mm). Each corpuscle consists of a terminal branch of a myelinated axon encased in several layers of flattened neurolemnocytes, surrounded by a fluid-filled space and multiple concentric layers formed by perineural epithelioid cells (Fig. 4-21). The layered lamellae of these corpuscles function as an extremely selective high-pass filters, which attenuate the large, dynamic stresses and strains applied to the skin. This specialization allows these receptors to be extremely sensitive to transient pressure, such as vibratory stimuli. Thus, these lamellar corpuscles are able to provide a neural representation of vibrations transmitted through the skin.

Bulbous corpuscles (Krause's corpuscles, Golgi-Mazzoni corpuscles, and genital corpuscles) vary in location, size, and shape. They are mechanoreceptors derived from myelinated axons that have highly coiled terminal branches enclosed in a relatively thin capsule derived from perineural epithelioid cells.

Neurotendinous spindles (Golgi tendon organs) are located at muscle-tendon junctions and are activated by tension. Derived from a large, myelinated axon, the receptor consists of terminal branches traveling along bundles of collagen fibers within a fluid-filled, thin capsule derived from perineural epithelioid cells (Fig. 4-21). Ruffini's corpuscle, a tonic mechanoreceptor found in the dermis, fascia, and ligaments, is structurally similar to the neurotendinous spindle.

Neuromuscular spindles (muscle spindles) are so elaborate that they could qualify as sense organs. These spindles are located in most skeletal muscles and have an elongated capsule (1.5 mm) derived from perineural epithelioid cells. The capsule encloses afferent and efferent innervation, along with two kinds of intrafusal muscle fibers: nuclear bag fibers and nuclear chain fibers (Fig. 4-22). A typical spindle has one or two **nuclear bag** fibers, each with a dilated middle zone filled with nuclei and striated polar ends that project beyond the spindle capsule. Also, several **nuclear chain** fibers are present, smaller than nuclear bag fibers, and entirely contained within the spindle capsule. These chain fibers have a chain of nuclei in the middle, lacking myofilaments in this region, which stretches when the striated polar regions contract. The striated regions of both types of intrafusal muscle fibers are innervated by fusimotor (γ) motor neurons that establish either end plate or trail-type neuromuscular synapses. Trail endings form multiple synaptic contacts as their terminal branches ramify on the surface of a muscle fiber.

Two types of receptors are found on intrafusal muscle fibers (Fig. 4-22). A **primary ending**, also called an **annulospiral ending**, is derived from a single large, myelinated axon. Its terminal branches spiral around the nuclear regions of intrafusal muscle fibers. A **secondary ending** is derived from a myelinated axon with dendritic branches arranged in a flower-spray configuration. These endings are situated on nuclear chain fibers adjacent to the annulospiral endings. Collectively, these receptors respond to the rate and degree of stretch experienced when either the polar ends of intrafusal muscle fibers contract or the whole muscle is stretched. The information conveyed by spindle receptors is primarily subconscious and important for regulating muscle tone, adjusting posture, and coordinating movements.

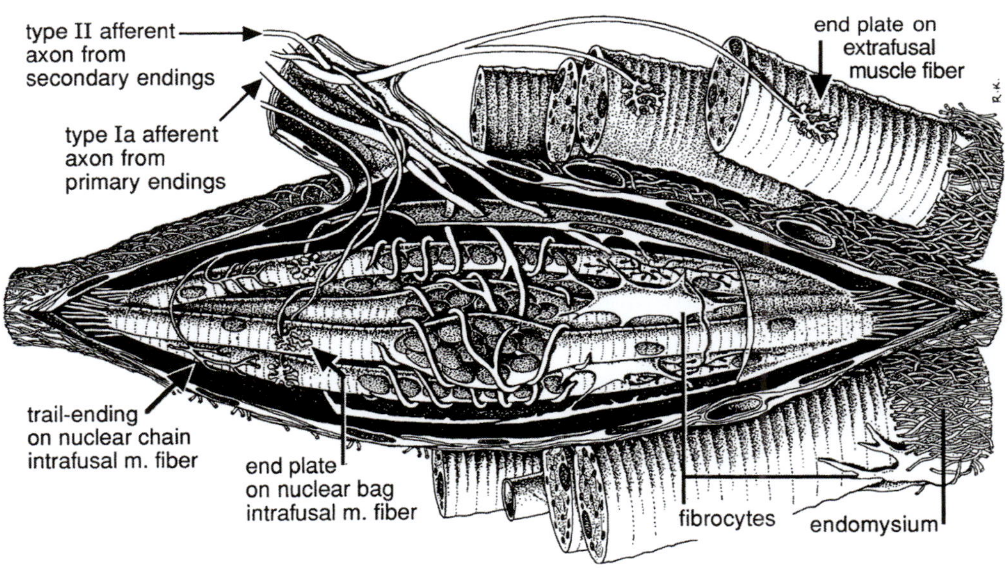

Figure 4-22 Schematic drawing of a muscle spindle and adjacent extrafusal muscle fibers connected by collagen fibrils of the endomysium. Perineural epithelioid cells continue to form the spindle capsule (shown cut open). The spindle contains nuclear bag and nuclear chain intrafusal muscle fibers, primary (annulospiral) and secondary (flower-spray) receptors, two types of neuromuscular synapses, and fibrocytes and collagen fibrils. Primary (annulospiral endings) spiral around nuclear bag and chain regions of intrafusal muscle fibers, arising from a large (myelinated) axon. Secondary receptors (flower-spray endings) contact nuclear chain fibers adjacent to the primary endings, arising from a medium-sized (myelinated) axon. Small (myelinated) axons of fusimotor (γ) neurons synapse on the polar regions of intrafusal muscle fibers, forming small end plates and trail endings. The trail endings are on nuclear chain fibers. Terminal branches of an α motor neuron form end plates on extrafusal muscle fibers. (From Krstić RV. General Histology of the Mammal. New York: Springer-Verlag, 1985).

Central Nervous Tissue

The CNS consists of the brain and spinal cord (plus the optic nerve and retina, which embryologically extend from the brain). The brain is divided into the brain stem, cerebellum, and cerebrum. Gross observation of the CNS reveals regions of white matter, gray matter, and regions where white and gray matter are mixed.

White matter is formed by dense accumulations of myelinated axons, whose lipid-rich myelin gives it a white appearance. Individual myelin sheaths are relatively thin in the CNS compared to the PNS. Nonmyelinated axons of the CNS lack myelin and are fully exposed to the CNS extracellular space. White matter is organized into tracts (called fasciculi or lemnisci in specific cases), each comprising nerve fibers that are functionally related, with similar origins and destinations.

In contrast, an absence or scarcity of myelin results in CNS tissue having a gray appearance. **Gray matter** is rich in neuronal cell bodies, glial cells, and neuropil. **Neuropil** refers to the axons, terminal branches, dendrites, and glial processes, forming a matrix background for the cell bodies visible with light microscopy. Most synapses occur within the neuropil. Neuropil appears dense because the CNS extracellular space is uniformly narrow (approximately 20 nm wide).

Gray matter on the surface of the cerebellum and cerebrum is called **cortex**. In contrast, the gray matter of the spinal cord is centrally located and therefore non cortical. Distinctive masses of gray matter within the CNS are typically referred to as **nuclei**. Generally, a nucleus receives input from one or more tracts and sends output to other tracts, which may in turn project to a different nucleus or to the cortex. For a given nucleus, incoming terminals typically synapse on small neurons with short axons, called **interneurons** because they are interposed between the input and output of the nucleus. Ultimately, the interneurons in a nucleus integrate incoming signals and determine the appropriate output for a particular input.

Nervous tissue exhibits a variety of configurations across different regions of the CNS. The features of gray and white matter in three major CNS regions will be presented: the cerebral cortex, cerebellum, and spinal cord.

Cerebral Cortex

The cerebrum of the brain is composed of paired cerebral hemispheres (Fig. 4-23). The surface of each hemisphere has **gyri** (ridges) demarcated by **sulci** (grooves). The outer layer of the hemisphere is coated by gray matter known as the cerebral cortex. The characteristic neuron of the cerebral cortex has a pyramid-shaped cell body oriented with its apex directed toward the surface (Fig. 4-24). Dendrites emerge from the apex and basal edges of the pyramidal cell, while the axon exits from the center of the base and extends into the white matter.

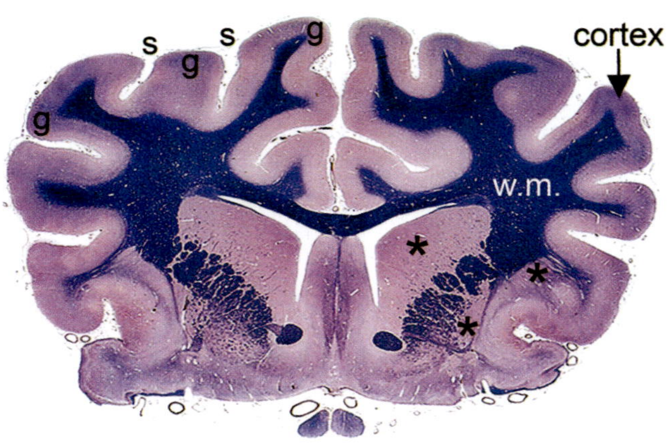

Figure 4-23 Transverse section through the cerebrum of a canine brain; dark staining indicates white matter. The cerebrum is composed of two hemispheres joined across the midline by white matter (corpus callosum). Surface elevations (gyri, g) are separated by grooves (sulci, s). Gray matter on the surface is cerebral cortex, with cerebral white matter (w.m.) beneath it. Internal masses of gray matter at the base of the cerebrum constitute basal nuclei (*). Luxol blue and hematoxylin. (Image by A.J. Beitz and T.F. Fletcher.)

In mammals, except for the ventral cerebral cortex, all areas are referred to as neocortex due to their recent evolutionary origin. The cerebral **neocortex** is divisible into six layers, although the layering is evident only in thick sections, and the prominence of individual layers varies between regions. From superficial to deep, the six layers are as follows (Fig. 4-24):

1) **Molecular layer**—predominantly oriented tangentially with neuropil, containing apical dendrites from pyramidal cells and terminal branches of superficial cortical afferent fibers.
2) **External granular layer**—predominantly composed of small neurons that serve as interneurons.
3) **External pyramidal layer**—contains small- and medium-sized pyramidal neurons that project axons to adjacent areas of the cerebral cortex.
4) **Internal granular layer**—thick layer with small stellate neurons that receive specific sensory inputs, particularly in sensory areas of the cortex (e.g., primary visual area).

5) **Internal pyramidal layer**—thick layer containing medium to large pyramidal neurons that project axons into the white matter, particularly prominent in motor areas of the cortex.
6) **Fusiform (multiform) layer**—has many spindle-shaped neurons that also project axons into the white matter. Beneath this layer, the cerebral white matter is composed of nerve fibers traveling to and from the cortex.

The basic functional unit of the neocortex is the 40- to 50-µm **minicolumn**, separated from adjacent minicolumns by vertical, cell-sparse zones that vary in size in different cortical areas. These minicolumns extend from the white matter to the cortical surface and are organized into larger units called **cortical columns** (approximately 0.3 mm in diameter). Cortical columns are formed by approximately 50 to 80 minicolumns bound together by shared inputs and short-range horizontal connections. Individual cortical columns are not histologically distinct. Physiologically, all neurons within a column become active in response to specific features of stimuli and are inactive in their absence. Pyramidal neurons are the anatomic basis for vertical column organization. They have basal dendrites for making radial connections within a column and establish vertical contact via superficially directed apical dendrites and deeply directed axons.

Two types of afferent fibers enter a cortical column from the white matter. Nonspecific afferents, which lack specific information content, ramify in all cortical layers, but especially in superficial layers. These fibers produce background excitation to alert cortical columns. The second type, specific afferents, convey modality-specific information relevant to the function of the column. These fibers synapse on the small neurons of the internal granular layer, which serve as interneurons to distribute excitation throughout the column.

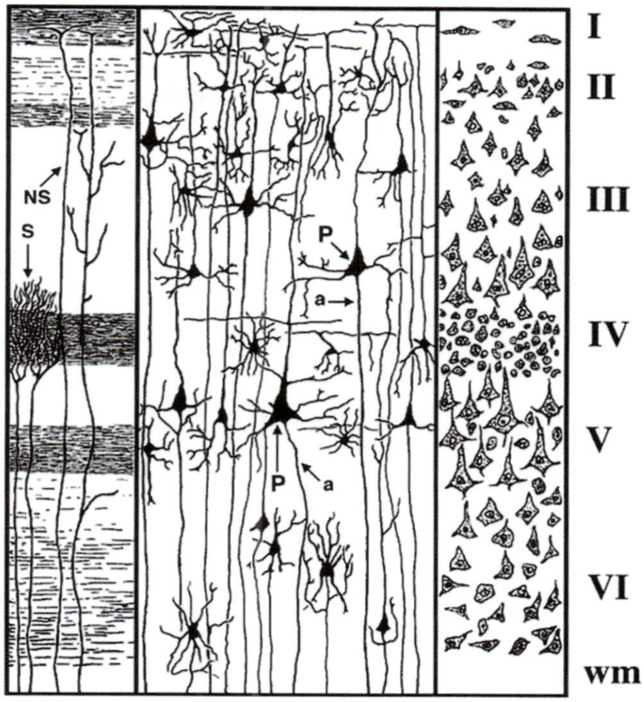

Figure 4-24 Schematic illustration of the six layers (I to VI) of cerebral cortex (neocortex), shown from three perspectives. The left panel illustrates nerve fibers (axons, telodendria, and dendrites) in the cortex. From the white matter (wm), modality-specific input fibers (S) terminate in layer IV, while nonspecific input fibers (NS) terminate predominantly in superficial layers. The middle panel displays individual neurons with Golgi stain, highlighting their characteristic pyramidal shape. Pyramidal neurons (P) have an apical dendrite ascending to the surface, radially oriented basal dendrites, and a single axon (a) extending into the white matter. The right panel shows neuron cell bodies in layers I to VI of the cerebral cortex, as seen with Nissl stain. (Modified from Crosby EC, Humphrey T, Lauer EW. Correlative Anatomy of the Nervous System. New York: The Macmillan Co., 1962).

Output from the cortical column is predominantly from pyramidal neurons, which send their axons into the white matter. Superficial neurons send axons to neighboring regions of cortex (short association fibers). Neurons in the deepest two layers of the cortex send long axons to the brain stem (projection fibers), to the contralateral cerebral hemisphere (commissural fibers), or to distant regions within the same hemisphere (long association fibers).

Cerebellum

The cerebellar surface features **folia** (narrow ridges) separated by **sulci** (grooves). Gray matter covering the surface is called **cerebellar cortex**. White matter is located deep to the cortex, and three bilateral pairs of cerebellar nuclei are embedded within the white matter (Fig. 4-25).

The cerebellar cortex is divisible into three layers (Fig. 4-26). The **molecular layer**, composed predominantly of neuropil, is most superficial. The **granule cell layer**, situated adjacent to white matter, features densely packed granule cells (small neurons with heterochromatic nuclei). Because of the extremely dense packing of the granule cells, the cerebellum contains about five times more neurons than the cerebral cortex. Finally, a single layer of large cell bodies is located at the interface of the molecular and granule cell layers. This is called the **piriform cell layer** (Purkinje cell layer).

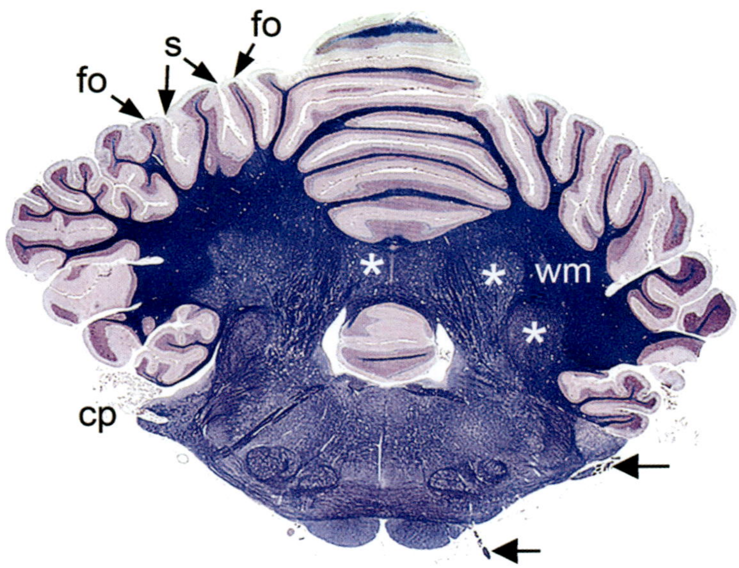

Figure 4-25 Transverse section through a canine hindbrain. The cerebellum (above) is connected to the brain stem (below). The cerebellar surface features elevations called folia (fo) separated by grooves called sulci (s). The cerebellar cortex, or surface gray matter, appears two-toned due to a cell-sparse molecular layer overlying a cell-dense granule layer. Three cerebellar nuclei (*) are located bilaterally deep to the white matter (wm). The brain stem exhibits white matter tracts, gray matter nuclei, regions with mixed white and gray matter, and emerging cranial nerve roots (arrows). On each side, the tip of a choroid plexus (cp) is seen within the surrounding subarachnoid space. Luxol blue and hematoxylin. (Image by A.J. Beitz and T.F. Fletcher).

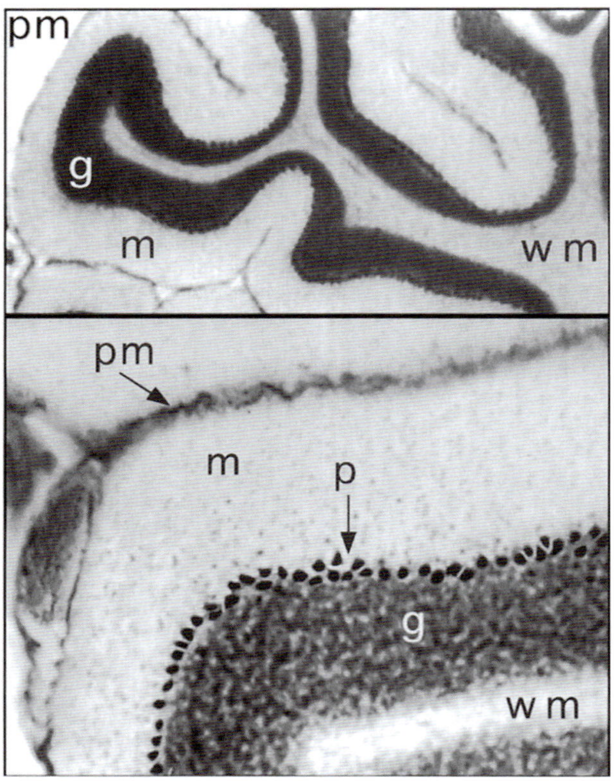

Figure 4-26 Two light micrographs at different magnification of cerebellar cortex (pig). **Top:** The white matter (wm) extends into the center of a cerebellar folium. The cortex covering the white matter exhibits a dense cell layer (g) and a relatively acellular layer (m). The pia mater (pm) covers the cerebellar surface and extends into sulci separating folia (×15). **Bottom:** The cerebellar cortex, situated between white matter (wm) and pia mater (pm), is composed of three layers. From deep to superficial: the granule cell layer (g), the Purkinje cell layer (p), and the molecular layer (m) (×55). Nissl stain.

The **piriform neurons (Purkinje cells)** send axons into the white matter to synapse on neurons of cerebellar nuclei. Each piriform neuron has an elaborate dendritic tree that projects into the molecular layer (Fig. 4-27) and makes more than 200,000 synaptic contacts with granule cell axons. Axons of **granule cells** enter the molecular layer, bifurcate, travel longitudinally within a folium, and synapse on numerous dendritic trees of the piriform neurons. Another neuron of the cerebellar cortex is called a **basket cell** because its terminal branches form "baskets" surrounding cell bodies of adjacent piriform neurons. The cell bodies of basket cells are found in the deep molecular layer; their axons course transversely in the folium and inhibit laterally positioned piriform neurons.

Two major types of input fibers enter the cerebellar cortex. One type (climbing fibers) has terminal branches that climb like vines on Purkinje dendritic trees, with each fiber making numerous synapses as it passes along a single dendritic tree. The other type of input fiber has terminal expansions (mossy endings) within the granule cell layer. Neighboring granule cells extend dendrites to synapse with each terminal expansion, thereby creating a synaptic complex known as a **glomerulus**.

The cerebellum regulates muscle tone, posture, and movement so that these are expressed in an appropriate, coordinated pattern. It operates as follows: neurons in the cerebellar nuclei are spontaneously active and send their axons out of the cerebellum to excite brain neurons responsible for initiating posture and movement. Input to the cerebellum comes from these brain neurons as well as from muscle and joint proprioceptors. These input fibers excite both the cerebellar nuclei and specific regions of the cerebellar cortex. Excitatory granule cells and inhibitory basket cells interact to produce a

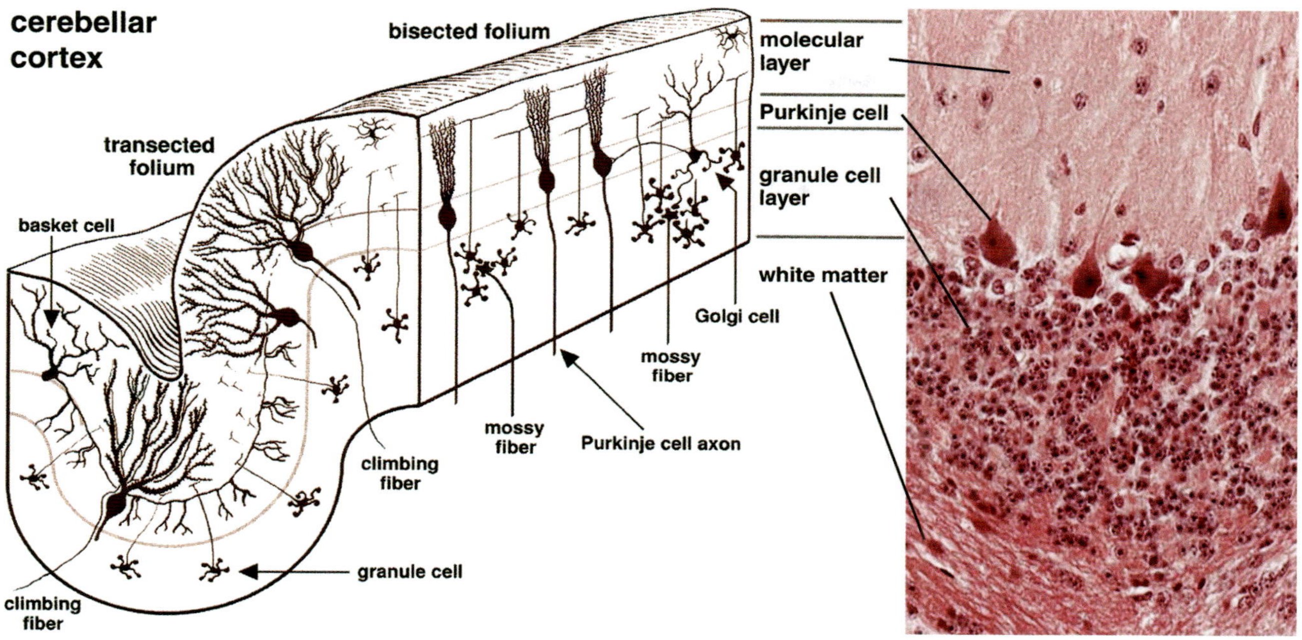

Figure 4-27 Schematic diagram of the cerebellar cortex. The three layers of cortex (labeled on the right) are shown in bisected (right side) and transected (left side) views of a folium. The H&E image on the right (×200) illustrates the histology of the three cortex layers. The molecular layer is composed of neuronal processes plus a few small stellate neurons (upper right and unlabeled). The *piriform (Purkinje) cell* layer features cell bodies of Purkinje neurons, whose axons project into the white matter. Purkinje cell dendrites are flattened and oriented perpendicular to the long axis of the folium. The granule cell layer is densely packed with small granule cell neurons that project axons into the molecular layer to synapse on Purkinje cell dendrites. Additional neurons include the *Golgi cell* (right edge), an inhibitory interneuron located in the upper granule cell layer, and the *basket cell* (left edge), another inhibitory neuron located deep within the molecular layer, forming axonal "baskets" around Purkinje cell bodies. Cerebellar white matter is composed of Purkinje cell axons leaving the cortex and two types of cortical afferents: mossy and climbing fibers. A mossy fiber makes synaptic contact with granule cell dendrites, with each mossy ending forming the center of a synaptic glomerulus. Climbing fibers make many synaptic contacts on a single Purkinje dendritic tree. (Modified from Jenkins TW. Functional Mammalian Neuroanatomy. 2nd Ed. Philadelphia, PA: Lea & Febiger, 1978).

localized pattern of active Purkinje neurons in the cerebellar cortex. The axons of these Purkinje neurons, the only output from the cortex, inhibit the neurons in the cerebellar nuclei. Thus, the cerebellar cortex continuously compares movement initiation with movement performance and regulates movement execution by selectively inhibiting the generalized excitatory influence of cerebellar nuclei.

Spinal Cord

The cylindrical spinal cord is divided into segments by the bilateral emergence of dorsal and ventral roots of spinal nerves. A transverse section of the spinal cord has a **central canal** surrounded by an H-shaped profile of gray matter, which is further surrounded by white matter (Fig. 4-28). The spinal cord is divided in the median plane by a **ventral median fissure** and a **dorsal median septum** (replaced by a fissure in the caudal half of the cord). Segments supplying limbs exhibit enlarged spinal gray matter due to increased nervous tissue needed for limb innervation.

Spinal gray matter contains three categories of neurons: *interneurons* (contained within the gray matter, connecting afferent and efferent neurons), *projection neurons* (which project axons through white matter tracts to the brain), and *efferent neurons* (which send axons into ventral roots). A group of related neuron cell bodies is designated as a **nucleus** (e.g., the intermediolateral nucleus comprises sympathetic preganglionic neuron cell bodies). Spinal gray matter is sometimes subdivided into 10 defined laminae, though these boundaries are often indistinct in ordinary tissue sections.

Bilaterally, spinal gray matter consists of dorsal and ventral gray columns connected by intermediate gray matter. In transverse sections, gray column profiles are usually called **horns**. The **ventral gray column** (horn) contains

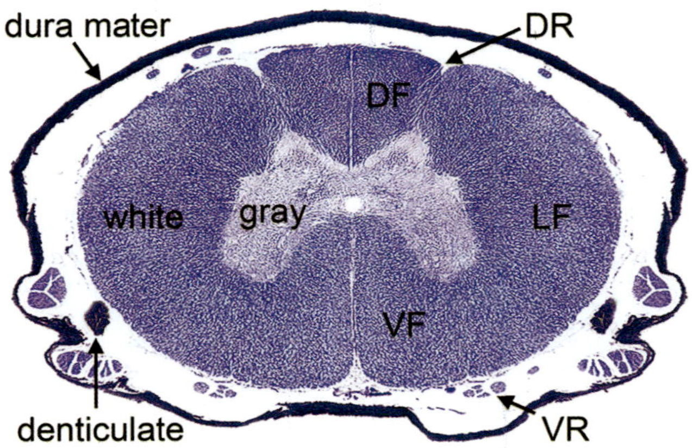

Figure 4-28 Transverse section through a canine spinal cord at the midthoracic region. The central canal (*) is surrounded by butterfly-shaped gray matter (gray), encased by darkly stained white matter (white). In this thoracic segment, gray matter features a small dorsal horn, a subtle lateral horn, and a large ventral horn, bilaterally. Meninges and transected nerve roots surround the white matter. Bilaterally, a process of denticulate ligament (denticulate) is evident between pia mater and dura mater. The spinal cord is divided into bilateral halves by a ventral median fissure and a dorsal median sulcus and septum. In each half, white matter is divided into three regions: dorsal funiculus (DF), lateral funiculus (LF), and ventral funiculus (VF). A prominent dorsolateral sulcus marks the entry of dorsal roots (DR), separating dorsal and lateral funiculi. The boundary between lateral and ventral funiculi is demarcated by the emergence of ventral roots (VR). Luxol blue and hematoxylin. (Image by A.J. Beitz and T.F. Fletcher.)

somatic efferent neurons that innervate skeletal muscle. The **dorsal gray column** (horn) contains interneurons and projection neurons where primary afferent neurons synapse, conveying sensory information such as pain, temperature, pressure, and touch. Intermediate gray matter features visceral neurons, while in thoracolumbar segments, a **lateral gray column** (horn) includes sympathetic preganglionic neurons (intermediolateral nucleus).

Spinal white matter is composed of fibers forming ascending and descending tracts plus fibers entering from dorsal roots or exiting to ventral roots. Ascending tracts terminate in the brain, while axons of descending tracts originate in the brain and mainly synapse on interneurons within the gray matter. Afferent axons of dorsal roots enter white matter at the dorsolateral sulcus and predominantly terminate in the dorsal gray column. Efferent neuron axons exit ventrolaterally as ventral root fibers.

Bilaterally, spinal white matter is divided anatomically into three regions: the **dorsal funiculus**, located between the midline and dorsal root attachments; the **ventral funiculus**, situated between the midline and ventral root attachments; and the **lateral funiculus**, positioned between dorsal and ventral root attachments.

Meninges, Blood Vessels, and Cerebrospinal Fluid

Meninges

The brain, spinal cord, and roots of peripheral nerves are enveloped by a series of CT sheaths termed **meninges**. Meninges also surround the entire optic nerve, which is CNS tissue. Meninges contain cerebrospinal fluid and constitute a protective barrier. Inflammation of the meninges results in a condition termed meningitis.

Traditionally, three meningeal layers are described from superficial to deep: dura mater, arachnoid, and pia mater (Fig. 4-29). The **dura mater** is sometimes called **pachymeninx** because it is thick and strong. The **arachnoid** and **pia mater** are collectively termed **leptomeninges** because they are delicate and connected both embryologically and physically. A **subarachnoid space** containing cerebrospinal fluid separates the arachnoid from pia mater.

The dura mater contains thick collagen bundles and elastic fibers, oriented longitudinally in the spinal dura and more irregularly in the cranial dura. It also contains fibrocytes, nerves, and lymph and blood vessels. The inner surface of the dura mater is lined by multiple layers of flattened fibrocytes, to which the outer cells of the arachnoid membrane adhere. Although there is no subdural space, hemorrhage can result in the accumulation of blood between these fibrocyte layers (subdural hematoma), giving the false impression of a subdural space.

The **spinal dura mater** is surrounded by an epidural space that separates the dura mater from the periosteum lining the vertebral canal. Collagen and elastic fibers within the spinal dura are oriented parallel to the long axis of the spine, providing the dura with longitudinal tensile strength, stiffness, and the property of relaxation.

The **cranial dura mater** is composed of two laminae. The internal lamina is comparable to spinal dura mater, while the external lamina serves as the periosteum of the cranial cavity. The two laminae are distinct only where the inner lamina separates from the outer one to form partitions within the brain (Fig. 4-29). Endothelium-lined spaces, called **dural venous sinuses**, are present where the internal and external laminae separate. Venous blood drains into these sinuses, which resist collapse because of their rigid walls.

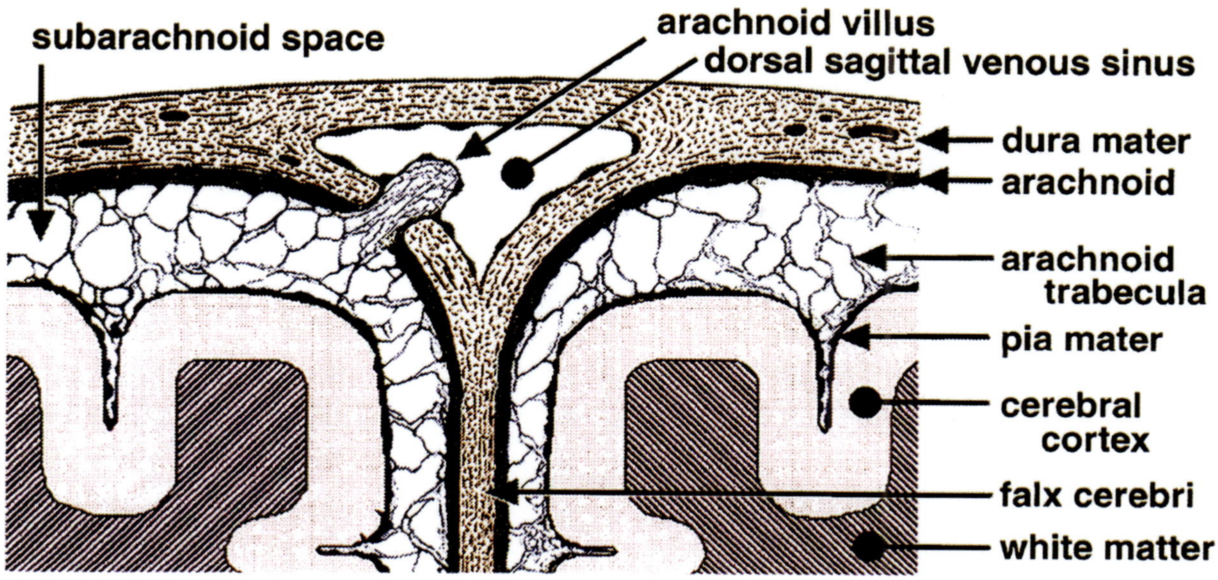

Figure 4-29 Schematic illustration of meningeal relationships at the dorsal midline of the cranial cavity. The internal lamina of dura mater separates from the external (periosteal) lamina to form the falx cerebri, dividing the cerebral hemispheres. This separation encloses a venous sinus lined with endothelial cells for venous drainage. Arachnoid tissue merges with flattened fibrocytes lining the internal surface of the dura mater. Arachnoid trabeculae connect to the pia mater by traversing the subarachnoid space filed with cerebrospinal fluid. The fluid drains into venous blood through arachnoid villi that expand or collapse according to the pressure differential across them. (Adapted from Weed LH. The absorption of cerebrospinal fluid into the venous system. Am J Anat 1923;31:191–221).

The arachnoid membrane consists of outer layers of flattened fibrocytes and inner fibrocytes arranged loosely around small bundles of collagen fibers. **Arachnoid trabeculae** are thin strands of the inner arachnoid that traverse the subarachnoid space and establish continuity with pia mater. **Arachnoid villi** are microscopic projections of arachnoid that penetrate the walls of dural venous sinuses and act as one-way valves for draining cerebrospinal fluid (Fig. 4-29). When cerebrospinal fluid pressure exceeds sinus blood pressure, arachnoid villi expand to facilitate fluid transfer into the bloodstream. The villi collapse to preclude blood reflux when venous pressure exceeds cerebrospinal fluid pressure. Cerebrospinal fluid can also drain into lymphatics of peripheral nerves.

The pia mater is a highly vascular layer that covers the spinal cord and brain, lining every sulcus and fissure. It is characterized by wide intercellular spaces containing variable amounts of interlacing collagen fibers and fine elastic networks, along with a few fibrocytes, lymphocytes, and mast cells. A basal lamina separates the collagen of the pia mater from the underlying glial-limiting membrane, which consists of astrocyte processes. The pia is covered on its outer surface by a layer of flat fibrocytes.

Together with arachnoid, pia mater bounds the subarachnoid space, which contains cerebrospinal fluid. The entire subarachnoid space, including the surfaces of nerves and vessels that traverse the space, is lined by flattened fibrocytes connected by zonulae adherens. These fibrocytes are capable of phagocytosis, and macrophages are sporadically found on the lining of the subarachnoid space. Since the fibrocytic layer lining the subarachnoid space lacks a basal lamina, there is limited exchange of fluid, small molecules, and immunocompetent cells between the cerebrospinal fluid and the arachnoid and pia compartments.

Along each midlateral surface of the spinal cord, an increase in the amount of pia mater collagen creates an elongated ligament called the **denticulate ligament**. This ligament extends laterally with periodic projections that attach to the spinal dura mater (Fig. 4-28). Thus, the bilateral denticulate ligaments suspend the spinal cord within the dura mater, ensuring it is surrounded by cerebrospinal fluid in the subarachnoid space.

As nerve roots converge to form cranial and spinal nerves at cranial and intervertebral foramina, there is a transition from meninges surrounding the nerve root to neural CT around the nerves. Flattened fibrocytes of the leptomeninges transition into the epithelioid cells of the perineurium. The dura mater continues as fibrous perineurium and epineurium. Pia mater collagen continues as the endoneurium.

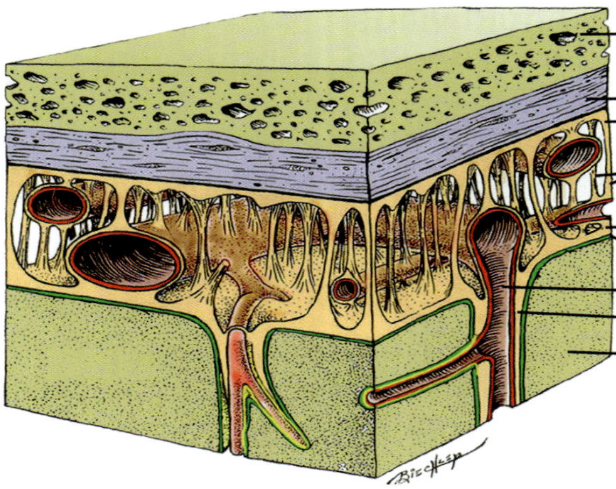

Figure 4-30 Schematic illustration showing cranial meninges and the perivascular space around vessels. The entire subarachnoid space, including the surfaces of vessels, is enveloped by leptomeninges (arachnoid and pia mater). The perivascular space, located between the glial-limiting membrane and the vessel wall, is filled with pia mater collagen fibers.

Blood Vessels

Blood vessels within the subarachnoid space are enveloped by leptomeningeal tissue derived from arachnoid trabeculae or pia mater (Fig. 4-30). When a vessel penetrates the CNS, it is surrounded by a **perivascular space** situated between the vessel wall and the glial-limiting membrane. This space extends to small vessels, where the basal lamina associated with the glial-limiting membrane merges with the vascular basal lamina. Leptomeninges, particularly pia mater collagen fibers, fill the perivascular space, making it less distinct unless filled with inflammatory cells under pathological conditions. Communication between perivascular spaces and the subarachnoid space is blocked by a continuous barrier of leptomeningeal cells, formed as cells on the vessel surfaces unite with those on the pia mater surface.

In contrast to most endothelial cells in the body, endothelial cells of CNS capillaries are generally nonfenestrated and connected by tight junctions. These unique endothelial features form the **blood–brain barrier**, which impedes the diffusion of hydrophilic molecules from the bloodstream into the CNS (polar molecules must be actively transported into the CNS). Astrocyte end feet, in contact with the basal lamina surrounding CNS capillaries, induce CNS endothelial cells to become nonfenestrated and form tight junctions. The blood–brain barrier is not present in neonates or at specific sites in the adult brain where modified ependymal cells are found (choroid plexuses and circumventricular organs).

A blood–brain barrier is also present in peripheral nerves. Capillaries within the endoneurium of peripheral nerves (excluding ganglia) exhibit zonulae occludens. Perineural epithelioid cells surrounding nerve fascicles also have zonulae occludens. These tight junctions establish a blood–nerve barrier that restricts the passage of hydrophilic molecules.

Cerebrospinal Fluid

Cerebrospinal fluid is produced by choroid plexuses located within the brain ventricles. A region of each ventricular wall is formed by **tela choroidea**, a term that refers to ependyma in direct contact with the pia mater, without intervening nervous tissue. Each **choroid plexus** arises from tela choroidea as a mass of villi, collectively forming a fuzzy tufted growth extending into the ventricle. Each villus consists of pial vasculature in loose CT covered by modified ependymal cells, called **chorioid plexus epithelium**. Although choroid plexus capillaries have fenestrated endothelial cells, the choroid plexus epithelial cells are joined by zonulae occludens near their luminal surfaces. These tight junctions contribute to the formation of the **blood–cerebrospinal fluid barrier**, regulating the entry of proteins and drugs into the cerebrospinal fluid.

Cerebrospinal fluid is produced by choroid plexus epithelium through a process that involves active Na^+ secretion. Choroid plexus epithelial cells exhibit pinocytotic vesicles, which originate at the base of each cell and migrate toward the luminal surface. In accordance with its location between two circulating fluid compartments (the blood and the cerebrospinal fluid), the choroid plexus epithelium facilitates numerous exchange processes. These processes supply the brain with nutrients and hormones while clearing deleterious compounds and metabolites from the brain. Choroid plexuses also participate in neurohumoral brain modulation and neuroimmune interactions, thereby greatly contributing to the maintenance of brain homeostasis.

Cerebrospinal fluid flows through the brain ventricles. The fluid exits these ventricles through the lateral apertures of the fourth ventricle and enters the subarachnoid space, where it surrounds the brain and spinal cord. Besides offering the physical protection of a fluid buffer, cerebrospinal fluid compensates for the lack of lymphatics in the CNS by allowing large molecules from the extracellular space of the CNS to pass between ependymal cells and into the cerebrospinal fluid.

Dendritic cells are a subclass of antigen-presenting cells critical in the initiation and regulation of adaptive immunity against pathogens and tumors (see Chapter 8). Recent studies have indicated that dendritic cells reside in normal meninges, choroid plexuses, and cerebrospinal fluid, but are absent from normal brain parenchyma. CNS inflammation is accompanied by recruitment of dendritic cells from the blood into the affected brain tissue. Dendritic cells located in different CNS compartments are likely to play an important role in the defense against CNS infections. However, they also may contribute to relapses or chronicity of CNS inflammation and the breakdown of tolerance to CNS autoantigens. Modulating dendritic cell recruitment and function within the CNS may represent a new strategy for treating neuroinflammatory diseases.

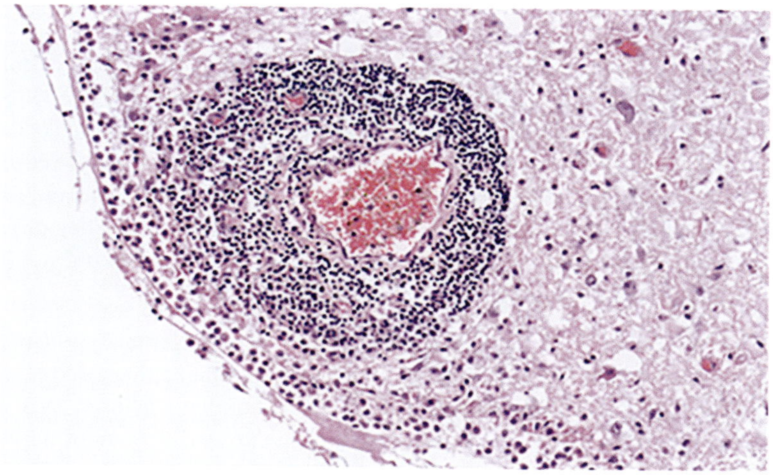

Figure 4-31 Inflammation presents microscopically as an influx of inflammatory cells in the affected brain and meninges, often forming perivascular accumulations of inflammatory cells (cuffing) around blood vessels. (Reproduced with permission from Salguero Bodes FJ, Pallares Martinez FJ. Aughey and Frye's Comparative Veterinary Histology with Clinical Correlates. 2nd ed. Boca Raton: CRC Press, 2023).

Clinical Correlations

Inflammatory, neoplastic, metabolic, and parasitic disorders affect the CNS, with certain species-specific characteristics. Feline parvovirus, which targets dividing cells, can attack the cerebellar germinal layer in young animals if the infection occurs before or shortly after birth. Primary CNS neoplasms are common in dogs and cats, originating from various cell types within the nervous system. Transmissible spongiform encephalopathies (TSE) such as prions enter through the oral route, proliferate in lymphoid tissues and the GI tract, with effects manifesting only upon reaching target areas of the CNS. Inflammation of the meninges (meningitis), the brain (encephalitis), or both simultaneously are frequent processes in animals caused by infections from bacteria, viruses, parasites, or fungi (Fig. 4-31).

Essentials

Neurons

- *Structure—Cell body*: It contains the nucleus and cytoplasm necessary for its metabolic functions. It integrates incoming signals from dendrites and generates outgoing signals along the axon. *Neuron processes*: The two main types are dendrites and axons. Dendrites: Short, branched extensions that receive signals (electrical and chemical) from other neurons or sensory receptors. Axon: A single elongated fiber that conducts electrical impulses or action potentials away from the cell body to target cells such as other neurons, muscle cells, or glands. *Terminal branches* (telodendrites): Fine branches at the end of the axon that synapse with other neurons or target cells.
- *Classification*: It is based on neuronal structure (multipolar, bipolar, and unipolar) and function (sensory, motor, and interneurons).
- *Regions of a neuron*: They include the input zone (dendrites), the integration zone (cell body), and the output zone (axon and terminal branches).
- *Neuronal communication*: Neurons communicate with each other and with other cells (such as muscle cells or glands) via specialized junctions called synapses. The synapse has a presynaptic terminal (containing synaptic vesicles with neurotransmitters), a synaptic cleft (a gap between pre- and postsynaptic membranes), and a postsynaptic membrane (with neurotransmitter receptors).

Neuroglia

CNS gliocytes include the following. (a) Astrocytes: They provide structural support to neurons, regulate the chemical environment, and participate in the repair process after injury. (b) Oligodendrocytes: They produce myelin in the CNS, which insulates axons and enhances the speed of electrical signal conduction. (c) Microglia: They act as immune cells in the CNS, involved in defense against pathogens plus removal of cellular debris. (d) Ependymal cells: They line the cavities of the brain and spinal cord, producing cerebrospinal fluid and assisting in its circulation.

PNS gliocytes include the following. (a) Ganglionic gliocytes: They provide support and protection to neurons in *ganglia* (clusters of nerve cell bodies outside the CNS). (b) Neurolemnocytes (Schwann cells): They form myelin sheaths around axons in the PNS, similar to oligodendrocytes in the CNS.

Myelin sheath. A fatty substance formed by neurolemnocytes (in the PNS) and oligodendrocytes (in the CNS) that wraps around axons, providing insulation and enhancing the speed of nerve impulse conduction.

Peripheral nervous tissue. *Nerves*: Axon bundles enclosed by CT that transmits sensory and motor information between the CNS and peripheral organs. *Ganglia*: Are clusters of nerve cell bodies located outside the CNS, involved in processing sensory information and coordinating reflexes. *Efferent Neurons*: They (motor neurons) carry signals from the CNS to muscles and glands, controlling movement and secretion. *Receptors*: Nonencapsulated receptors are distributed throughout tissues and respond to stimuli such as temperature, pain, and pressure, whereas encapsulated receptors are found in CT capsules and respond to more specific stimuli (touch, vibration, and stretch).

Central nervous tissue. *Cerebral cortex*: It is an outer layer of the cerebrum responsible for higher cognitive functions. *Cerebellum*: It is involved in coordinating voluntary movements and maintaining balance and posture. *Spinal cord*: It connects the brain to the PNS, serving as a pathway for sensory and motor information.

Meninges and cerebrospinal fluid. The meninges include dura mater, arachnoid mater, and pia mater—protective membranes that surround the brain and spinal cord, providing physical protection and support. Blood vessels supply oxygen and nutrients to the brain and spinal cord. Cerebrospinal fluid is a clear, colorless fluid that circulates around the brain and spinal cord, providing cushioning, buoyancy, and chemical stability to the nervous system.

Suggested Readings

Alabi AA, Tsien RW. Synaptic vesicle pools and dynamics. *Cold Spring Harbor Perspect Biol* 2012;4(8):a013680.

Allen NJ, Lyons DA. Glia as architects of central nervous system formation and function. *Science* 2018;362(6411):181–185.

Bergman RA, Afifi AK, Heidger PM Jr. Atlas of Microscopic Anatomy. 4th Ed. Lippincott Williams and Wilkins, 1996.

von Bernhardi R, Eugenín-von Bernhardi J, Flores B, et al. Glial cells and integrity of the nervous system. *Adv Exp Med Biol.* 2016;949:1–24.

Bettio LE, Rajendran L, Gil-Mohapel J. The effects of aging in the hippocampus and cognitive decline. *Neurosci Biobehav Rev* 2017;79:66–86.

Choquet D, Triller A. The dynamic synapse. *Neuron* 2013;80(3):691–703.

Cooper JR, Bloom FE, Roth RH. The Biochemical Basis of Neuropharmacology. 8th Ed. New York: Oxford University Press, 2003.

Deng S, Gan L, Liu C, et al. Roles of ependymal cells in the physiology and pathology of the central nervous system. *Aging Dis* 2023;14(2):468–483.

Dyer CA. The structure and function of myelin: from inert membrane to perfusion pump. *Neurochem Res* 2002;27:1279–1292.

Fawcett DW. A Textbook of Histology. 13th Ed. Chapman & Hall, 1994.

Gibbins I. Functional organization of autonomic neural pathways. *Organogenesis* 2013;9(3):169–175.

Gu C. Rapid and reversible development of axonal varicosities: a new form of neural plasticity. *Front Mol Neurosci* 2021;14:610857.

Hansson E, Ronnback L. Glial neuronal signaling in the central nervous system. *FASEB J* 2003;17:341–348.

Heck N, Benavides-Piccione R. Editorial: dendritic spines: from shape to function. *Front Neuroanat* 2015;9:101.

Jänig I. Sympathetic nervous system and inflammation: a conceptual view. *Auton Neurosci* 2014;182:4–14.

Jensen CJ, Massie A, De Keyser J. Immune players in the CNS: the astrocyte. *J Neuroimmune Pharmacol* 2013;8(4):824–839.

Jones EG. The nervous tissue. In: Weiss L, ed. Cell and Tissue Biology. 7th Ed. Raven Press, 1988.

Junqueira LC, Carneiro J, Kelly RO. Basic Histology. 13th Ed. McGraw-Hill Education, 2013.

Kratzer I, Ek J, Stolp H. The molecular anatomy and functions of the choroid plexus in healthy and diseased brain. *Biochim Biophys Acta Biomembr* 2020;1862(11):183430.

Krstić RV. General Histology of the Mammal. 2nd Ed. New York: Springer-Verlag, 1995.

Marina N, Christie IN, Korsak A, et al. Astrocytes monitor cerebral perfusion and control systemic circulation to maintain brain blood flow. *Nat Commun* 2020;11:131.

Matejuk A, Vandenbark AA, Offner H. Cross-talk of the CNS with immune cells and functions in health and disease. *Front Neurol* 2021;31(12):672455.

Morgan CW. Axons of sacral preganglionic neurons in the cat: I. Origin, initial segment, and myelination. *J Neuro-Oncol* 2001;30:523–544.

Mountcastle VB. Introduction. Computation in cortical columns. *Cereb Cortex* 2003;13:2–4.

Neurocytology PE. Fine structure of neurons, nerves processes, and neuroglial cells. 2nd Ed. New York: Thieme Medical Publishers, 1994.

Orlin JR, Osen KK, Hovig T. Subdural compartment in pig. A morphologic study with blood and horseradish peroxidase infused subdurally. *Anat Rec* 1991;230:22–37.

Ozgen H, Baron W, Hoekstra D, et al. Oligodendroglial membrane dynamics in relation to myelin biogenesis. *Cell Mol Life Sci* 2016;73:3291–3310.

Peters A, Palay SL, Webster HD. The Fine Structure of the Nervous System: Neurons and Supporting Cells. 4th Ed. New York: Oxford University Press, 1991.

Rasband MN, Peles E. Mechanisms of node of Ranvier assembly. *Nat Rev Neurosci* 2021;22(1):7–20.

Sie C, Korn T. Dendritic cells in central nervous system autoimmunity. *Semin Immunopathol* 2017;39:99–111.

Sternberg SS. Histology for Pathologists. 5th Ed. Wolters Kluwer, 2019.

Stevens B, Porta S, Haak LL, et al. Adenosine: a neuron-glial transmitter promoting myelination in the CNS in response of action potentials. *Neuron* 2002;36:855–868.

Varga V, Mravec B. Chapter 8—Nerve Fiber Types. In: Tubbs RS, Rizk E, Shoja MM, et al., eds. Nerves and Nerve Injuries. Academic Press, 2015: 107–113.

Yasuda R. Biophysics of biochemical signaling in dendritic spines: implications in synaptic plasticity. *Biophys J* 2017;113(10):2152–2159.

5

Muscle

Craig McGowan

CHAPTER MENU

Overview

Muscle is the principal tissue responsible for generating movements of and within the body. Muscle tissue is found throughout the body and is divided into three basic types. **Skeletal muscle**, associated with voluntary movement, is found in the limbs, trunk, and head. **Cardiac muscle** is exclusively found in the heart. **Smooth muscle** lines the walls of hollow organs such as blood vessels, the gastrointestinal tract, and the urogenital tract. All three types of muscles share common features, but they also have distinct differences that are suited to their functional roles. These features can be identified in gross and histological preparations. Skeletal and cardiac muscles have a characteristic striped appearance due to the underlying filament structure that stains highly eosinophilic and are thus termed **striated muscles**. Smooth muscle has a more random organization and lacks the striated appearance.

Muscle tissue is comprised of specialized muscle cells known as **myocytes** or **myofibers** that are often referred to simply as **muscle fibers**. Myocytes are elongated and taper at the ends, giving them a fusiform shape, and the cells tend to be aligned with the direction of contraction. This fusiform shape is clear in longitudinal sections, whereas myocytes have

Dellmann's Textbook of Veterinary Histology, Seventh Edition. Edited by Marxa L. Figueiredo and John J. Turek.

Companion website: www.wiley.com/go/figueiredo/vethistology7e

a polygonal shape in cross-section. It should be noted that muscle fibers differ from connective tissue (CT) fibers, which are made up of extracellular substances. All myocytes share an excitable membrane that depolarizes to propagate action potentials along the length of the cell, and they all convert chemical energy into mechanical energy to generate movement.

Skeletal Muscle

Function and Structure

The primary function of skeletal muscle is to produce voluntary movements. Under the control of the nervous system, skeletal muscles are recruited to perform a wide range of movements, from the large-scale swinging of limbs during running to the fine-scale subtle movements of the eyes. Muscles may also simply resist movement when an external load is applied, such as when maintaining posture. While the largest and strongest muscles are located in the limbs, skeletal muscle is found throughout the body. In addition to producing movements, skeletal muscle can also generate heat through shivering.

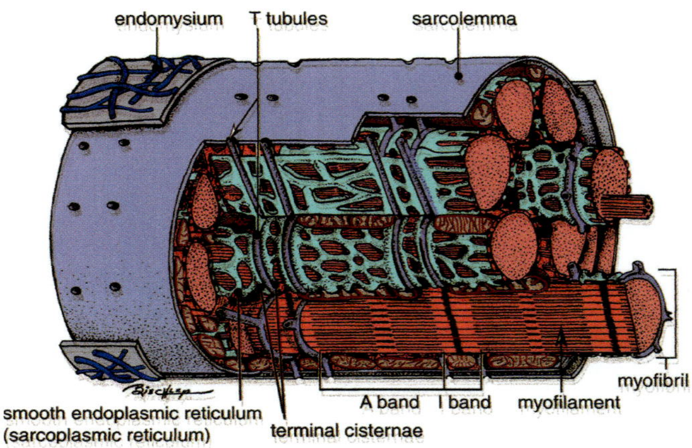

Figure 5-1 The myofibrils of skeletal muscle are comprised of myofilaments. Smooth endoplasmic reticulum surrounds each myofibril and forms terminal cisternae near the T tubule. T tubules extend into the cytoplasm from the cell membrane and surround the myofibrils at the A–I junction. A T tubule, along with two terminal cisternae, forms a triad structure. Peripheral nuclei of the skeletal muscle myofiber are not shown in this illustration.

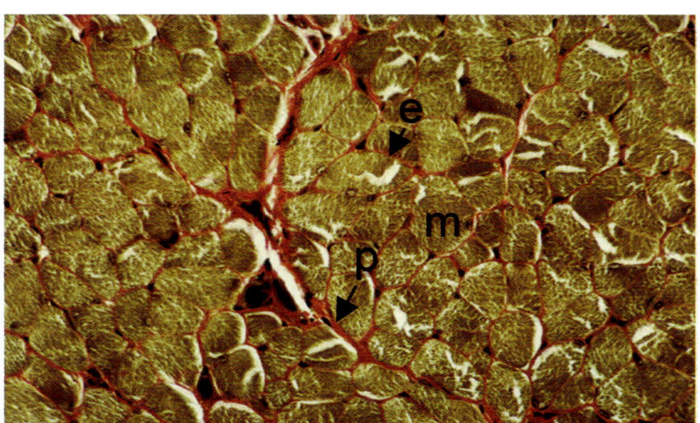

Figure 5-2 Connective tissue (CT) is stained red, and fibers are gold. Individual skeletal muscle myofibers (m) are surrounded by fine CT called endomysium (e). Bundles of myofibers, or fascicles, are surrounded by perimysium (p), which consists of dense irregular CT. The epimysium (not shown) is CT that covers the entire gross muscle. Soft palate, cat, Verhoeff-van Gieson (×250). (Image by W.E. Haensly.)

Skeletal muscles are organized in a hierarchical fashion (Fig. 5-1). Individual myocytes range from 10 to 110 µm in diameter and can extend up to several centimeters in length. These myocytes are densely packed with myofilaments organized into **myofibrils** within the cell. Each myocyte is surrounded by a layer of CT called **endomysium**, which contains nerve fibers and a network of capillaries supplying the myocytes (Fig. 5-2). Groups of muscle cells are organized into bundles called muscle fascicles. Each fascicle is surrounded by a second, denser layer of CT called the **perimysium**, which also houses nerves and blood vessels. The perimysium also contains muscle spindles, sensory organs that detect changes in muscle length. Finally, the collection of muscle fascicles that make up the whole muscle is wrapped in another layer of dense CT called the **epimysium**. All layers of CT throughout the muscle are interconnected and provide a mechanism to transmit force from the muscle to its point of attachment.

Light Microscope Structure

Myocytes are formed by the prenatal fusion of many myoblasts, which leads to each myocyte having multiple nuclei. The nuclei are located peripherally within the cell because the majority of the cell is occupied by a dense packing of myofibrils (Fig. 5-3). Because of the distribution of nuclei along the length of the myocyte, they may not be visible in all cross-sections (Fig. 5-4). In longitudinal sections, each cell will generally have several oval-shaped peripheral nuclei. **Satellite cells** are found between the basement membrane and the plasma membrane of myocytes. These cells form during development from undifferentiated progenitor cells and are crucial for muscle maintenance and growth in response to exercise, injury, or disease. Satellite cells contain a single nucleus that is heterochromatic, in contrast to the lighter staining nuclei of the myocyte, and are best visualized with electron microscopy.

The characteristic striped pattern seen in longitudinal sections of striated muscles arises from the highly ordered myofilaments making up **sarcomeres**. These sarcomeres are arranged in series within myofibrils that run longitudinally through the muscle cell (Fig. 5-5). Each single sarcomere spans between two **Z disks** and can be divided into distinct bands based on its structure. The Z disks appear as dark lines perpendicular to the muscle fiber and serve as anchor points for thin filaments and the elastic protein titan. At the center of the sarcomere is the **M line**, which is the anchor point for the thick filaments. The **I band**, adjacent to the Z disks, includes only thin filaments and appears lighter in color. The **A band** spans the length of the thick filaments and appears darker, especially in the region where thick and thin filaments overlap. The **H zone** is within the A band, adjacent to the M line, where thick and thin filaments do not overlap and thus appear slightly lighter. In cross-section, each thick filament is surrounded by six thin filaments forming a hexagonal lattice.

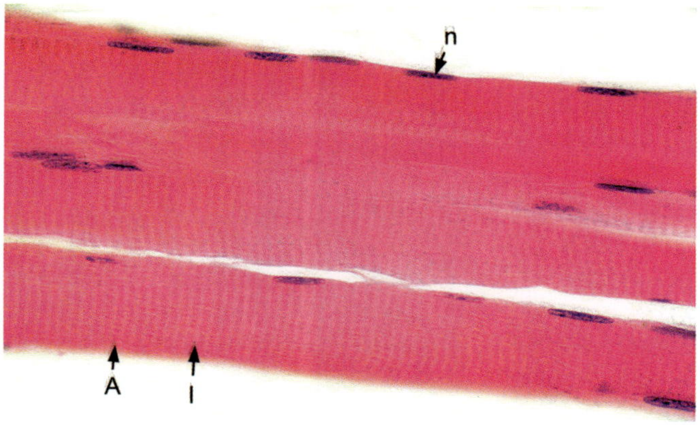

Figure 5-3 The cross-striations of skeletal muscle fibers are clearly visible when the fiber is cut longitudinally. Light-staining I bands (I) alternate with dark-staining A bands (A). Multiple nuclei (n) are located at the periphery of the fiber. Hematoxylin and Eosin (H&E) (×400). (Image by W.E. Haensly.)

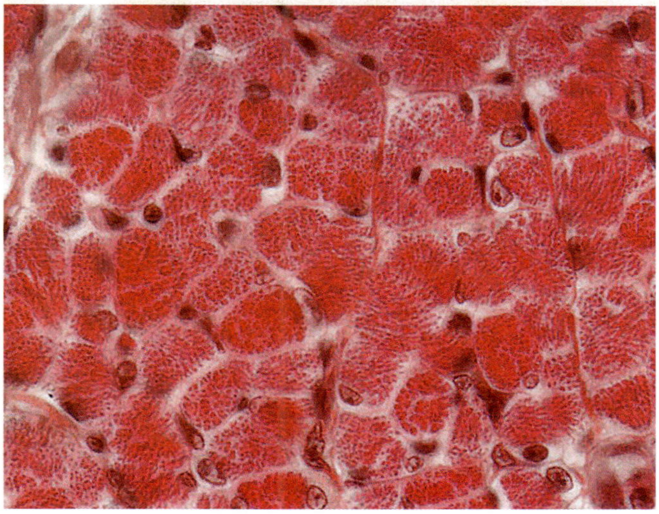

Figure 5-4 Cross-section of skeletal muscle fiber or myofiber. The cytoplasm is filled with contractile myofibrils (small pink dots). The nuclei of each myofiber are located at the periphery of the cell. Diaphragm muscle. H&E (×400). (Image by John J. Turek.)

Fine Structure

The contractile proteins of skeletal muscle are primarily composed of thin and thick myofilaments. **Thin filaments** are made up of **actin** and the regulatory proteins **troponin** and **tropomyosin**. The thin filament is formed by two strands of F-actin, arranged in a double helix. F-actin is a polymer of the globular molecule, G-actin, each of which has a binding site for myosin cross-bridges from the thick filament. A filamentous strand of tropomyosin runs in the groove formed between the F-actin strands and covers the myosin binding sites. Troponin, a globular three-unit protein, attaches to tropomyosin at intervals along the thin filament. When the muscle is activated, calcium binds to troponin and causes a conformational change that moves tropomyosin to uncover the myosin binding sites. **Thick filaments** are composed of the protein **myosin** and include two heavy chains and four light chains of amino acids. The heavy chains are wound in a double helix to form a rod-like tail. At one end, each of the heavy chains folds to form a protruding globular head that contains two of the light chains in each head. These myosin heads have binding sites for actin and adenosine triphosphate (ATP), facilitating the formation of **cross-bridges** between the thick and thin filaments during muscle contraction.

In addition to the contractile filaments, myocytes contain several structural proteins that contribute to maintaining their striated appearance. The giant protein **titan** spans from the Z disk to the M line and has multiple functions, including maintaining sarcomere integrity, contributing to passive tension, contributing to myofibrillar assembly, and cell signaling. Titan also is sensitive to calcium and thus may play a role in active muscle function. **Desmin** links adjacent myofibrils together at the Z disks and connects myofibrils to the cell membrane at rib-like structures called **costameres**. **Nebulin** is associated with actin and acts to stabilize the thin filaments. **Dystrophin** is a transmembrane protein complex that attaches

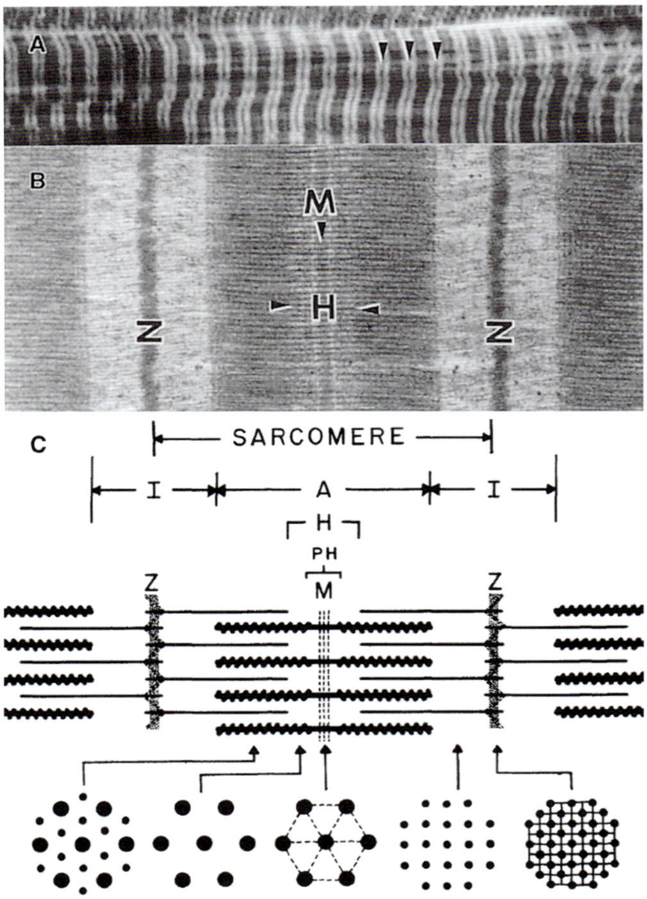

Figure 5-5 Light micrograph **(A)** and electron micrograph **(B)** of longitudinally oriented skeletal muscle, along with **(C)** a schematic representation of a sarcomere. In panel **A**, transverse striations show that alternating light bands (I bands) and dark bands (A bands) are present. Each I band is bisected by a Z line (arrowheads) (×1150). In panel **B**, the transverse striations can be further resolved into Z lines (Z) that define a sarcomere and bisect the light I band (not labeled). The A band is electron dense and is bisected by the M line (M, arrowhead), which connects adjacent thick myofilaments. On either side of the line, an electron-lucent area represents the H band (H), where thick and thin myofilaments do not overlap (×22,500). In panel **C**, the arrangement of myofilaments is shown in relation to the electron micrograph. PH is the pseudo-H zone, a more electron-lucent region in which thick myofilaments lack cross-bridges. The bottom diagram represents a cross-section of the region indicated by the arrows, with large dots representing thick myofilaments and small dots representing thin myofilaments.

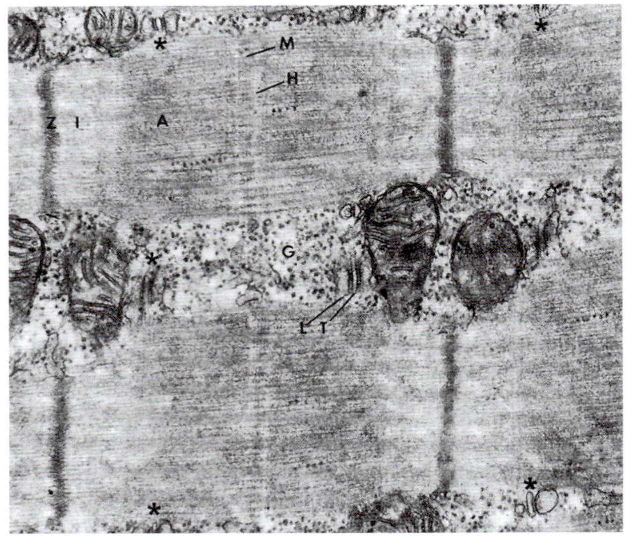

Figure 5-6 Electron micrograph of a longitudinal section through a skeletal muscle cell. Structures identified include the following: A band (A), I band (I), Z line (Z), M line (M), pseudo-H band (H), glycogen (G) adjacent to mitochondria in the cytoplasm, terminal cisternae (L), T tubule (T), and additional triads (*) located at the A–I junction (×34,000).

myofibrils to the myocyte cell membrane and provides stability. Mutations in dystrophin can lead to muscular dystrophies in both animals and humans.

The plasma membrane of myocytes, often referred to as the **sarcolemma**, is an excitable membrane that acts to propagate action potentials along the fiber and into the cell via transverse tubules or **T tubules** (Fig. 5-1). T tubules are invaginations of the cell membrane that penetrate into the cell at regular intervals. Within the myocyte, each myofibril is surrounded by a network of specialized smooth endoplasmic reticulum known as the **sarcoplasmic reticulum (SR)**, which stores and releases calcium ions. At the A–I band junction, the SR expands into terminal cisternae that have voltage-gated channels and act as reservoirs for calcium (Fig. 5-6). Each T tubule is associated with two terminal cisternae, forming what is referred to as a **triad**. When the muscle is activated, action potentials travel down the T tubules and trigger the release of calcium from the SR. This calcium release initiates muscle contraction.

Contraction

Muscles contract when an action potential from a motor neuron reaches the myocyte. One motor neuron may innervate many myocytes within a muscle (termed a motor unit), but each myocyte is innervated by only one motor neuron. Motor neurons branch within the muscle and form **motor end plates** where they meet individual myocytes (Fig. 5-7). When the motor neuron is stimulated, acetylcholine is released from the motor end plate into the synaptic cleft between the end plate and the myocyte. Acetylcholine binds to receptors on the myocyte cell membrane, opening channels that allow sodium to enter and depolarize the cell. The action potential spreads along the cell membrane and down the T tubules as adjacent voltage-gated channels open in response to the depolarization. Depolarization of the T tubules causes the

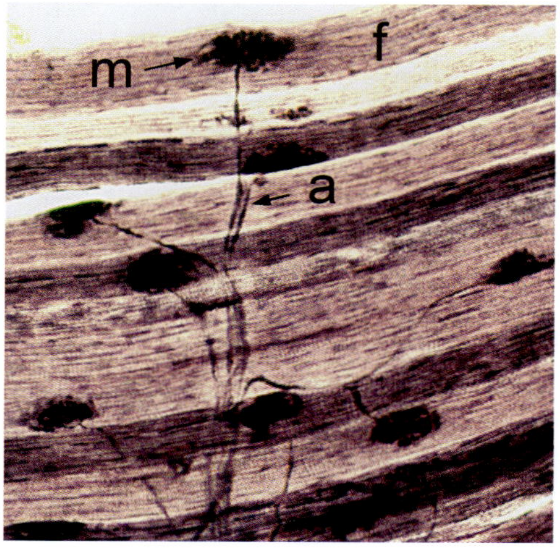

Figure 5-7 Axon (a) of a motor neuron ending at a motor end plate (m) on a skeletal muscle fiber (f). Silver stain (×200). (Image by John J. Turek.)

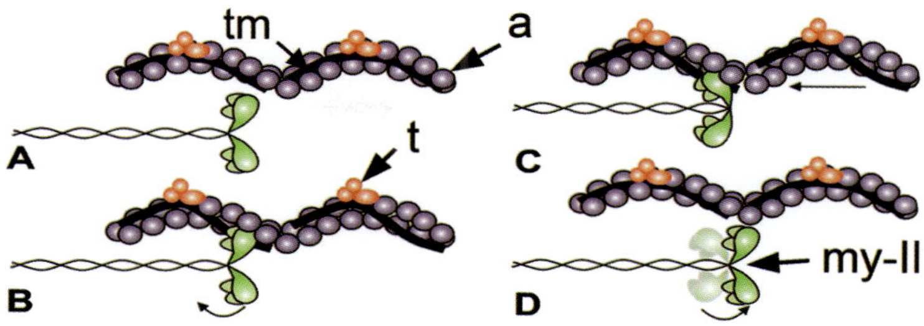

Figure 5-8 Schematic representation of a thin myofilament [actin (a), troponin (t), tropomyosin (tm), and a myosin-II molecule (my-II)]. Several myosin-II molecules aggregate to form a thick myofilament. **A.** The muscle is relaxed; actin and myosin-II are not linked. **B.** As contraction begins, the troponin–tropomyosin complex moves off the actin-binding site and allows myosin-II to bind. The myosin-II head then bends. **C.** The thin myofilament is pulled toward the center of the sarcomere (to the left in this drawing). **D.** The actin–myosin complex then dissociates, troponin–tropomyosin covers the actin-binding site again, and the myosin head swings forward to repeat the cycle.

release of calcium from the terminal cisternae, which then bathes the myofilaments. On the thin filament, calcium binds to troponin, causing a conformational change that moves the tropomyosin strand and exposes myosin binding sites, leading to cross-bridge cycling. Cross-bridge cycling is the process by which actin and myosin generate tension and create movement.

The cross-bridge cycle involves a series of steps (Fig. 5-8). (A) The muscle is relaxed, and myosin is not bound to actin. (B) The myosin head, energized by ATP hydrolysis, binds to the actin thin filament. (C) The myosin head undergoes a power stroke, in which the head swivels to pull the Z disk toward the M line, and the hydrolyzed ATP is released. (D) A new ATP molecule binds to the myosin head, and the myosin head detaches from the actin filament. Rigor mortis sets in when ATP is depleted postmortem, preventing the myosin heads from detaching from actin filaments. When the cell is no longer depolarized, calcium is actively transported back into the SR and the contraction ends. Contractions result in the Z disks moving closer to one another, and the I and H bands becoming narrower due to increased overlap between thick and thin filaments. The width of the A band remains constant as this is determined by the length of the thick filaments.

Muscle Fiber Types

Skeletal muscle fiber types are characterized based on their contractile (twitch) properties and metabolic characteristics. A range of histochemical and immunohistochemical techniques have been developed that differentiate between slow and fast twitch fibers, and between fatigue-resistant and fast-fatiguing fibers (Fig. 5-9). In general, **Type I** fibers contract slowly, produce relatively low forces, and have a high mitochondrial density supporting aerobic metabolism and fatigue resistance. **Type II** fibers, known as fast twitch fibers, are further subdivided into **Type IIa** and **Type IIb** fibers. Both Type IIa and IIb fibers have fast contraction speeds and produce higher forces compared to Type I fibers. However, Type IIa fibers have moderately high levels of mitochondria, while Type IIb fibers have very low levels of mitochondria. Therefore, Type IIb fibers produce high forces quickly but also fatigue quickly, whereas Type IIa fibers are somewhat fatigue resistant. Slow and fast twitch muscles also differ in their gross appearance. Due to their high concentration of mitochondria and the presence of myoglobin, a protein that transports oxygen, slow muscles tend to appear as **red** or dark, whereas fast twitch muscles tend to be **white** or light in color. Most muscles are composed of a mix of fiber types that are distributed randomly throughout the muscle. Additional subtypes of muscle fibers have also been characterized (e.g., Type IIx), and it is likely that more will be identified with ongoing advances in detection techniques.

Myogenesis, Hypertrophy, Atrophy, and Regeneration

During development, multiple myoblasts fuse to form elongated myotubes. Contractile myofibrils are formed within the myotube, and as additional myoblasts fuse to the myotube, more myofibrils are added. Each myoblast contributes one nucleus, which is pushed to the periphery by densely packed myofibrils, forming multinucleate myocytes. Satellite cells,

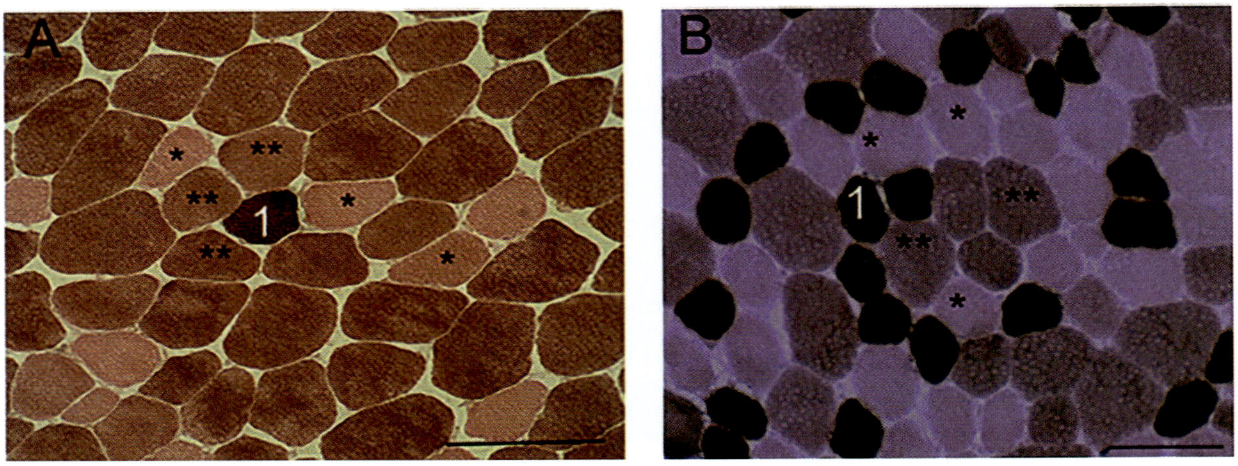

Figure 5-9 Cross-section of gluteal muscle from a Quarter Horse and a Thoroughbred stained with myosin ATPase at pH 4.4 and counterstained with eosin. **A.** The Quarter Horse has a low proportion of Type I (1) and IIa (*) fibers and a high proportion of Type IIx (**) fibers. **B.** The Warmblood has a high proportion of Type I (1) and IIa (*) fibers and a low proportion of Type IIx (**) fibers. (Reproduced with permission from Valberg et al., *Journal of Equine Veterinary Science*, vol. 118, 2022, article 104123).

which are Pax3+ and Pax7+ potential myogenic cells, remain within the basal lamina next to the mature myocyte. Pax transcription factors are essential for satellite cell maintenance and activation during muscle growth and repair.

Skeletal muscles increase in size primarily by **hypertrophy** (enlargement of myocytes) rather than **hyperplasia** (increased number of myocytes). Hypertrophy of mature skeletal myocytes occurs through the activity of satellite cells, which divide to form two daughter cells. One of the daughter cells remains a satellite cell, while the other fuses with the myocyte, adding additional nuclei. These new nuclei direct the synthesis of more myofibrils and other cytoplasmic elements. Neither the myocyte nor its nuclei divide during hypertrophy. In contrast, during atrophy of skeletal muscle, myofibrils and nuclei are lost.

Regeneration of muscle is dependent on the extent of the injury. Small areas of muscle can be regenerated through the fusion of satellite cells with existing myocytes or with each other to form new myocytes. However, if damage is extensive, the muscle tissue may be replaced by CT scars instead.

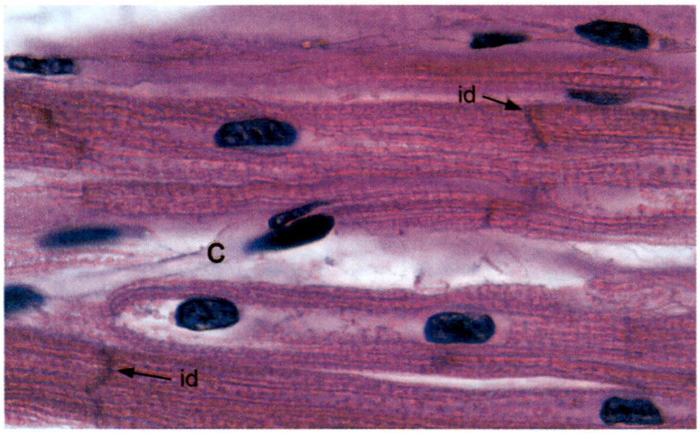

Figure 5-10 Cardiac muscle cells are long, branching fibers with distinct striations. Note the centrally located nucleus. Adjacent myocytes are connected by specialized intercellular junctions called intercalated disks (id). This tissue has many capillaries (c). Heart, dog. H&E (×700). (Image by J. Eurell).

Cardiac Muscle

Function

Cardiac muscle is found exclusively in the heart. **Cardiac myocytes**, or cardiomyocytes, are specialized to produce highly synchronized activation patterns that generate rhythmic contractions to pump blood through the body. As striated muscle cells, cardiac myocytes share many similarities with skeletal muscle, yet several key differences enable cardiac myocytes to perform their specialized functions.

Light Microscope Structure

Cardiac myocytes have a striated appearance similar to skeletal myocytes but have a variable branching morphology (Fig. 5-10). On average, cardiac myocytes measure 100 to 150 μm in length and 20 to 35 μm in width. At the ends of the branches, cardiac myocytes are interconnected by **intercalated disks**. Each muscle cell has a single, centrally located nucleus (Fig. 5-11). Layers of CT analogous to the endomysium and perimysium of skeletal muscles, surround individual cardiac myocytes and groups of myocytes, respectively. However, the heart lacks tissue analogous to the epimysium of skeletal muscles. Consistent with the high aerobic demands of the heart, cardiac myocytes are surrounded by extensive networks of capillaries.

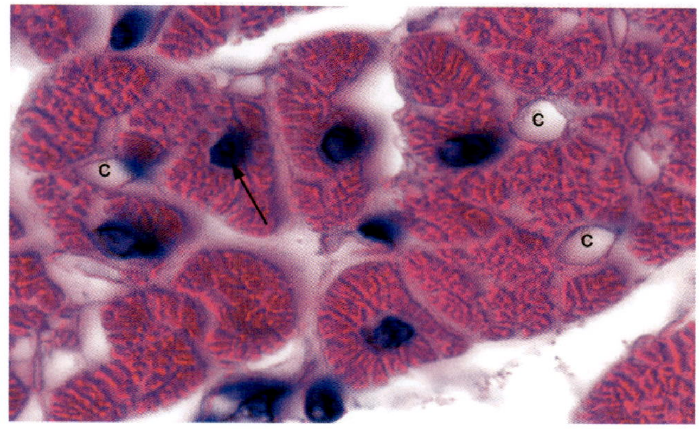

Figure 5-11 Cardiac muscle cross-section. Note the centrally located nuclei (arrow) and numerous capillaries (c). H&E (×800). (Image by J. Eurell).

Fine Structure

The myofibrils of cardiac myocytes are similar in structure and appearance to skeletal myocytes. A system of regularly spaced T tubules penetrates from the cell membrane adjacent to the Z disks (Fig. 5-12). Each myofibril is surrounded by SR that expands to terminal cisternae near the Z disks and closely associates with the T tubules. In cardiac myocytes, each T tubule is paired with only one terminal cisterna, forming a **diad** structure, unlike the triads found in skeletal myocytes. The myofibrils are held in place by a network of desmin filaments that are anchored at multiple points on the cell membrane, including at costameres. The mitochondria are larger and more densely packed in cardiac myocytes (Fig. 5-13) compared to skeletal myocytes. The cytoplasm of cardiac myocytes also contains lipid droplets and glycogen, which serve as fuel for aerobic metabolism. Atrial myocytes tend to be long and thin compared to myocytes in the ventricles, and they have fewer or no T tubules.

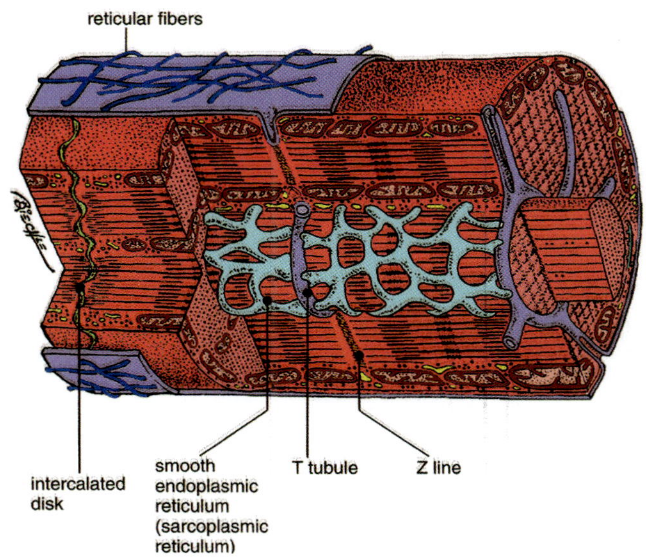

Figure 5-12 The T tubules of cardiac muscle are located at the Z line. Smooth endoplasmic reticulum surrounds the myofibrils and makes contact with the T tubules, forming a diad structure. The ends of the adjacent muscle fibers are joined by an intercalated disk. A nucleus, which is centrally located in the cardiac muscle fiber, is not shown in this drawing.

The intercalated disks play a significant role in the structure and function of cardiac muscle (Fig. 5-14). These disks provide both a physical connection and a means for rapid communication between the adjacent cell membranes of branching myocytes. On the transverse surface of the intercalated disk, **desmosomes** and **fascia adherens** form mechanical connections. Desmosomes create a strong link between cells by anchoring intermediate filaments that span the cell membranes and extend into the cytoplasm. Desmosomes are also another anchor point for the desmin filaments. Fascia adherens provide an anchor point for the actin filaments of the myofibrils, facilitating the transmission of contractile forces across the cellular junction. **Gap junctions** are located on the longitudinal surface of the intercalated disk, running parallel to the axis of the myofibrils. These junctions contain clusters of channels that allow for direct transmission of chemical signals and rapid conductions of action potentials from one cell to the next.

Cardiac Nodes and Impulse Conduction Fibers

Modified cardiac myocytes form the **cardiac nodes** and **impulse conduction fibers** that generate synchronized, rhythmic contractions of the heart. The contraction cycle is initiated in the sinoatrial (SA) node and triggers the contraction of the atria. The impulse then passes to the atrioventricular node and enters a specialized conduction system that includes the bundle of His, main branch bundles, and the Purkinje fiber network, stimulating ventricular contraction beginning from

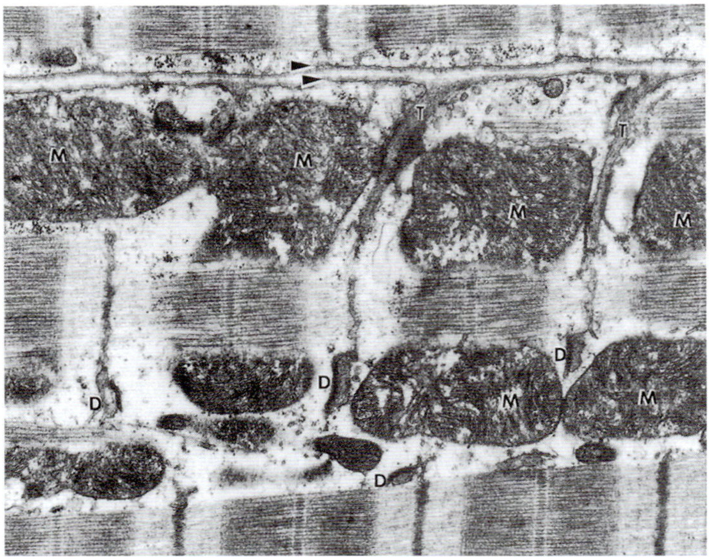

Figure 5-13 Electron micrograph of a longitudinal section of cardiac muscle. The cell membrane and basement membrane of each myocyte are indicated with arrowheads. Large mitochondria (M) with densely packed cristae are located just below the cell membrane. Note the two large T tubules (T) entering the lower myocyte at the Z lines. Diads (D), composed of a T tubule and smooth endoplasmic reticulum, are present deeper in the cell between the myofibrils (×22,500). (Courtesy of W.S. Tyler).

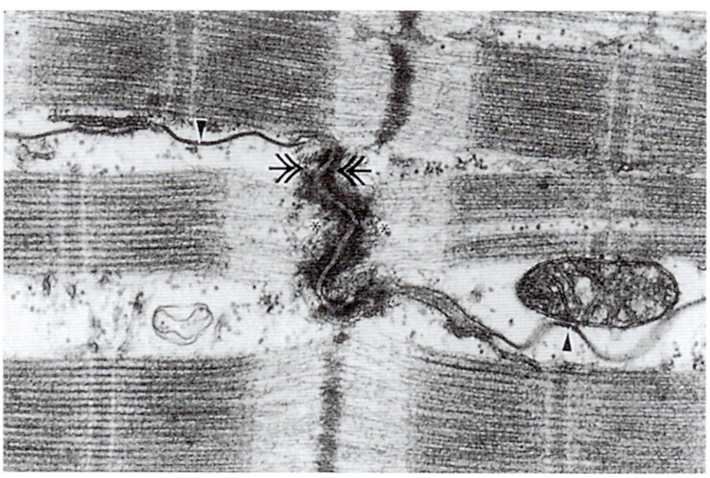

Figure 5-14 Electron micrograph of an intercalated disk from cardiac muscle. The fascia adherens junction (*) is oriented transversely to the long axis of the myofibril. Desmosomes are indicated by the double arrow. Gap junctions (arrowheads) are oriented parallel to the long axis (×42,100). (Courtesy of W.S. Tyler).

the apex of the heart. The cardiac node cells tend to be small, with few myofibrils and dispersed gap junctions. They stain positive for acetylcholinesterase due to their conduction function. These cells have mitochondria and SR but lack T tubules. The impulse conduction fibers (Fig. 5-15) are similar to nodal cells but have abundant gap junctions for rapid transmission of action potentials. These cells tend to be larger than adjacent cardiac myocytes, especially toward the apex of the heart.

Contraction

The mechanism of contraction in cardiac myocytes is very similar to that of skeletal muscle. Action potentials propagate down T tubules and trigger the release of calcium for the SR, leading to cross-bridge cycling between the thick and thin myofilaments. The wave of action potentials, initiating in the SA node, spreads between myocytes via gap junctions in the intercalated disks.

Myogenesis, Hypertrophy, and Regeneration

Cardiac myocytes develop from splanchnic mesoderm surrounding the endocardial tube. These fibers arise by differentiation and growth of single cells. As the cells grow, new myofilaments form. The ability of cardiac myocytes to divide is lost shortly after birth. Enlargement of the heart wall due to exercise or disease is primarily through hypertrophy rather than hyperplasia. Damage to the heart wall that results in cell death is repaired primarily by CT leading to scar tissue, rather than regeneration of new myocytes.

Smooth Muscle

Function

Smooth muscle is found throughout the body. For example, it is present in the walls of blood vessels, airways, the gastrointestinal tract, and the bladder. It is in the skin (for hair erection) and in the eye (for pupil constriction). Smooth muscle is not under voluntary control and is generally regulated by the autonomic nervous system. Smooth muscle serves many functions, such as changing shape to regulate pressure within a blood vessel or creating waves to facilitate the movement of food through the digestive tract.

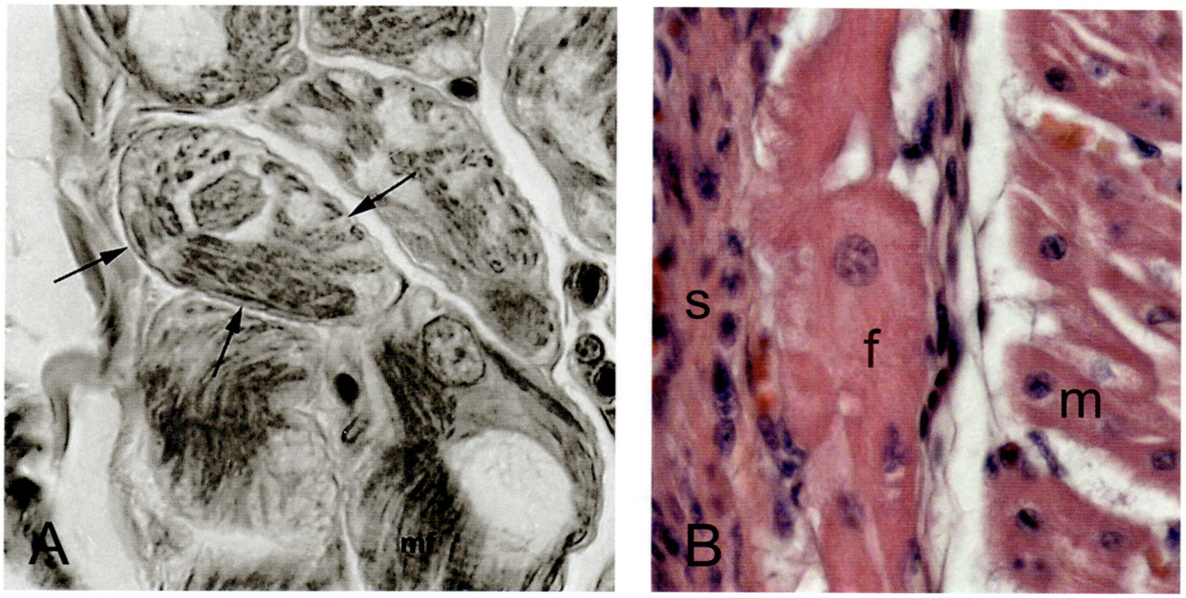

Figure 5-15 **A.** Cardiac impulse conduction fibers (one is outlined by arrows) are larger than myocytes. They have a centrally located nucleus and sparse myofibrils (mf) in their cytoplasm. Phosphotungstic Acid Hematoxylin (PTAH) stain (×1200). **B.** Conduction fiber or Purkinje fiber (f) in the interventricular septum. Smooth muscle of adjacent artery (s) and cardiac myocytes (m) (H&E).

Light Microscope Structure

Smooth muscle myocytes are elongated, fusiform cells with a single large centrally located nucleus (Fig. 5-16). The nucleus is surrounded by mitochondria, rough endoplasmic reticulum, and Golgi apparatus indicating a high capacity for protein synthesis. These myocytes range from 20 μm to 1 mm in length and 5 to 20 μm in width. Due to their tapered shape, there is substantial variation in cell size in cross-sections, and the nucleus may not be visible in all cells (Fig. 5-16B). Smooth muscle myocytes lack the highly structured myofibril arrangement of striated muscles, and consequently, they do not exhibit the characteristic banding pattern. Individual myocytes are surrounded by a network of reticular fibers, blood vessels, and nerves, but lack the hierarchical CT structure seen in skeletal and cardiac muscles.

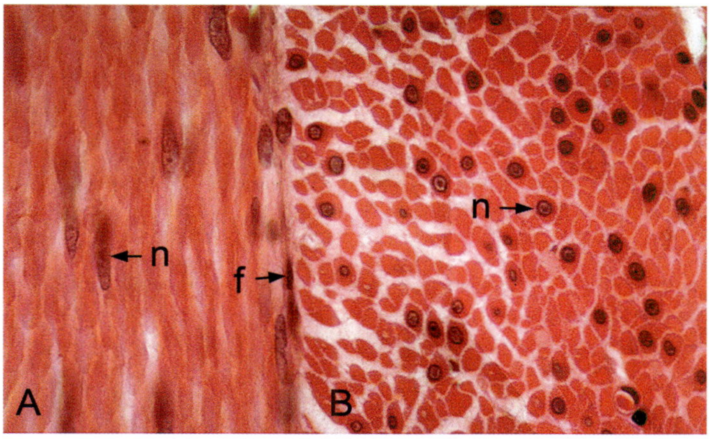

Figure 5-16 Smooth muscle fibers are long, spindle-shaped cells **(A)** with a centrally located nucleus (n). The nuclei are absent in several cross-sections of fibers **(B)** due to sectional geometry. Fibrocytes within the CT between the muscle layers have smaller, darker nuclei (f). Tunica muscularis of the jejunum, dog. H&E (×1000). (Image by W.E. Haensly).

Fine Structure

Unlike striated muscle, myofilaments in smooth muscle myocytes are dispersed throughout the cytoplasm at various angles (Fig. 5-17). The thin myofilaments contain actin and tropomyosin but lack troponin, while the myosin thick filaments are relatively sparse. On average, the ratio of actin to myosin is 15:1 in smooth muscle myocytes compared to 6:1 in striated muscle. Instead of Z disks, the myofibrils are anchored to **dense bodies** distributed throughout the cell, linked together by a network of intermediate filaments composed of **desmin** and **vimentin**.

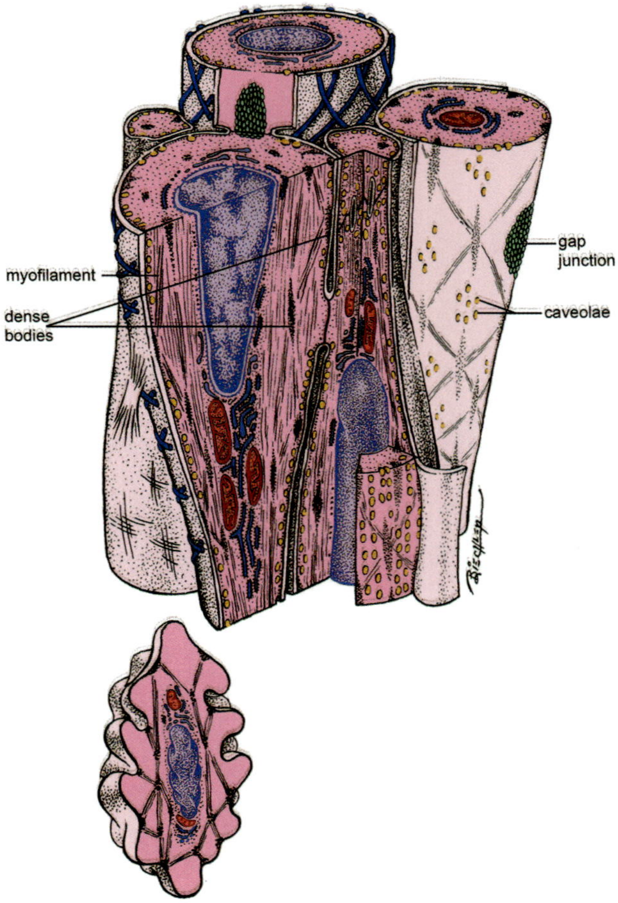

Figure 5-17 The smooth muscle cell has a centrally located nucleus surrounded by cytoplasm containing myofilaments in various orientations. The contractile myofilaments anchor into dense bodies on the cell membrane and within the cytoplasm of the smooth muscle cell. When the myofilaments contract, the cell shortens (lower diagram). Numerous caveolae, vesicles, and gap junctions are present along the cell membrane.

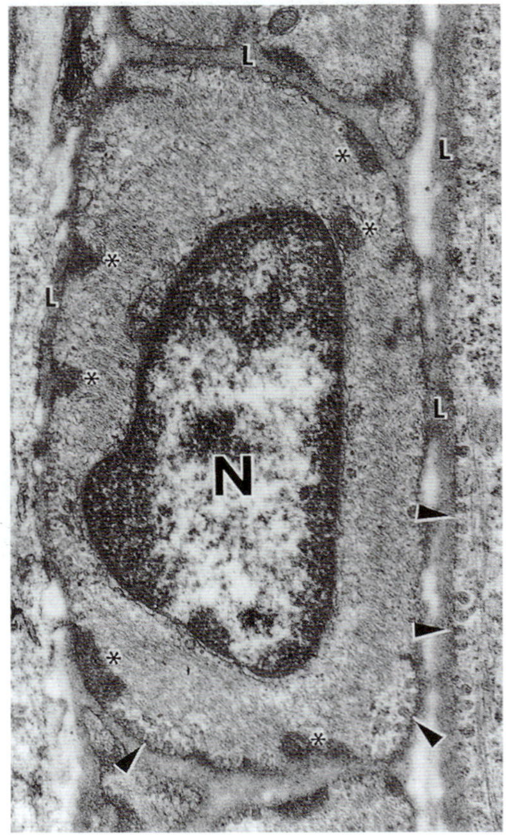

Figure 5-18 Electron micrograph of a cross-sectioned smooth muscle cell. The nucleus (N) is centrally located, and the cytoplasm contains numerous myofilaments. Electron-dense bodies (*) serve as attachment sites for the myofilaments. Numerous caveolae (arrowheads) are present along the plasma membrane of an adjacent cell. The basal laminae (L) are visible between the two cells and appear fused at points (×23,900). (Courtesy of W.S. Tyler).

Smooth muscle myocytes contain limited SR and lack T tubules but have calcium channels along the cell membrane which open in response to an action potential. **Caveolae**, which are flask-shaped invaginations arranged in rows along the cell membrane (Fig. 5-18), substantially increase the overall surface area and may increase the proximity of the cell membrane to the SR.

Contraction

Contractions of smooth muscle myocytes are initiated by an increase in calcium in the cytoplasm via an influx through voltage-gated calcium channels on the cell membrane or by inositol 1,4,5-triphosphate-induced release from the SR. Unlike in striated muscle, where calcium directly binds to the thin filament to trigger cross-bridge formation, in smooth muscle myocytes, calcium binds to **calmodulin**. The calcium–calmodulin complex activates myosin light chain kinase, which phosphorylates the myosin light chain in the thick filament head, enabling cross-bridge cycling with actin and resulting in muscle contraction. Slower rates of ATPase and other factors contribute to the slower contractions of smooth muscle compared to striated muscles.

Smooth muscle contractions are involuntary and can be triggered in a number of ways. Neurotransmitters from the autonomic nervous system can cause cell membranes to depolarize. Hormones can have varied effects, leading to contraction in some muscles and relaxation in others. Some smooth muscle cells have stretch-activated calcium release, quickly responding to changes in length and regulating internal pressure autonomously. Smooth muscles such as those found in the wall of the visceral organs tend to act in a networked fashion and are referred to as **single-unit smooth muscles**. The myocytes in these muscles are connected by gap junctions but are sparsely innervated. **Multiunit smooth muscles**, such as those in the iris of the eye, have individual innervation to the myocytes, giving fine motor control. These myocytes lack gap junctions.

Myogenesis, Hypertrophy, and Regeneration

Smooth muscle myocytes arise from both mesoderm and neural crest cells, reflecting their diverse locations throughout the body. Smooth muscle tissue increases in size by both hypertrophy (enlargement of existing cells) and hyperplasia (formation of new cells). New smooth muscle cells can arise via mitosis or differentiation from pericytes. However, the formation of new myocytes is limited, so healing of smooth muscle is mainly through the formation of CT scars rather than the regeneration of new myocytes.

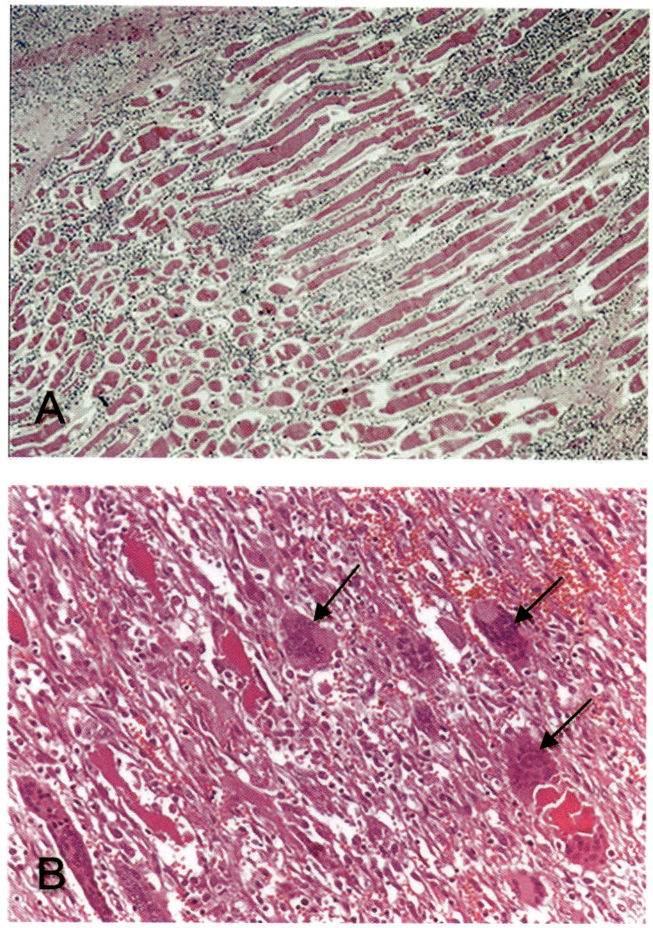

Figure 5-19 **Myositis. A.** The production of abnormal antibodies attacks the masticatory muscles, and the tissue becomes dominated by a cellular response, with progressive muscle destruction and fixation of the jaws. German Shepard dog. **B.** Multinuclear giant cells (arrows) can be seen between muscle fibers in a skeletal muscle from porcine. (Reprinted with permission from Salguero Bodes FJ, Pallares Martinez FJ. Aughey and Frye's Comparative Veterinary Histology with Clinical Correlates. 2nd ed. Boca Raton: CRC Press, 2023).

Clinical Correlations

Myopathies may be congenital, metabolic, or inflammatory, caused by a variety of agents including viral, bacterial, fungal, and parasitic. When there is inflammation, the condition would be called a myositis. In eosinophilic myositis, the masticatory muscles of dogs can be infiltrated by numerous eosinophils, and to a lesser extent, lymphocytes and other inflammatory cells. There is muscle degeneration and atrophy, as illustrated in Fig. 5-19A. Pigs also can have a granulomatous myositis in different skeletal muscles, with invasion of the space between muscle fibers by multinuclear giant cells. This finding has been related to infection by type 2 porcine circovirus (Fig. 5-19B). Other non-neoplastic conditions may involve neuropathies from disturbance of innervation and myasthenic conditions of the motor end plate.

Essentials

Skeletal (striated) muscle has three layers of CT: the outer *epimysium*, *perimysium* around muscle fascicles, and *endomysium* around muscle fibers. Muscle cells (fibers) are multinucleated and surrounded by a basal lamina. The plasma membrane (sarcolemma) invaginates into cells to form T tubules, which interact with adjacent SR. T tubules carry depolarization into the cell and trigger the release of calcium from the SR. Calcium binds to troponin-C and unmasks myosin binding sites on actin, facilitating sarcomere contraction via myosin–ATPase.

The functional unit of contraction is the sarcomere, which extends from Z disk to Z disk. The Z disk anchors actin filaments primarily via α-actinin. Myosin filaments are located only in the A band, where actin is also present. The I bands contain actin and shorten during muscle contraction.

Muscle fibers are innervated by myelinated axons at the motor end plate. The basal laminae of the Schwann cell and muscle fiber fuse at the motor end plate. Acetylcholine released at the axon terminal binds to receptors on junctional folds in the postsynaptic cleft.

Muscle spindles are encapsulated intrafusal muscle fibers that function as *stretch* receptors. The **myotendinous junction** connects muscle to tendon, where a highly folded muscle cell membrane interdigitates with tendon collagen. The **Golgi tendon organs** are located on tendons where muscle attaches to bone and detect *tension* in the muscle-tendon. ***Healing***: Satellite cells are stem cells located between the basal lamina and sarcolemma, and they proliferate in response to injury. The healing process is regulated by various transcription and growth factors.

Cardiac Muscle: Cells contain a single central nucleus and branch, joined together by intercalated disks containing fascia adherens, desmosomes, and gap junctions. They contain more mitochondria and larger T tubules compared to skeletal muscle. SR is less organized than the triad system of skeletal muscle. Sarcomere contraction is regulated by intracellular calcium releasing from the SR and extracellular calcium entering the cell via ion channels. ***Healing***: Poor capacity to heal and the response to injury is typically fibrosis.

Smooth Muscle: Under *involuntary* control via sympathetic and parasympathetic innervation, smooth muscle cells are spindle shaped and surrounded by a basal lamina and contain many gap junctions. Smooth muscle is organized as sheets in various portions of respiratory, digestive, and reproductive systems, or occurs as single cells aiding in exocrine gland secretions.

Smooth muscle lacks sarcomeres and troponin. Actin filaments anchor to *cytoplasmic dense bodies* that contain α-actinin. Myosin filaments in the soluble form are not visible by electron microscopy in relaxed cells. Calcium triggers contraction by interaction with *calmodulin*, leading to myosin phosphorylation and filament assembly. Smooth muscle contraction or relaxation can be triggered by drugs or hormones altering intracellular calcium levels. ***Healing***: Smooth muscle cells divide and form new cells after injury.

Suggested Readings

Alberts B, Bray D, Lewis J, et al. Molecular Biology of the Cell. 6th Ed. Garland Science, 2014.

Bloch RJ, Gonzalez-Serratos H. Lateral force transmission across costameres in skeletal muscle. *Exerc Sport Sci Rev* 2003;**31**:73–78.

Calderón JC, Bolaños P, Caputo C. The excitation-contraction coupling mechanism in skeletal muscle. *Biophys Rev.* 2014 Mar;6(1):133–160.

Cardinet GH III, Leong DL, Means PS. Myocyte differentiation in normal and hypotrophied canine pectineal muscles. *Muscle Nerve* 1982;5:665.

Dellmann HD, Carithers JR. Cytology and Microscopic Anatomy. 8th Ed. Lippincott Williams & Wilkins, 2007.

Fu X, Wang H, Hu P. Stem cell activation in skeletal muscle regeneration. *Cell. Mol. Life Sci.* 2015;72:1663–1677.

Gillies AR, Lieber RL. Structure and function of the skeletal muscle extracellular matrix. *Muscle Nerve* 2011 Sep;44(3):318–331.

Guyton AC, Hall JE. Textbook of Medical Physiology. 14th Ed. Elsevier, 2020.

Huxley HE. Electron microscopy studies of the structure of natural and synthetic protein filaments from striated muscle. *J Mol Biol* 1963;7:281–308.

Jones DA, Round JM. Skeletal Muscle in Health and Disease. 2ndEd. Human Kinetics, 2005.

Murray IR, Baily JE, Chen WCW, et al. Skeletal and cardiac muscle pericytes: functions and therapeutic potential. *Pharmacol Ther.* 2017 Mar;171:65–74.

Pardo JV, Siliciano JD, Craig SW. A vinculin-containing cortical lattice in skeletal muscle: transverse lattice elements ("costameres") mark sites of attachment between myofibrils and sarcolemma. *Proc Natl Acad Sci U S A* 1983;80:1008–1012.

Paulin D, Li Z. Desmin: a major intermediate filament protein essential for the structural integrity and function of muscle. *Experimental Cell Research* 2004;301(1):1–7.

Pollard TD, Earnshaw WC. Cell Biology. 3rd Ed. Elsevier, 2017.

Salguero Bodes FJ, Pallares Martinez FJ. Aughey and Frye's Comparative Veterinary Histology with Clinical Correlates. 2nd ed. Boca Raton: CRC Press, 2023

Severs NJ. Cardiac muscle cell interaction: from microanatomy to the molecular make-up of the gap junction. *Histol Histopathol* 1995;10:481–501.

Squire JM, Paul DM, Morris EP. Myosin and actin filaments in muscle: structures and interactions. In: Parry D, Squire J, eds. Fibrous Proteins: Structures and Mechanisms. Subcellular Biochemistry. Vol. 82. Cham: Springer, 2017.

Valberg SJ. Skeletal muscle function. In: Kaneko J, ed. Clinical Biochemistry of Domestic Animals. New York: Academic Press, 2008: 459–484.

Webb RC. Smooth muscle contraction and relaxation. APS Refresher Course Report. *The American Physiological Society* 2003;17:4.

Willingham TB, Kim Y, Lindberg E, et al. The unified myofibrillar matrix for force generation in muscle. *Nat Commun* 2020;**11**:3722.

6

Blood and Bone Marrow

Joanne B. Messick

CHAPTER MENU

Blood

Composition and Function of Blood

The blood consists of specialized cells derived from the bone marrow that are suspended in a light, yellowish-colored fluid known as plasma. Water and salts absorbed through the digestive tract are the major source of plasma in the blood. An animal's total blood volume is the sum of cellular and plasma volumes within the circulatory system. The plasma component represents

Dellmann's Textbook of Veterinary Histology, Seventh Edition. Edited by Marxa L. Figueiredo and John J. Turek.

Companion website: www.wiley.com/go/figueiredo/vethistology7e

Table 6-1 Circulating blood volume of animals

Animal	Average Blood Volume (ml/kg)
Cat	55
Dog	86
Horse	76
Cow	55
Pig	65
Sheep	60
Goat	70
Rabbit	56
Mouse	79
Rat	64

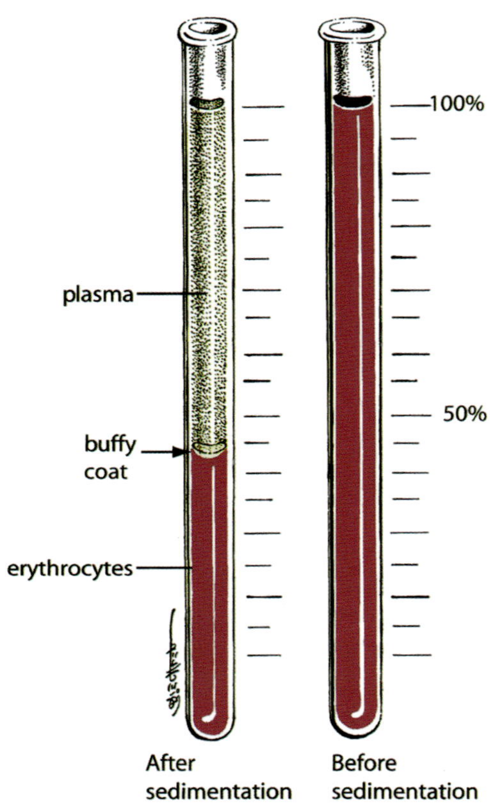

Figure 6-1 Blood before and after sedimentation. The volume of packed erythrocytes constitutes almost 45% of the total blood volume. The leukocytes and platelets form a buffy coat, accounting for approximately 1% of the blood volume. The remainder of the blood is the supernatant plasma.

about 55% of the blood volume, with the formed or cellular elements (red blood cells or erythrocytes, white blood cells or leukocytes, and platelets) making up the remaining 45%. Red blood cells are the major contributor to cellular volume with white blood cells and platelets accounting for less than 1%. In an adult animal, the blood volume typically ranges from 8 to 10% of the body weight in kilograms or approximately 28 to 40 mL of blood for each lb (0.454 kg) of body weight. Thus, the total blood volume in a 454-kg/1000-lb horse is estimated at 35 L, whereas that of a 4.54-kg/10-lb dog is only about 350 to 400 mL. The blood volume of some laboratory animals such as rats may be as low as 6% of body weight. Table 6-1 shows the circulating blood volume, given in volume per kg, for various healthy adult animals. However, the blood volume in obese and old animals may be reduced by as much as 15% compared to the standard volume for their species.

It is extremely important that an animal's blood volume be maintained within a critical range, ensuring the constant perfusion of all tissues of the body. The maintenance of blood volume serves several important functions. First, the hemoglobin contained within red blood cells carries oxygen to the tissues and collects carbon dioxide to facilitate its removal. Blood also conveys nutrients such as amino acids, sugars, and minerals to the tissues. Further, it serves as a conduit for byproducts and toxic substances that may be removed by the liver and kidneys. Hormones, enzymes, and vitamins make their way to tissue targets by means of the blood. As a result of the phagocytic activity of leukocytes, the killing potential of their granules, and the humoral and cell-mediated immune responses mounted by lymphocytes, the blood provides a defense system for the animal. Finally, platelets are tiny cellular elements that play a major role in hemostasis, preventing excessive blood loss during hemorrhage. When a tissue loses its blood supply, ischemia occurs, and the tissue may die.

Plasma

When blood is freshly drawn into a test tube without anticoagulants, platelets and coagulation factors in the fluid portion are responsible for the formation of a clot. Fibrinogen is consumed in this process, and the fluid portion in clotted blood is known as serum. The addition of an anticoagulant such as ethylene diamine tetra-acetic (EDTA) acid to a test tube of freshly drawn blood will prevent the formation of a clot. Plasma, the fluid portion of anticoagulated blood, can be separated from its cellular components by centrifugation, resulting in plasma at the top of the centrifuged blood and cellular components on the bottom of the tube (Fig. 6-1). The plasma is colorless to lightly yellow, depending on the animal species, and is a slightly alkaline fluid consisting of approximately 92% water and 8% dissolved substances (solids or dry matter). About 90% of the dissolved substances in plasma are organic molecules such as glucose, lipids (cholesterol, triglycerides, phospholipids, lecithin, and fats), proteins (albumin, globulins, fibrinogen, and others), glycoproteins, hormones, amino acids, and vitamins. An inorganic or mineral portion (sodium, potassium, calcium, chloride, bicarbonate, sulfate, and phosphate) is dissolved in plasma in ionic forms that can dissociate into positive and negative ions. Albumin is the most abundant of the plasma proteins. While albumin plays an important role in transporting substances in the plasma, it also plays a critical role in maintaining the oncotic pressure of blood. Oncotic pressure is the driving force exerted by albumin that pulls water into the vasculature from surrounding tissues through osmosis. This movement of fluid contributes to the maintenance of blood volume.

Cellular Elements

The cellular elements of blood form distinct layers following centrifugation. The lowest layer is red in color and represents about 45% of the blood volume. This layer consists of red blood cells or erythrocytes and represents the packed cell volume (PCV) or hematocrit. The PCV is a measure (%) of the volume of erythrocytes relative to the total volume of whole blood in a sample. The buffy coat is a small off-white layer identified on top of the packed red cells. In the normal patient, the buffy coat accounts for about 1% of the total blood volume and consists of platelets and leukocytes (neutrophils, eosinophils, basophils, monocytes, and lymphocytes). The platelet layer is whiter and is located on top of the buffy coat. This thin layer can sometimes be distinguished from the underlying leukocyte layer, which is slightly pink due to an admixture with erythrocytes of low specific gravity, including reticulocytes. Although the numbers of leukocytes and platelets vary in domestic animals, 8000 to 12,000 leukocytes/μL of blood and 200,000 to 400,000 platelets/μL are typical.

Erythrocytes

Erythrocytes are derived from a pluripotent stem cell population in the bone marrow. They undergo a series of differentiation stages, developing into cells morphologically recognizable as immature erythroid cells or erythroid precursors. In the final stages of maturation, these precursors become progressively smaller, acquiring hemoglobin in their cytoplasm, before they extrude their nucleus and are released from the bone marrow into circulation. The process of red cell development is known as erythropoiesis.

Hemoglobin is the oxygen-carrying protein of red cells. It binds oxygen in the lungs, where it is most abundant, and delivers it to the tissues. The lack of a nucleus and the biconcave shape of mature red blood cells contribute to their increased oxygen-carrying capacity. The latter is likely related to an increase in the cell's surface area. Reticulocytes, or polychromatophilic red blood cells, are partially hemoglobinized, immature, non-nucleated red cells that develop into mature erythrocytes within 1 to 3 days.

A few reticulocytes are normally found in peripheral blood smears of certain species. In contrast, these cells are normally absent from the blood of healthy adult horses, cows, and goats. Reticulocytes appear slightly bluish compared to mature red blood cells in a Wright–Giemsa-stained blood smear due to the presence of residual ribonucleic acid. The ribosomes, polyribosomes, and mitochondria retained in these cells aggregate into a reticular mesh when stained with vital stains such as new methylene blue (NMB). Enumeration of reticulocyte numbers in peripheral blood using the NMB stain is an indication of bone marrow erythropoietic activity. Within a few days, reticulocytes lose their reticular structures to become mature erythrocytes.

In general, the size of an erythrocyte, or red blood cell, in domestic animal species ranges from 3 to 7 μm. The red blood cells of dogs are largest at about 7 μm in size, whereas those of sheep and goats are only 4.5 and 3.2 μm, respectively. The shape of the erythrocyte and the presence of a nucleus vary among animal species. Although mammalian red cells are reported to have a biconcave disk shape that results in a slight central pallor visible with light microscopy, this feature is only easily seen in the red blood cells of the dog (Fig. 6-2). The erythrocytes of the Camelidae family, including camels, llamas, and alpacas, have a characteristic oval shape. Red blood cells of amphibians, reptiles, and birds are also oval and, unlike mammalian cells, retain a nucleus in maturity. Fragments of the nucleus, or Howell–Jolly bodies, are normally observed in a few circulating red cells of horses and cats. An increased number of circulating red cells with nuclei or Howell–Jolly bodies in other animal species may suggest abnormal splenic function or a history of splenectomy.

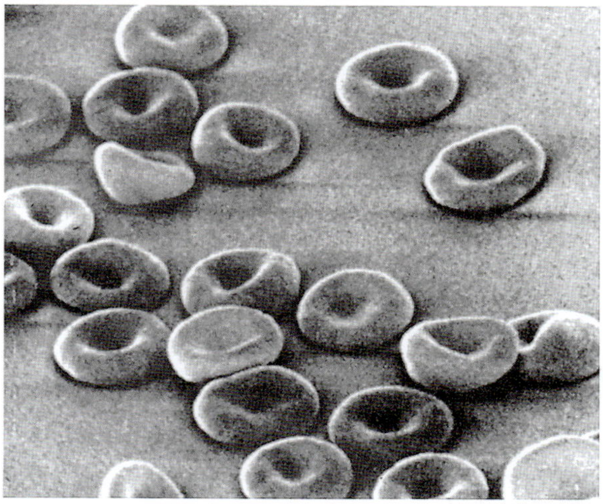

Figure 6-2 Scanning electron micrograph of erythrocytes from a clinically normal dog. The erythrocytes are biconcave disks. (From Jain NC. Schalm's Veterinary Hematology. 4th Ed. Philadelphia: Lea & Febiger, 1983.)

A slight variation in the size of red blood cells, or anisocytosis, is a common finding in peripheral blood smears. Although the presence of poikilocytosis, or variation in the shape of red blood cells, is a normal finding in goats, sheep, and pigs, it is uncommon in most other animal species. Crenated red blood cells, which have numerous short, evenly spaced, blunt, or sharp projections, are also a common finding. Although these changes are usually artifacts, they may occur in animals with lymphoma or uremic patients. Rouleau formation, or aggregates of red blood cells resembling "stacked coins," is a common finding in the blood smear of horses and cats. In dogs and other animal species, the presence of rouleau may suggest that certain total protein concentrations, such as immunoglobulins or fibrinogen, are increased. However, agglutination, the irregular clumping of red blood cells, in any species, rather than "coinlike" stacking, is abnormal and must be distinguished from rouleau formation. This problem may be caused by coating of red blood cells with antibodies and is often associated with a condition known as immune-mediated hemolytic anemia (IMHA). Further, red blood cells in IMHA typically lose their bioconcave disk shape, becoming spherocytic (lacking central pallor).

About 1 to 3 million red blood cells are produced by the bone marrow every second and released into circulation. Erythrocytes are the most numerous of the formed elements in the blood. About 5 to 10 million red blood cells are typically present in every microliter of blood in a healthy adult animal. In contrast, in sheep and goats, the number of red blood cells may be as high as 12 to 15 million/μL of blood.

The lifespan of the red blood cells in circulation is variable in veterinary species. In mice, the lifespan of red blood cells is about 30 days, while those of cats and dogs are reported to survive 68 and 110 days, respectively. A longer lifespan has been reported in adult goats, cows, and horses, approaching 115, 130, and 145 days, respectively. The loss of these cells is continually balanced by the release of reticulocytes and mature red blood cells from the bone marrow. Old or damaged red blood cells are removed from the circulation by macrophages, primarily in the spleen and liver.

Leukocytes

As with the red blood cells, leukocytes, or white blood cells, begin their life in the bone marrow. They too are derived from pluripotent hematopoietic stem cells (HSCs) and undergo lineage-specific differentiation to become mature leukocytes, a process known as leukopoiesis. A continual release of leukocytes from the bone marrow into circulation is essential to meet the peripheral demand for these cells, with an estimated 10^{10} to 10^{11} cells exiting the marrow daily.

Blood leukocytes are divided into two categories: *granulocytes* and *agranulocytes*. The term granulocyte relates to the presence of specific granules in the cytoplasm of these cells, which can be used to differentiate the neutrophil (neutral or pale pinkish granules), eosinophil (reddish-orange granules), and basophil (dark blue or purplish granules). The differing affinity of the granules for neutral, acidic, and basic stains gives them their characteristic color. Agranulocytes, which include lymphocytes and monocytes, lack distinctive granules. Leukocytes mount the body's response to tissue injury and infection. In general, these cells are integral to the immune system, participating in both innate (nonspecific) and adaptive (specific) immune responses.

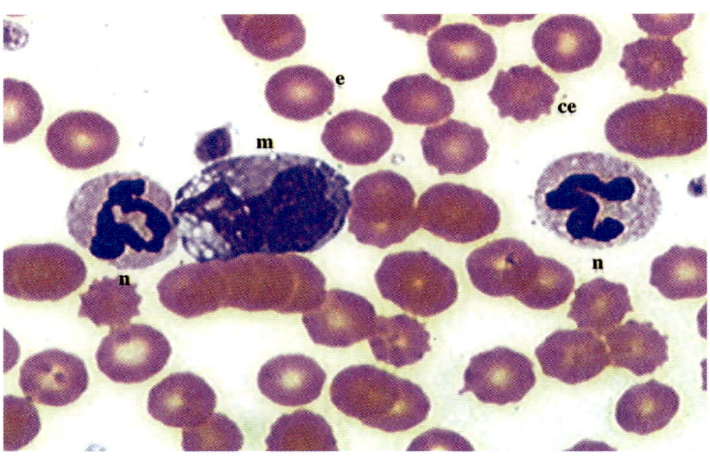

Figure 6-3 Two neutrophils (n) and one monocyte (m) are surrounded by erythrocytes (e) in this smear of canine blood. The neutrophil is characterized by a segmented nucleus and neutral-staining cytoplasm. Neutrophils are the most numerous circulating granulocytes and rapidly invade tissues in response to microbial infection. Monocytes are the largest circulating leukocyte; they have a pleomorphic nucleus and gray-blue cytoplasm with vacuoles. Erythrocytes, or red blood cells, have a biconcave shape, resulting in a pale-staining center. Crenated erythrocytes (ce) display short surface projections; this alteration in cell shape is an artifact. (Image by J. Messick).

Neutrophil

The primary function of neutrophils is to capture and kill invading organisms, particularly bacteria, within the bloodstream or tissues through a process called phagocytosis. Neutrophils can exit the vasculature, navigating to the site of an insult where they subdue the invader. These cells also have the ability to re-enter the bloodstream after inspecting the tissues.

In response to granulocyte colony-stimulating factor (G-CSF) and other cytokines, neutrophils are produced in the bone marrow and released into the blood once they mature. The mature neutrophil is approximately 12 to 15 μm in diameter and is distinguished by a segmented nucleus, often comprised of three to four lobes containing clumped or heterochromatic chromatin (Fig. 6-3). The granules within neutrophils contain many hydrolytic enzymes and antibacterial substances needed to inactivate and digest phagocytosed microorganisms. The cytoplasm of neutrophils is rather transparent because the granules are small and neutral-staining in most mammalian species. In contrast, the cytoplasmic granules of neutrophils in rabbits, guinea pigs, birds, amphibians, and reptiles are large and red, and the cell is called a heterophil (Fig. 6-4).

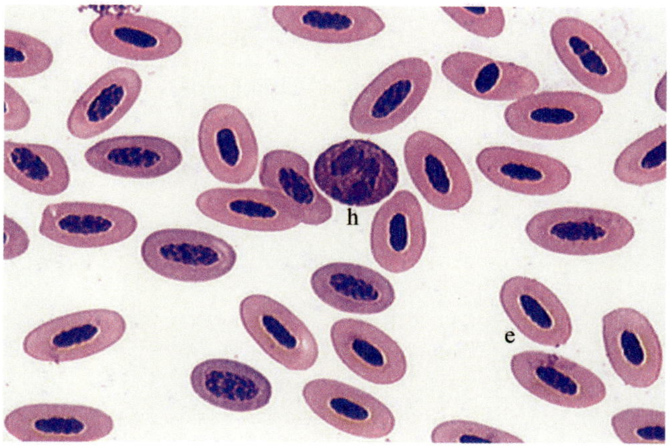

Figure 6-4 Heterophil and erythrocytes, avian blood. Avian erythrocytes (e) are oval, and mature cells retain their nucleus, unlike mammalian erythrocytes. Heterophils (h) have large, red cytoplasmic granules. The heterophil is analogous in function to the mammalian neutrophil, which lacks prominent granules. (Image by J. Messick).

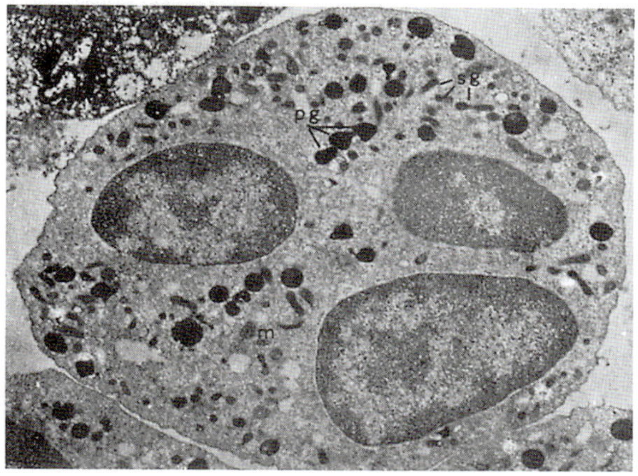

Figure 6-5 Electron micrograph of a mature neutrophil from canine bone marrow stained for peroxidase. The neutrophil contains large, spherical, peroxidase-positive primary granules (pg) and small, pleomorphic, peroxidase-negative secondary granules (sg). Some mitochondria (m) are present. The nuclear lobes show chromatin condensation. (From Jain NC. Schalm's Veterinary Hematology. 4th Ed. Philadelphia: Lea & Febiger, 1983.)

Electron microscopic and cytochemical studies have revealed that neutrophils contain an active Golgi complex but few mitochondria. The cytoplasmic granules of the neutrophil vary in size and peroxidase activity. Primary granules (azurophilic granules) are larger and peroxidase-positive, whereas secondary granules (specific granules) are smaller and lack peroxidase activity (Fig. 6-5). The primary granules are membrane-bound and contain enzymes such as acid hydrolases, neutral proteases, and elastase. Microbicidal elements, including myeloperoxidase, lysozyme, defensins, and bactericidal permeability-inducing protein, are also contained in primary granules. Interspecies variation in the cytochemical reactivity and content of the primary granules has been reported. Secondary (specific) granules of neutrophils contain enzymes such as alkaline phosphatase, collagenase, and C5a-splitting enzymes. Neutrophils possess both oxygen-dependent and oxygen-independent systems for destroying internalized microorganisms within their secondary granules. These antimicrobial elements include cationic proteins and enzymes such as hydrolases, proteases, lactoferrin, lysozyme, and defensins, along with enzymes that generate toxic metabolites of oxygen.

In most animal species, neutrophils are the most numerous circulating white cells, accounting for 40 to 80% of the total white cell count. They function as the body's first line of defense against microbial infections. After spending a brief time of approximately 8 hours circulating in the blood, neutrophils migrate into surrounding tissues and body cavities to carry out their specific functions. Thus, the entire circulating pool of neutrophils is turned over about three times daily. Physiologic stimuli, such as stress (corticosteroids) or fear (epinephrine), can increase neutrophil numbers, either by enhancing bone marrow release or redistributing these cells in the blood. Both the production and release of neutrophils from the bone marrow contribute to the increased neutrophil count in blood associated with inflammatory conditions such as infection, infarction, or trauma.

The circulating neutrophilic cells in a normal, healthy animal typically include mature, segmented neutrophils along with a few band neutrophils. The band neutrophil, a slightly less mature neutrophil, is approximately the same size or slightly larger (12 to 15 μm) than the mature segmented neutrophil. The nuclear chromatin pattern of the band is less condensed, and the nucleus appears nonsegmented with a smooth contour and parallel-appearing sides. The mature neutrophil (segmented neutrophil) shares features with the band neutrophil, but its nucleus typically has 2 to 5 distinct lobes connected by fine nuclear filaments. The cytoplasm of both band and segmented neutrophils is clear and contains pale- or neutral-staining granules. The numbers of band neutrophils and less mature cells of the neutrophilic series may increase in response to an inflammatory disease process. If the numbers of bands increase, but remain less than the numbers of mature neutrophils, this blood count is referred to as a "left shift." Other morphologic indications of an inflammatory blood picture may include the presence of blue cytoplasmic inclusions known as Döhle bodies (aggregates of ribosomes and endoplasmic reticulum), cytoplasmic basophilia, and cytoplasmic vacuoles.

Eosinophil

Eosinophils develop and mature in the bone marrow under the influence of specific cytokines and growth factors. Interleukin-5 (IL-5) is a key cytokine essential for the final stage of eosinophil differentiation acts as trigger for their release into the bloodstream. Furthermore, IL-5 promotes the survival of eosinophils once they migrate into the tissues.

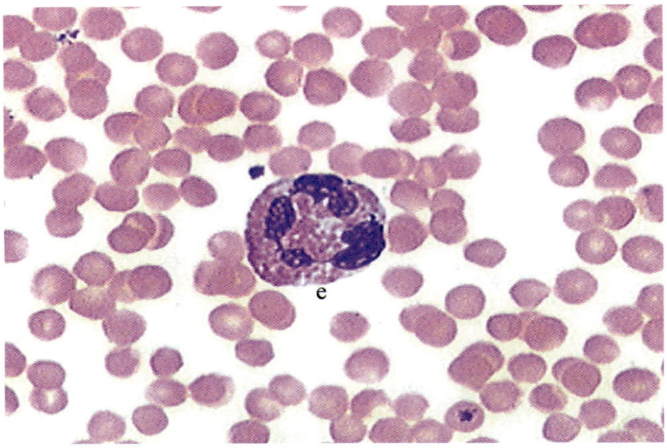

Figure 6-6 Eosinophil, bovine. Eosinophils (e) have red granules in their cytoplasm. These cells play an important role in acute inflammatory, allergic, and anaphylactic responses. (Image by J. Messick).

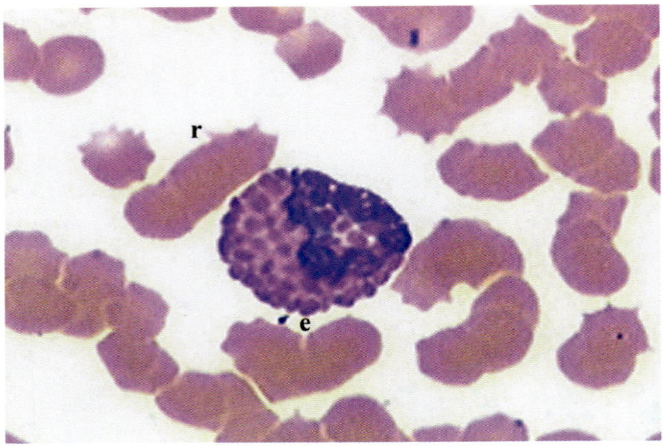

Figure 6-7 Eosinophil, equine. The bright reddish granules in the equine eosinophil (e) are larger than those of other species. The eosinophil nucleus rarely has more than two lobes, in contrast to the three or four lobes of the neutrophil nucleus. Stacking of red blood cells or rouleaux formation (r) is a common finding in the blood of horses. (Image by J. Messick).

Eosinophils are approximately the same size as neutrophils but are easily distinguished by the presence of bright reddish granules in their cytoplasm. The granules of the eosinophil have an affinity for eosin, a red acidophilic dye found in the Wright stain. This staining characteristic is attributed to a high content of arginine-rich, highly basic proteins that attract the acidic dye. Another feature that is helpful in identifying the eosinophil is the presence of a nucleus that rarely has more than two lobes, whereas the neutrophil nucleus usually has three or four lobes.

The size, shape, number, and staining characteristics of the granules in eosinophils vary among the different animal species. In dogs, the granules rarely fill the cytoplasm of the cell and may vary from small, homogeneous pinkish orange to vacuolated granules. The granules in the eosinophil of cats are rod-shaped and numerous, staining reddish. Large, bright reddish granules are found in horses, whereas smaller, less intensely stained granules that almost completely fill the cytoplasm are seen in sheep, goats, cows, and pigs (Figs. 6-6 and 6-7).

Ultrastructural studies of the eosinophil have shown that the Golgi complex elaborates many primary granules (azurophilic granules). These granules are larger than primary granules in neutrophils. The secondary granules (specific granules) of canine eosinophils vary from dense homogenous granules surrounded by a narrow rim of lighter matrix to a clear vesicle with only a cap of dense material. A few mitochondria and remnants of rough endoplasmic reticulum are also found in mature eosinophils (Fig. 6-8). Feline and guinea pig eosinophils have characteristic crystalloid specific granules, whereas other species, including cows and horses, have only homogenous granules.

Eosinophils usually account for only 0 to 8% of the total leukocyte count, giving absolute numbers of 0 to 500 eosinophils/μL of blood. The intravascular lifespan of the eosinophil is extremely short, estimated at less than 1 hour in dogs. Eosinophils play important roles in acute inflammatory, allergic, and anaphylactic reactions, and in controlling infestations by helminthic parasites. In the process of regulating allergic and inflammatory responses, these cells phagocytize immune complexes and inhibit the release and replenishment of histamine and other vasoactive amines. The phagocytic and bactericidal capabilities of eosinophils are limited when compared to those of neutrophils. It has been demonstrated that eosinophils may also induce damage in tissues and play a role in fibrosis when present in excessive numbers. Substances such as antigen–antibody complexes, fibrin, fibrinogen, and factors released from stimulated T-lymphocytes, basophils, or mast cells may act as chemotactic factors for eosinophils. Histamine, released by both mast cells and basophils in response to tissue injury or allergic reactions, is the major chemotactic factor for eosinophils.

Basophil

Basophils, the rarest granulocytes in blood, are mainly involved in hypersensitivity and anaphylactic reactions. They are derived from stem cell progenitors in the bone marrow. Although several cytokines and growth factors contribute to the differentiation of basophils, interleukin-3 (IL-3) is the key driver. Basophils are released into circulation as mature cells and are easily recognized by their characteristic deep-purple cytoplasmic granules. Upon stimulation, these cells exert powerful immunoregulatory functions through the release of effector molecules and cytokines from their granules.

The basophil measures 10 to 15 μm and has a segmented nucleus. Characteristic deep-purple granules often fill the cytoplasm and obscure the nucleus. The purplish staining of the granules is ascribed to their content of sulfated glycosaminoglycans. Granules of feline basophils are rod-shaped and usually stain dull purplish gray due to lack of sulfated glycosaminoglycans, whereas granules of canine basophils stain reddish violet (Fig. 6-9) Basophil granules in dogs do not fill the cytoplasm of the cell, in contrast to the granules in basophils from cows, horses, and cats. In some species, the granules are water-soluble and may be partially dissolved or lost during the process of staining the blood smear.

Basophils rarely account for more than 0 to 1.5% of the total leukocyte count or 0 to 200 basophils/μL of blood. Evidence supports the role of basophils in allergic conditions, including urticaria, allergic rhinitis, allergic conjunctivitis, asthma, allergic gastroenteritis, and anaphylaxis caused by drug reactions or insect stings. Another function of basophils is to promote lipolysis. Heparin released from the granules of basophils promotes the release of lipoprotein lipase from endothelial cells of the blood vessel wall. This process causes clearing of chylomicrons from the blood and facilitates the metabolism of triglycerides. Basophils also play a major role in mediating inflammatory responses. The anticoagulant actions of heparin and the procoagulant effects of protease-generated kallikreins that are secreted by basophils may antagonize and promote hemostasis, respectively.

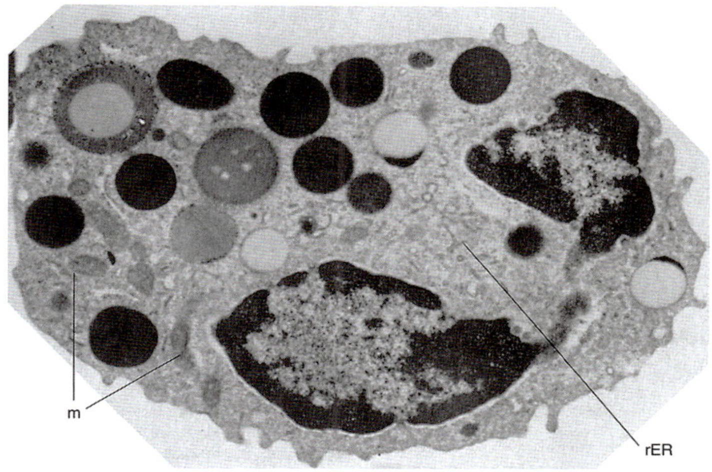

Figure 6-8 Electron micrograph of a canine eosinophil. The cell contains pleomorphic granules. Dense and light homogeneous granules and clear vesicles are present. A few mitochondria (m) and remnants of rough endoplasmic reticulum (rER) are scattered throughout the cell. (From Jain NC. Schalm's Veterinary Hematology. 4th Ed. Philadelphia: Lea & Febiger, 1983.)

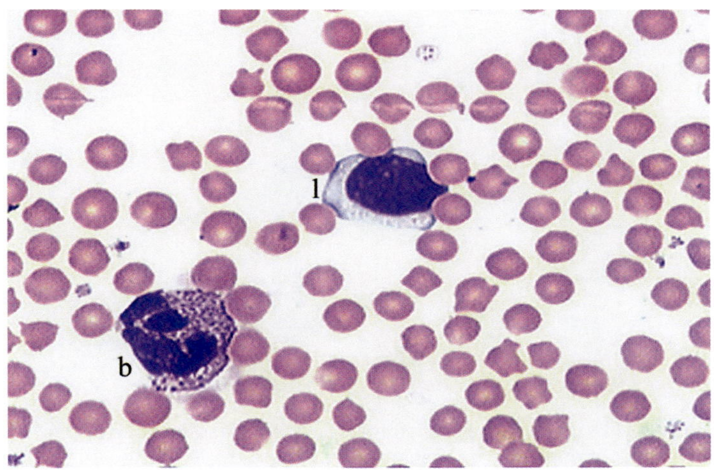

Figure 6-9 Basophil and lymphocyte, ovine. Lymphocytes (l) have a round to slightly indented nucleus. The nuclear-to-cytoplasmic ratio is higher than in other leukocytes. The cytoplasm of lymphocytes is generally agranular. Lymphocytes play a key role in the immune response. A basophil (b) is also present in this blood smear. (Image by J. Messick).

Monocyte

The mononuclear phagocyte system (MPS) consists of three types of cells: monocytes, dendritic cells (DCs), and tissue macrophages (fetal- and HSC-derived). Monocytes and DCs arise from HSCs in the bone marrow and are closely related to neutrophils, sharing the same progenitor cell population (common myeloid progenitor) in their differentiation pathway. Upon release from the bone marrow, monocytes and DCs only transiently circulate in the peripheral blood. They exit the vasculature, either randomly or in response to an inflammatory stimulus, and monocytes become tissue macrophages. While macrophages remove apoptotic cells and microbes by phagocytosis, DCs are professional antigen presenting cells and contribute to the activation of T cells. A population of fetal-derived macrophages is also found in tissues; these resident macrophages have a high self-renewal capacity. Thus, both fetal- and HSC-derived macrophages may coexist in various tissues and contribute functionally at those sites. Cells of the MPS are found in the blood and are widely distributed in various tissues throughout the body. Specific cells such as stellate macrophages (Kupffer cells) in the liver, alveolar and interstitial macrophages in the lung, and synovial cells in the joints are part of the MPS.

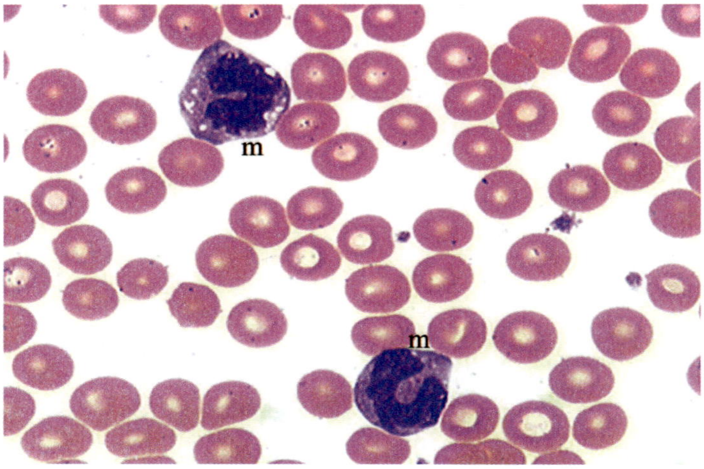

Figure 6-10 Monocyte, canine blood. Note the large size of monocytes (m) by comparing them to surrounding erythrocytes. The dark purple nucleus is horseshoe-shaped. Characteristic cytoplasmic vacuoles are visible in the upper cell. (Image by J. Messick).

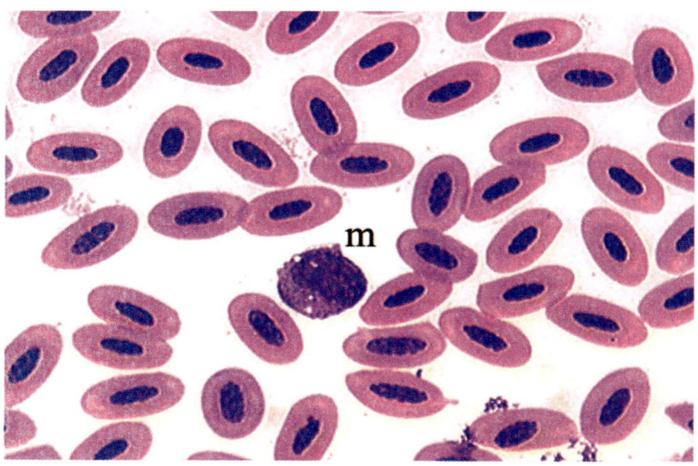

Figure 6-11 Monocyte and erythrocytes, avian. Avian monocytes (m) are similar in appearance to mammalian monocytes. Note the nucleated erythrocytes surrounding the monocyte. (Image by J. Messick).

Monocytes are the largest leukocytes in the blood. They vary from 12 to 20 μm in diameter and have a pleomorphic nucleus, which may appear elongated, folded, indented, horseshoe-shaped, or even lobed. The nuclear chromatin of monocytes is lacy or reticular with some areas of condensation, and nucleoli are inconspicuous. The cytoplasm is abundant and grayish blue in color, often containing a few discrete vacuoles and/or fine azurophilic granules (Figs. 6-10 and 6-11). Monocytes account for 3 to 8% of the total leukocyte count. Thus, the absolute number of monocytes is approximately 200 to 1000 cells/μL of blood. Increased numbers of monocytes in the blood may be associated with chronic infectious or inflammatory conditions, trauma, autoimmune diseases, and some malignancies. The circulating half-life of monocytes in the blood varies among species.

Upon leaving the blood, monocytes differentiate into long-lived macrophages under the influence of specific tissue factors. The young macrophage is similar in morphology to circulating monocytes, but with time, they become activated, increasing in size, phagocytic activity, and lysosomal enzyme content. Electron micrographic studies (Fig. 6-12) often show many short microvillus-like projections along the surface of the macrophages, and the cytoplasm is frequently vacuolated. Although tissue macrophages are capable of cell division, most of the macrophages at an inflammatory site are recruited from the blood. The exact lifespan of macrophages in tissues is unknown. It appears that resident macrophages are long-lived; however, macrophages that accumulate in response to inflammatory stimuli are shorter-lived.

Monocyte/macrophages are functionally and phenotypically a heterogeneous population of cells. At least two subsets (classical and nonclassical) are recognized; however, there are significant overlaps and conflicting reports regarding their functions. Classical monocytes can differentiate into macrophages in the tissue and play a critical role in the initial inflammatory response. Phagocytosis and digestion of cellular debris, microorganisms, and particulate matter are major functions of classical monocytes. These cells express various pattern recognition receptors or toll-like receptors (TLRs) on their surface, which detect invading microbes by recognizing specific pathogen-associated molecular pattern molecules (PAMPs). Thus, they initiate the body's immune response to the pathogen and produce cytokines and growth factors that drive the production and recruitment of more monocytes and other inflammatory cells to the site of the intruding pathogen. Further, classical monocytes are capable of presenting antigen to lymphocytes, which initiates specific humoral and cellular immune responses. On the other hand, nonclassical monocytes appear to be sentinels, serving as a first line of defense in recognition and clearance of pathogens and damaged or neoplastic cells, as well as playing a role in maintaining vascular endothelial homeostasis. Although they are widely recognized to be more involved in promoting the resolution of inflammation, in some cases they may contribute to disease progression.

Lymphocyte

Lymphocytes, a key component of the adaptive immune response, develop in the bone marrow from a pluripotential HSC. While B-lymphocytes mature in the marrow, a subset of lymphocytes exits the marrow and matures in the thymus gland. The latter cells are known as T-lymphocytes. B-lymphocytes express surface immunoglobulin (Ig) receptors and play a role in antibody-mediated or humoral immunity, whereas T-lymphocytes express T-cell receptors and are involved in cell-mediated immunity. Development of B- and T-lymphocytes is largely dependent on the unique microenvironment provided by stromal cells in the bone marrow and thymus, respectively.

Lymphocytes are variable in size. The smaller cells are 6 to 9 μm in diameter, which is only slightly larger than a red blood cell, while larger lymphocytes measure up to 15 μm in diameter (Figs. 6-13 and 6-14). Small lymphocytes are the most numerous and may be found in the blood, lymphatic circulation, and lymphatic tissue. In the blood of dogs and cats, most lymphocytes are small, whereas both small and large lymphocytes are present in the blood of cows, sheep, and goats. These large lymphocytes are mature and lack nucleoli.

The cell profile of lymphocytes is normally round and smooth with light microscopy, whereas short microvilli may be observed on their surface with electron microscopy (Fig. 6-15). Lymphocytes have a round to slightly indented nucleus with clumped heterochromatin. Although classified as agranular, some lymphocytes may have a few azurophilic granules in their cytoplasm. The nuclear-to-cytoplasmic ratio of small lymphocytes is high, with only a modest amount of pale blue cytoplasm.

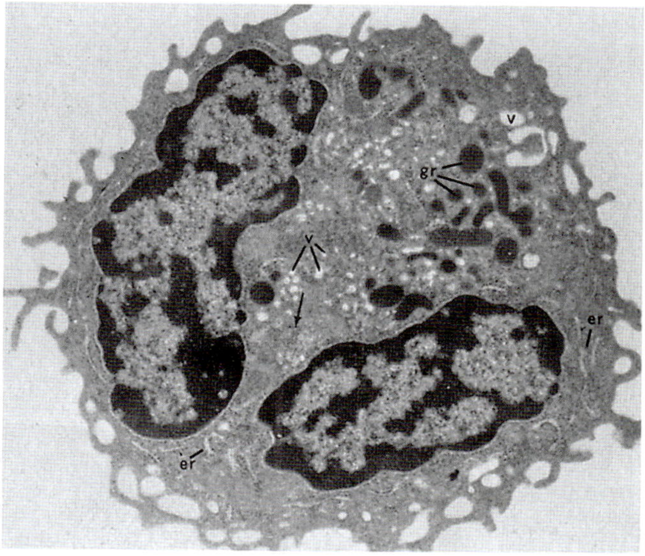

Figure 6-12 Electron micrograph of a canine monocyte. The cell contains many lysosomal granules (gr), several small to large vesicles (v), abundant ribosomes (arrow), and prominent rough endoplasmic reticulum (er), especially along the cell periphery. This cell also has many microvillus-like projections along the cellular outline. The nucleus appears bilobed and shows areas of chromatin condensation. (From Jain NC. Schalm's Veterinary Hematology. 4th Ed. Philadelphia: Lea & Febiger, 1983.)

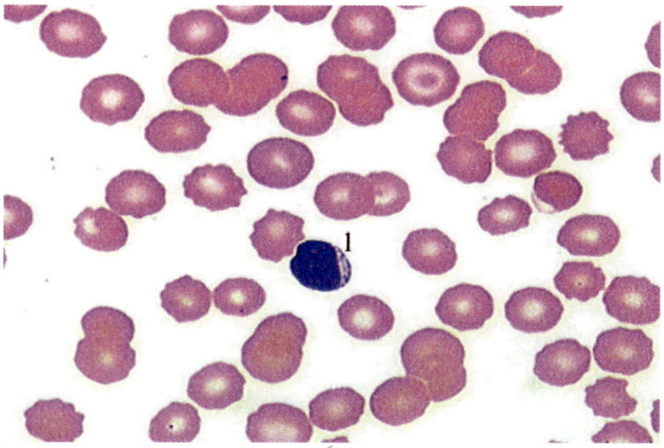

Figure 6-13 Lymphocyte, canine. Lymphocytes (l) vary considerably in size. Compare this small canine lymphocyte with the larger lymphocyte in Fig. 6-9. Note that this small lymphocyte is similar in size to the neighboring erythrocytes, which measure 6–8 μm. (Image by J. Messick).

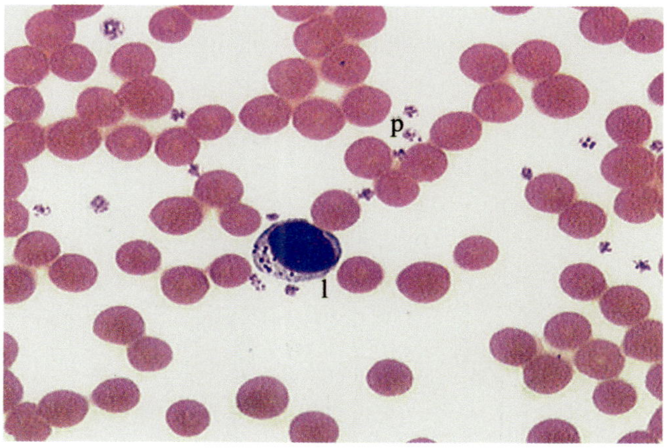

Figure 6-14 Lymphocyte with granules and platelets, bovine. Although lymphocytes (l) are generally agranular, azurophilic granules are occasionally present in the cytoplasm, as in this bovine cell. Several platelets (p) are scattered among the erythrocytes. (Image by J. Messick).

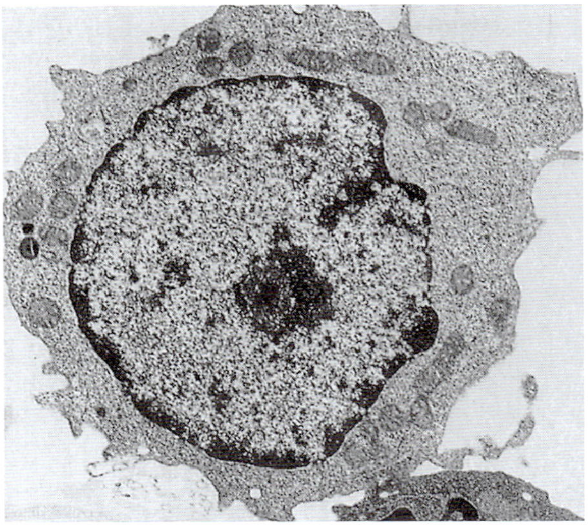

Figure 6-15 Electron micrograph of a canine lymphocyte. The cell has a moderate amount of cytoplasm surrounding a large nucleus with a nucleolus. The cytoplasm is rich in free ribosomes, has some profiles of rough endoplasmic reticulum and scattered mitochondria, and contains dense granules (azurophilic granules). (From Jain NC. Schalm's Veterinary Hematology. 4th Ed. Philadelphia: Lea & Febiger, 1983.)

The number of lymphocytes in the peripheral circulation varies among the species. These cells account for 20 to 40% of the total leukocyte count in dogs, cats, and horses but may be 50 to 60% of the leukocyte differential in cows, mice, and pigs. Most of the lymphocytes in the bloodstream are T-lymphocytes.

Platelets/Thrombocytes

In the bone marrow, megakaryocytes are responsible for the formation and release of platelets into the bloodstream. These cells arise from pluripotent stem cells, developing into a bipotential progenitor cells (megakaryocyte-erythroid progenitor), before starting their lineage-specific differentiation. The mature megakaryocyte is the largest hematopoietic cell in the bone marrow, yet it comprises less than 1% of all the nucleated cells in this tissue. Thrombopoietin (TPO) is the primary regulator of platelet production or thrombopoiesis.

Platelets vary in size from 5 to 7 µm in length and 1.3 to 4.7 µm in width among animal species. A slight variation in platelet size is present in most species but is greatly accentuated in cats (Fig. 6-16). Larger platelets, or proplatelets, up to 20 µm in length can be occasionally observed in the blood of horses. In stained blood smears, platelets are discoid, oval, or elongated fragments of cytoplasm that lack a nucleus and have fine, reddish-purple granules. The terms platelet and thrombocyte are often used interchangeably; however, when describing the nucleated platelet in fish, reptiles, and birds, the term thrombocyte is preferred (Fig. 6-17).

When observed by electron microscopy, resting platelets have a smooth surface with random indentations that represent the membranous invaginations of the open canalicular system (OCS) (Fig. 6-18). This system opens to the platelet surface and is used for externalization of platelet secretory products and internalization of substances from plasma into the platelet. Bovine platelets are devoid of an OCS and secrete their contents directly to the exterior. Normal platelets are covered with amorphous material that forms a thin external glycocalyx. This glycoprotein-rich layer is responsible for the platelet's adhesive properties.

Beneath the surface membrane of the platelet, some microfilaments and a bundle of microtubules are observed by electron microscopy. These cytoskeletal elements maintain normal platelet shape and make up the contractile system. Thus, they are responsible for the change in shape of platelets following activation and the subsequent secretion of

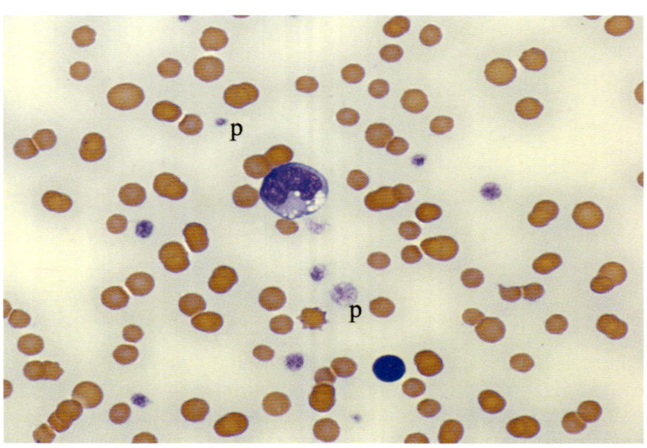

Figure 6-16 Platelets of cat. Platelets (p) vary in size, which is typical for this species.

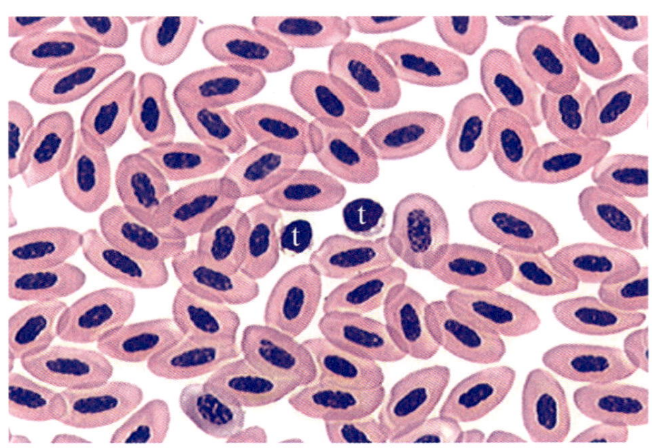

Figure 6-17 Thrombocyte, avian. Avian thrombocytes (t) retain their nuclei. These cells perform the same function as smaller, anucleate mammalian platelets. (Image by J. Messick).

platelet granules. Another series of channels, the dense tubular system (DTS), is found deep to the superficial cytoskeleton. The DTS provides a site for sequestration of calcium and localization of enzymes for prostaglandin synthesis. The internal structure of the platelet is composed of many α-granules, electron-dense granules, and glycogen particles, with only a few mitochondria and lysosomes. The α-granules are membrane-bound and contain platelet factor 4, coagulation factors I (fibrinogen) and V (proaccelerin), platelet-derived growth factor, and many other components. Electron-dense granules are a storage pool for adenine nucleotides, histamine, serotonin, catecholamines, and calcium.

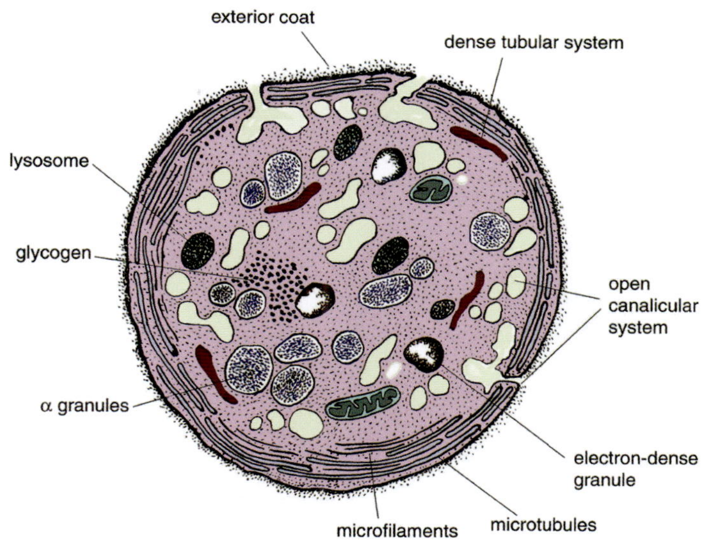

Figure 6-18 Schematic drawing of the fine structure of a platelet.

The number of platelets in circulation ranges from about 200,000 to 400,000/μL of blood. In general, the lifespan of circulating platelets in domestic animal species is about 8 to 12 days. A key role of platelets is maintenance of primary (platelet plug formation) and secondary (coagulation) hemostasis. Following blood vessel damage, platelets become activated and adhere to the exposed tissues, forming a platelet plug. Coagulation factors aggregate on the surface of the plug, ultimately stabilizing the plug and transforming it into a clot that stops the bleeding.

Bone Marrow

Structure and Function

Bone marrow is the site of hematopoiesis, a process by which highly differentiated cells in the peripheral blood are produced. The marrow is surrounded by cortical bone that transitions inward in some areas to form a network of interconnected rods and plates called trabeculae. The spaces or pores formed between these trabeculae are filled with bone marrow; this is the marrow space, the primary site of hematopoiesis. It consists of hematopoietic cellular elements and a complex microenvironment (Fig. 6-19).

In the adult animal, bone marrow is contained within the medullary cavity of flat and proximal portions of long bones, representing almost 5% of total body weight. It is a soft, gelatinous tissue that is divided into irregular, interconnected spaces by bony trabeculae. The rapidly dividing, hematopoietic precursor cells (erythroid, myeloid, and megakaryocytic lineages) are an extremely labile population that continuously undergoes a process of self-replication and/or differentiation. These precursor cells produce all the peripheral blood cells, including erythrocytes, leukocytes, and platelets.

Cells of the bone marrow microenvironment, which include stromal cells (fibroblast-like reticular cells, endothelial cells, adipocytes, and macrophages), accessory cells (T-lymphocytes, natural killer cells, and monocytes/macrophages), and their products [extracellular matrix (ECM) and cytokines], are distributed throughout the bone marrow space. These components provide a scaffold as well as nutrient support for the developing hematopoietic cells. The supporting cells also play an active role in the regulation of hematopoiesis by direct cell-to-cell contact and/or by secreting regulatory molecules that either positively or negatively influence the growth of hematopoietic precursor cells. ECM molecules, such as collagen, fibronectin, laminin, thrombospondin, hemonectin, and proteoglycans, produced by stromal cells, bind and present growth factors to hematopoietic precursors cells. In addition, osteoblasts and osteoclasts associated with adjacent trabecular bones are part of the marrow microenvironment. These cells are responsible for the formation and resorption of bone, respectively.

Blood Supply

The bone marrow receives arterial blood from two major sources. One primary source is the nutrient artery, which penetrates the bony shaft at the nutrient foramen and branches to run parallel to the long axis of the bone in the central part of the marrow cavity (central artery). This artery then gives off several branches that extend throughout the marrow cavity and feed a branching network of arterioles and sinusoids that are intimately associated with the hematopoietic spaces. The second source

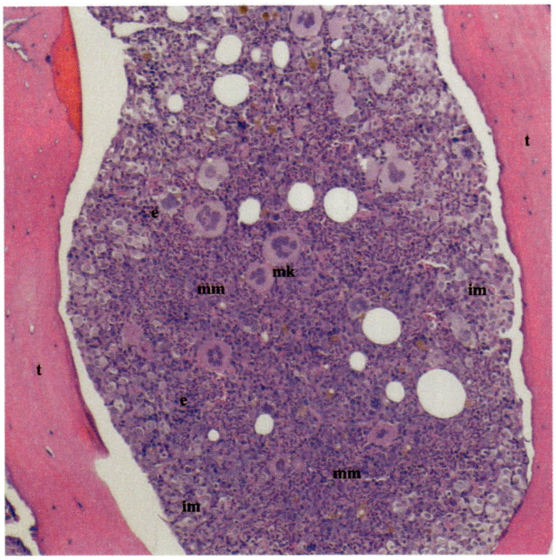

Figure 6-19 Bone marrow core biopsy of dog stained with hematoxylin and eosin (H&E). Trabecular bone (t) surrounds the marrow space filled with immature and mature myeloid (im and mm), erythroid (e), and megakaryocytic (mk) cellular elements. Fat content is minimal, and sinusoids are obscured by the hematopoietic precursors.

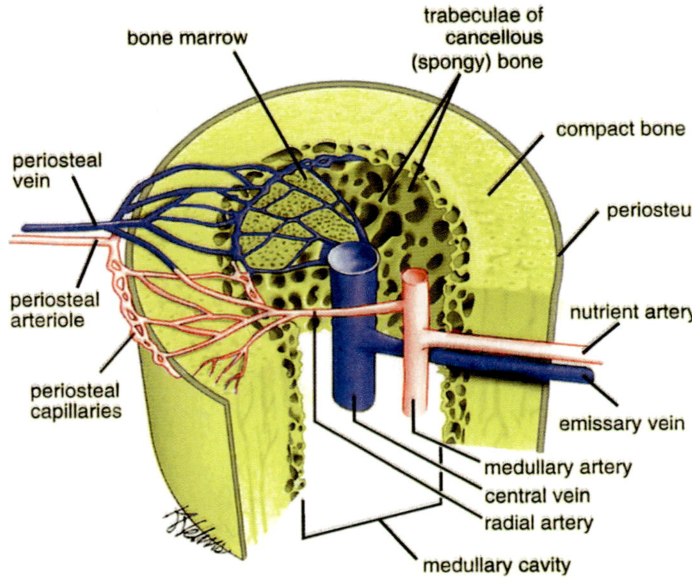

Figure 6-20 Schematic drawing of the microcirculation of the bone marrow. The sinusoids receive blood from two sources: the nutrient artery and a periosteal capillary network, both of which penetrate the cortical bone through numerous osteal canals.

of blood supply to the bone marrow comes from the periosteal network that sends small vessels into perforating canals in the cortical bone (Fig. 6-20). These transosteal vessels branch and join with the blood supply that feeds the sinusoids of the bone marrow. Blood drains from the sinusoids in the marrow into the longitudinal central vein, which empties into veins within the perforating or nutrient canals. These veins form the major vascular outflow tracts from the marrow.

The perfusion of bone marrow space by an extremely dense and highly interconnected microvascular network is essential for supplying oxygen and nutrients and for eliminating metabolic wastes. While the concentration of small arterioles and sinusoids is highest near the bone, in central areas of the marrow, the density is less. This pattern parallels the distribution of hematopoiesis, which is greater in areas near bone and lowest in the vicinity of the central artery. Experimental studies in various animal species estimate the proportion of cardiac output received by bone and marrow compartments ranges from 10 to 15%. Although the bone marrow is devoid of lymphatics, it has a rich nerve supply that accompanies the blood vessels. These nerve fibers respond to intramedullary pressure resulting from cellular proliferation, transmitting signals to the vessel walls. This signaling mechanism results in adjustments of blood flow and release of hematopoietic cells into the circulation.

Sinusoids

The walls of sinusoids within the bone marrow space are thin and lined by a single layer of endothelial cells on the inside (vascular space), called sinusoidal endothelial cells (SECs). Outer layers, including a basement membrane and supporting reticular cells, are either discontinuous or completely absent in the sinusoids. A selective barrier between the blood and bone marrow results from the loose intercellular junctions created by the overlap of adjacent endothelial cells. (Fig. 6-21). As a result of the unique structure of the wall, the sinusoid may dilate readily to accommodate a highly active, hyperplastic bone marrow. The reticular cells covering the outer surface of the sinusoid wall appear to control access of cells from the marrow space into the circulation. When there is massive demand for peripheral blood cells, the amount of surface covered by these cells is markedly reduced. Reticular cells of the bone marrow are also phagocytic and can accumulate a substantial amount of fat, thereby reducing the marrow space available for hematopoiesis.

During development, a stratification of hematopoietic cells in the marrow space occurs, with immature cells in areas nearest the trabecular bone and mature cells at the vascular interface. Upon reaching maturity, hematopoietic cells migrate from the marrow space across the endothelium into the lumen of the sinusoid, thereby gaining access to the vascular or blood compartment. The bone marrow endothelium was once thought to have intracellular pores but is now recognized to be continuous. Red blood cells and leukocytes migrate through attenuated areas of the endothelium (transcellular migration or diapedesis), particularly near their intercellular junctions. A high steady state of diapedesis is essential to maintain peripheral blood levels of these cells. In addition to the transcellular migration of mature blood cells, the cytoplasmic processes of megakaryocytes penetrate the sinusoid wall. These projecting portions of the megakaryocyte dribble small cell fragments known as platelets into the circulation.

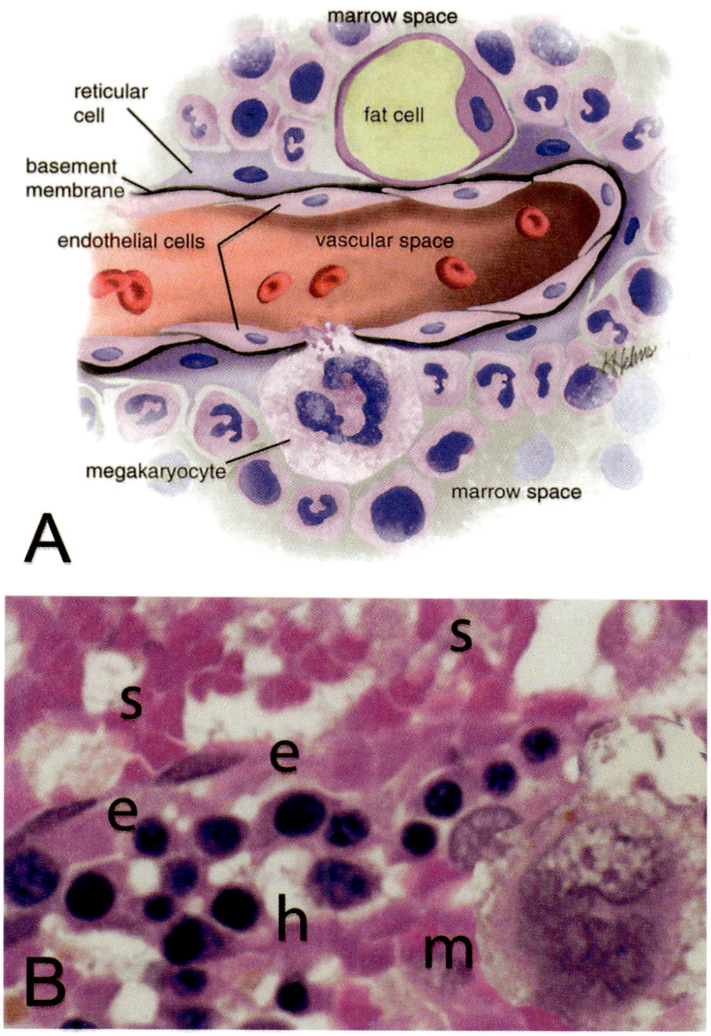

Figure 6-21 **A.** Schematic drawing of the bone marrow, showing the vascular (sinusoid) and marrow (hematopoietic) compartments. The hematopoietic cells are closely associated with thin-walled venous sinusoids. The sinusoid walls consist of a single layer of endothelial cells with a discontinuous or absent basement membrane. The reticular cells branch into the marrow spaces and come in intimate contact with hematopoietic precursors. **B.** Histologic section of a bone marrow core biopsy stained with H&E, showing (s) sinusoid or vascular spaces and (h) hematopoietic or marrow space. The epithelial lining cells of the sinusoid (e) and a megakaryocyte (m) adjacent to the sinusoid are also shown.

Stromal Cells

Endothelial Cells

Endothelial cells of the bone marrow sinusoids have been shown to support the proliferation and differentiation of myeloid and megakaryocytic progenitors. The primary function of SECs includes regulating the trafficking (outgoing) and homing (incoming) of hematopoietic cells into and out of the marrow. One consequence of this unique function is that only selected cells may gain access to a recipient's bone marrow after a bone marrow transplant. Endothelial cells and fibroblast-like cells are often indistinguishable in a Wright's-stained marrow smear.

Reticular Cells

Fibroblast-like reticular cells support the walls of the bone marrow sinusoids and make up the "web" within the marrow space on which the hematopoietic cells grow. These supporting cells may be further categorized based on their location. Fibroblast-like cells occupying interstitial spaces are referred to as reticular cells, whereas those found in the periphery of small vessels are called adventitial cells. Collectively, these supporting cells are also known as adventitial reticular cells. The morphology of these cells is somewhat variable. Because of their elongated processes, the cells may range up to 30 μm in overall diameter. A few primary granules and vacuoles are commonly found within the cytoplasm. The cell nucleus is typically spherical to ovoid in shape with a fine chromatin pattern and a variable number of nucleoli. Fibroblast-like cells are part of the marrow stromal microenvironment and induce the proliferation of early myeloid and B-lymphoid progenitor cells.

Branching from the sinusoid wall into the marrow space, fibroblast-like reticular cells may completely encircle developing hematopoietic precursor cells. These cells are tightly associated with the marrow vasculatures and assist in hematopoiesis by binding essential growth factors. Excessive proliferation of reticular or stromal cells (myelofibrosis) in the sinusoid wall and/or within the marrow space may result in the failure of mature hematopoietic cells to gain access to the circulation. The peripheral blood of patients with myelofibrosis is often characterized by a severe pancytopenia (reduction in the number of circulating blood cells). Myelofibrosis has been recognized in dogs and cats with underlying myeloproliferative diseases, as a terminal event in dogs with a red cell metabolic defect (pyruvate kinase deficiency), and in feline leukemia–infected cats; however, most cases in animals are idiopathic.

Adipocytes

The adipocyte is a prominent component of the marrow stroma. Its nucleus is often eccentric and compressed by fat-laden cytoplasmic vacuoles. The number of adipocytes in the bone marrow space depends on the age of the individual animal and the location of the marrow. Marrow cellularity approaches 100% (red marrow) at birth, and hematopoiesis may extend into the diaphysis of long bones in neonatal animals. In contrast, the marrow cavity of long bones in adult animals contains mostly fatty tissue (yellow bone marrow). Active bone marrow is found only in the sternum, ribs, vertebrae, scapulae, skull, pelvis, and proximal ends of the femur and humerus in adult animals. The proportion of fatty tissue may increase dramatically with age, and cellularity declines, such that hematopoietic cells may occupy as little as 10 to 20% of the marrow space in geriatric animals. The diaphysis of long bones in the adult and older animals is typically filled with yellow marrow. These age-related differences are important when interpreting marrow cellularity.

Proliferating hematopoietic cells may rapidly replace marrow adipose tissue when there is increased demand for blood cell production. Animals with certain diseases, such as severe hemolytic anemia or chronic hypoxia, may have a markedly reduced bone marrow fat content. In contrast, in other diseases such as aplastic anemia, excessive infiltration of yellow marrow has been reported. This condition is characterized by extremely low numbers of hematopoietic precursors, replacement of areas of active hematopoiesis by adipocytes, and peripheral blood pancytopenia. Certain therapeutic drugs also influence the amount of fat in the bone marrow (adipogenesis), in particular, steroidal anti-inflammatory agents are known to suppress bone formation while stimulating adipocyte production in the marrow.

Adipocytes not only act as a passive storage site for energy in the bone marrow but also secrete cell-signaling molecules known as adipokines. These cytokines can function locally, contributing to the promotion of hematopoiesis and bone remodeling. However, there is evidence that adipocytes are also involved in controlling adipose mass and inflammatory responses, and they may be involved in regulating glycolipid metabolism at distant sites.

Osteoblasts and Osteoclasts

In bone marrow biopsy specimens, osteoblasts and osteoclasts are found adjacent to bony trabeculae (Fig. 6-22). Osteoblasts, like stromal cells, are derived from a specific mesenchymal stem cell line that is distinct from the HSC. The osteoblast has a large, eccentric nucleus with prominent nucleoli and abundant basophilic cytoplasm. These cells are involved in the deposition of osteoid and formation of new bone. Osteoblasts may be seen lining trabecular bone in bone marrow biopsies of young animals but are rare in biopsies from adults. The osteoclast is involved in resorption and remodeling of bone. These cells are derived from the monocytic lineage and are multinucleated cells. The nuclei of osteoclasts are discrete and individual, which distinguishes them from the single, hyperlobulated nucleus of the megakaryocyte.

Hematopoiesis

Hematopoiesis is the process by which highly differentiated cells in the blood (erythrocytes, leukocytes, and platelets) develop from a pluripotent HSC. In the embryo and fetus, HSCs move from blood islands in the yolk sac to developing organs. Primitive nucleated red blood cells that produce embryonic hemoglobin are released into the circulation early in gestation. The hematopoietic activity of the yolk sac is short-lived, and its declining production of blood cells is accompanied by a sharp increase in hematopoiesis by the liver. It is unclear whether hematopoiesis begins in the liver through differentiation of primitive mesenchymal cells into HSCs or by colonization with stem cells that migrate from the yolk sac. Definitive hematopoiesis, which develops in the liver, is characterized by HSCs capable of self-renewal and the generation of progenitors committed to erythroid, myeloid, megakaryocytic, and lymphoid lineages. The spleen, lymph nodes, and thymus may contribute to hematopoiesis during this phase, but these organs generally are more active in lymphocyte production. The liver and spleen retain their potential for hematopoiesis throughout life. When hematopoiesis is present in these organs in the adult animal, the process is termed extramedullary hematopoiesis (EMH) and is considered an abnormal finding. EMH, for the most part, is a compensatory response to insufficient bone marrow production of blood cells. The most common conditions associated with marked splenic EMH in the dog are myelofibrosis, marrow failure or hypoplasia, and myeloproliferative disorders. Severe anemia in both dogs and cats may also play a role in the development of EMH in the spleen. Rodents are notable exceptions since their spleen normally serves as a hematopoietic organ.

It is likely that the concentration of growth factors and selective ECM components in organs supporting the production of blood cells changes with time. This alteration may explain the shifting of hematopoiesis from one organ to another during fetal life. The bone marrow begins to produce blood cells late in gestation and becomes the primary site of hematopoiesis at birth, continuing to increase cell production thereafter. The bone marrow in the adult animal is an extremely active tissue with a daily output of blood cells approaching 2.5 billion red cells, an equivalent number of platelets, and 1 billion granulocytes per kilogram of body weight.

Although not evident in routine histologic sections, the bone marrow microenvironment is highly organized. The functional unit of erythropoiesis, the **erythroblastic island**, consists of a central macrophage (nurse cell) encircled by erythroid precursor cells. The macrophage provides iron to the developing erythroid cells. Erythroblastic islands are usually located away from the bone trabeculae and near vascular structures (sinusoids), where mature erythrocytes have ready access to the blood. The sinusoids are often indistinct or obscured by the developing hematopoietic cells within the marrow space. Other components of the microenvironment, including the ECM, stromal cells, and a variety of regulatory cytokines, play an important role in supporting the proliferation and/or differentiation of hematopoietic progenitor cells. For example, in the ECM, certain proteoglycans (heparan sulfate, chondroitin sulfate, and hyaluronic acid) bind growth factors and present them to the progenitor cells. The modulation of erythropoiesis by fibronectin, particularly in disease, involves the attachment of this ECM component to early erythroid progenitors, whereas hemonectin participates in the maturation and release of granulocytic cells from the bone marrow. These complex interactions also lead to distinct topographic patterns in the bone marrow. For example, granulopoiesis takes place primarily in subtrabecular areas where the concentration of hemonectin and alkaline phosphatase–producing stromal cells is higher. In addition, stromal cells produce other growth factors that regulate granulopoiesis, including granulocyte–macrophage colony stimulating factor (GM-CSF), granulocyte colony–stimulating factor (G-CSF), and macrophage colony–stimulating factor (M-CSF).

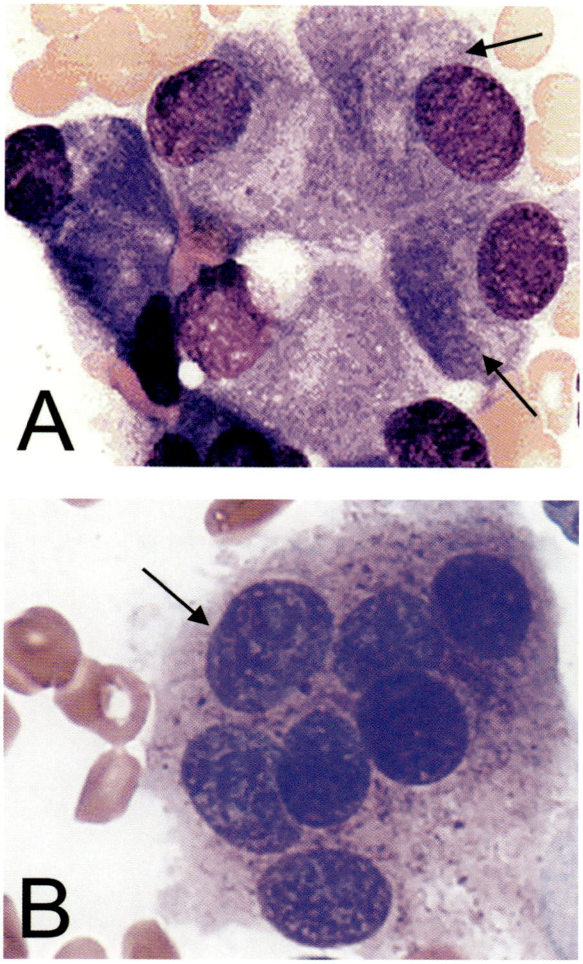

Figure 6-22 Bone marrow smears. **A.** Osteoblasts (arrows). **B.** A single multinucleated osteoclast (arrow).

Hematopoietic Stem Cells

Hematopoietic stem cells primarily reside within the bone marrow. Recent studies suggest that HSCs are enriched in two regions or niches: the arteriolar niche and the sinusoidal-megakaryocytic niche. Both niches localize to highly vascular endosteal regions of the bone marrow. A dense network of stromal cells within these niches is implicated in HSC maintenance, including a population of reticular cells known as CXC chemokine ligand 12-abundant reticular cells. These are the major cellular component of HSC niches.

All cells in the bone marrow, including erythroid, granulocytic–monocytic, lymphoid, and megakaryocytic lineages, originate from HSCs (Fig. 6-23). Over the years, these cells have been given various names, including pluripotent or uncommitted stem cells. The HSCs are rare with an estimated frequency of 0.01% of all the nucleated cells in the marrow and are not morphologically distinct. However, these cells have highly specific homing properties for the bone marrow and can undergo either self-renewal or differentiation into hematopoietic precursor cells. The HSCs may differentiate into two types of primitive multipotent committed precursor cells: colony-forming unit–lymphoid (CFU-L) and colony-forming unit–granulocyte, erythrocyte, monocyte/macrophage, and megakaryocyte (CFU-GEMM). The term colony-forming unit

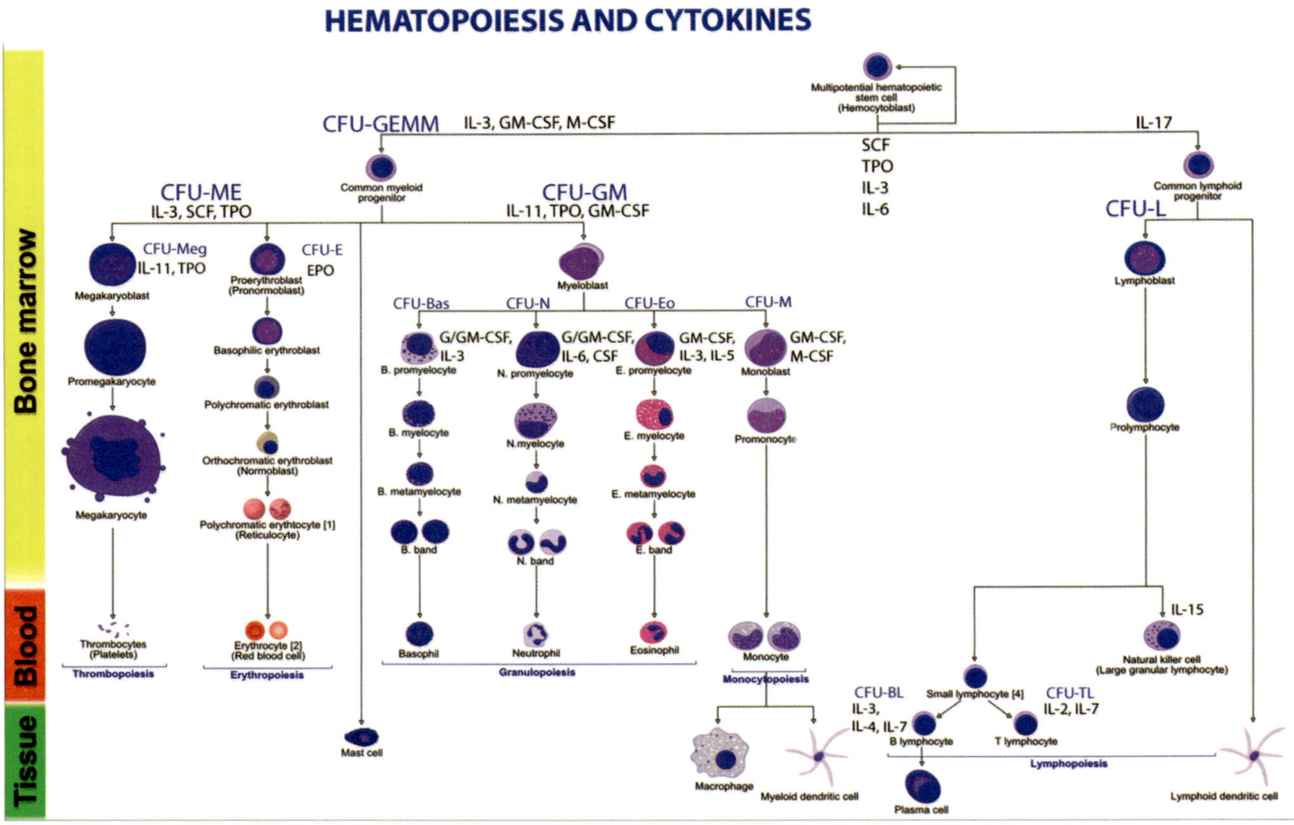

Figure 6-23 Hematopoiesis and cytokines. The hematopoietic stem cell gives rise to all blood cell in the peripheral blood, including myeloid cells (granulocytic, monocytic, erythrocytic, and megakaryocytic lineages) and lymphoid cells (T cells, B cells, and natural killer cells). Cytokines involved in hematopoiesis are also shown. (https://commons.wikimedia.org/wiki/File:Hematopoiesis_(human)_diagram_en.svg / CC BY 3.0)

(CFU) has been adopted to describe an individual cell capable of giving rise to a colony of hematopoietic cells. With further differentiation, multipotent CFUs give rise to committed progenitors that proliferate and mature along restricted pathways. Thus, a bipotent progenitor cell for granulocytes and monocytes (CFU-GM) is derived from the multipotent precursor cell CFU-GEMM, which undergoes further proliferation and differentiation to result in an even more restricted progeny. Thereafter, some progenies can differentiate along the neutrophilic (CFU-N), eosinophilic (CFU-Eo), and basophilic (CFU-Bas) lineages while others differentiate along only the monocytic lineage (CFU-M). Megakaryocytes and erythrocytes are derived from a bipotent erythroid/megakaryocytic progenitor (CFU-ME). In addition, progenitors that are committed solely to the development of erythrocytes (CFU-E) and megakaryocytes (CFU-Meg) have been described. Similarly, further differentiation of CFU-L results in progeny committed to becoming T-lymphocytes (CFU-TL) and B-lymphocytes (CFU-BL). The development of unipotent progenitor cells (CFU-N, etc.) has been characterized both functionally and by membrane antigen expression. Ultimately, the commitment of progenitor cells to specific hematopoietic lineages is controlled through cell-specific transcription factors that initiate a pathway of distinct cellular signals.

Cytokines and Regulation of Hematopoiesis

Several cytokines, including colony-stimulating factors (CSFs), interleukins (ILs), and growth factors, are involved in the regulation of hematopoiesis. The primary effects of these cytokines at different levels in the developmental pathways of blood cells and their progenitors have been extensively studied. There is often a broad and overlapping spectrum of action for various hematopoietic target cells. Whether there is a stimulatory or inhibitory effect of the regulator on the target depends on the concentration and duration of exposure to the cytokine. The maturation stage of the target cell, existing cytokine milieu, and the physical relationship of the target cell to the marrow microenvironment may also influence this response.

For the most part, CSF and ILs are growth-stimulatory cytokines. Synergy between stimulatory cytokines may result in important biologic responses. For example, stem cell factor (SCF), an essential growth factor in normal hematopoiesis, exerts potent effects when combined with granulocyte CSF (G-CSF). IL-3 also demonstrates synergistic effects with interleukin-1 (IL-1) and EPO in the generation of erythroid progenitors, whereas IL-3 and IL-5 promote the development of eosinophils. In normal animals, the effect of TPO primarily is directed at increasing the number of platelets. However, the administration of TPO to an animal with a suppressed bone marrow is associated with greatly accelerated recovery in all three cell lineages. The latter reflects an essential role that TPO plays in the maintenance of HSC within the bone marrow.

Cytokines that primarily act as negative regulators of hematopoiesis include tumor necrosis factor-α (TNF-α), interferon-γ (IFN-γ), transforming growth factor-β, and lactoferrin. There is strong evidence that TNF-α and IFN-γ play a role in the development of anemia of chronic disease. However, the role of lactoferrin in the negative feedback regulation of granulopoiesis is controversial.

Granulopoiesis

Granulopoiesis in the bone marrow shows a distinct pattern of maturation with immature granulocytic precursors in the paratrabecular area and progressive maturation toward the central marrow space. Normal bone marrow has a heterogenous population of hematopoietic cells at various stages of differentiation; however, the most mature cells of a given lineage are present in the greatest numbers, with neutrophilic granulocytes being the most prominent cell lineage. The individual pathways and major cytokines involved in the production of each type of mature blood cell from a precursor or stem cell population are shown in Fig. 6-23 and described in detail hereafter. The characteristic heterogeneity of the marrow may be altered in various hematologic disorders, including inflammation, myelodysplastic syndromes, and hematopoietic neoplasia.

The process of granulopoiesis, or white blood cell formation, begins with the proliferation and differentiation of the myeloblast, which is a progeny of the CFU-GM (Fig. 6-23). The transit time from the myeloblast stage to release of mature granulocytes into the circulation may be as short as 4 to 5 days or as long as 10 days. In general, as these cells mature, their size decreases progressively, their nuclear chromatin condenses, and nucleoli disappear. Ultimately, the nucleus of the granulocyte becomes lobulated or segmented, the cytoplasm gradually loses basophilia, and specific or secondary granules accumulate.

The morphology and development of granulocytes in the bone marrow have been extensively studied. The first three cells of the myeloid lineage, the myeloblast, promyelocyte, and myelocyte, are capable of mitotic cell division. The myeloblast undergoes division and differentiates to produce two promyelocytes, each of which then multiplies and differentiates into two myelocytes (Fig. 6-24). The myelocyte may undergo two or three successive mitotic cell divisions, without significant differentiation, to replicate additional myelocytes. One consequence of multiple successive divisions is that the generation of granulocytes may be amplified at this step. On the other hand, successive divisions may be skipped to expedite the production of mature granulocytes when there is great demand. Each myelocyte undergoes maturation without further cell division, generating the metamyelocyte, band, and mature segmented granulocyte.

Once released into the circulation, the mature granulocytes, which are mostly segmented neutrophils, are distributed between two peripheral blood pools. The marginal granulocytic pool (MGP) consists of granulocytes that line the walls of capillaries and venules, whereas the circulating granulocyte pool (CGP) consists of cells that are more centrally located and free-floating in the vessels. The total and differential cell counts in the complete blood count reflect the CGP. The MGP and CGP are approximately equal in size but may freely exchange cells, thus altering the size of these pools. In cats, the marginal pool of neutrophils is threefold that of the circulating pool. Granulocytes remain in the blood for a brief period, randomly leaving the circulation and moving into the tissues where they perform their specific functions.

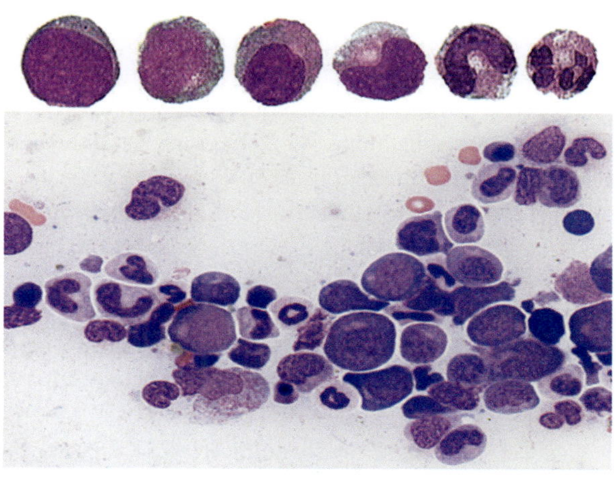

Figure 6-24 Granulocytic lineage (upper figure, left to right): myeloblast, promyelocyte, myelocyte, metamyelocyte, band, and neutrophil. Bone marrow smear (lower figure) showing various stages of granulocyte differentiation.

Granulocytes can also be specifically attracted to tissues that are infected by microorganisms. This process is known as chemotaxis. Under inflammatory conditions, the production and release of granulocytic precursors, predominately neutrophilic, from the bone marrow is increased to meet peripheral demands. Cytokines generated at the site of inflammation, such as G-CSF and GM-CSF, are critical to driving granulopoiesis. The function of the neutrophil is to phagocytize, digest, and kill the invading bacteria. Although the eosinophil is also phagocytic, this cell is primarily involved in limiting hypersensitivity reactions and defending against parasitic infections. The basophil is the source of mediators that promote immediate (allergic and anaphylactic) and delayed hypersensitivity reactions.

Neutrophilic Precursors

Neutrophilic precursors (myeloblasts, promyelocytes, and myelocytes) are the mitotic or proliferating cells of this lineage. The earliest granulocytic precursor that can be morphologically identified is the myeloblast. This cell ranges in size from 15 to 20 μm and is characterized by a spherical nucleus with finely stippled chromatin, one or two nucleoli, and lightly to moderately basophilic cytoplasm. The cytoplasm of the myeloblast lacks or has few primary granules. Typically, myeloblasts lack a prominent light-staining perinuclear region, indicating a poorly developed Golgi complex.

Promyelocytes are slightly larger than myeloblasts and may range up to 25 μm in diameter. The nucleus is often eccentric and has slightly coarser chromatin and prominent nucleoli. A conspicuous light-staining Golgi zone is characteristic of the promyelocyte. The cell cytoplasm is lightly basophilic, more abundant than the cytoplasm of the myeloblast, and contains numerous primary granules. The nucleus of the myelocyte is spherical to ovoid, has coarse chromatin, and lacks distinct nucleoli. In most animal species, the synthesis of primary granules ceases at the myelocyte stage, and the number of these granules decreases during subsequent cell divisions. The appearance of secondary or specific granules in the myelocyte indicates a commitment to development along a specific cell lineage (neutrophilic, eosinophilic, and basophilic myelocytes).

The postmitotic neutrophilic precursor cells include the neutrophilic metamyelocytes and bands, which mature to become segmented neutrophils. In general, as the cell matures, its nucleus varies from indented to band-shaped to a cell with definite lobes. The nucleus of the mature segmented neutrophil has 2–5 lobes with an average of 3; these lobes are connected by a thin strand of nuclear material. The chromatin is bluish-purple and becomes progressively coarser with some clumping; nucleoli are not seen in any of these post mitotic cells. Specific granules are not easily resolved at the light microscopic level, giving the cytoplasm a pale pinkish color. On average, the postmitotic neutrophilic precursors are 10 to 18 μm in size, tending to be smallest when fully mature.

Eosinophilic and Basophilic Granulocytes and Mast Cells

The stages of maturation of eosinophilic and basophilic granulocytes are similar to those of neutrophilic granulocytes. However, the size, shape, color, and number of specific or secondary granules vary greatly among animal species. In general, the secondary granules of the eosinophil are lysosomes, containing enzymes such as peroxidase, acid phosphatase, and arylsulfatase. These granules also contain a variety of highly toxic proteins, such as major basic protein, eosinophil peroxidase, and eosinophilic cationic protein. Based on their affinity for anionic dyes such as eosin, the granules are reddish when stained with routine hematologic stains. The contents of the granules are released directly onto helminthic and protozoan targets to assist in killing the parasites. Eosinophils play a role in anaphylactic and allergic reactions and can phagocytize particles such as immune complexes.

The primary substances stored in granules of the basophil include biogenic amines, heparin, hydrolytic enzymes, proteoglycans, and major basic protein. These granules are dark purple with routine hematologic stains, and they obscure the nucleus in some species. The basophil is mainly involved in allergic and anaphylactic reactions. This process is mediated by cross-linking of surface Ig E antibodies on the basophil, which results in the release of the contents of the granules into the environment. Histamine, a major biogenic amine, contributes to local increases in vascular permeability, smooth muscle contraction, and bronchoconstriction. The basophil may also play a role in host defense against bacterial and viral infections, in some chronic and fibrotic disorders, and possibly in tumor initiation and progression. However, it is controversial whether the secretion of cytokines and chemokines by basophils may result in tumor-promoting or tumor-protecting activities.

Mast cells are traditionally believed to originate from a pluripotent hemopoietic stem cell, a lineage distinct from monocyte and granulocyte precursors. Marrow-derived mast cells mature under the influence of c-kit ligand, SCF, and other cytokines. Mature mast cells are not found in the blood under normal circumstances but migrate into tissues where their maturation is completed. However, recent studies have revealed a distinct population of fetal-derived mast cells present in the tissues. These cells are capable of self-replication and persist in adult animals. Mast cells produced through waves of bone marrow hematopoiesis may contribute to tissue numbers of these cells.

The mast cell is larger than the basophil and has more abundant purplish granules and a spherical nucleus. Although mast cells are normal residents of the bone marrow, only a few are normally present. The committed mast cell precursors move from marrow to blood and then into various tissues, especially respiratory and mucosal tissues. In these locations, the functions of mast cells include promoting hypersensitivity reactions, modulating immune responses, defending against tissue parasites, and promoting acute and chronic inflammatory responses. A subset of mast cells, often found adjacent to microvasculature and neural tissues, may also be involved in angiogenesis and tissue repair.

Monocytopoiesis

Monocytes are produced from HSCs and committed progenitors in the bone marrow known as the granulocyte–monocyte colony-forming unit. The stages of monocyte maturation in the bone marrow progress through an undetermined number of mitotic cell divisions. Monocytes are innate immune cells, playing a key role in host defenses, including the initiation, orchestration, and resolution of inflammation and tissue repair. They represent about 5% of the nucleated blood cells in circulation, with a half-life of 1 to 3 days.

Monocytes migrate from the bloodstream into the tissues in response to stimuli, where they become tissue macrophages. However, recent studies have shown there is a diverse population of tissue macrophages; some macrophages arise from yolk sac progenitors, while others are derived from HSCs. It is recognized that monocytes and macrophages are heterogeneous and functionally diverse, yet our understanding of mechanisms controlling this programming is incomplete.

The monoblast is a morphologically distinguishable, committed progenitor cell of the monocyte/macrophage lineage. It has a spherical to slightly indented nucleus with a fine chromatin pattern and nucleoli but is not easily distinguished from the promonocyte. The mature monocyte is characterized by its indented, often reniform or folded nucleus and an abundant amount of bluish-gray cytoplasm. Generally, monocytes do not have nucleoli but sometimes have small, indistinct primary granules and variable cytoplasmic vacuolation. The cytokines principally involved in the regulation of monocyte development and function include IL-3, GM-CSF, and M-CSF. Canine and bovine GM-CSFs have been produced as recombinant proteins, which, following administration, produce a dose-dependent neutrophilia and monocytosis.

Erythropoiesis and Erythroid Precursors

The differentiation of erythroid precursors in the bone marrow takes place in the erythroblastic islands. These structures consist of a central macrophage surrounded by erythroid precursors at various stages of differentiation. Iron is supplied by the central macrophage to the developing erythroid precursors for hemoglobin synthesis. The central macrophage also provides proliferative and survival signals to the developing precursors and phagocytizes the extruded nuclei at the final stage of erythroid maturation. Typically, the erythroblastic islands are randomly distributed throughout the marrow spaces.

Erythropoiesis, the production of erythrocytes or red blood cells, is controlled by growth factors that permit cellular survival and proliferation, as well as by nuclear regulators that activate lineage-specific genes. Erythropoietin, a hormone produced mainly by the kidney, is the primary physiologic regulator of red cell production. The apoptosis of newly formed erythroid progenitor cells is inhibited by EPO, thereby allowing the cells to differentiate into mature erythrocytes. Erythropoietin also plays a role in the proliferation and differentiation of committed erythroid progenitor cells, and it enhances the release of more mature cells into the blood.

The rubriblast (erythroblast), which is derived from the colony-forming units–erythroid (CFU-E), is the earliest recognizable erythroid precursor (Fig. 6-25). The cell ranges in size from 15 to 25 μm and is characterized by a spherical nucleus, stippled chromatin, one or two nucleoli, and deeply basophilic cytoplasm with a perinuclear pale area and no granules. A single rubriblast undergoes division and differentiates to produce two prorubricytes or basophilic rubricytes (or basophilic erythroblasts). Although similar in appearance to the rubriblast, the nuclear chromatin of the prorubricyte shows some condensation, nucleoli are indistinct, and its overall size is smaller. The prorubricyte undergoes successive mitotic cell divisions and continues to mature, producing polychromatophilic rubricytes (polychromatic erythroblasts). The nuclear chromatin of the polychromatophilic rubricytes is condensed but separated by light streaks, and the cell is slightly smaller in size than the prorubricyte. In the polychromatophilic rubricyte, the change in color of the cytoplasm to a grayish blue indicates that hemoglobin synthesis

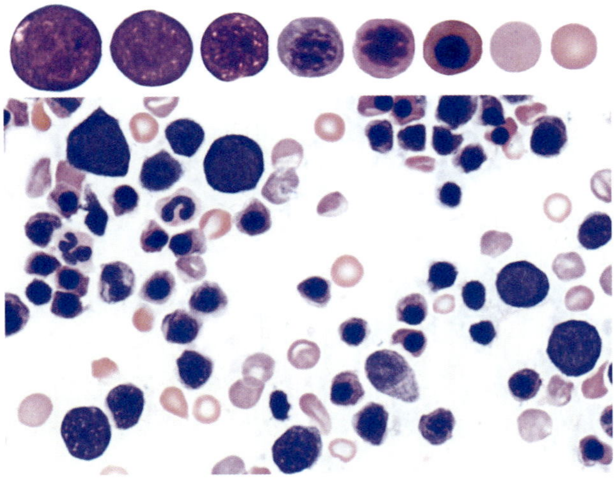

Figure 6-25 Erythrocytic lineage (upper figure, left to right): rubriblast, two basophilic rubricytes—early and late, two polychromatophilic rubricytes—early and late, metarubricyte, reticulocyte, and erythrocyte. Bone marrow smear (lower figure) showing the various stages of erythroid differentiation.

is well under way. Polychromatophilic rubricytes are the last stage in red cell maturation capable of mitotic division, giving rise to the orthochromatic rubricytes or metarubricytes (or orthrochromatic erythroblasts). Metarubricytes are the smallest nucleated erythrocytes, having condensed nuclear chromatin and slightly gray, pink to reddish, almost fully hemoglobinized cytoplasm. A reticulocyte is formed when the metarubricyte expels its nucleus. However, the reticulocyte still contains a significant number of ribosomes, and thus, its cytoplasm stains grayish or a dull bluish pink in Romanowsky stains. While most reticulocytes mature in the bone marrow, some may be released into the circulation alongside fully mature erythrocytes or red blood cells. Within 1 to 2 days, the reticulocytes lose their ribosomes and become mature, circulating erythrocytes.

In general, erythroid precursors become smaller with each successive mitotic division. Their chromatin continues to condense until the nucleus becomes pyknotic and is eventually extruded from the cell. After 3 to 5 days, the rubriblast matures into the reticulocyte, and after an additional 1 to 2 days, the reticulocyte is released into the circulation. When senescent, red blood cells are removed from circulation by the MPS. The lifespan of erythrocytes in circulation varies from about 70 to 160 days in domestic animals.

Thrombopoiesis and Platelet Precursors

Megakaryopoiesis, the differentiation process resulting in platelet production, is highly regulated. Megakaryoblasts are the earliest recognizable precursor cell in this lineage and arise from a multipotent progenitor cell, CFU-GEMM (Fig. 6-23). SCF, IL-3, GM-CSF, and other factors stimulate the production of megakaryoblasts (Fig. 6-26), whereas thrombopoietin (TPO), a hormone produced by the liver, promotes the proliferation and differentiation of megakaryocytic progenitors. TPO also enhances the release of platelets from mature megakaryocytes into the circulation. In response to these factors, the megakaryoblast undergoes endomitosis, a process of nuclear division and cytoplasmic maturation without cellular division. The process of megakaryocytic maturation occurs adjacent to vascular sinusoids in the marrow. During maturation, there is a progressive increase in cell size, nuclear ploidy (number of nuclei), and cytoplasmic volume. The cytoplasm becomes progressively less basophilic and acquires primary granules. The mature cell may contain as many as 16 to 32 nuclei that are discrete but connected.

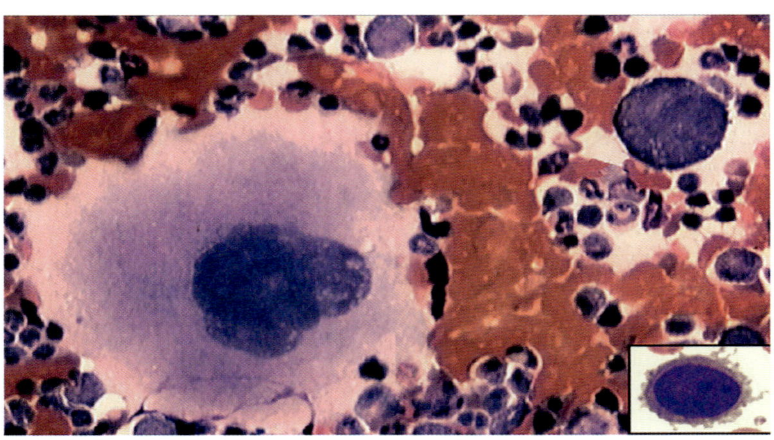

Figure 6-26 Megakaryocytic lineage: bone marrow smear showing a mature, granular megakaryocyte and a promegakaryocyte. A megakaryoblast is shown in the inset.

Platelets are the end product of the megakaryocytic cell lineage. The formation of platelets involves the extension of cytoplasmic projections of the megakaryocyte through the sinusoid endothelium, dribbling platelets (fragments of their cytoplasm) into the vascular space. It is unclear what role TPO and other humoral regulators play in the final stages of platelet formation. Each megakaryocyte is estimated to release 1000 to 3000 platelets into the bloodstream. About two-thirds of the total body platelet mass is found in the circulation, whereas the remaining one-third is present in the spleen.

Lymphopoiesis and Lymphoid Precursors

Lymphocytes, like other hematopoietic cells, originate from a population of pluripotent stem cells (Fig. 6-23). The earliest progenitor cell in this lineage, the lymphoblast, is present in low numbers in the marrow and is difficult to distinguish from rubriblasts and early myeloblasts. A spherical nucleus, fine chromatin, variable number of nucleoli, and a thin rim of deeply basophilic, agranular cytoplasm characterize this cell. The lymphoblast undergoes division and differentiates to produce prolymphocytes that subsequently divide and differentiate into mature lymphocytes. The exact number of mitotic cell divisions that occur between the progenitor and mature stage is not known. Most of the marrow lymphocytes are small with clumped nuclear chromatin and no apparent nucleoli. Up to 20% of the nucleated cells in feline bone marrow are mature lymphocytes, whereas less than 10% are mature lymphocytes in dogs and other species.

There are two populations of mature lymphocytes: T-lymphocytes and B-lymphocytes that function in cell-mediated and humoral immunity, respectively. B- and T-lymphocytes cannot be distinguished by their morphology alone; rather special staining techniques, such as immunophenotyping, are required. While terminal differentiation of B-lymphocytes is known to occur in the bone marrow, immature cells may also migrate to peripheral nodes, spleen, and other lymphoid tissues, where they populate these sites and may mature into small lymphocytes that express cell surface Ig receptors. B-lymphocytes may undergo further differentiation to become antibody secreting B cells known as plasma cells. Plasma cells are distinguished from resting lymphocytes by the presence of more abundant, deeply basophilic cytoplasm, a prominent light-staining perinuclear Golgi zone, and an eccentric nucleus. In birds, the process of B-lymphocyte maturation occurs in the cloacal bursa (bursa of Fabricius).

Some lymphoid precursors leave the marrow and seed the thymus, where they differentiate into thymic or T-lymphocytes. In the bone marrow, a small population of lymphocytes with an abundant amount of lightly basophilic cytoplasm and azurophilic granules is often present. These cells are large granular lymphocytes and function as either natural killer cells or cytotoxic T-lymphocytes. They play an important role in tumor resistance and host immunity to viral and other microbial infections.

Clinical Correlations

An inflammatory condition associated with injury to the pancreas is known as **pancreatitis**. In this case, the bone marrow response (Fig. 6-27) is to produce and release increased numbers of granulocytes to meet tissue (pancreas) demands. Systemic G-CSF and GM-CSF dramatically increase, driving the bone marrow to produce more neutrophils and monocytes. The function of these leukocytes is to phagocytize and kill invading bacteria and clear tissue debris, respectively.

The bone marrow is unable to produce enough hematopoietic cells (erythroid, myeloid, and megakaryocytic cells) in this condition known as **aplastic anemia** (Fig. 6-28). It is caused by damage to the HSCs. The numbers of red blood cells, white blood cells, and platelets are extremely low in the peripheral blood. Most cases of this condition have no known cause but have been reported in association with infectious causes, drug therapy, toxins, and total body irradiation.

Essentials

1) **Blood:** It consists of plasma, a light, yellow-colored liquid with proteins and dissolved substances, and cellular elements, including red blood cells, white blood cells, and platelets.
2) **Erythrocytes or red blood cells:** They are non-nucleated, biconcave cells in the blood carrying hemoglobin, which bind oxygen in the lungs and carry it to the tissues and play a primary role in the transport of carbon dioxide from the tissues back to the lungs to be eliminated. They are produced in the bone marrow from erythroid progenitor cells; EPO is the primary regulator of red cell production (erythropoiesis).
3) **Leukocytes or white blood cells:** Nucleated blood cells are involved in both innate (nonspecific) and humoral/cellular (specific) immune responses. They are classified as granulocytes (neutrophils, eosinophils, and basophils) and agranulocytes (lymphocytes and monocytes). These cells are produced in the bone marrow from myeloid or lymphoid progenitor cells.
4) **Platelets:** Non-nucleated cytoplasmic fragments released into the bloodstream by precursor cells known as the megakaryocytes. Megakaryocytes are produced in the bone marrow from megakaryocytic progenitor cells; TPO is the primary regulator of platelet production (thrombopoiesis).

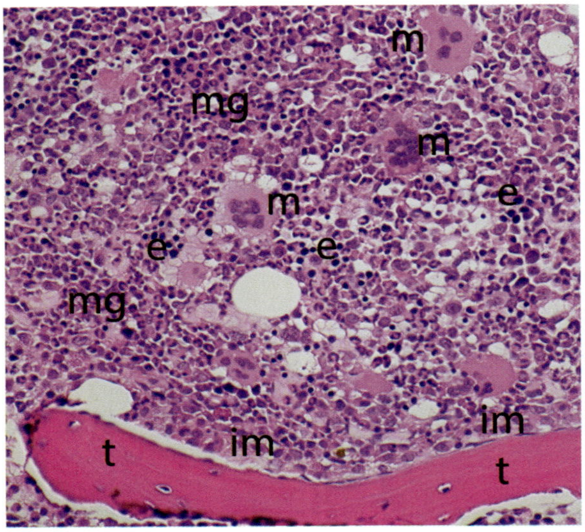

Figure 6-27 Bone marrow core biopsy from a dog with pancreatitis. Marrow cellularity is high, approaching 100% (few adipocytes). There are increased numbers of immature granulocytes (im) close to the trabecular bone (t) with progressive maturation to mature granulocytes (mg) away from the bone and toward central marrow areas. A few erythroid islands (e) and several megakaryocytes (m) are also noted. The expansion of leukocytes at all stages of maturation and the presence of other hematopoietic precursors (erythroid and megakaryocytic) are important features for recognizing this reactive bone marrow response. H&E (×20).

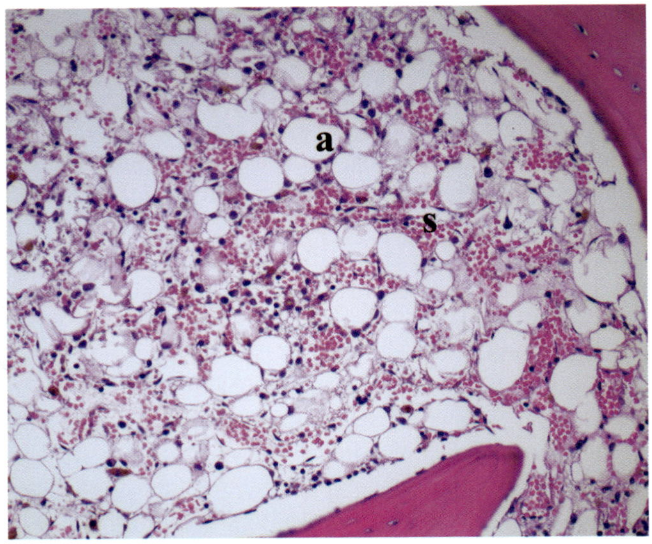

Figure 6-28 Bone marrow core biopsy from a dog with aplastic anemia. Marrow cellularity is profoundly decreased. The hematopoietic marrow spaces are replaced by fat or adipocytes (a). While the sinusoids (s) are not typically visible in a normal marrow, they are easily identified by the mature red blood cells present within them in an aplastic marrow. The dog had very few red cells, white cells, and platelets in its blood. No potential etiology was identified in this case. H&E (×20).

5) **Hematopoiesis:** This is the process by which precursor and mature blood cells of the erythroid, myeloid, and megakaryocytic lineages are produced from pluripotent cells known as hematopoietic stem cells or HSC. Hematopoiesis occurs within bone marrow spaces created by adjacent trabecular bones in an extravascular location.
6) **Bone marrow blood supply**: The two major blood supplies of the bone marrow are the branching nutrient and periosteal arterial networks.
7) **Sinusoids:** Vascular structures, lined by a single layer of endothelium, serve as the site for large-scale cellular trafficking between the extravascular hematopoietic compartment of the bone marrow and the bloodstream.
8) **Bone marrow microenvironment:** It includes stromal cells, accessory cells, and products of these cells including cytokines and ECM. These microenvironmental components provide a scaffold and nutrient support for developing hematopoietic cells.
9) **Cytokines:** These are substances secreted by certain cells, which regulate hematopoiesis, including ILs, CSFs, interferons, EPO, and TPO.

Suggested Readings

Andreasen CB. Neutrophil structure and biochemistry. In: Brooks MB, Harr KE, Seelig DM, et al., eds. Schalm's Veterinary Hematology. New York, NY: Willey Blackwell, 2022: 333–338.

An X, Mohandas N. Erythroblastic islands, terminal erythroid differentiation and reticulocyte maturation. *Int J Hematol* 2011;93(2):139–143.

Aulbach AD, Weiss DJ. Chronic inflammation and secondary myelofibrosis in domestic and laboratory animals. In: Brooks MB, Harr KE, Seelig DM, et al., eds. Schalm's Veterinary Hematology. New York, NY: Willey Blackwell, 2022: 138–143.

Barger AM. Erythrocyte morphology. In: Brooks MB, Harr KE, Seelig DM, et al., eds. Schalm's Veterinary Hematology. New York, NY: Willey Blackwell, 2022: 188–197.

Boudreaux MK, Christopherson PW. Platelet structure. In: Brooks MB, Harr KE, Seelig DM, et al., eds. Schalm's Veterinary Hematology. New York, NY: Willey Blackwell, 2022: 658–666.

Boudreaux MK, Christopherson PW. Thrombopoiesis. In: Brooks MB, Harr KE, Seelig DM, et al., eds. Schalm's Veterinary Hematology. New York, NY: Willey Blackwell, 2022: 651–657.

Cenariu D, Iluta S, Zimta AA, et al. Extramedullary hematopoiesis of the liver and spleen. *J Clin Med* 2021;10(24):831.

Ciofani M, Zúñiga-Pflücker JC. The thymus as an inductive site for T lymphopoiesis. *Annu Rev Cell Dev Biol* 2007;23:463–493.

Dean, L. Blood Groups and Red Cell Antigens (2005). Bethesda (MD): National Center for Biotechnology Information (US); Chapter 1, Blood, and the cells it contains.

Dos Santos AP, Christian JA. Erythrokinetics and erythrocyte destruction. In: Brooks MB, Harr KE, Seelig DM, et al., eds. Schalm's Veterinary Hematology. New York, NY: Willey Blackwell, 2022: 172–180.

Dzierzak E, Philipsen S. Erythropoiesis: development and differentiation. *Cold Spring Harb Perspect Med* 2012;3(4):a011601.

Florencio-Silva R, Sasso GR, Sasso-Cerri E, et al. Biology of bone tissue: structure, function, and factors that influence bone cells. *Biomed Res Int* 2015;2015:421746.

Garden OA, Kidd L, Mexas AM, et al. ACVIM consensus statement on the diagnosis of immune-mediated hemolytic anemia in dogs and cats. *J Vet Intern Med* 2019;33(2):313–334.

Graham GJ, Pragnell IB. Negative regulators of haemopoiesis—current advances. *Prog Growth Factor Res* 1990;2(3):181–192.

Guilliams M, Mildner A, Yona S. Developmental and functional heterogeneity of monocytes. *Immunity* 2018;49(4):595–613.

Harrier CM, Bennett PM, Gascoyne SC, et al. Erythrocyte size, number and haemoglobin content in vertebrates. *Br J Haematol.* 1991;77(3):392–397.

Harvey JW. Veterinary Hematology: A Diagnostic Guide and Color Atlas. Philadelphia: Saunders, 2012.

Hassanshahi M, Hassanshahi A, Khabbazi S, et al. Bone marrow sinusoidal endothelium as a facilitator/regulator of cell egress from the bone marrow. *Crit Rev Oncol Hematol* 2019;137:43–56.

Hawk CT, Leary S, Morris T. Formulary for Laboratory Animals. 3rd Ed. Wiley-Blackwell, 2005.

Holinstat M. Normal platelet function. *Cancer Metastasis Rev* 2017;36(2):195–198.

Iijima T, Brandstrup B, Rodhe P, et al. The maintenance and monitoring of perioperative blood volume. *Perioper Med (Lond)* 2012;2:9.

Joles JA, Rabelink TJ, Braam B, et al. Plasma volume regulation: defences against edema formation (with special emphasis on hypoproteinemia). *Am J Nephrol* 1993;13:399–412.

Kastl BC, Pohlman LM. Basophils, mast cells, and their disorders. In: Brooks MB, Harr KE, Seelig DM, et al., eds. Schalm's Veterinary Hematology. New York, NY: Willey Blackwell, 2022: 373–380.

Kaushansky K. Historical review: megakaryopoiesis and thrombopoiesis. *Blood* 2008;3:981–986.

Klamer S, Voermans C. The role of novel and known extracellular matrix and adhesion molecules in the homeostatic and regenerative bone marrow microenvironment. *Cell Adh Migr* 2014;8(6):563–577.

Krystel-Whittemore M, Dileepan KN, Wood JG. Mast cell: a multi-*functional master cell. Front Immunol* 2016;6:620.

Lawrence SM, Corriden R, Nizet V. The Ontogeny of a neutrophil: mechanisms of granulopoiesis and homeostasis. *Microbiol Mol Biol Rev* 2018;82(1):e00057–e00017.

Levine DN, Andreasen CB. Neutrophil function and responses. In: Brooks MB, Harr KE, Seelig DM, et al., eds. Schalm's Veterinary Hematology. New York, NY: Willey Blackwell, 2022: 339–346.

Lucas D. Structural organization of the bone marrow and its role in hematopoiesis. *Curr Opin Hematol* 2021;28(1):36–42.

Marenzana M, Arnett TR. The key role of the blood supply to bone. *Bone Res* 2013;1(3):203–215.

Mathew J, Sankar P, Varacallo M. Physiology, blood plasma. In: StatPearls [Internet]. Treasure Island (FL): StatPearls Publishing, 2023.

Mayer P, Werner FJ, Lam C, et al. In vitro and in vivo activity of human recombinant granulocyte-macrophage colony-stimulating factor in dogs. *Exp Hematol* 1990;18(9):1026–1033.

McCourt MR, Rizzi TE. Hematology of dogs. In: Brooks MB, Harr KE, Seelig DM, et al., eds. Schalm's Veterinary Hematology. New York, NY: Willey Blackwell, 2022: 971–982.

Metcalf D. Hematopoietic cytokines. *Blood* 2008;111(2):485–491.

Messick JB. A primer for the evaluation of bone marrow. *Vet Clin North Am Small Anim Pract* 2023;53(1):241–263.

Newcomer BW, Cebra C, Chamorro MF, et al. Diseases of the hematologic, immunologic, and lymphatic systems (multisystem diseases). *Sheep, Goat, and Cervid Med* 2021:405–438.

Nichols BA, Bainton DF, Farquhar MG. Differentiation of monocytes. Origin, nature, and fate of their azurophil granules. *J Cell Biol* 1971;50(2):498–515.

Olsen Saraiva Camara N, Lepique AP, Basso AS. Lymphocyte differentiation and effector functions. *Clin Dev Immunol* 2012;2012:510603.

Olver CS. Erythropoiesis. In: Brooks MB, Harr KE, Seelig DM, et al., eds. Schalm's Veterinary Hematology. New York, NY: Willey Blackwell, 2022: 151–157.

Olver CS. Erythrocyte structure and function. In: Brooks MB, Harr KE, Seelig DM, et al., eds. Schalm's Veterinary Hematology. New York, NY: Willey Blackwell, 2022: 158–165.

Passegué E, Jamieson CH, Ailles LE, et al. Normal and leukemic hematopoiesis: are leukemias a stem cell disorder or a reacquisition of stem cell characteristics? *Proc Natl Acad Sci U S A.* 2003;100(Suppl 1):11842–11849.

Radin MJ, Wellman ML. Granulopoiesis. In: Brooks MB, Harr KE, Seelig DM, et al., eds. Schalm's Veterinary Hematology. New York, NY: Willey Blackwell, 2022: 325–332.

Rieger MA, Schroeder T. Hematopoiesis. *Cold Spring Harb Perspect Biol* 2012;4(12):a008250.

Rodnan GP, Ebaugh FG Jr, Fox MR. The life span of the red blood cell and the red blood cell volume in the chicken, pigeon and duck as estimated by the use of Na2Cr51O4, with observations on red cell turnover rate in the mammal, bird and reptile. *Blood* 1957;12(4):355–366.

Rosales C. Neutrophil: a cell with many roles in inflammation or several cell types? *Front Physiol* 2018;9:113.

Sage PT, Carman CV. Settings and mechanisms for trans-cellular diapedesis. *Front Biosci (Landmark Ed)* 2009;14(13):5066–5083.

Sarkaria SM, Decker M, Ding L. Bone marrow micro-environment in normal and deranged hematopoiesis: opportunities for regenerative medicine and therapies. *Bioessays* 2018;40(3):10.

Sebo ZL, Rendina-Ruedy E, Ables GP, et al. Bone marrow adiposity: basic and clinical implications. *Endocr Rev* 2019;40(5):1187–1206.

Sharma R, Sharma S. Physiology, blood volume. In: StatPearls [Internet]. Treasure Island. (FL): StatPearls Publishing, 2023.

Souza CD, Weiss DJ. Monocytes, macrophages, and dendritic cell production. In: Brooks MB, Harr KE, Seelig DM, et al., eds. Schalm's Veterinary Hematology. New York, NY: Willey Blackwell, 2022: 381–394.

Stegner D, vanEeuwijk JMM, Angay O, et al. Thrombopoiesis is spatially regulated by the bone marrow vasculature. *Nat Commun* 2017;8(1):127.

Tvedten H, Moritz A. Reticulocyte and Heinz body staining and enumeration. In: Brooks MB, Harr KE, Seelig DM, et al., eds. Schalm's Veterinary Hematology. New York, NY: Willey Blackwell, 2022: 181–187.

Ushach I, Zlotnik A. Biological role of granulocyte macrophage colony-stimulating factor (GM-CSF) and macrophage colony-stimulating factor (M-CSF) on cells of the myeloid lineage. *J Leukoc Biol* 2016;100(3):481–489.

Warren AL, Yates RM. Lymphocyte ontogeny and lymphopoiesis. In: Brooks MB, Harr KE, Seelig DM, et al., eds. Schalm's Veterinary Hematology. New York, NY: Willey Blackwell, 2022: 395–401.

Wasserkrug-Naor A. Platelet kinetics and laboratory evaluation of thrombocytopenia. In: Brooks MB, Harr KE, Seelig DM, et al., eds. Schalm's Veterinary Hematology. New York, NY: Willey Blackwell, 2022: 971–1033.

Weiss DJ, Smith SA. A retrospective study of 19 cases of canine myelofibrosis. *J Vet Intern Med* 2002;16(2):174–178.

Yoder MC. Blood cell progenitors: insights into the properties of stem cells. *Anat Rec A Discov Mol Cell Evol Biol* 2004;276(1):66–74.

Young KM, Layne EA. Eosinophils and their disorders. In: Brooks MB, Harr KE, Seelig DM, et al., eds. Schalm's Veterinary Hematology. New York, NY: Willey Blackwell, 2022: 363–372.

Yu VW, Scadden DT. Hematopoietic stem cell and its bone marrow niche. *Curr Top Dev Biol* 2016;118:21–44.

Zahr AA, Salama ME, Carreau N, et al. Bone marrow fibrosis in myelofibrosis: pathogenesis, prognosis and targeted strategies. *Haematologica* 2016;101(6):660–671.

7

Cardiovascular System

Ji-Ming Feng

CHAPTER MENU

Most tissues and organs of domestic animals are permeated by a network of tubular passages that conduct the more fluid components of the body. Highly cellular and viscous blood flows through the **blood vascular system**, while the relatively acellular and watery lymph passes through the **lymphatic vascular system**. In domestic mammals, the blood vascular system forms circulatory arcs emanating from and returning to the heart. The lymphatic vascular system forms drainage channels, which join the major veins at the thoracic inlet, facilitating the return of accumulating tissue fluid to the circulating blood.

Dellmann's Textbook of Veterinary Histology, Seventh Edition. Edited by Marxa L. Figueiredo and John J. Turek.

Companion website: www.wiley.com/go/figueiredo/vethistology7e

Blood and lymph flow because of the pressure gradients within the lumina of their respective vascular networks. These pressure gradients arise from several forces, including gravity, the pumping action of the heart, and the movements of musculoskeletal body parts. The pressure inside the vascular tubes differs from the pressure outside, and the resulting pressure gradients, coupled with the shearing forces of fluid flow, likely determine the structure of the various tubular portions comprising the vascular system.

Blood Vessels

Structure–Function Relationships of Blood Vessels

The blood vessels of the **macrovasculature**, including elastic and muscular arteries, as well as accompanying veins, are visible to the naked eye. Arteries of the macrovasculature carry blood from the heart to the **microvasculature**, which includes arterioles, metarterioles, capillaries, venules, and arteriovenous anastomoses. Veins serve as return vessels, transporting blood from the microvasculature back to the heart.

Blood vessels are commonly categorized by their position in the vascular circuit and are histologically characterized by their individual structure, which reflects the particular forces withstood during blood flow and the mechanisms controlling vascular function. Arteries control blood flow to the microvasculature, where blood moves at a slow pace and may pause intermittently due to the delicate balance between blood pressure and the surrounding tissue pressure. In veins, the velocity of the blood flow returns to at least half that of the corresponding arteries, but the blood pressure is reduced.

The contractions of the heart ventricles are the primary force driving blood circulation. Upon each contraction, the thick conducting **elastic arteries**, such as the aorta, receive the initial surge of blood, leading to peak velocities and pressures. The high pressure generated by the blood pumped out of the heart ventricles during contraction (systole) is largely absorbed by the stretch of the highly elastic arterial walls. At the time of ventricular dilation (diastole), arterial wall tension decreases while still maintaining blood pressure, facilitating the distribution of blood into numerous **muscular arteries**. These vessels lead to specific organs or body parts and eventually drain into the **arterioles**, the smallest branches of the arterial tree. The velocity of flow is gradually reduced as additional distributive branches greatly expand the total blood vessel volume, but the pressure in the muscular arteries remains high. Peripheral outflow is regulated by the sympathetic division of the autonomic nervous system, which determines the contraction or relaxation of the smooth muscle cells within the arterial walls.

Frequently, the elastic, muscular, and arteriolar arteries are classified as **large**, **medium**, or **small arteries**, respectively. However, on a comparative anatomic basis, the latter nomenclature can be confusing because an elastic artery in one species, such as a cat, may have a smaller caliber than a muscular artery in another species, such as a large ruminant. Nonetheless, within a single species, the assumption of a relationship between structure and relative size is valid.

From the arterial tree, the vessels open into expansive networks of small, uniformly thin-walled tubules called **capillaries**. In specific organs, such as the liver, bone marrow, and certain endocrine glands, the capillaries are called **sinusoids**. The total blood volume within capillaries and sinusoids significantly surpasses that in arterioles, resulting in a decrease in blood flow velocity from meters per second in the arterial tree to less than 1 mm/second in capillaries. The shearing forces generated by viscous blood flowing through the narrow arterioles reduce the blood pressure until it slightly exceeds the pressure of the surrounding tissue fluid by 10 mmHg or less. Thus, capillaries mainly counter small-scale forces and, therefore, can have thin walls structured from single cells. Blood–tissue exchanges take place within the capillary network, as well as across the walls of postcapillary venules, which share a comparable structure.

Blood from the capillaries and sinusoids returns to the heart via the **veins**. Veins, categorized as **small**, **medium**, or **large veins**, progressively increase in size. They form inverse vascular trees that are analogous to, and in most instances parallel with, the arterial trees. Consequently, arteries and their accompanying veins are commonly seen adjacent to each other in most tissue sections. Usually, a nerve, and sometimes a lymphatic vessel, accompanies the paired blood vessels. However, there are specific exceptions, such as in the lung, where arteries and veins group independently.

Because veins receive blood from low-pressure capillaries, they oppose little residual pressure from the pumping action of the heart. They do, however, withstand pressures caused by gravity and surrounding tissues, such as muscle. The flow of blood through the veins is caused by the minimal pressure of blood flowing from the capillaries into the veins and by pressure differences with surrounding tissues. This flow is augmented by a series of **valves** in the long veins of the extremities that facilitate the movement of blood toward the heart.

The small pressure gradients within the veins result in relatively lower flow velocities compared to arteries. However, despite this, venous channels are larger in comparison to companion arteries; consequently, the rate of flow through the two vessel types is equal. Due to their larger size, veins accommodate nearly half of the total blood volume in the body. The contractile state of the walls of the larger veins plays an important role in determining the total vascular volume.

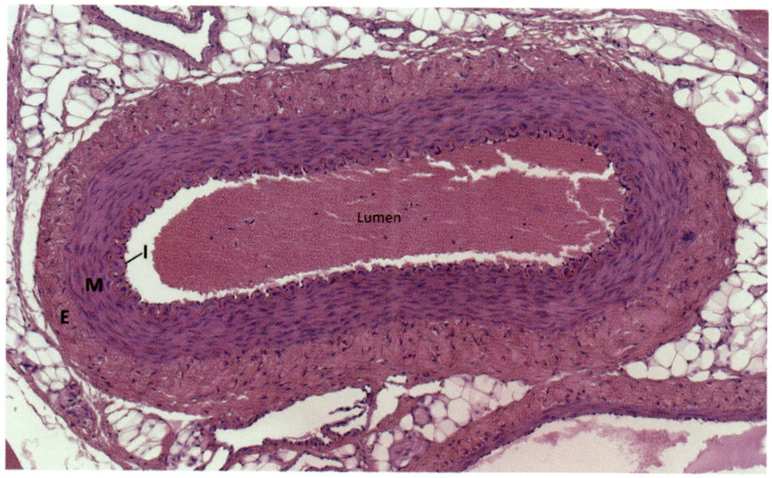

Figure 7-1 Cross-section of a muscular artery. The tunica interna (I) has a prominent wave-shaped internal elastic membrane in arteries. The tunica media (M) consists of several layers of smooth muscle cells. The tunica externa (E) contains many elastic and collagen fibers, which are gradually blended with its surrounding connective tissues. The lumen is filled with blood cells. Hematoxylin and eosin (H&E) (×400). (Image by J. Feng.)

General Structural Organization of Blood Vessels

The walls of all blood vessels larger than capillaries are composed of three concentric layers or tunics: the inner **tunica interna** (intima), the middle **tunica media**, and the external **tunica externa** (adventitia) (Fig. 7-1). Arteries and veins are distinguished from each other based on the thickness of the vascular wall and differences in the composition of the various tunics. Particularly, the tunica media of arteries is much thicker than that of veins (Fig. 7-2).

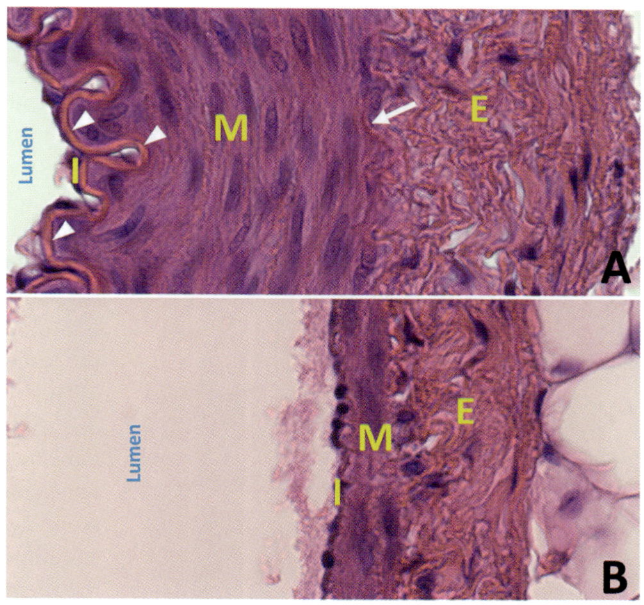

Figure 7-2 Cross-section through part of a muscular artery **(A)** and its companion, a medium vein **(B)**. Arteries have a much thicker smooth muscle layer in the tunica media (M) than in their companion veins. Note the distinguishable, wavy, refractive internal elastic membrane (arrowheads) in the tunica interna (I) and the less clear external elastic membrane (arrow) in the tunica externa (E) of the arterial wall. H&E (×800). (Image by J. Feng.)

The **tunica interna** (tunica intima) is lined with a simple squamous epithelium known as **endothelium**, along with its underlying basal lamina. This vascular endothelium serves as a barrier between the circulating blood and the surrounding tissues or organs. Endothelial cells not only provide a smooth surface but also actively secrete collagens, endothelin, nitric oxide, and von Willebrand factor (vWF). They also have membrane-bound enzymes on the surface, such as **angiotensin-converting enzyme**, which converts **angiotensin I** into **angiotensin II**, and **lipoprotein lipase**, which degrades lipoproteins. Vascular endothelial cells exhibit structural heterogeneity, such as the presence or absence of certain cellular organelles like **Weibel–Palade bodies** (Fig. 7-3). These membrane-bound storage granules are often present in arterial endothelial cells and harbor densely packed tubular elements containing vWF, a regulatory factor for platelet coagulation during clot formation, and P-selectin, an important adhesion molecule involved in the selective seeding of metastatic cells from tumors and the site-specificity of lymphocyte homing. The **subendothelial layer**, which exhibits considerable variation in thickness ranging from inconspicuous in small vessels to visible in large vessels, contains collagen and elastic fibers, fibrocytes, and sometimes smooth muscle cells. The outermost layer of the tunica interna is the **internal elastic membrane (lamina)**. This membrane consists of elastin and contains gaps that permit diffusion of nutrients into the tunica media. In arteries, it is often observed as the highly wavy, strongly refractive membrane (Figs. 7-1 and 7-2A), but it is absent in smaller veins and thinner or inconspicuous in larger veins. The internal elastic membrane can be identified readily by electron microscopy

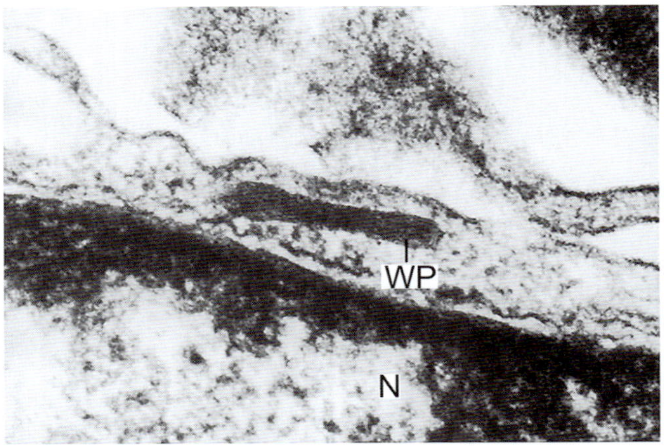

Figure 7-3 Electron micrograph of a part of a porcine endothelial cell of the choroid containing the so-called Weibel–Palade body (WP), longitudinally cut. These are specialized storage granules for von Willebrand factor and P-selectin in the cytoplasm of vascular endothelial cells. Cell nucleus (N) (×150,000).

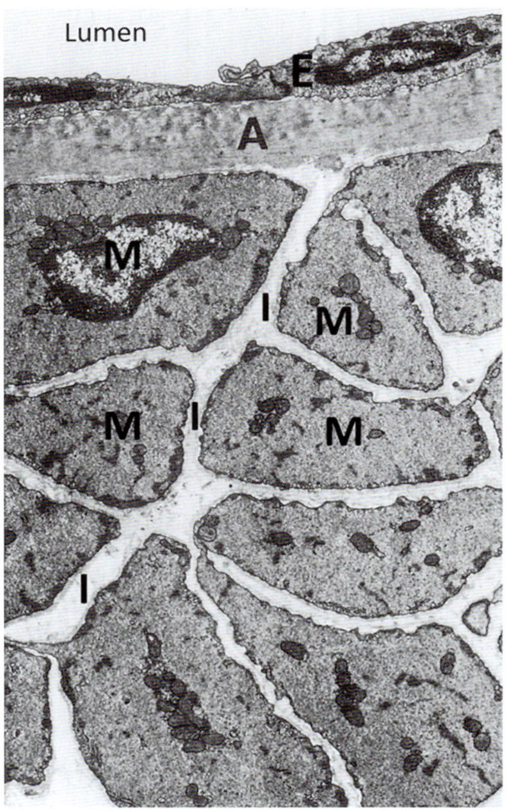

Figure 7-4 Electron micrograph of a part of the wall of a muscular artery. The endothelium (E) rests on a thick internal elastic membrane (A). The smooth muscle cells (M) of the tunica media are surrounded by a basal lamina, and collagen fibrils are present in the intercellular spaces (I) (×7800).

(Fig. 7-4). The tunica interna is avascular and is nourished through the transendothelial transport of substances from the circulating blood.

The **tunica media** consists of several layers of smooth muscle arranged helically, interspersed with varying numbers of elastic laminae, elastic fibers, and collagen fibers. Most of the inner half of the tunica media receives nutrients from the tunica interna, while the remainder is supplied by **vasa vasorum**, which are small blood vessels that nourish the vessel wall. An **external elastic membrane (lamina)**, similar in structure to the internal elastic membrane, is less distinguishable and is only present in the largest muscular arteries (Fig. 7-2A).

In the outermost layer, the **tunica externa** (adventitia), collagen and elastic fibers are predominant, and smooth muscle cells may also be present. This layer also contains vasa vasorum (Fig. 7-5), which extend into the outer layers of the tunica media. Vasomotor nerves **(nervi vasorum)** form plexuses in the adventitia of most large blood vessels, with a few axons penetrating the tunica media and terminating near smooth muscle cells (Fig. 7-6).

Arteries

Elastic Arteries

The tunica interna of elastic arteries, particularly the subendothelial layers, is often thicker than that of other types of arteries (Fig. 7-7). The endothelial cells often have a brick-like shape. The subendothelial layer contains smooth muscle cells, fibroblasts, primarily longitudinally oriented collagen fibers, and numerous fine elastic fibers. In large domestic mammals, this layer is particularly thick (Fig. 7-8). The internal elastic membrane often splits and merges with the elastic lamellae of the tunica media.

The tunica media is the thickest of the three tunics of the vessel wall and consists primarily of concentrically arranged, fenestrated elastic lamellae (Figs. 7-5 and 7-7). Smooth muscle cells lie between adjacent lamellae, to which they are attached by collagen fibrils. The amorphous ground substance is basophilic due to the high quantity of sulfated glycosaminoglycans. All intercellular fibers and ground substance within the media are synthesized by the smooth muscle cells. As the distance from the heart increases, the number of smooth muscle cells in the tunica media of elastic arteries increases, while the amount of elastic tissue decreases. The external elastic membrane is either absent or indistinct.

In the tunica externa, longitudinally arranged bundles of collagen fibers predominate and are intermixed with a few elastic fibers and fibroblasts. The interlacing of the collagen fibers limits the elastic expansion of the vessel.

The transition from elastic to muscular arteries may occur gradually or abruptly. In dogs, typical muscular renal arteries arise immediately at right angles from the elastic abdominal aorta. On the other hand, carotid, femoral, vertebral, and brachial arteries commonly begin as elastic arteries and gradually transform into the muscular type in peripheral regions. The location of the transitional zone for each vessel varies among species and individual animals.

Muscular Arteries

The tunica interna of muscular arteries consists of the endothelium with an underlying thin subendothelial layer composed of collagen and elastic fibers. In large muscular arteries, a few fibroblasts and smooth muscle cells are present. With decreasing vessel size, the subendothelial layer gradually becomes thinner. The prominent, thick internal elastic membrane (Figs. 7-1, 7-2A, and 7-4) has fenestrations through which cytoplasmic processes of endothelial cells contact the smooth muscle of the tunica media. Blood vessel tone is determined by both smooth muscle and endothelial function. These two cell types interact in a dynamic manner to regulate blood vessel diameter.

Muscular arteries are characterized by a thick tunica media, composed mainly of smooth muscle cells arranged in circular or helical wrappings, ranging from 3 to more than 40 cell layers (Figs. 7-1, 7-2A, and 7-4). The external elastic membrane adjacent to the tunica externa is often discontinuous and not always clearly defined.

The tunica externa is primarily composed of collagen fibers, fibroblasts, and elastic fibers, with the number of elastic fibers decreasing as the size of the vessel decreases.

When living tissues are prepared for fixation or when an animal dies, muscular arteries contract considerably,

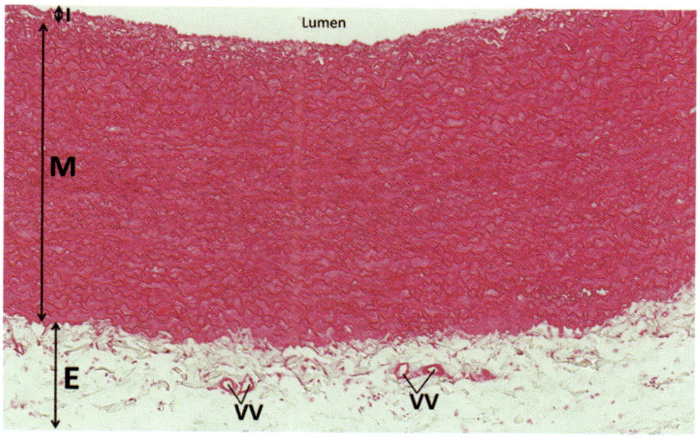

Figure 7-5 Cross-section through part of an elastic artery. Several small branches of the vasa vasorum (VV) are shown in the tunica externa (E). The tunica media (M) is very thick and contains many wave-shaped elastic lamellae. Tunica interna (I). H&E (×150). (Image by J. Feng.)

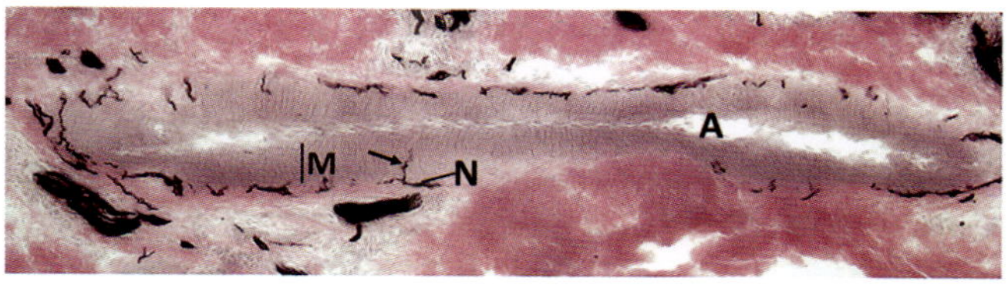

Figure 7-6 Longitudinal section through a bovine pododermal arteriole (A). Nervi vasorum (N) form a plexus around the vessel, and a few axons (arrow) penetrate the tunica media (M). The nerve plexuses and fibers showing acetylcholinesterase activity (black) are highlighted in a histochemistry method, counterstained with nuclear fast red (×100). (Courtesy of Dr S. Buda, Berlin.)

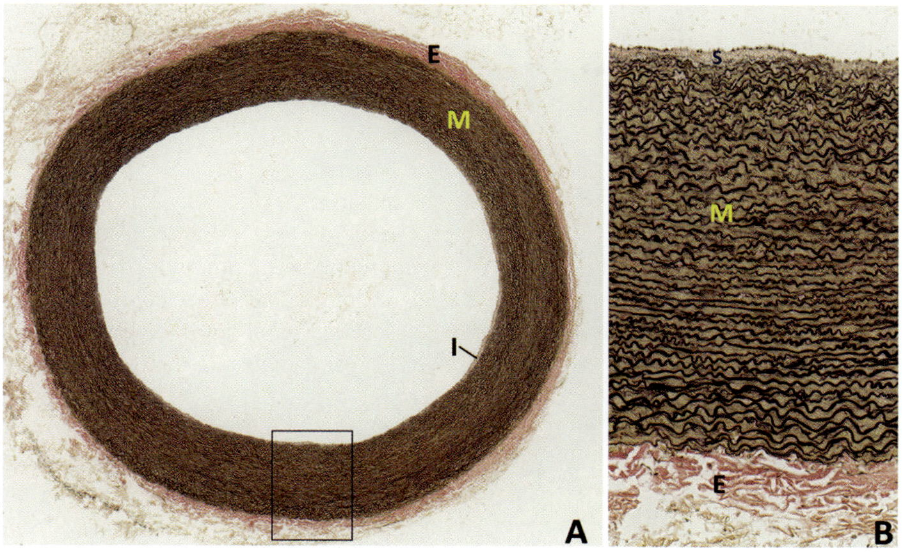

Figure 7-7 Cross-section through the cat carotid artery, an elastic artery at low magnification (**A**, ×25). The tunica media (M) is the thickest layer and rich in concentrically arranged elastic laminae (black). A part of the wall (the boxed region) is enlarged (**B**, ×100) to show the relatively thicker subendothelial layer (S) of the tunica intima (I) compared to other types of arteries. The collagen fiber bundles are stained pink in the tunica externa (E). Verhoeff's elastin stain. (Image by J. Feng.)

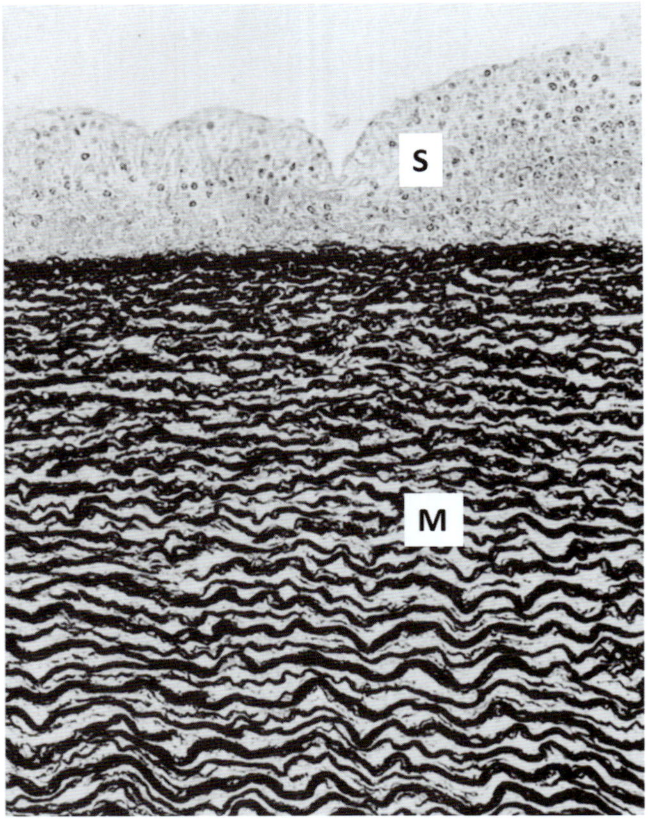

Figure 7-8 Cross-section through part of the wall of the equine thoracic aorta. A particularly thick subendothelial layer (S) contains many longitudinally oriented elastic fibers. In the tunica media (M), elastic laminae predominate. Resorcin–fuchsin–van Gieson's stain (×50). (Courtesy of A. Hansen.)

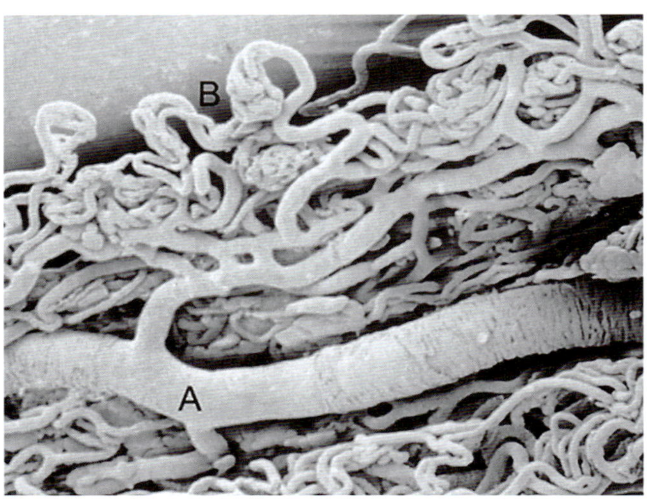

Figure 7-9 Scanning electron micrograph of a microcorrosion cast of a bovine pododermal arteriole (A) with branching convoluted capillaries (B) (×70). (Courtesy of Dr R. Hirschberg, Berlin.)

forcing blood out of the lumina into the more expandable venous circulation. As a result, the tunica interna, including the underlying internal elastic membrane, and the external elastic membrane are thrown into longitudinal folds. Consequently, the cross-sectional profiles of muscular arteries in most histologic preparations show relatively small lumina containing little blood, and the elastic membranes appear scalloped (Figs. 7-1 and 7-2A).

Microvasculature

In its simplest form, the microvasculature comprises afferent arterioles leading to capillary networks drained by efferent venules. Shunts may exist between arterioles and venules, either in the form of arteriovenous anastomoses or central channels that create preferential flow through capillary beds. In many organs, the microvasculature has unique architectural and structural characteristics. Examples of exceedingly intricate and extremely convoluted microcirculation are found in the lung, hoof, and claw (Fig. 7-9).

Arterioles

The tunica interna of arterioles consists of endothelium, a thin subendothelial layer of collagen and elastic fibers (which is absent in the smallest arterioles), and an internal elastic membrane. The internal elastic membrane is fenestrated and eventually disappears in the smallest arterioles, allowing basal processes of the endothelial cells to establish direct contact with the underlying smooth muscle cells of the tunica media. The tunica media typically contains one to three layers of smooth muscle cells (Fig. 7-10), and an external elastic membrane is absent. The tunica externa consists of loose connective tissue (CT).

Capillaries

Capillaries are tubules of uniform diameter that are approximately 8 µm wide (ranging from 5 to 10 µm). The walls of capillaries are composed of endothelial cells, an associated basal lamina, pericytes, and a thin adventitial CT layer. Notably, this adventitial layer is absent around brain capillaries (Figs. 7-11 to 7-15). A tunica media is absent.

Pericytes (Figs. 7-11 and 7-12) are cells enclosed within the basal lamina of capillaries and postcapillary venules and characterized by numerous processes. They are considered to be undifferentiated mesenchymal cells that can be readily stimulated to divide mitotically and to migrate around or away from vessels. Pericytes may play a critical role in blood vessel development and maturation, with the potential to transform into other cell types, especially fibroblasts and smooth muscle cells. Apparently, a capillary can transform by this means into other types of vascular tubes if the internal flow characteristics change. Indeed, this concept is compatible with the embryogenic development of arteries and veins, which originate as simple endothelium-lined capillary-like tubes during **vasculogenesis** or **angiogenesis**. Recent research indicates that various soluble factors can either activate or inhibit capillary growth in certain tissues.

Capillaries form networks called **capillary beds**, the density of which is a reflection of the metabolic requirements of different organs. For example, capillary beds are most densely packed in cardiac and skeletal muscle but are relatively sparse in tendons. Capillaries are absent in many tissues, including most epithelia, dental enamel, dentin, cementum, most cartilage, the cornea, vitreous body, and lens. In fibrocartilaginous articular menisci, both vascular and avascular zones have been identified.

Within the capillary beds, exchange takes place between the circulating blood and interstitial fluid, allowing water and water-soluble substances to exit at the arterial end of the capillaries. These fluids then reenter at the venous end of the capillary, as well as in postcapillary venules further downstream. Plasma molecules may exit the capillary lumen by transcytosis, temporary transendothelial channels, monolayered diaphragms, or by free diffusion, especially lipid-soluble substances.

Three types of capillaries (Fig. 7-11) can be distinguished by fine-structural characteristics of the capillary wall: (a) **continuous capillaries**, (b) **fenestrated capillaries**, and (c) **sinusoids**. These structural differences correspond to measurable differences in capillary permeability. Fenestrated capillaries have the highest permeability, while continuous neural capillaries have the least permeability. The permeability of continuous muscular capillaries lies between these extremes.

Continuous capillaries are virtually ubiquitous throughout the organism. Individual endothelial cells are interconnected by tight junctions (Figs. 7-11A to 7-13). Usually, these cells contain only a few mitochondria and ribosomes, limited endoplasmic reticulum, and small Golgi complexes. The presence of transcytotic vesicles varies; they may be numerous, as seen in muscular capillaries, or scarce to nonexistent, as observed in neural capillaries.

Fenestrated capillaries have pores (fenestrae) in their walls and are commonly found in visceral organs such as the gastrointestinal tract (Figs. 7-11B and 7-14). These capillaries have a larger diameter, and their shape is adapted to the surrounding parenchymal cells, which are separated from them by a basal lamina and a small amount of adventitial CT. In these capillaries, portions of the endothelial cells are attenuated and have circular fenestrae that are 60 to 80 nm in diameter. The fenestrae are closed by monolayered **diaphragms** that are thinner than the cell membrane (Figs. 7-11B and 7-14). An exception is seen in the renal glomerulus, where the fenestrated capillaries lack diaphragms (Figs. 7-11B and 7-15). Fenestrations facilitate the passage of substances across the endothelium.

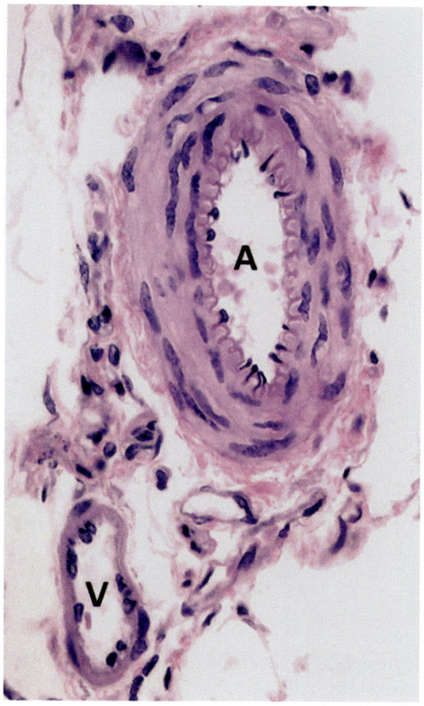

Figure 7-10 Cross-sections through an arteriole (A) show a prominent internal elastic membrane, whereas the venule (V) lacks such a feature. Note that the arteriole has a thicker wall composed of three layers of smooth muscle. In contrast, the venule has a thinner wall, containing only one smooth muscle layer. H&E (×400).

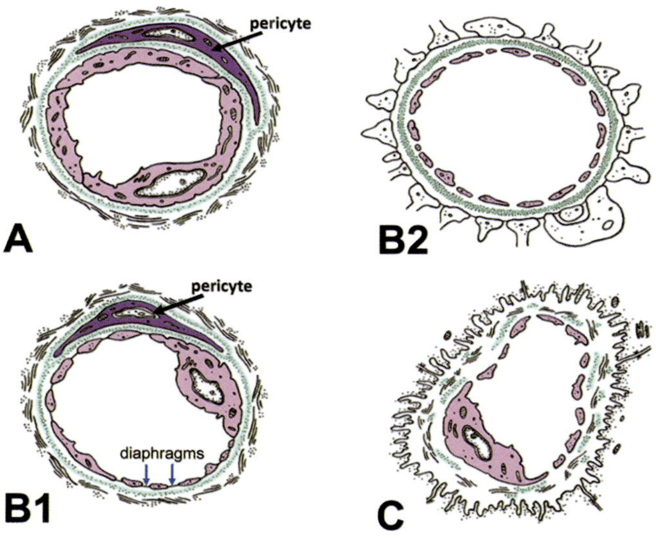

Figure 7-11 Drawing illustrating the fine-structural characteristics of three types of capillaries: (A) continuous capillary, (B1) fenestrated capillary with diaphragms or (B2) without diaphragms, and (C) sinusoid. Pericytes are indicated in A and B1. The fine dots surrounding the endothelial cells and pericytes indicate the basal lamina, which is particularly thick in the fenestrated capillaries lacking diaphragms (B2) and discontinuous in sinusoids (C).

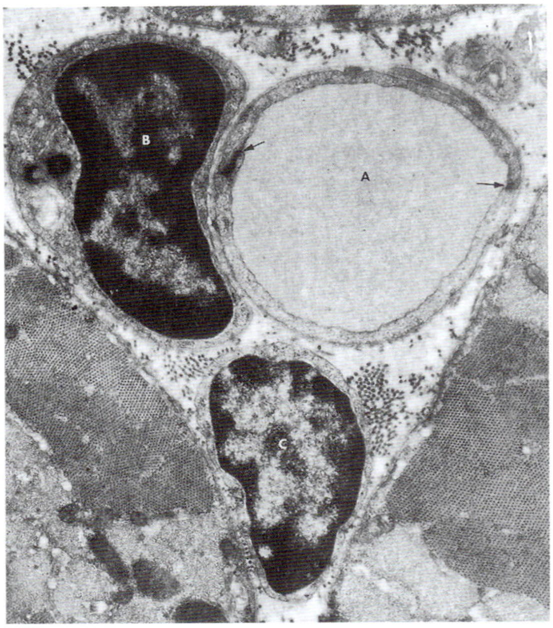

Figure 7-12 Electron micrograph of a continuous (muscular) capillary (A). Tight junctions (arrows) are present between the endothelial cells. The basal lamina of the endothelium extends around the adjacent pericyte (B). Cell C is either a fibrocyte or another pericyte. The black dots between the cells represent cross-sections of collagen fibrils (×16,000).

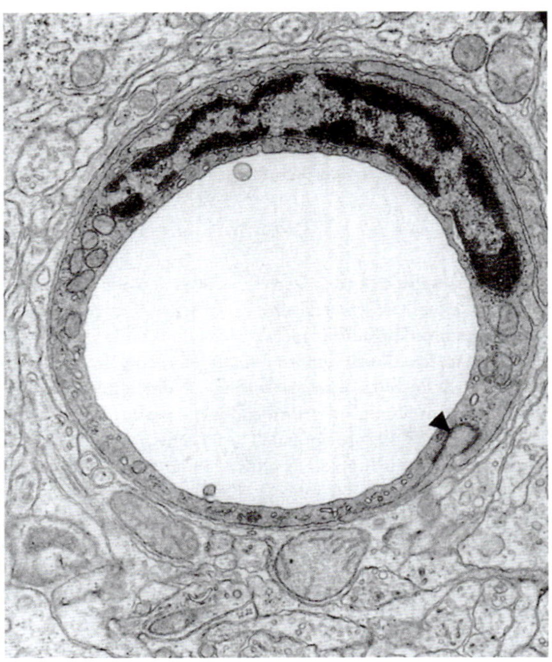

Figure 7-13 Electron micrograph of a continuous (neural) capillary. Tight junctions (arrowhead) are present between adjacent endothelial cells (×21,000).

Sinusoids are present in the liver, bone marrow, and certain endocrine glands (Fig. 7-11C). These capillaries are larger than others, lack uniformity in diameter, and conform to the space within the confines of the surrounding parenchyma. Large intercellular openings and pores through the endothelial cells, along with the discontinuity or absence of the surrounding basal lamina, facilitate maximum exchange between blood and surrounding tissues. Phagocytic cells often traverse the lumen of sinusoids or reside just outside the endothelium.

Arterioles extend into capillary beds (Fig. 7-16). Each capillary bed has a wide **central channel**, ensuring continuous blood flow. Capillaries branching off from this central channel experience more intermittent blood flow. The proximal portion of the central channel, the **metarteriole**, is a narrow vessel surrounded by large, isolated bundles of smooth muscle. The initial portion of the metarteriole is encircled by additional smooth muscle cells, which form a **precapillary sphincter** that regulates blood flow through the capillary bed. The distal portion of the central channel is similar in structure to other capillaries but lacks the smooth muscle found in the wall of the metarteriole. This portion of the central channel empties into the venule.

Venules

Immediate **postcapillary venules** are similar in structure to capillaries but are larger in diameter (10 to 30 μm) (Fig. 7-10). The tunica interna is formed by either continuous or fenestrated endothelial cells connected by incomplete tight junctions, a basal lamina, and a thin subendothelial layer of longitudinal collagen fibers. Pericytes are occasionally present.

Postcapillary venules have a functional significance that is not evident through simple morphologic studies. The junctions between endothelial cells are more permeable than those in capillaries and are particularly sensitive to leakage induced by such agents as serotonin and histamine. These compounds play an important role in the inflammatory reaction, leading to the accumulation of excessive extravascular fluid, soluble substances, and blood cells. Immediate postcapillary venules, referred to as **high endothelial venules**, are prevalent in most lymphoid tissues and are characterized by specialized endothelial cells crucial for the migration of lymphocytes (see Chapter 8).

As venules increase in diameter (30 to 50 μm), they are called **pericytic venules** or **collecting venules**, where pericytes form a continuous layer (Fig. 7-16). Fibrocytes and collagen fibers form a thin tunica externa. With further dilation (50 to 100 μm), pericytes gradually give way to circularly arranged muscle cells (Fig. 7-16). When these cells form one to two complete layers, the venule is referred to as a **muscular venule** (Figs. 7-10 and 7-16). The tunica externa, containing elastic and collagen fibers along with scattered fibrocytes, becomes more prominent. Pericytic venules serve as a definite site for large molecular exchange between the vascular and CT spaces.

Arteriovenous Anastomoses

Direct connections between arterioles and venules without an intervening capillary bed are called **arteriovenous anastomoses** (Fig. 7-16). These anastomoses are typically short, nonbranched, and often coiled vessels. They possess a thick smooth muscle layer in the subendothelium, receiving a dense vasomotor nerve supply. Often, longitudinally oriented smooth muscle fibers form cushions or sleeves. When arteriovenous anastomoses are open, blood essentially bypasses capillary beds and is shunted directly into the venous system. Conversely, when they are closed, blood flow to capillary beds increases. Arteriovenous anastomoses are abundant in the skin, lips, intestine, salivary glands, nasal mucosa, and male and female reproductive tracts. They function in the regulation of blood pressure and blood flow into capillary beds, thermoregulation, and erection.

A highly convoluted arteriovenous anastomosis surrounded by a thick CT capsule is called a **glomus**. The vessel of the glomus is distinguished by numerous longitudinal, subendothelial epithelioid muscle cells surrounded by circularly arranged muscle cells in the media. An internal elastic membrane is absent. Glomera are especially abundant in digital pads and the external ear, where they serve a thermoregulatory function.

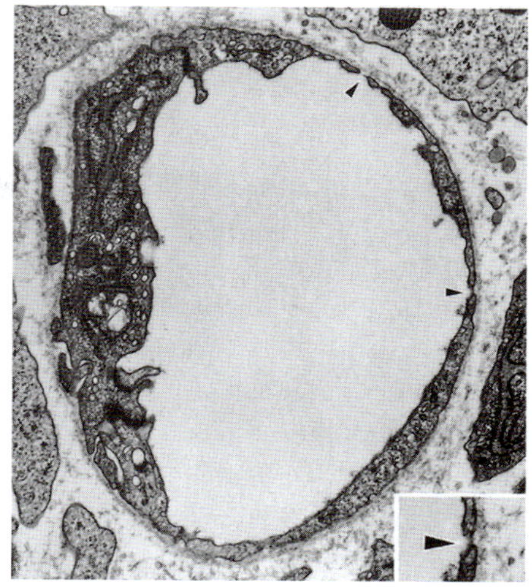

Figure 7-14 Electron micrograph of a fenestrated capillary in the lamina propria of the small intestine (rat). The fenestrations (arrowheads) are sealed by a monolayered diaphragm (×15,600). The inset (lower right) provides a detailed view of a pore with a diaphragm (×45,000).

Veins

Blood courses through venous trees in a direction opposite to that in arterial trees. The structure of veins varies widely and appears to be influenced by local mechanical conditions. Consequently, the classification of veins is challenging, especially because layers in their walls are often absent or difficult to distinguish.

The terms **small**, **medium**, and **large veins** have only relative meaning within a particular animal. For instance, the large veins of a cat may be smaller than the medium-sized veins of a cow. Small veins continue from muscular venules, while medium-sized veins function as collecting veins and are comparable in function and location to medium or muscular arteries. Veins equivalent to the aorta are referred to as the great veins, large veins, or simply by their gross anatomic names such as the vena cava.

All veins that carry blood against gravity, ranging from venules to small and medium veins in the extremities, are equipped with flap-like, semilunar **valves**. These venous valves consist of paired folds of the intima composed of endothelium covering a core of collagen fibers (Fig. 7-17). Proximal to the attachment of the valves, the wall of the vein is slightly distended to form a valve sinus. The free margins of the valves are oriented toward the heart. When closed, the valves prevent the backflow of blood.

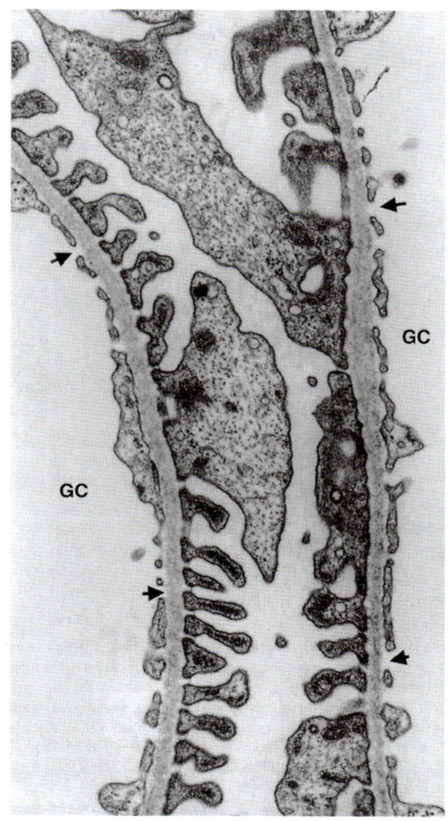

Figure 7-15 Electron micrograph showing part of the walls of two glomerular capillaries (GC) in the kidney. The endothelial cells have fenestrae or pores (at arrows) without diaphragms (×27,600).

Small Veins

As venules further increase in diameter, they transition into **small veins**. The endothelium and the associated basal lamina lining a small vein are surrounded by a distinct media. The media has two to four continuous layers of circularly oriented smooth muscle cells interspersed with varying amounts of CT that blend with the surrounding tunica externa.

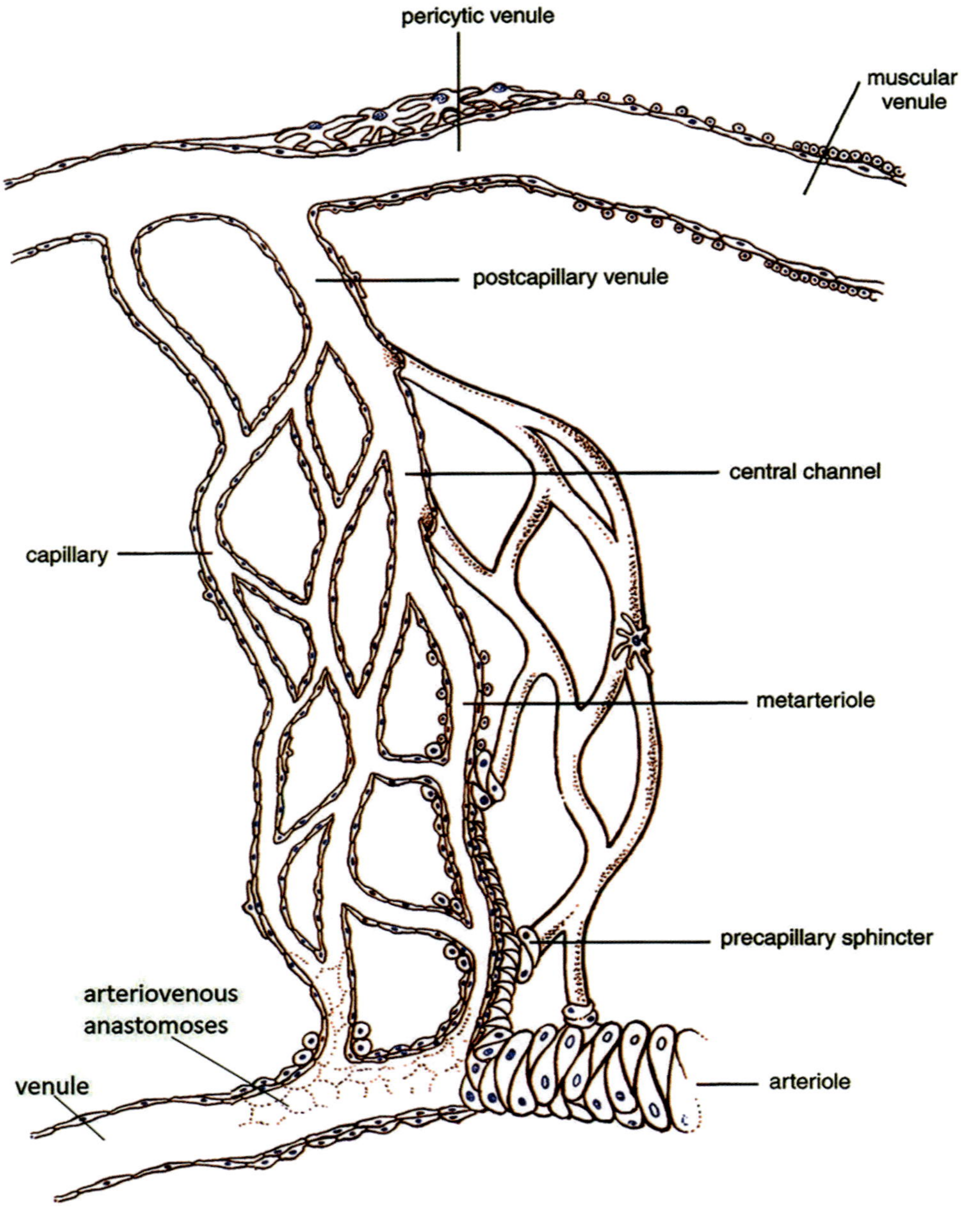

Figure 7-16 Schematic drawing of the microvasculature. Capillaries arise from both an arteriole and a metarteriole, with precapillary sphincters present. The metarteriole continues into a central channel, followed by a postcapillary venule, pericytic venule, and muscular venule, linked by a venule with an incomplete layer of smooth muscle. Arteriovenous anastomoses are direct connections between arterioles and venules without an intervening capillary bed.

Medium Veins

The wall structure of the **medium veins** reflects the physical stresses of gravity and the centrifugal forces of locomotion that they must withstand. Because the variation in position and orientation of smooth muscle components is considerable in different veins within the various species, inclusive descriptions are difficult.

The tunica interna consists of an endothelial lining and a thin subendothelial layer of collagen and elastic fibers. In larger vessels, an internal elastic membrane may be present. Usually, the tunica media consists of several layers of smooth muscle with associated collagen and elastic networks, commonly arranged in circular or spiral fashion. In the outer tunica media, smooth muscle cells may be longitudinally oriented. The tunica externa is composed predominantly of collagen networks anchored to both the tunica media and the surrounding CT, with longitudinally oriented elastic fibers.

Large Veins

The tunica interna of **large veins** has essentially the same structure as that of medium veins. However, the endothelium is often slightly thicker and blocklike, smooth muscle cells are present occasionally, and the internal elastic membrane is more prominent.

The tunica media is thin when compared to the relative size of the vessel or the diameter of the lumen. It consists of collagen, elastic fibers, and smooth muscle cells in varying proportions. In most large veins, the amount of smooth muscle is insignificant (Fig. 7-18).

Conversely, the tunica externa is prominent, composed of longitudinally or spirally oriented bundles of smooth muscle cells (Fig. 7-18), along with collagen and elastic fibers. These components maintain the proper tension of the wall. The thickness of this layer varies depending on the location of the vein and is more pronounced in veins subjected to a greater pressure from the surrounding environment, such as those within the thoracic and abdominal cavities.

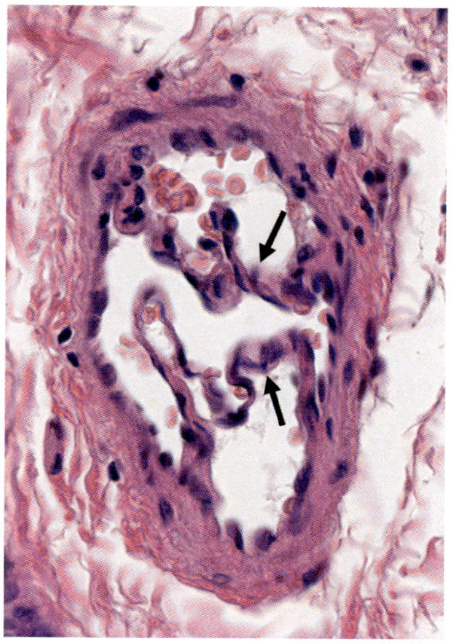

Figure 7-17 A cross-section through a small vein in the dermis of palm skin (monkey). In the lumen, a pair of folded venous valves (arrows) is shown extending from the intima. H&E (×200). (Image by J. Feng.)

Specialized Blood Vessels

Many blood vessels have special structural features that fulfill specific functions in regulating blood flow. An increase in wall thickness is observed in vessels subjected to unusual blood pressures, such as the arteries and veins of the teat, veins of the glans penis, and coronary arteries. Conversely, a reduction in wall thickness occurs in protected, low-pressure areas such as the skull (e.g., arteries of the brain and dural venous sinuses), bones, and lungs. Longitudinal muscle bundles, capable of halting blood flow through the vessel, are present in the tunica interna in both arteries and veins of the penis, ovary, and uterus. Additionally, circular sphincter-like thickenings of the tunica media in veins serve similar functions in the large intestine, liver, and skin.

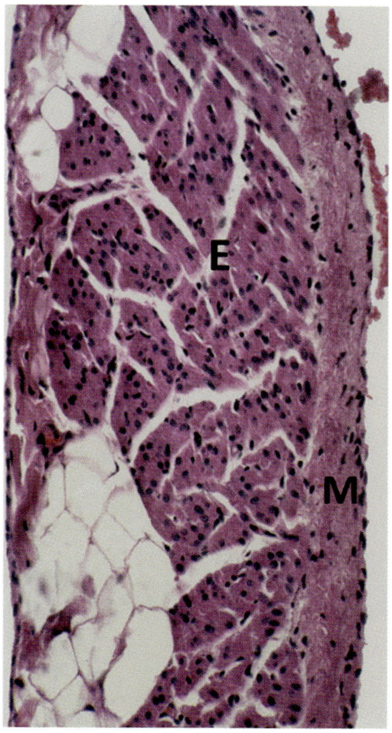

Figure 7-18 Cross-section through a segment of the ovine vena cava. The thin tunica media (M) consists of a few bundles of smooth muscle cells. The tunica externa (E) is the most prominent layer and contains many bundles of longitudinally oriented smooth muscle. H&E (×40).

Specialized Sensory Receptors

Three types of specialized sensory receptors are present in the walls of major arteries: the **carotid bodies**, **aortic bodies**, and **carotid sinuses**. Nerve endings in these structures monitor changes in blood chemical composition (chemoreceptors) and blood pressure (baroreceptors).

Carotid Bodies

The **carotid body** (carotid glomus or glomus caroticum) is a bilateral arterial chemoreceptor located in the adventitia at the bifurcation of the common carotid artery. It is a small, oval structure enclosed by a CT capsule and consists of a dense sinusoidal capillary network surrounding clusters of cells. Two cell types are present within these clusters: **glomus cells** (type I cells, granular endocrine cells, or chemoreceptor cells), which contain many granules rich in catecholamines and serotonin, and **sheath cells** (type II cells or sustentacular cells), which have few or no granules. The sheath cells incompletely invest several glomus cells (Fig. 7-19). Nonmyelinated afferent and efferent nerve terminals synapse on granular endocrine cells. Changes in oxygen and carbon dioxide tension, as well as blood pH, generate action potentials in afferent nerve fibers. These action potentials then travel to the central nervous system (CNS) and trigger responses primarily in the respiratory and cardiovascular systems.

Aortic Bodies

The **aortic bodies** are scattered around the inferior surface of the aortic arch. Their structure and function resemble those of the carotid bodies.

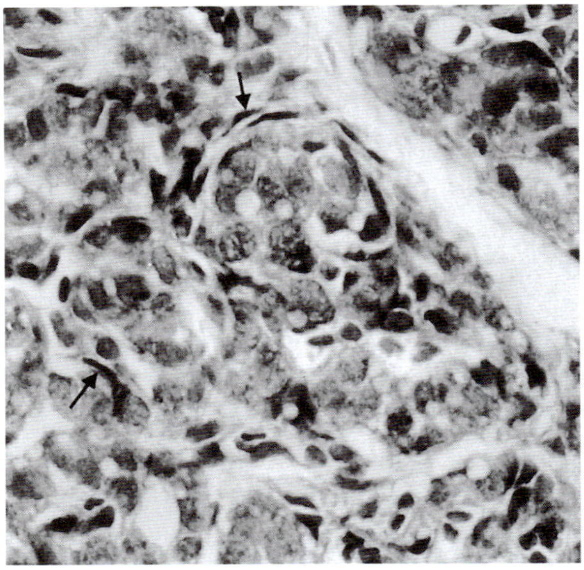

Figure 7-19 Ovine carotid body. Groups of glomus cells are invested by flatter sheath cells (arrows). H&E (×350). (Courtesy of J. H. Riley.)

Carotid Sinuses

The **carotid sinus** (or carotid bulb) is a bilateral baroreceptor that appears as a dilation of the internal carotid artery just superior to the bifurcation of the common carotid artery. At this point, the tunica media of the artery is thin and surrounded by a thick tunica externa that contains numerous terminals from the carotid sinus branch of the glossopharyngeal nerve (cranial nerve IX). These terminals function as mechanoreceptors that elicit reflex bradycardia (a decrease in heart rate) and dilation of the splanchnic blood vessels when stimulated by increased blood pressure.

Heart

The thick wall of the heart is primarily composed of cardiac muscle cells capable of spontaneous rhythmic contractions, which pump blood into the vascular system. The inner layer of the heart, referred to as the endocardium, is continuous with the tunica interna of the large blood vessels entering and leaving the heart. The middle contractile muscular layer is called the **myocardium** and is by far the thickest layer of the organ. Finally, the outermost layer is the **epicardium**.

Endocardium

The endocardium completely lines the ventricles and atria, covering the cardiac valves and associated structures. The endocardium usually consists of three layers (Fig. 7-20). The innermost layer comprises a continuous **endothelium**. Beneath the endothelium lies the **subendothelial layer**, composed of dense irregular CT containing collagen, elastic fibers, and occasional smooth muscle cells. Elastic fibers are particularly abundant in the atrial walls and are usually arranged parallel to the endocardial surface.

The **subendocardial layer** is predominantly composed of loosely arranged collagen and elastic fibers. Adipose cells may be present, along with a rich supply of blood and lymph vessels, and CT continuous with that of the myocardium. In some locations, modified cardiac muscle cells of the cardiac impulse conduction system are present in the subendocardial layer (Fig. 7-20).

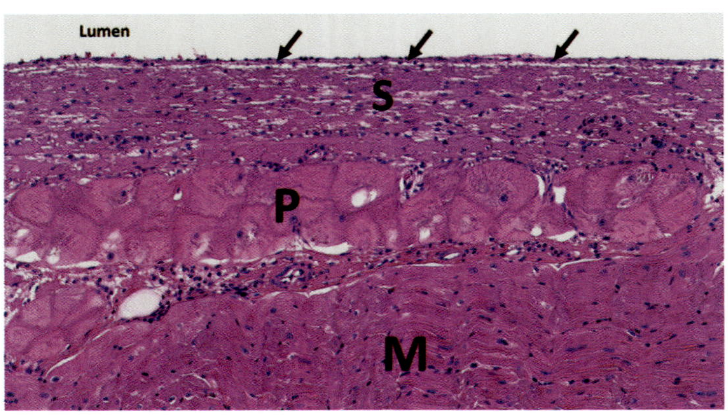

Figure 7-20 Horizontal section through a portion of the bovine heart wall. The continuous endothelium (arrows) forms the innermost layer. Peripheral to the subendothelial layer (S) lies the subendocardial layer, containing many large Purkinje fibers (P), specialized modified cardiac muscle fibers responsible for conducting impulses, and the myocardium (M). H&E (×200). (Image by J. Feng.)

The **cardiac valves** are endocardial folds covered by endothelium. The subendothelial layer is rich in elastic and collagen fibers. The **atrioventricular valves** consist of a **stratum spongiosum** located toward the atrial side and a **stratum fibrosum** on the ventricular side (Fig. 7-21). In the stratum spongiosum, elastic and collagen fibers are loosely arranged, and blood vessels are located exclusively within it. In the stratum fibrosum, collagen fibers predominate and connect with the fibrous rings surrounding the atrioventricular openings. These fibers also extend to the fibrous cords (**chordae tendineae**), which arise from the endomysium of the papillary muscles. In the **semilunar valves** of the aorta and the pulmonary trunk, the central collagen fibers have a predominantly circular

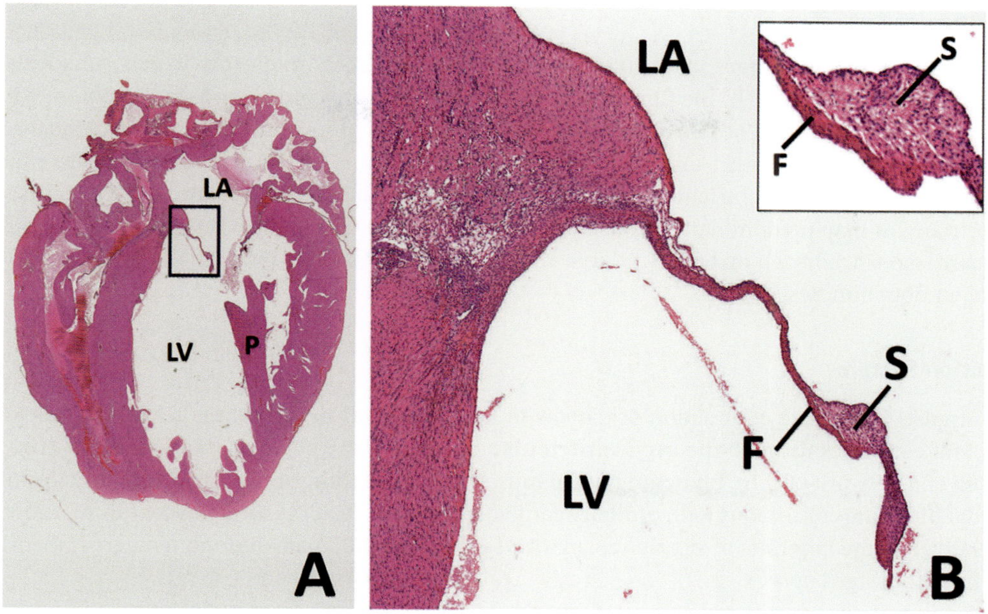

Figure 7-21 Sagittal section through the heart of a rat at low magnification (**A**, ×8). The boxed region is enlarged (**B**, ×50) to illustrate the atrioventricular valve (bicuspid valve), situated between the left atrium (LA) and ventricle (LV). The valve is covered by endothelium and consists of a stratum fibrosum (F) and a stratum spongiosum (S), with details shown in the inset (upper right). Papillary muscle (P) is also visible. H&E (Image by J. Feng.)

arrangement and are reinforced by a thin layer of elastic fibers near the vessel and a thicker layer of elastic fibers on the ventricular side. The thickening of the free edge of the semilunar valves is caused by the presence of loose connective and cartilaginous tissues.

Myocardium

The middle and thickest layer of the heart is the **myocardium**, composed of bundles of cardiac muscle cells, branches of cardiac conduction fibers, an extensive capillary network, and the cardiac skeleton.

Bundles of cardiac muscle cells are embedded in loose CT containing a dense capillary network, lymph vessels, and autonomic nerve fibers. The amount of interstitial CT is subject to local variations and is greater in the myocardium of the right ventricle compared to that of the left ventricle. The atrial cardiac muscle cells are usually smaller than the ventricular cardiac muscle cells. In atrial cardiac muscle cells, numerous specific **atrial granules** containing atrial natriuretic peptide (ANP) are present. ANP plays an important role in fluid homeostasis, such as diuresis, natriuresis, and vasodilation.

Epicardium and Pericardium

The myocardium is covered externally by the **epicardium**, also known as the visceral serous pericardium. The outermost layer consists of mesothelial cells, which line the pericardial cavity. Beneath this epithelium lies a layer of loose CT rich in elastic fibers, which forms protective sheaths around blood vessels and nerves. This CT, which is often rich in adipocytes, is particularly abundant around the large coronary blood vessels.

The epicardium reflects off the surface of the heart to form the **parietal serous pericardium**. The parietal pericardium consists of an innermost layer of mesothelial cells resting on a thin layer of loose CT, which fuses with the **fibrous pericardium**—a thick layer of collagen fiber bundles and elastic fibers. Located between the visceral and parietal serous pericardium, the **pericardial cavity** contains serous fluid that lubricates the mesothelial surfaces, allowing frictionless cardiac movement.

The pericardium can readily adapt to normal continual changes in the size of the heart and can also limit overfilling of the heart. However, cardiac tamponade (compression of the heart) may result if the pericardial cavity fills with excessive fluid.

Cardiac Skeleton

The musculature of the atrial and ventricular walls is inserted into the **cardiac skeleton**, which is made up of three parts: (a) the fibrous rings (annuli fibrosi), (b) the fibrous triangles (trigona fibrosa cordis), and (c) the fibrous (or membranous) part of the interventricular septum. The **fibrous rings** consist of intermingling bundles of collagen and a few elastic fibers surrounding the atrioventricular, aortic, and pulmonary trunk openings. The **fibrous triangles** are small areas of CT, filling the spaces between the atrioventricular openings and the base of the aorta. The nature of this CT is species and age dependent. The triangles may predominantly consist of dense, irregular CT (in pigs, cats, and rabbits), fibrocartilage (in dogs), hyaline cartilage (in horses), or bone (in large ruminants). The **fibrous part of the interventricular septum** consists of collagen fiber bundles.

Cardiac Conduction System

The electrical impulse for cardiac contraction originates in the **sinoatrial node**, subsequently spreads to the **atrioventricular node**, and continues through the **atrioventricular bundle** (also known as the **bundle of His**). The sinoatrial node is composed of a network of thin, branching nodal muscle cells containing scarce myofibrils and lacking intercalated disks. These nodal fibers are continuous with ordinary cardiac muscle fibers of the atrial myocardium. Individual fibers are separated by relatively large amounts of highly vascularized CT containing many autonomic nerve fibers and occasional ganglion cells (from the vagus nerve).

The atrioventricular node is composed of irregularly arranged, small, branching nodal muscle fibers, which exhibit a morphology similar to those of the sinoatrial node. These nodal muscle fibers are interposed between atrial myocardial fibers and the impulse-conducting fibers that form the atrioventricular bundle.

The cardiac conduction fibers in the atrioventricular bundle pass down the interventricular septum and travel within the subendocardial CT as **Purkinje fibers**, transmitting impulses to the cardiac muscle cells at the apex of the heart. These Purkinje fibers are readily identified by their large diameter, large central spherical nucleus, and scarce peripheral myofibrils. The central area of the cytoplasm is rich in glycogen, creating a light-staining halo around the nucleus (Fig. 7-20). In longitudinal sections, characteristic cross-striations and intercalated disks typical of cardiac muscle cells are visible. The conducting fibers connect with smaller transitional cells lacking intercalated disks, which in turn connect with ordinary myocardial cells.

Cardiac Blood Vessels, Lymph Vessels, and Nerves

The coronary arteries are thick muscular arteries that often contain bundles of longitudinal smooth muscle and epithelioid muscle cells in the interna. This muscle component regulates the blood flow within these vessels. Originating from the coronary arteries, a dense capillary network supplies the myocardium, epicardium, cardiac skeleton, and peripheral portions of the cardiac valves. Blood from the cardiac capillary beds is collected by venules and veins that open into the right atrium either through the coronary sinus or through direct openings in the endocardium (venae cordis minimae).

Lymph capillaries form a network in the cardiac CT. These small lymphatics are continuous with larger lymph vessels, especially in the subendocardial layer and the subepithelial CT of the epicardium.

Both sympathetic and parasympathetic nerves innervate the heart, with a greater abundance in the atria compared to the ventricles, where mainly sympathetic fibers are represented. These nerves form extensive plexuses, particularly dense around the sinoatrial and atrioventricular nodes. Parasympathetic (vagus) fibers terminate on ganglion cells, which contribute fibers to the aforementioned plexuses. Additionally, both the myocardium and epicardium receive sensory fibers that terminate with club-shaped or plate-like enlargements.

Lymph Vessels

The lymphatic vascular system is an integral part of both the circulatory system and the defense systems. It originates as a network of anastomosing lymph capillaries in the CT of the organism. These capillaries are continuous with larger lymphatic vessels that pass through at least one lymph node on their way to larger collecting ducts that drain the lymph into the venous system.

Lymph Capillaries

Lymph capillaries are endothelium-lined tubes that are usually larger in diameter than blood capillaries and variable in shape (Fig. 7-22). It is often difficult to distinguish between lymph and blood capillaries in histologic sections; however, recently described histochemical markers that discriminate between vascular and lymphatic endothelium may aid in this distinction. The endothelial lining of lymph capillaries is usually thin and contains many pinocytic vesicles (Fig. 7-23). Adjacent endothelial cells are joined by intimate interdigitations, simple overlapping without tight junctions. Frequently, variably sized gaps are observed between adjacent cells (Fig. 7-23), likely temporary as they appear or disappear continuously. Permeability is facilitated by pinocytosis and the presence of gaps between endothelial cells.

Lymph capillaries lack associated pericytes, and their basal lamina is either discontinuous or absent (Fig. 7-23). Fine, extracellular matrix–anchoring filaments link the outer surface of the endothelial cells to pericapillary collagen fibrils and elastic fibers. These filaments are responsible for keeping the lumina of the capillaries open, especially when the tissues are edematous.

Valves may be present occasionally in lymph capillaries and are a constant feature of all other lymph vessels (Fig. 7-24). They are composed of an endothelial fold with little intervening CT, except at the junction with the vessel wall, where it is more abundant. Occasional smooth muscle fibers are found in the valves of the larger lymph vessels.

As a general rule, lymph capillaries are found in conjunction with loose CT, where they drain excess interstitial fluid containing fat, proteins, cells, and particulate matter. They are absent in the CNS, certain structures within the eye, bone marrow, cartilage, red pulp of the spleen, and liver lobules.

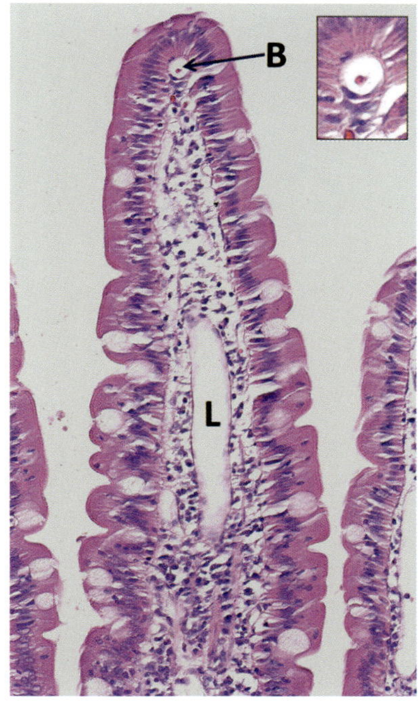

Figure 7-22 Sagittal section through a cat intestinal villus, showing the central lacteal as an example of a lymph capillary (L). A blood capillary (B) is also visible, with details shown in the inset (upper left). H&E (×330). (Image by J. Feng.)

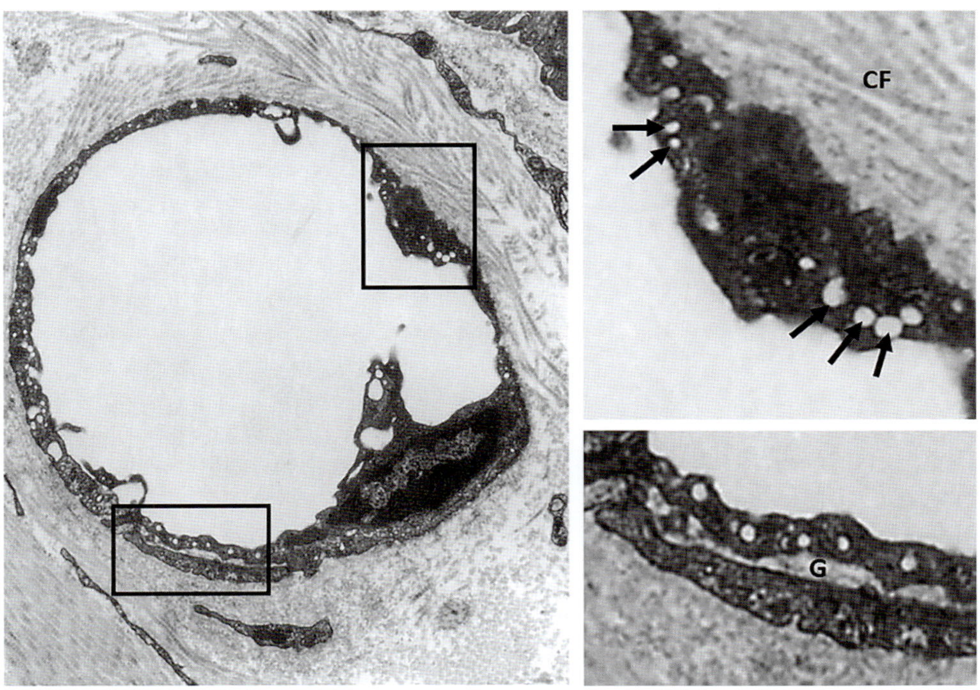

Figure 7-23 Electron micrograph of a lymph capillary. The lymph capillary lacks a basal lamina and associated pericytes. The thin endothelium contains many pinocytotic vesicles (arrows), and the pericapillary collagen fibrils (CF) are visible in the upper right inset. A gap (G) is present between endothelial cells in the lower right inset. (×16,000).

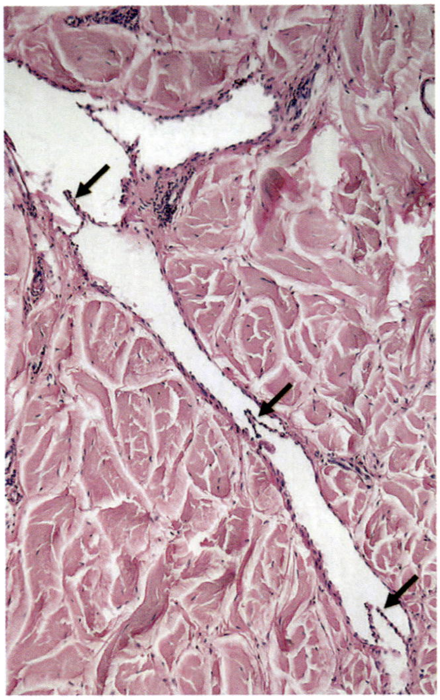

Figure 7-24 Lymph vessels of the bovine dermis cut longitudinally. The lymph vessels have valves (arrows) and display very large caliber lumina compared to the thickness of the wall. H&E (×100).

Small and Medium Lymph Vessels

The structure of the wall of small and medium lymph vessels varies greatly according to the location and the species involved. These vessels differ from lymph capillaries by their larger diameter and the presence of a continuous basal lamina. As the vessel diameter increases, a thin subendothelial CT layer appears. In larger vessels, one or two layers of smooth muscle and elastic fibers are subsequently added. The tunica externa is indistinguishable from the CT surrounding the lymph vessel.

Large Lymph Vessels (Ducts)

They are the final two collecting ducts of lymph vascular system. The short **right lymph duct** drains its contents into the venous system at the junction of the right internal jugular and subclavian veins. Meanwhile the longer and larger **thoracic duct** originates from the **cisterna chyli** in the abdomen and ascends through the thorax and neck to drain at the junction of the left internal jugular and subclavian veins. The right lymph duct collects lymph from the upper right quadrant of the body, while the thoracic duct collects lymph from the remainder of the body.

Similar to blood vessels, the walls of these large lymph vessels (ducts) comprise three tunics; however, the layers are not always distinctly delineated. The tunica interna consists of endothelium and a layer of longitudinal, interlacing collagen and elastic fibers. An internal elastic membrane is usually absent. The tunica media contains smooth muscle cells, surrounded by numerous elastic and collagen fibers, with the variation in number and orientation depending on the location and species. The tunica externa is composed of collagen and elastic fibers and may also contain muscle cells.

Clinical Correlations

A range of cardiovascular diseases is significant in veterinary medicine. The heart can be affected by congenital, degenerative, inflammatory, and neoplastic conditions, each with various causes. In adult animals, primary cardiac diseases often manifest as cardiomyopathy or degenerative changes in the heart muscle or valves. For instance, *myxomatous degeneration* in the mitral valve of a 12-year-old dog with heart failure is depicted in Fig. 7-25.

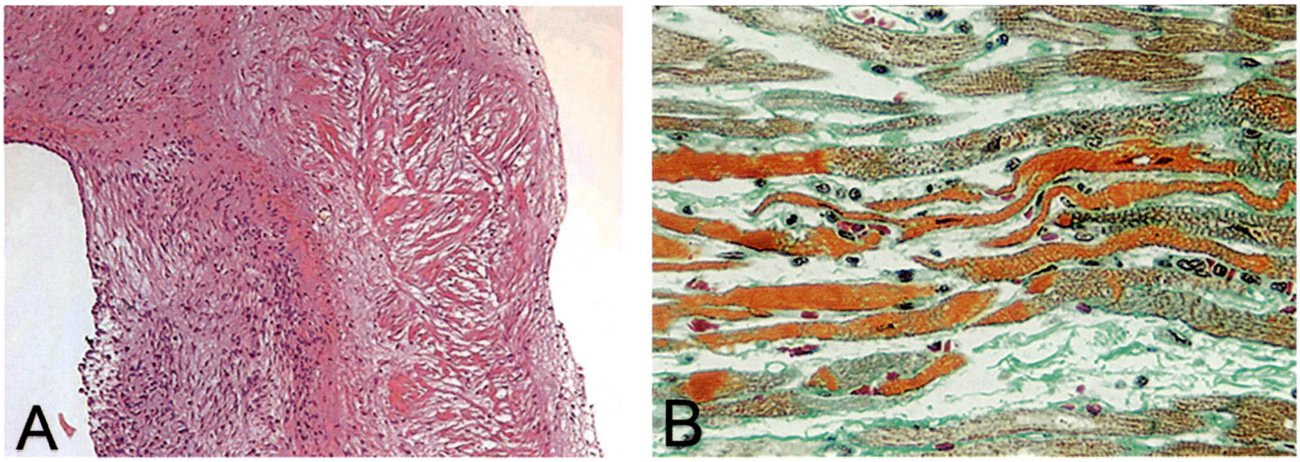

Figure 7-25 **A.** Mitral valve, H&E. **B.** Masson's trichrome stain highlights muscle fibers (red/orange) undergoing degeneration and being replaced by collagen material (blue). Reproduced with permission from Salguero Bodes FJ, Pallares Martinez FJ. Aughey and Frye's Comparative Veterinary Histology with Clinical Correlates. 2nd ed. Boca Raton: CRC Press, 2023.

Essentials

1) **Blood vessels:** They have three tunics or layers: endothelium-lined *tunica intima*, smooth muscle–containing *tunica media*, and an outer CT layer—*tunica adventitia*.
2) **Arteries:** *Elastic arteries*: They are major heart-associated vessels with thick tunica media containing elastic tissue bands and smooth muscle. They lack a complete internal elastic lamina but ensure blood flow in diastole through elastic rebound. *Muscular arteries*: They have a well-developed internal elastic lamina, containing tunica media of smooth muscle with some elastic fibers. The external elastic lamina marks tunica media boundary. Tunica adventitia may be as thick as tunica media.
3) **Arterioles:** They include one to three smooth muscle layers. Tunica adventitia primarily loose CT merging with surrounding tissues. Vasodilation and vasoconstriction in arterioles are important for *blood pressure regulation*.
4) **Capillaries:** (a) *Continuous*: No fenestrae, tight junctions, and pinocytic vesicles for transcytosis are present; found in muscle, central nerve system, and CT. (b) *Fenestrated*: They have endothelial cells with small gaps (fenestrae), which regulate permeability, found in endocrine glands and the gastrointestinal (GI) tract. (c) *Discontinuous (sinusoidal)*: These have large gaps between endothelial cells and incomplete basal lamina, facilitating the passage of cells and large molecules; found in liver, bone marrow and spleen.
5) **Postcapillary venules:** They contain the highest concentration of *pericytes*, a key site for *inflammatory response* (fluid extravasation and migration of inflammatory cells into tissue).
6) ***Venules* and *muscular venules*:** Both have one to two layers of smooth muscle, with muscular venules being larger.
7) **Veins:** They are larger but with a well-developed tunica adventitia. Tunica media acquires some elastic fibers but not much more smooth muscle. The *largest veins* (i.e., vena cava) can have three to five layers of smooth muscle and semilunar *valves* to prevent retrograde flow.
8) **Lymphatics:** They start as blind-end capillaries lacking basal lamina or tight junctions. Endothelial cells attach to surrounding CT by fine anchoring filaments. The basal lamina is poorly developed. They collect extracellular fluid, filter through lymph nodes, and recycle back to venous blood circulation. Lymphatics entering lymph nodes have valves to prevent retrograde flow.
9) **Endothelial cell function:** Endothelial cells have a role in (a) the regulation of *inflammation* by facilitating diapedesis of inflammatory cells into tissues, (b) blood pressure regulation via production of vasodilators (nitric oxide) and vasoconstrictors (endothelin-1), and (c) the regulation of clotting via production of prostacyclin, which inhibits platelet adhesion and clot formation.
10) **Heart**. It contains three wall layers: (a) *endocardium* lined by endothelium, homologous to the tunica intima of blood vessels; (b) *myocardium*: contractile muscle cells; (c) *epicardium*: outer layer covered by mesothelial cells. *Cardiac skeleton*: It is composed of dense irregular CT surrounding the base of major vessels and valves. It not only provides structural support but also helps to isolate atria from ventricles electrically. *Valves* have a two-layered structure of dense irregular CT fibrosa and a loose CT spongiosa, with the fibrosa layer continuous with the cardiac skeleton. *Conducting fibers*: They originate at the sinoatrial node, extend along the interventricular septum, and terminate as Purkinje fibers located between the endocardium and myocardium of the ventricles. Modified *atrial muscle cells* produce the key blood-pressure regulating hormone, *atrial natriuretic factor (ANF)*. In response to high blood pressure (stretch in the atrium), ANF increases sodium and water secretion from the kidney.

Suggested Readings

Bannykh S, Mironov Jr A, Bannykh G. The morphology of valves and valve-like structures in the canine and feline thoracic duct. *Anatomy and embryology.* 1995;192(3):265–74.

Boyett MR, Honjo H, Kodama I. The sinoatrial node, a heterogeneous pacemaker structure. *Cardiovascular research.* 2000;47(4):658–87.

Caporali A, Martello A, Miscianinov V, Maselli D, Vono R, Spinetti G. Contribution of pericyte paracrine regulation of the endothelium to angiogenesis. *Pharmacology & therapeutics.* 2017;171:56–64.

Castenholz A. Structure of initial and collecting lymphatic vessels. In *Lymph stasis: pathophysiology, diagnosis and treatment* 2019 Jun 4 (pp. 15–42). *CRC Press.*

Gonzalez C, Almaraz L, Obeso A, Rigual R. Carotid body chemoreceptors: from natural stimuli to sensory discharges. *Physiological reviews.* 1994;74(4):829–98.

Iturriaga R, Alcayaga J, Chapleau MW, Somers VK. Carotid body chemoreceptors: physiology, pathology, and implications for health and disease. *Physiological reviews.* 2021;101(3):1177–235.
Mehta D, Malik AB. Signaling mechanisms regulating endothelial permeability. *Physiological reviews.* 2006;86(1):279–367.
Minami T, Muramatsu M, Kume T. Organ/tissue-specific vascular endothelial cell heterogeneity in health and disease. *Biological and Pharmaceutical Bulletin.* 2019;42(10):1609–19.
Noorman M, van der Heyden MA, van Veen TA, Cox MG, Hauer RN, de Bakker JM, van Rijen HV. Cardiac cell–cell junctions in health and disease: electrical versus mechanical coupling. *Journal of molecular and cellular cardiology.* 2009;47(1):23–31.
Patan S. Vasculogenesis and angiogenesis as mechanisms of vascular network formation, growth and remodeling. *Review. J Neurooncol.* 2000;50:1–15.
Racker DK, Kadish AH. Proximal atrioventricular bundle, atrioventricular node, and distal atrioventricular bundle are distinct anatomic structures with unique histological characteristics and innervation. *Circulation.* 2000;101(9):1049–59.
Salguero Bodes FJ, Pallares Martinez FJ. *Aughey and Frye's Comparative Veterinary Histology with Clinical Correlates.* 2nd ed. Boca Raton: CRC Press, 2023.
Simionescu M, Simionescu N, editors. Endothelial cell biology in health and disease. *Springer Science & Business Media*; 2013 Nov 11.
Stone EA, Stewart GJ. Architecture and structure of canine veins with special reference to confluences. *Anat Rec.* 1988;222:154–163.
Thaemert JC. Atrioventricular node innervation in ultrastructural three dimensions. *Am J Anat.* 1970;128:239–263.
Tse D, Stan RV. Morphological heterogeneity of endothelium. In *Seminars in thrombosis and hemostasis* 2010 Apr (Vol. 36, No. 03, pp. 236–245). *Thieme Medical Publishers.*
Vanhoutte PM, Shimokawa H, Tang EH, Feletou M. Endothelial dysfunction and vascular disease. *Acta physiologica.* 2009;196(2):193–222.
Verna A. Ultrastructure of the carotid body in mammals. *Int Rev Cytol.* 1979;60:271–330.
Wiedeman MP. An introduction to microcirculation. *Elsevier*; 2012 Dec 2.

8

Immune System

Charles McLean Press

CHAPTER MENU

Dellmann's Textbook of Veterinary Histology, Seventh Edition. Edited by Marxa L. Figueiredo and John J. Turek.

Companion website: www.wiley.com/go/figueiredo/vethistology7e

The immune system comprises organs, aggregated lymphatic tissue, and cells that collectively work to maintain the integrity of the body. Cells and tissues of the immune system have the task of identifying and protecting against pathogenic organisms and processes. They ensure that the body's response to these destructive agents is appropriate. The immune system must locate sites of tissue damage or infection and mediate effective host defense against insults occurring sporadically and without warning. To meet these challenges, the immune system has developed a mixture of fixed cells distributed sparsely in tissues and migratory cells that leave the blood circulation under the direction of signals from these fixed sentinel cells as well as from parenchymal elements. The rapid growth rate and adaptability of microbes require the immune system to employ multiple defense strategies to prevent their evasion of immune control. The immune system has developed two broad categories of immune effector responses: *innate* and *adaptive*. Innate responses involve immune cells responding directly to broad categories of microbes or host products triggered by specific sensors for microbial material. Adaptive immune effectors arise via the proliferation of small numbers of precursor lymphocytes, each carrying a clonally distributed receptor specific for a defining constituent of a pathogen (antigen receptors and antigens, respectively). This diversity of lymphocytes is generated in primary lymphoid organs. Given the rare nature of precursor lymphocytes specific for any one pathogen and the unpredictable nature of pathogen appearance, the immune system employs a body-wide surveillance strategy. Lymphocytes regularly enter and exit the bloodstream, migrating through organized lymphoid structures, such as lymph nodes, spleen, or Peyer's patches in the gut. The spleen surveys the blood for evidence of pathogen spread, whereas other secondary lymphoid tissues concentrate pathogen information from local regions of the body (skin or internal organs). This searching process may take several days for rare lymphocytes to locate antigens, become activated, proliferate to adequate numbers, and develop effector functions for pathogen clearance. It is the role of the innate immune system to hold pathogens in check while the adaptive system is mobilized. The organs and tissues of the immune system house both arms of the immune system, directing microbial defense to prevent pathogen spread and mobilizing adaptive immunity for efficient pathogen elimination and the generation of memory responses for protecting against future related challenges.

Cells of the Immune System

The cellular participants of the immune response can be categorized as either migratory cells or fixed cells. Lymphocytes, granulocytes, and monocytes are migratory cells that are free to move anywhere in the body. The recirculation of lymphocytes through the lymph or blood is a prominent feature of the immune system, ensuring effective surveillance of the tissues. Fixed cells, on the other hand, are either mesenchymal or epithelial cells that establish a scaffold within the stromal matrix of lymphatic tissue. These cells create a supportive framework that sustains the lymphocytes during different phases of development and function. Additionally, these cells can serve as sentinel cells to recognize and respond to invading microbes when the opportunity arises. The remarkable diversity exhibited by both migratory and fixed cells contributes to the unique character of lymphatic tissue.

Lymphocytes

The histology of lymphocytes is described in detail in Chapter 6. For an in-depth exploration of lymphocyte function, the reader is referred to standard veterinary immunology textbooks. Lymphocytes are migratory cells of the immune system that control adaptive immunity by initiating specific responses upon encountering antigens. Antigens consist of molecular components derived from exogenous agents, such as bacteria, viruses, protozoa, or toxins, as well as endogenous agents, such as tumor cells. The lymphocytic lineage gives rise to two major cell types: B cells (*b*ursa-dependent) and T cells (*t*hymus-dependent). These cells and their subpopulations are distinguished by different surface molecules that recognize antigens, including antigen receptors and coreceptors, which play key roles in signal transduction and cell cooperation. B and T cells cannot be identified using standard histologic stains such as hematoxylin and eosin (H&E).

B and T cells differ in the way that they effect an immune response. Each B cell can bind to and respond to a single antigen, and with appropriate costimulation, it will respond by secreting its receptors into body fluids (immunoglobulins, also known as antibodies). T cells recognize antigens when displayed in the context of major histocompatibility complex (MHC) molecules on the surface of antigen-presenting cells. After antigen stimulation, both lymphocyte types undergo proliferation and differentiation, giving rise to either memory cells or effector cells. Memory cells are long-lived and can mount an enhanced response upon re-encounter with antigen. Effector B-cell function is mediated by antibodies. During their active secretory phase, B effector cells typically manifest as plasma cells (refer to Chapter 3 for the histology of plasma cells). Since antibodies circulate in the extracellular fluids ("humors"), B cells are said to be responsible for the humoral immune response. Antigens attached to antibodies are more easily recognized by phagocytes and eliminated. Additionally, the antigen–antibody complex triggers a collection of plasma proteins called the complement system. The complement system is an important component of innate defense, with wide-ranging effects that include the ability to kill microorganisms.

Effector T cells, on the other hand, act more directly on adjacent cells within tissues. The two major subsets of effector T cells mediate their effects in different ways. T helper cells act through the secretion of soluble, locally acting molecules called cytokines, whereas T cytotoxic cells attach to antigens on target cells to kill them. Since these cell-killing actions require close cell-to-cell contact, T cells are said to be responsible for the cell-mediated immune response.

A third category of lymphocytes lacks the typical antigen receptor found in either B or T cells. These cells, known as innate lymphoid cells, rapidly respond to foreign antigens or destroy abnormal cells immediately after they are encountered. This category includes innate helper cells that can regulate responses to intestinal microbiota, allergic diseases, and autoimmunity. Additionally, it includes innate cytotoxic cells called "natural killer" (NK) cells, which rely on an antigen recognition system less specific than that used by B and T cells. The cell-mediated killing mechanism of NK cells is similar to that of T cytotoxic cells. In some species, NK cells appear as large granular lymphocytes. Natural killer T cells (NKT cells) are innate-like T cells that express both NK cell markers and a T cell receptor of limited diversity. NKT cells mount rapid responses relative to conventional T cells, producing cytokines to modulate immunity across a broad spectrum of diseases. NKT cells trigger chemokine and cytokine release, enhance NK function, and promote dendritic cell (DC) maturation and B cell responses.

Lymphocyte Diversity The antigen diversity of microbial and pathogenic agents is vast, yet the antigen receptor of a lymphocyte has a unique antigen specificity, i.e., an individual lymphocyte can only be activated by the antigen that can be recognized by its antigen receptor. To address this diversity, the immune system generates a population of lymphocytes with a diverse repertoire of antigen receptors. The diversification of the pre-immune antigen-receptor repertoire occurs in primary lymphoid organs through a process of gene rearrangement events in T or B cells. T and B cell populations can be divided further into subpopulations and subsets based on the functional capabilities of their antigen receptor, associated coreceptor molecules, and cytokine profiles.

Lymphocyte Recirculation

Lymphocytes circulate continuously from the blood through lymphatic and nonlymphatic tissues, subsequently returning to the blood either directly or via the lymphatic system. This process, called lymphocyte recirculation, facilitates the dissemination of an immune response throughout the body and enables effective immune surveillance for foreign invaders and alterations in the body's own cells. Most lymphocytes enter organs, such as the lungs, liver, and bone marrow, and return to the blood via venules. Some lymphocytes leave these organs via the lymphatic vessels and drain to lymph nodes via afferent lymphatic vessels. Tissue fluid from large peripheral areas also drains into regional lymph nodes, further enhancing the likelihood of an encounter between a lymphocyte and its target antigen. Additionally, some lymphocytes migrate directly from the blood into lymphatic tissues through specialized postcapillary venules called high endothelial venules (see the "Lymph Nodes" section below [Fig. 8-13]). High endothelial venules have cuboidal lining cells, in contrast to the flattened endothelial cells of other blood vessels. These specialized venules are abundant in lymphatic tissue and serve as entry sites for both T and B cells from the blood circulation. The spleen is an exception as it lacks postcapillary venules or afferent lymphatics. Lymphocytes migrate into the spleen via blood capillaries in the marginal zone (see the "Spleen" section below). Normally, relatively few lymphocytes migrate into organs such as the skin, synovia, muscle, and brain; however, during acute and chronic inflammation, an influx of large numbers of lymphocytes can occur.

Antigen Presentation

For antigen recognition and the initiation of an immune response to occur, B cells can recognize antigens either directly or as complexes presented by an antigen-presenting cells such as follicular dendritic cells (DCs). On the other hand, T cells require antigens to be presented on the surface of antigen-presenting cells, such as DCs, in association with MHC molecules. Most nucleated cells express MHC class I and can present antigens to cytotoxic T cells. B cells, macrophages, and DCs constitutively express MHC class II and can present antigens to T helper cells. In contrast to macrophages, which ingest most foreign substances, B cells bind a specific single antigen through surface immunoglobulin. The bound molecule is then endocytosed, fragmented, and presented by MHC-II molecules. Other cell types that can take up and process antigens, such as granulocytes, endothelial cells, fibroblasts, smooth muscle cells, and some epithelial cells, can be induced to express MHC-II under certain conditions, such as inflammation or infection. The functional role of MHC-II upregulation in these cells is incompletely understood.

Phagocytes

Phagocytes are specialized cells that function to detect, ingest, and eliminate foreign material, including bacteria, harmful particles or substances, and dead or dying cells. Common phagocytes include macrophages, monocytes, neutrophils, and DCs. These cells possess cell surface receptors for recognizing foreign agents, are effective at phagocytosis, and produce an array of cytokines to regulate inflammatory and immune responses. In contrast, other cell types such as epithelial cells, endothelial cells, fibroblasts, and mesenchymal cells have limited or less effective phagocytic capability.

Macrophages

Macrophages, also known as mononuclear phagocytes, are found in various tissues and are active in the phagocytosis and degradation of foreign substances (see Chapter 3 for the histology of macrophages). The processing of foreign substances into short peptides is essential for antigen presentation to T cells via the peptide-binding groove of the MHC-II molecule. Tissue-resident macrophages in lymphoid tissues include marginal zone and red pulp macrophages in the spleen, subcapsular sinus and medullary sinus macrophages in the lymph nodes, and tingible body macrophages in germinal centers and the thymus. Monocytes arise from bone marrow precursor cells, circulate in the blood, and upon exiting the blood vessels, differentiate into macrophages. However, it is important to note that not all tissue-resident macrophages are derived from monocytes or have a bone marrow origin. They can arise from embryonic precursors, yolk sac-derived macrophages, fetal liver precursors, and also undergo local proliferation and maintenance within tissues.

Dendritic Cells

DCs, along with monocytes and tissue macrophages, comprise the mononuclear phagocyte system. While macrophages are predominantly effector cells of the innate immune system, DCs are specialized to induce adaptive immunity. Most DCs, including interstitial DCs, interdigitating DCs, veiled cells, and intraepidermal macrophages, are derived from hematopoietic stem cells. These cells typically have numerous long cytoplasmic processes. Functionally, DCs bind antigens and cluster lymphocytes on their surface in tissues throughout the body. Once antigens are bound, phagocytosed, and processed, DCs become antigen-presenting cells to activate T cells by presenting the processed antigen on MHC-II molecules. In stratified squamous epithelia, DCs localize in the upper spinous layer and are termed intraepidermal macrophages or Langerhans cells (see Chapter 16). When they are in lymph and blood, DCs possess prominent surface folds and are referred to as veiled cells. Interstitial DCs are located in various organs such as the heart, kidney, gut, and lung.

Interdigitating Dendritic Cells Interdigitating DCs are primarily found in lymph nodes, the thymic medulla, and the spleen. Cytoplasmic granules are characteristic features of these DCs, which also have numerous MHC-II molecules on their surface. Interdigitating DCs present antigens to T lymphocytes (helper cells), which in turn stimulate a cellular immune response.

Other Leukocytes and Mast Cells

The histology of leukocytes is described in detail in Chapter 6. In addition to lymphocytes, other white blood cells actively participate in both innate and adaptive immunity. Neutrophils, for instance, are prominent in the clearance of bacteria and microbes and contribute to shaping the host response to infection and immune system homeostasis. Eosinophils, basophils, and mast cells, on the other hand, are phagocytic cells that can engulf and destroy foreign organisms and substances. They also play prominent roles in allergic reactions and defense against parasites.

Stromal Cells

Stromal cells are nonhematopoietic connective tissue (CT) cells. These fixed cells of the lymphatic system form a tissue reticulum and support the immune response. The major stromal cell types that can be distinguished by morphology and function include fibroblastic reticular cells, marginal reticular cells, lymphatic endothelial cells, blood endothelial cells, and follicular dendritic cells. In the thymus, epithelial cells create a supportive mesh or stroma for the lymphocytes comprising the parenchyma of this lymphatic organ.

Fibroblastic Reticular Cells

Fibroblastic reticular cells, originating from mesenchymal cells and exhibiting a fibroblast-like structure, form a reticulum in all lymphatic organs except the cortex of the thymus and cloacal bursa (see the "Lymph Nodes" section below [Fig. 8-11]). Because of their numerous long and branching processes, these cells have a stellate appearance. They synthesize reticular fibers closely associated with or invaginated into their cell surface. Fibroblastic reticular cells establish an interconnected network, known as the conduit system, within lymphoid tissues, facilitating the rapid transmission of molecular signals, including antigens and fluid distribution. This conduit network is dense in areas rich in T cells, such as the deep cortex of the lymph node, but it shows reduced branching and is less common in B cell-rich areas such as the primary and secondary nodules of lymph nodes (Fig. 8-14).

Follicular Dendritic Cells Follicular dendritic cells are specialized stromal cells localized within the B-cell areas (nodules) of lymphatic tissue. Despite their name, follicular dendritic cells are not related to DCs and are not derived from bone marrow. Follicular dendritic cells are part of the network of fibroblastic reticular cells in lymphatic tissues. In contrast to dendritic cells, follicular dendritic cells can trap and retain antigens in a complex for long periods of time, enabling the presentation of unprocessed antigens. Importantly, follicular dendritic cells lack the MHC-II surface molecules typically found in interdigitating DCs.

Thymic and Bursal Epithelial Cells

In the thymus and cloacal bursa, stellate epithelial cells form a reticulum that supports developing lymphocytes and macrophages (see the "Thymus" section below [Fig. 8-4]). Unlike fibroblastic reticular cells, thymic epithelial cells (TECs) do not produce reticular fibers (Fig. 8-14).

Endothelial Cells and Sinus-Lining Cells

Lymphatic endothelial cells line the branched sinus system of lymph nodes and form a continuous barrier with the afferent and efferent lymphatic vessels, which convey lymph to and from the lymph node. The endothelial cells facing the capsule are called the ceiling lymphatic endothelial cells, while those overlaying the lymphocyte-containing lymph node parenchyma are called floor lymphatic endothelial cells. Sinusoidal lymphatic endothelial cells are active in the sorting of lymph-borne macromolecules and in controlling the entry and exit of cellular traffic across the subcapsular floor of the lymph node.

Organization of Cells to Form Lymphatic Tissues and Organs

As the fetus develops, the immune system is molded into two principal types of tissues: diffuse and organized lymphatic tissues. Diffuse lymphatic tissues are scattered throughout loose connective tissues of the gut, respiratory tract, urogenital system, and skin, as well as in extra-nodular areas of lymphatic organs. Organized lymphatic tissues include encapsulated organs such as the thymus, lymph nodes, and spleen, as well as nodular aggregates of the mucosa-associated lymphoid tissue (MALT).

Diffuse Lymphatic Tissue

Diffuse lymphatic tissue comprises a variable number of small lymphocytes, often mingled with lymphoblasts undergoing mitosis, and macrophages. The stroma of diffuse lymphatic tissue consists of a three-dimensional network formed by reticular cells, DCs, and CT.

Organized Lymphatic Tissue

Organized lymphatic tissue contains accumulations of B cells arranged in primary and secondary nodules.

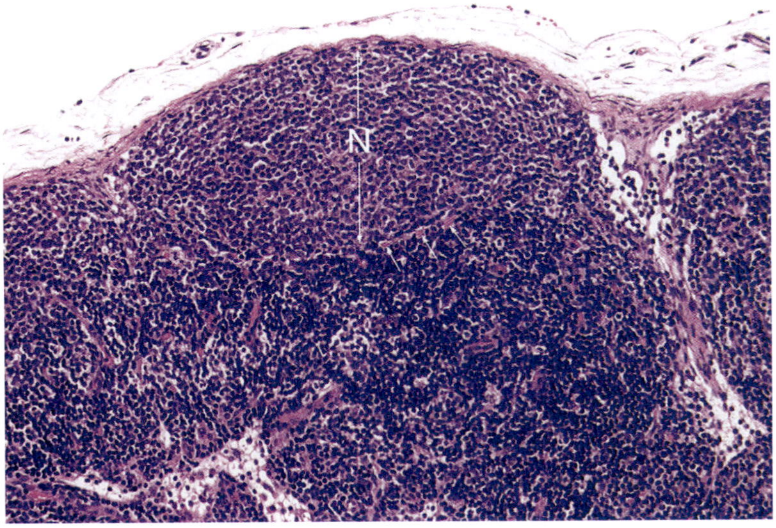

Figure 8-1 Lymph node (fetal lamb at 140 days of gestation). The primary lymphatic nodule (N) in the outer cortex consists of an aggregate of small-to medium-sized lymphocytes and some follicular dendritic cells. Note the presence of a capillary network outlining the primary nodule (arrows). Hematoxylin and eosin (H&E).

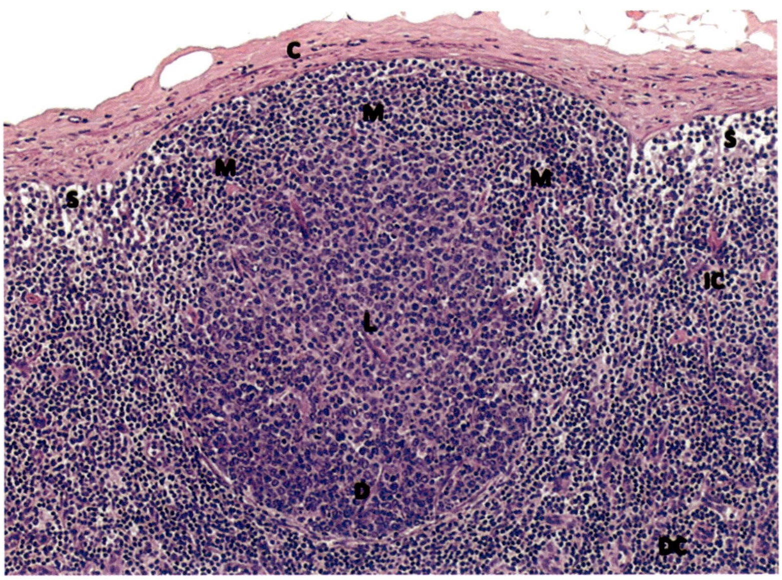

Figure 8-2 Lymph node (goat). Secondary lymphatic nodule with germinal center. Dark zone (D), light zone (L), mantle (M), capsule (C), subcapsular sinus (S), internodular cortex (IC), and deep cortex (DC). H&E.

Primary Lymphatic Nodules

Primary lymphatic nodules consist of a stromal network of CT and immature follicular dendritic cells (Fig. 8-1). Within this stromal network, small, tightly packed lymphocytes along with some medium lymphocytes are distributed, predominantly representing naive recirculating B cells. Primary nodules do not contain germinal centers.

Secondary Lymphatic Nodules

Secondary lymphatic nodules are characterized by a light-staining germinal center within the nodule (Fig. 8-2). The formation of the germinal center begins in a primary nodule with an accumulation of large, euchromatic lymphoblasts and tingible body macrophages. Differentiated reticular cells form the stroma of the secondary nodules. An established germinal center consists of a central light zone and an adjacent dark zone. Follicular dendritic cells are localized in the light zone of the germinal center. The light zone is populated by B lymphocytes with euchromatic, light-staining nuclei. Along the periphery of the light zone is a thin layer of small heterochromatic lymphocytes that often form a thicker cap, called the mantle, over the apex of the germinal center. The dark zone is composed of B-cell lymphoblasts engaged in intense mitotic activity. Typically, the germinal center is oriented such that the light zone is closest to the subcapsular sinus in lymph nodes, the surface epithelium in mucosal nodules, or the marginal zone in the spleen. The germinal center regresses when cellular activity declines late in an immune response.

Germinal Center Reaction Activated B cells migrate to the T cell–B cell border of the nodule, where they present antigens to T helper cells and receive costimulation. Selected B cells then migrate to the center of the nodule, initiating a cycle of proliferation and hypermutation in the dark zone before undergoing antigen-driven selection by follicular dendritic cells in the light zone. After selection by the follicular dendritic cell, the B cell can either re-enter the dark zone of the germinal center for further proliferation and hypermutation or, with the assistance of T follicular helper cells, exit the germinal center as either a memory B cell or as a plasma cell. B cells that do not receive survival signals will undergo apoptosis.

Primary Lymphatic Organs

During fetal development, the unique identity of T and B lymphocytes is first established within primary lymphatic organs. These organs include the bone marrow (in mammals), ileal Peyer's patch (in sheep and cattle), cloacal bursa (in birds), and thymus (in both mammals and birds). Stem cells within these organs reside in specialized environments isolated from circulating antigens and foreign substances to avoid interference in the education and development of lymphocytes (see the "T Lymphocyte Development" section below). Intense cell proliferation is accompanied by random rearrangement of genes responsible for the antigen receptor and the expression of accessory molecules facilitating interactions with other cells and conferring effector functions. Lymphocytes leaving a primary lymphatic organ are classified as naive or virgin cells because they have not been exposed to foreign antigens. Scrutiny of the emerging lymphocytes is followed by the elimination of more than 90% of the cells that are identified as unsuitable, largely because of their reaction with the body's own molecules (autoreactivity). These lymphocytes are eliminated by apoptosis, a mechanism that involves the activation of a genetic pathway ensuring the rapid disintegration of selected cells with minimal harm to surrounding tissues.

Despite the elimination of most of their cells, primary lymphatic organs still continue to produce vast numbers of B and T cells with a diverse repertoire of non-self-antigen specificities. These cells are released and disseminated throughout the body, populating diffuse lymphatic tissue, secondary lymphatic tissue (i.e., MALT), and secondary lymphatic organs (e.g., lymph nodes). In these locations, they will encounter antigen and initiate immune responses.

Bone Marrow

The structure and major hematopoietic functions of the bone marrow are detailed in Chapter 6. In mammals, the bone marrow is the source of pluripotent stem cells, including B- and T-cell precursors, and facilitates B-cell differentiation. B cells are located adjacent to the endosteum of bone and undergo differentiation and selection as they migrate centrally toward the venous sinuses within the hematopoietic space. B-cell maturation occurs in close association with stromal reticular cells and macrophages within the bone marrow.

Thymus

The thymus originates as a solid outgrowth from the epithelium (endoderm) of the third pharyngeal pouch. The proliferation of epithelial cells gives rise to a thymic epithelial reticulum, which is subsequently invaded by blood vessels from the surrounding mesenchyme. Migration of lymphocytic progenitor cells from the bone marrow into the thymus occurs early in ontogeny, likely in response to chemotactic signals produced by the developing thymic tissue (thymic anlage). The lymphocytic progenitor cells invade the interstices, filling the spaces between the epithelial cells. The thymus is therefore often referred to as a "lymphoepithelial organ."

The thymus comprises right and left lobes, each encased in a capsule of CT that extends into thin septa, dividing the lobes into partially separated lobules. Each lobule contains a central medulla, branching from a central stalk within the lobe, and is surrounded by a cortex (Fig. 8-3).

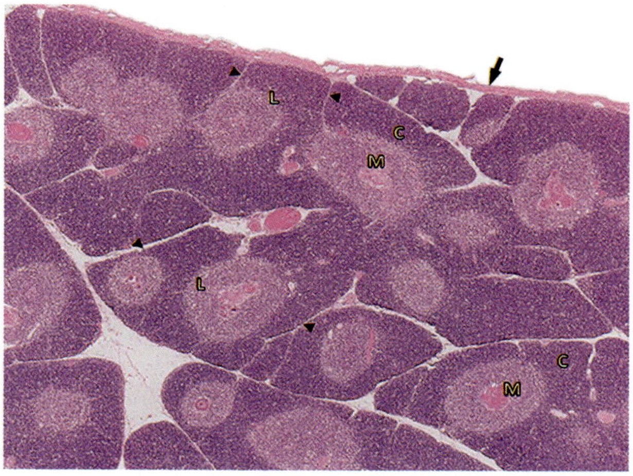

Figure 8-3 Thymus (cat). The thymic lobules (L) consist of a light medulla (M) surrounded by a dark cortex (C) and are partially separated by thin septa of connective tissue (CT) (arrowheads). Capsule (arrow). H&E.

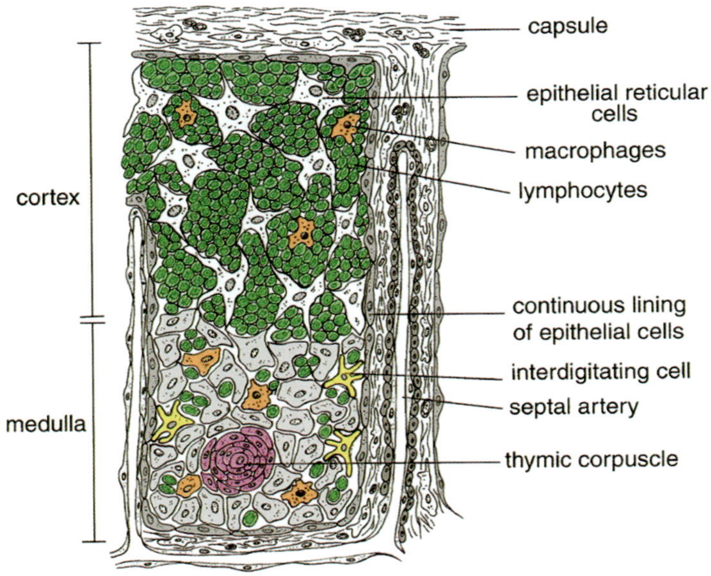

Figure 8-4 Schematic drawing of a portion of a thymic lobule. The lobule consists of a cortex and medulla and has a border of flattened epithelial cells. The epithelial reticulum of the cortex is heavily infiltrated by lymphocytes undergoing cell division and differentiation. The epithelial cells of the medulla may form concentric arrangements called thymic corpuscles or Hassall's corpuscles. Blood vessels supply the lobule via the capsule and thin CT septa to reach the corticomedullary junction.

Cortex

The thymic cortex consists mainly of an epithelial reticulum and lymphocytes (Fig. 8-4). Stellate TECs have large, pale, ovoid nuclei and long, branching cytoplasmic processes containing numerous intermediate filaments; their cellular organelles are inconspicuous. Adjacent TECs are interconnected by desmosomes, forming a cellular stromal network. A continuous lining of long, flattened epithelial cells surrounds the periphery of the lobules and perivascular spaces. Lymphoblasts and medium-sized lymphocytes predominate in the meshes of the peripheral epithelial reticulum, undergoing mitotic divisions to produce small lymphocytes that differentiate in the deep cortex. Tingible body macrophages, frequently found near the medulla, phagocytize and eliminate dead T lymphocytes, often containing lymphocyte remnants. The thymic cortex appears darker stained than the medulla because it contains a greater concentration of lymphocytes (Fig. 8-5).

Medulla

Many of the TECs in the medulla have the same structure as those found in the cortex. However, some are much larger, with their epithelial nature more pronounced. These larger cells contain more mitochondria, an extensive rough endoplasmic reticulum, a well-developed Golgi complex, and granules compared to cortical TECs.

Certain medullary TECs contribute to the formation of thymic corpuscles, also called Hassall's corpuscles (Fig. 8-6). These corpuscles comprise one to several calcified or degenerated large central cells, surrounded by flat keratinized cells in a concentric arrangement. The corpuscle cells are interconnected by desmosomes and contain bundles of intermediate filaments. There is evidence that these corpuscles are not entirely degenerative structures and may have a role in the development of regulatory T cells.

Interdigitating DCs, similar to those present in the T-cell areas of secondary lymphatic organs, are also present in the medulla. The cellular composition within the meshes of the thymic epithelial network primarily consists of small lymphocytes, accompanied by a small number of macrophages.

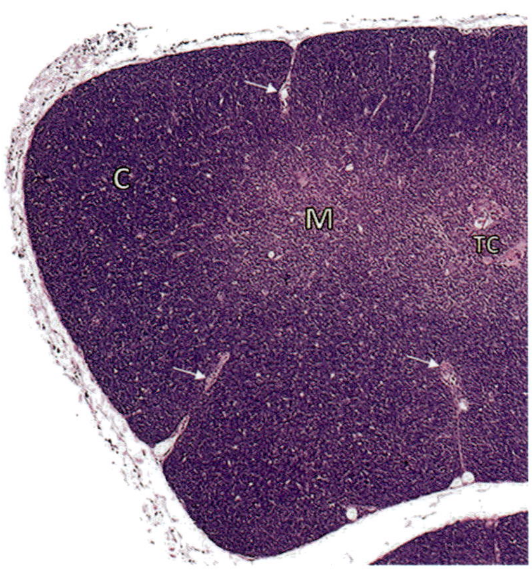

Figure 8-5 Thymus (lamb). The dark cortex (C) is clearly distinguishable from the light medulla (M), in which large thymic corpuscles (TC) are readily identified. Blood vessels are visible in thin CT septa (arrows). H&E.

T Lymphocyte Development Within the thymus, lymphocytic progenitor cells develop into T cells. Originating from the cortical-medullary junction, lymphocyte progenitor cells from the bone marrow are termed "double negative" (DN) thymocytes because they do not express CD4 and CD8 coreceptors, characteristic of mature T cells. These DN thymocytes migrate to the subcapsular cortical region, where they undergo proliferation and differentiation into "double positive" (DP) thymocytes, expressing both coreceptors. DP cells constitute the majority of thymocytes in early thymic development. The mature T cell receptor complex is formed during the DP stage. DP thymocytes expressing mature T cell receptors subsequently undergo positive selection, recognizing peptides in the context of self-MHC. The recognition of signals results in survival, while the lack of recognition leads to death by apoptosis. The recognition of self-peptides is governed by the coreceptors and results in the choice to be "single positive" (SP) thymocytes expressing either the CD4 or CD8 coreceptor. SP cells migrate to the medullary region for negative selection, where self-reactive T cells are deleted, establishing central tolerance. An important function of medullary TECs is the promiscuous expression of tissue-restricted antigens and nuclear autoimmune regulator protein, pivotal for central tolerance development. Medullary TECs also transfer antigen to DCs, establishing an additional pathway for negative selection. During negative selection, SP T cells are presented with tissue-restricted antigens by medullary thymic epithelial cells and DCs, testing their affinity toward self-antigens. Strong recognition of self-peptides will lead to apoptosis. The majority (>90%) of developing T cells "fail" positive or negative selection and die or fail to be exported. Even so, a full complement of diverse naive CD4+ and CD8+ T cells is released from this selection process, capable of recognizing millions of different antigenic epitopes. Naive CD4+ T cells recognize epitopes presented by MHC class II molecules and differentiate into T-helper effector cells, coordinating cellular immunity against diverse pathogens. Naive CD8+ T cells recognize epitopes presented by MHC class I molecules and differentiate into cytotoxic T cells. Negative selection in the medulla is also important for the generation of regulatory T cells and unconventional T cell lineages, including gamma-delta ($\gamma\delta$) T cells, NKT cells, and intraepithelial lymphocytes of the gut.

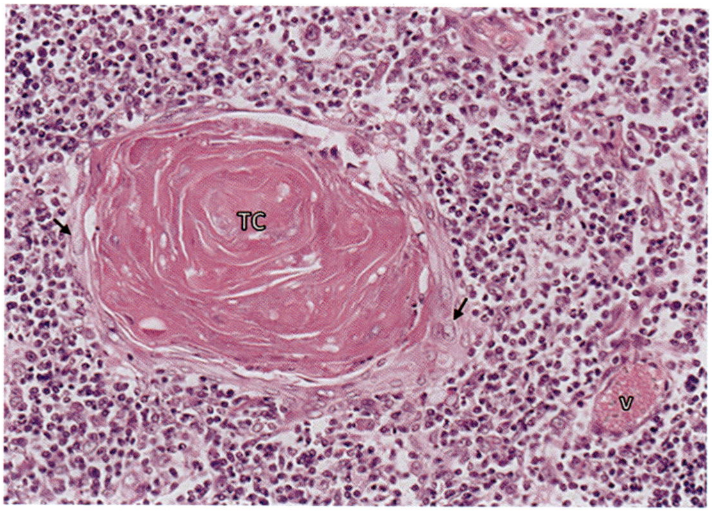

Figure 8-6 Thymic corpuscle, thymus (cat). Notice the arrangement of the cells in concentric layers and enlarged thymic epithelial cells (arrows) in a large thymic corpuscle (TC). Blood vessel (v). H&E.

Blood Vessels, Lymph Vessels, and Nerves

The blood supply of the thymus is derived from arteries that penetrate the parenchyma at the corticomedullary junction by way of the CT septa (Fig. 8-5). These arteries branch into arterioles that traverse along the junction and give rise to a capillary network within the cortex. Capillaries then drain into postcapillary venules located either at the corticomedullary junction or within the medulla, where they join veins within the CT septa. Cortical capillaries are characterized by a continuous endothelium, surrounded by perivascular CT and enveloped by a sheath of TEC processes. Together, these layers form the blood–thymus barrier, which restricts the access of circulating antigens that might interfere with the positive selection of lymphocytes in the cortical tissue. Conversely, the absence of such a barrier at the corticomedullary junction allows circulating antigens to participate in the negative selection processes of lymphocytes.

T cells exit the thymus by crossing the endothelium of postcapillary venules located at the corticomedullary junction. The T cells released from the thymus migrate to settle within the T-cell areas of diffuse lymphatic tissue, secondary lymphatic tissue, and various organs.

The thymus is particularly active in young animals, with normal involution of the organ occurring after sexual maturity. Involution of the thymus is characterized by a gradual depletion of lymphocytes (especially from the cortex), accompanied by the enlargement of the TECs. Additionally, white adipocytes originating from the interlobular CT invade the parenchyma. In adult animals, the thymus consists of narrow cords of lymphocytes, predominantly surrounded by enlarged TECs amid adipose tissue.

Primary Lymphatic Organs at Mucosal Surfaces

Ileal Peyer's Patch of Ruminants

Most organized lymphatic tissue associated with the gut has been attributed to functions related to mucosal and systemic immunity (see the "Gut-Associated Lymphatic Tissue" section below). In young ruminants, pigs, horses,

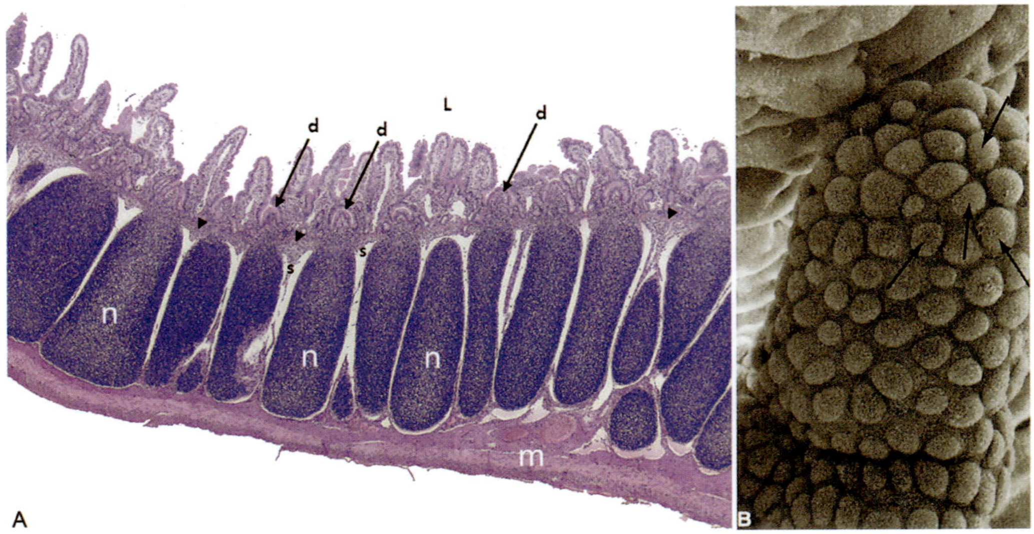

Figure 8-7 Ileal Peyer's patch. **A.** Goat kid. The submucosa contains many closely apposed large lymphatic nodules (n) that are separated by lymphatic sinuses (s) and small triangular internodular (T-cell) regions (arrowheads). Small conical domes (d) protrude through the tunica mucosa to contact the gut lumen (L). Tunica muscularis (m). H&E. **B.** Calf. Nodule-associated epithelium. A homogenous population of modified epithelial cells possessing surface folds (arrows) overlies the dome. Scanning electron microscopy.

and carnivores, a single large aggregate of lymphatic nodules (the ileal Peyer's patch) is present in the distal jejunum/ileum. A specific role for the ileal Peyer's patch in the diversification of the pre-immune antigen-receptor repertoire and expansion of early B-cell populations has been defined in sheep and cattle (Fig. 8-7). The intense cell division in the aggregated nodules is independent of foreign antigen. As with the avian bursa described below, the processes of positive and negative lymphocyte selection likely occur, ensuring the suitability of the lymphocytes that exit into the blood and lymphatic circulations. In rabbits and pigs, the diversification of the primary antibody repertoire occurs after birth in gut-associated lymphatic tissue, with exogenous factors derived from microbial flora being required. In rabbits, organized gut-associated lymphatic tissue (GALT) consists of Peyer's patches in the small intestine, the *sacculus rotundus* at the ileo-cecal junction, and the appendix extending from the distal end of the cecum.

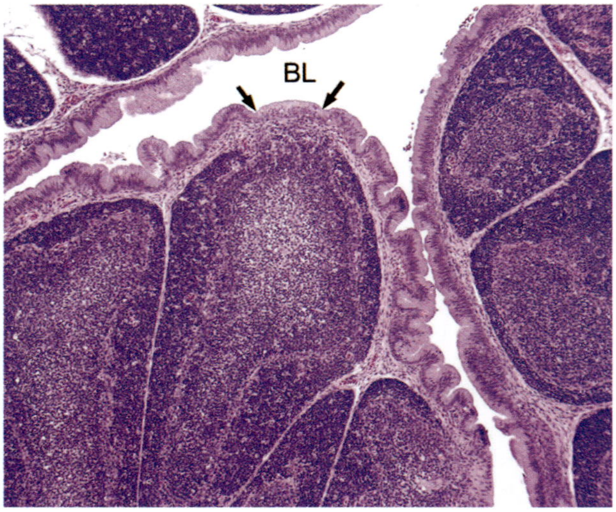

Figure 8-8 Cloacal bursa (chicken). The modified epithelium (between arrows) overlies a lymphatic nodule that contains a dark peripheral zone and a light central zone. The bursal lumen (BL) is also visible. H&E.

It should be noted that both the single large aggregate of lymphatic nodules in the distal small intestine of sheep and the avian bursa receive B cells that are already committed to the B-cell lineage. Thus, neither organ strictly functions as a primary lymphatic organ, where B cells develop de novo from uncommitted precursors.

Similar to the thymus, the ileal Peyer's patch in sheep and cattle, as well as the avian bursa, undergoes involution. Conversely, the GALT in rabbits and pigs does not undergo involution and continues in the adult as secondary lymphatic tissues.

Cloacal Bursa of Birds

The dichotomy of the T- and B-cell lineages was first revealed in birds, where B cells were discovered in association with the avian cloacal bursa. The cloacal bursa (bursa of Fabricius) is a lymphatic organ located in the dorsal wall of the cloaca (Fig. 8-8). It plays a key role in the differentiation of B cells and the generation of antibody diversity.

From day 8 to day 15 of chicken embryo development, precursor cells committed to the B-cell lineage migrate into the developing organ. Lymphatic nodules begin to form as invaginations of the cloacal epithelium into underlying tissues of the cloaca at approximately day 12 of incubation. Longitudinal folds containing the nodules and a stroma of epithelial cells then protrude into the bursal lumen, followed by the formation of light central and dark peripheral zones, initiating lymphocyte differentiation within the nodules. The simple columnar or pseudostratified epithelium overlying the nodules within the folds has a remarkable capacity for transcytosis of macromolecules, including antigens, from the bursal lumen into the nodules.

Secondary Lymphatic Tissues and Organs

Secondary lymphatic tissues and organs are strategically situated to monitor and respond to foreign organisms and substances entering the host. They collect immunological information from peripheral tissues through immune cells and soluble mediators. These lymphatic tissues and organs are equipped with specialized microenvironments to enact innate responses for immediate protection against harmful agents and initiate adaptive responses to mobilize immune protection. Unlike primary lymphatic organs where exposure to foreign material is tightly regulated, secondary lymphatic tissues and organs are routinely exposed to the microbial products and inflammatory mediators. Invading pathogens, along with foreign antigens, are transported from their site of entry into the body to the secondary lymphatic tissues via blood or lymph, often associated with cells such as DCs and/or macrophages. The secondary lymphatic tissues associated with mucosal surfaces are termed mucosa-associated lymphatic tissue, while lymph nodes, spleen, and hemal nodes are examples of secondary lymphatic organs.

Tertiary lymphatic structures, resembling secondary lymphatic organs, develop in nonlymphatic tissues in response to chronic inflammation. They lack capsules but can be divided into T and B cell areas.

Lymph Nodes

Lymph nodes, situated along the extensive drainage system of lymph vessels, filter foreign material from the lymph before returning lymph to the bloodstream. They are the only lymphatic organs with both afferent and efferent lymph vessels and sinuses. These organs usually have a slight indentation known as the hilus, where blood and lymph vessels enter or exit the lymph node. The parenchyma is organized into a cortex of lymphatic nodules and diffuse lymphatic tissue, and a medulla of lymphatic tissue arranged in cords (Fig. 8-9).

Lymph nodes are surrounded by a capsule composed primarily of dense irregular CT. In ruminants, smooth muscle cells are also present. Trabeculae extend from the capsule into the parenchyma as irregular septa that are distributed throughout the cortex and medulla (Fig. 8-10). The trabeculae provide support for the entire node, carry blood vessels and nerves, and are surrounded by sinuses. The stroma of the lymph node is composed of reticular cells and fibers. Lymphocytes, macrophages, and plasma cells are supported by this reticular meshwork.

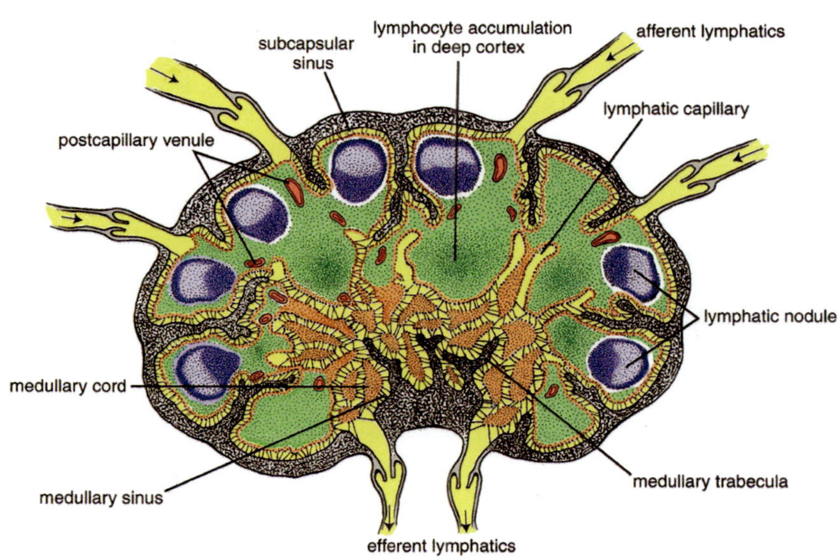

Figure 8-9 Schematic drawing of a lymph node. The direction of lymph flow is shown with arrows. Lymph enters the node through afferent lymph vessels that penetrate the capsule and open into the subcapsular sinus. Efferent lymph vessels collect drained lymph and leave the node at the hilus.

Lymphatic Vessels and Sinuses

Afferent lymph vessels penetrate the capsule at several different sites and open into the subcapsular sinus (Fig. 8-9). Valves are present in both afferent and efferent lymphatic vessels,

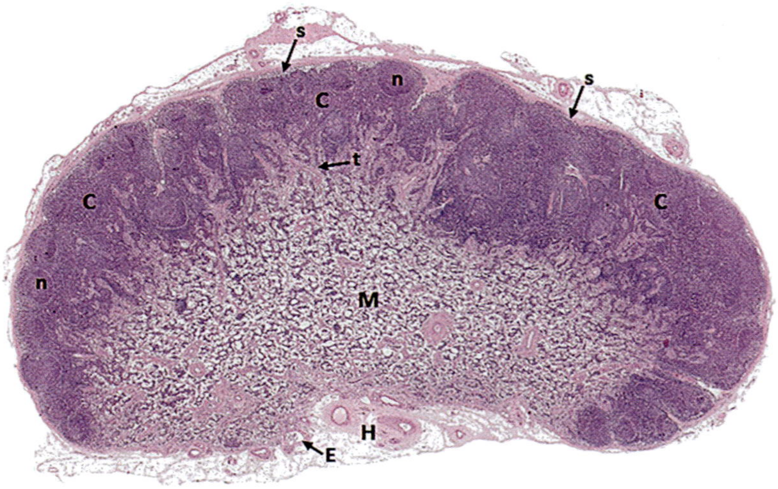

Figure 8-10 Lymph node (goat). The dark cortex (C) with lymphatic nodules (n) lies adjacent to the lighter-appearing medulla (M). Subcapsular (s) and trabecular (t) sinuses are continuous with sinuses in the medulla that drain toward the hilus (H) to empty into efferent lymph vessels (E). H&E.

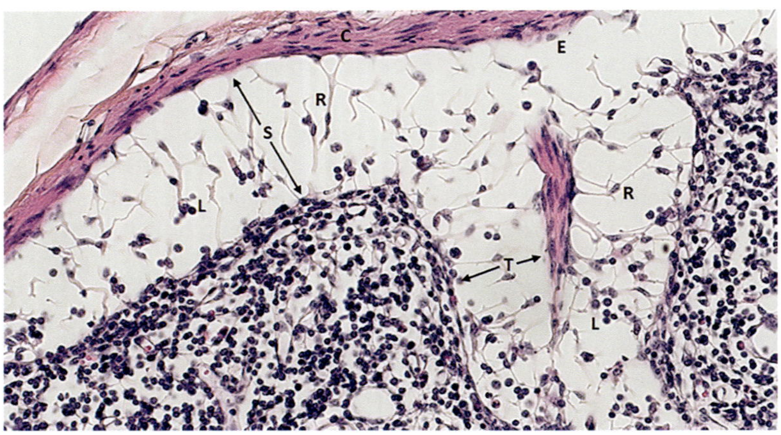

Figure 8-11 Lymph node, perfused (cow). Beneath the CT capsule (C) is the subcapsular sinus (S), lined by flattened lymphatic endothelial cells (E). The cortical (trabecular) sinus (T) accompanies a CT trabecula into the outer cortex of the lymph node. Fibroblastic reticular cells (R) and lymphocytes (L) are present in the sinus. Note that the lymph node was perfused during fixation, resulting in the washing out of many cells from the parenchyma and the expansion of the sinuses, which are clearly visible. H&E.

thereby ensuring a unidirectional flow of lymph. Cortical sinuses originate from the subcapsular sinus to accompany the CT trabeculae and extend into medullary sinuses. These sinuses form a network of branching and anastomosing channels that converge toward the hilus to open into the efferent lymph vessels. All lymph exits the node through the efferent lymphatic vessels (Fig. 8-9).

The sinuses are lined by flattened lymphatic endothelial cells, forming a continuous lining in the proximal portion adjacent to the capsule and trabeculae. Toward the parenchyma, this lining becomes more discontinuous. The lumina of the sinuses are traversed by a dense network of interconnected reticular cells attached to the sinus walls through numerous slender processes (Fig. 8-11). Many sinus macrophages are attached to this network. Lymphocytes, macrophages, and DCs are found both freely within the stromal mesh and within the sinus lumen. The reticular cells function as a baffle to slow lymph flow within the sinuses to facilitate both antigen–cell interactions and the phagocytic activities of macrophages.

Cortex

Most of the outer cortex of the lymph node consists of primary and secondary lymphatic nodules separated by diffuse lymphatic tissue (Fig. 8-10). The deep cortex also is composed of diffuse lymphatic tissue and is drained by lymphatics (Fig. 8-10). Because most lymphocytes in the deep cortex originate from the thymus, this area is referred to as a T-cell or thymus-dependent zone. The term paracortex has been applied variably to the deep cortex or to the diffuse lymphatic tissue of both the deep and outer regions of cortex.

Medulla

The medulla of the lymph node is much less organized than the cortex. Lymphatic tissue extends from the cortical T-cell areas as medullary cords, which branch and anastomose throughout the medulla (Fig. 8-9). These cords are separated by a network of sinuses and CT trabeculae. Within the stromal mesh of the medullary cords, plasma cells are prominent, alongside lymphocytes and macrophages (Fig. 8-12).

Blood Vessels and Nerves

The major arteries enter the lymph node at the hilus, whereas smaller vessels penetrate the capsule at various sites. Upon entering the hilus, some arteries branch to supply the medullary cords directly, while other branches enter the trabeculae to supply the CT and capsule. Vessels supplying the medullary cords distribute capillaries along their course, with the main vessels continuing into the cortex, where branches feed capillary networks between and within the nodules. Internodular branches form capillary arcades below the subcapsular sinus and then extend inward to the deep cortex, forming postcapillary venules lined by a cuboidal endothelium in most species (Fig. 8-13). These postcapillary venules, also called high endothelial venules, join veins in the medullary trabeculae, which subsequently empty into veins exiting at the hilus.

Nerve fibers supply the capsule and trabeculae, and vasomotor nerves form perivascular networks throughout the lymph node.

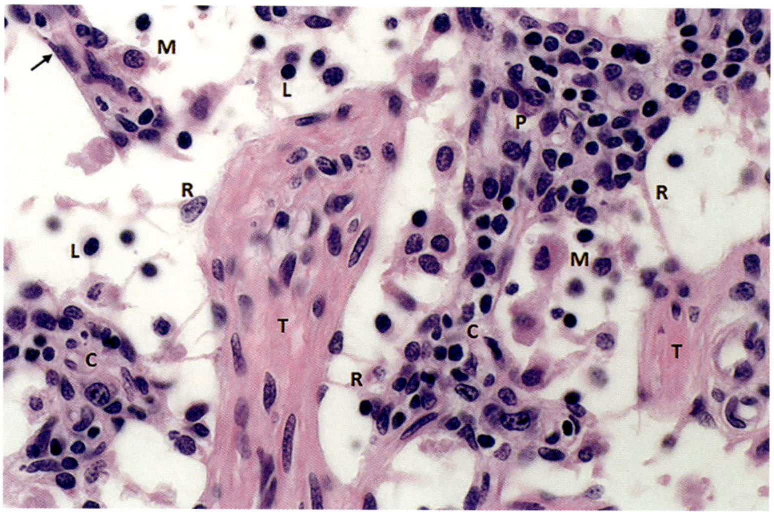

Figure 8-12 Lymph node, medulla (goat). Flattened lymphatic endothelial cells (arrow) line the medullary sinus, which contains lymphocytes (L), macrophages (M), plasma cells, and reticular cells (R). Medullary cords (C) are composed of lymphocytes, macrophages, and plasma cells (P). Trabecula (T) are also visible. H&E.

Stromal Network

The lymphatic parenchyma of the lymph node is supported by a stromal network of reticular fibers primarily composed of bundles of type III collagen fibers (Fig. 8-14). The spaces within this three-dimensional reticulum are filled with lymphocytes and antigen-presenting cells. The reticular fibers originate from the CT capsule and trabeculae and extend across the subcapsular and trabecular sinus into the diffuse lymphatic tissue of the outer cortex, further penetrating into the deep cortex and medulla. Fibroblastic reticular cells produce these reticular fibers, surrounding them and the extracellular matrix with a basement membrane, forming an interconnected system of tubes known as the conduit system. This system functions as a molecular sieve. Most fluid that enters the lymph node via afferent lymph and the subcapsular sinus is directed through the sinus system to the medulla, exiting the lymph node through efferent lymph vessels. The sinus lining cells form a basement membrane, preventing fluid entry into the lymphatic parenchyma. Particles and larger molecules are removed from the lymph by sinus macrophages. Fluid and smaller molecules can permeate the lymphatic parenchyma through the tubes of the reticular fiber network, passing between the sinus-lining cells. This conduit system functions to transport small antigens from the subcapsular sinus to areas of the cortex containing high endothelial venules and populations of circulating lymphocytes and antigen-presenting cells.

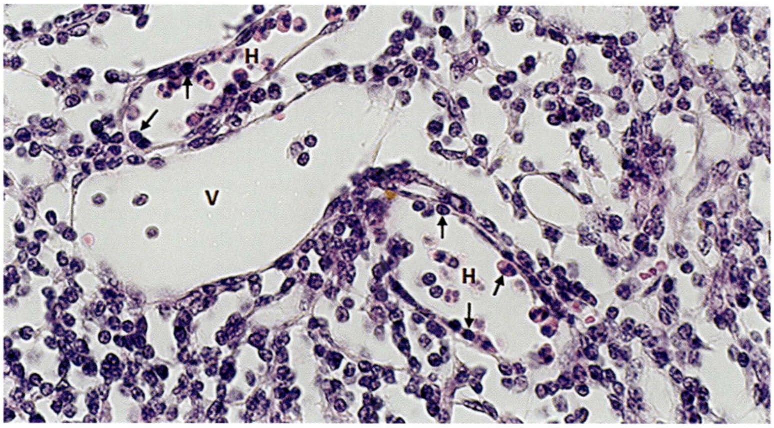

Figure 8-13 Lymph node, perfused (cow). High endothelium in postcapillary venules (H) with numerous migrating lymphocytes and granulocytes (arrows). A larger venule (V) is also observed. Note that the lymph node was perfused during fixation, resulting in the washing out of many cells from the parenchyma and the expansion of the blood vessels, which are clearly visible. H&E.

Immune Response Development Information about the state of peripheral tissues is delivered to the draining lymph node via afferent lymph vessels, either through direct drainage into lymph or active transport by migratory DCs. Macrophages and resident DCs located within or near lymphatic sinuses efficiently capture antigens and inflammatory mediators. Innate and adaptive immune cells positioned near the subcapsular sinus initiate early inflammatory responses to promote pathogen containment and clearance. Upon reaching the lymphatic sinuses, proteins and particles are physically separated.

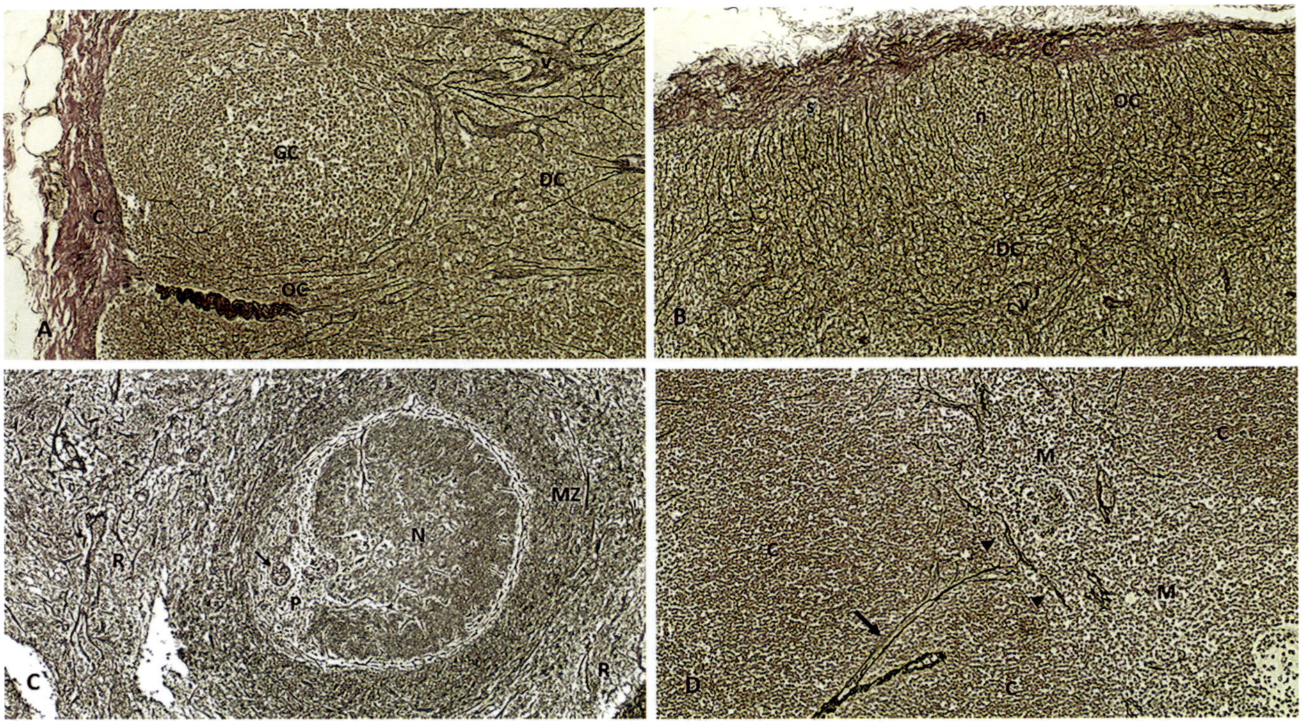

Figure 8-14 Reticular fiber network of lymphatic tissues. Gomori's silver impregnation procedure stains reticular fibers that appear black, while nuclei appear grey, and CT is stained reddish. **A.** Lymph node (sheep). The internodular region of the outer cortex (OC) and the deep cortex (DC) contains a rich network of black reticular fibers. Reticular fibers are sparse in the germinal center (GC) of a secondary nodule. Blood vessels (v) are also visible. **B.** Lymph node (sheep). Reticular fibers arise from the CT capsule (C), extend across the subcapsular sinus (s), and enter the internodular region of outer cortex (OC), continuing into the deep cortex (DC). Small nodule (n) and a blood vessel (v) are indicated. **C.** Spleen (goat). The red pulp (R) contains a network of black reticular fibers, while reticular fibers are scant in marginal zone (MZ) and in the germinal center of a spleen nodule (N). A distinct network of reticular fibers is present in the periarterial lymphatic sheath or PALS (P). A central artery is indicated (arrow). **D.** Thymus (sheep). Black reticular fibers follow CT septa (arrow) to the cortico-medullary junction (arrowheads) and branch into the medulla (M). The cortex (C) of the thymus lacks reticular fibers. Gomori's silver impregnation.

Smaller antigens (<70 kDa) and fluids enter the lymph node conduit network and distribute throughout the diffuse lymphatic tissue of the outer cortex and the deep cortex (T cell areas). These conduits guide fluid-borne antigens, cytokines, and chemokines to blood vessels, thereby enhancing the trafficking of immune cells through high endothelial venules into the lymph node. Large antigens and pathogens are retained within the lymphatic sinuses and can directly traverse the sinus wall into the lymph node parenchyma, either by passive diffusion via local fenestrations or by active transcytosis by lymphatic endothelial cells. Most lymph node macrophages, including subcapsular sinus macrophages and medullary macrophages, are localized within the lymphatic sinuses, facilitating the rapid capture of pathogens arriving via lymph. Innate lymphoid cells, including NK cells, $\gamma\delta$T cells, NKT cells, and innate-like CD8 T cells, are positioned near subcapsular sinus macrophages to respond rapidly to macrophage-derived inflammatory signals and to help initiate early immune responses.

Upon encountering foreign antigens or mediators sampled from the conduit system, resident DCs undergo maturation and migrate into the deep cortex (T cell area). Meanwhile, inflammatory monocytes infiltrate the lymph node from the blood via high endothelial venules. These two cell types cooperate to initiate early T cell activation and effector differentiation. Migratory DCs bearing antigens and mediators of tissue damage and cell death relocate to the border between T cell areas and B cell areas (nodules) to induce T cell differentiation. Naive B cells, circulating through high endothelial venules, encounter antigen and are activated in the diffuse lymphatic tissue of the cortex by antigen-bearing DCs or sinus macrophages. Activated B cells interact with T cells to receive the necessary signals to relocate to the center of the nodule, where they form the initial germinal center cluster and sustain a successful germinal center reaction (see above for a detailed description).

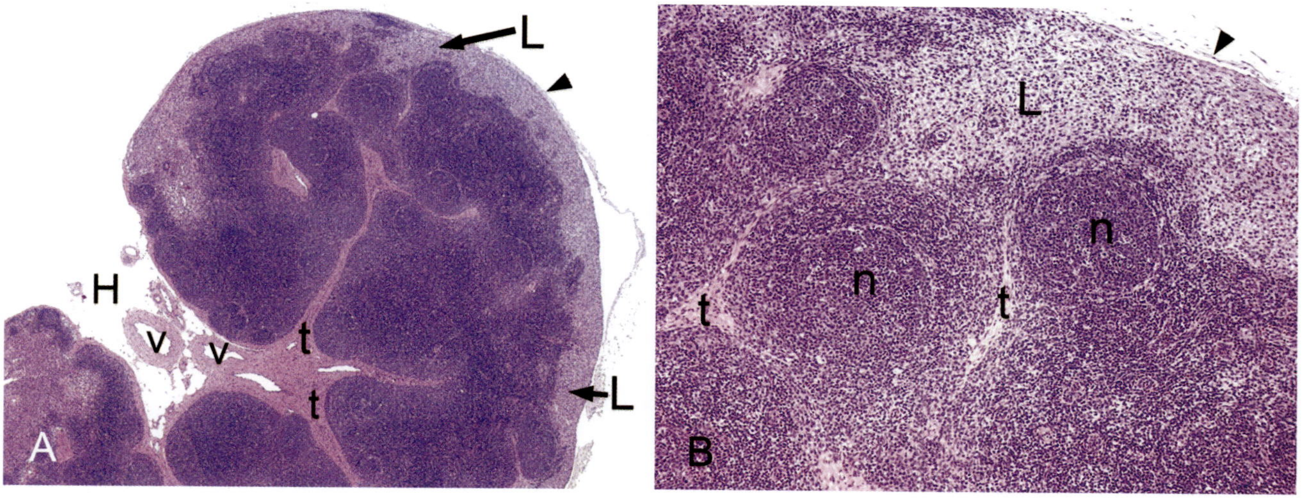

Figure 8-15 Lymph node (pig). **A.** Afferent lymphatic vessels (v) enter the node at a hilus (H) and accompany trabeculae (t) to penetrate deeply into the parenchyma, reaching central tissue containing lymphatic nodules. Capsule (arrowhead). Loose peripheral tissue (L). H&E. **B.** Higher magnification showing the arrangement of lymphatic nodules (n) along trabeculae (t). Loose peripheral tissue (L). Capsule (arrowhead). H&E.

Species Differences

Porcine lymph nodes are different from those of most other mammals (Fig. 8-15). The majority of nodules are situated deep within the center of the node along trabecular sinuses. Areas similar to the deep cortex in conventional lymph nodes, containing many postcapillary venules, are observed near clusters of nodules. However, the periphery of the node is occupied primarily by loose lymphoreticular tissue containing macrophages and only a few plasma cells. Afferent lymph vessels penetrate the capsule at one or more sites and extend deep into the area occupied by the lymphatic nodules via the trabeculae, where they open into the trabecular sinuses. The lymph then filters into the peripheral sinuses, which converge and give rise to several efferent vessels at the periphery of the node. Functionally, the flow of the lymph in the porcine lymph nodes is identical to that in other animals because the incoming lymph initially reaches the region of the node rich in lymphatic nodules. However, the efferent lymph in pigs contains fewer lymphocytes compared to other species, and recirculating lymphocytes exit porcine lymph nodes via the blood.

Arteries enter the porcine lymph nodes with the afferent lymph vessels, while veins exit with the efferent lymph vessels. As a result, a distinct hilus may not always be visible; instead, microscopic hilus-like indentations are apparent wherever afferent lymph vessels enter. Many small lymph nodes may fuse, thereby forming a large cluster of nodes, which often contributes to the difficulty in locating a hilus in porcine lymph nodes.

In contrast, chickens lack encapsulated lymph nodes typical of mammals, although a rudimentary lymph node has been described. Mural lymph nodes associated with deep lymphatic vessels emerge after 6 weeks of age and persist in the adult. These nodes are embedded in the lateral wall of lymphatic vessels and do not obstruct lymph flow. Lymph sinuses within mural lymph nodes lack reticular fibers and macrophages. Germinal centers are present in the dense lymphoid tissue occupied by B and T cells. High endothelial venules are absent in mural lymph nodes. "Conventional" encapsulated lymph nodes have been described in some avian species including ducks, geese, and swans.

Spleen

The spleen is the main secondary lymphatic organ responsible for filtering the blood and mounting immune responses against blood-borne antigens. Erythrocytes are stored in the red pulp of the spleen, while platelets are stored in the splenic cords.

As erythrocyte cell membrane elasticity declines with age, old erythrocytes are unable to traverse the narrow spaces of the splenic cords and interendothelial slits of venous sinuses or venules within the red pulp. Macrophages then remove the damaged erythrocytes from circulation.

The ability of the spleen to filter the blood is enhanced by a reticular fiber network filled with reticular cells and macrophages. Virtually every section of the red pulp contains numerous macrophages filled with engulfed red blood cell fragments and an iron pigment called hemosiderin.

Capsule and Supportive Tissue

The spleen is surrounded by a thick CT capsule invested by the peritoneum. This capsule consists of two layers: a dense irregular CT layer and a layer of smooth muscle. The total thickness and proportion of smooth muscle present may vary across species. Trabeculae, composed of collagen, elastic fibers, and smooth muscle cells, extend from the capsule and the hilus into the parenchyma. The trabeculae contain arteries, veins, lymph vessels, and nerves. Together, the capsule, trabeculae, and reticular fibers provide structural support to the splenic parenchyma. The splenic parenchyma is composed of the red pulp, involved in the storage of red blood cells, and the white pulp, rich in lymphocytes and actively engaged in immune responses.

Red Pulp

Most of the splenic parenchyma is composed of red pulp, owing its name to the vast amount of blood held within its reticular network (Figs. 8-14 and 8-16). The red pulp is composed of venous sinuses or venules and splenic cords. In mammalian spleens, two primary types of red pulp are present, distinguished by the type of postcapillary vessels present: sinusal or nonsinusal. Among domestic animals, only dogs possess typical venous sinuses, similar to those found in human and rat spleens.

The splenic sinuses are wide vascular channels lined with elongated, longitudinally oriented endothelial cells that contain contractile microfilaments aligned in bands parallel and adjacent to the lateral cell margins. Gaps or slits in the sinus wall are created upon contraction of these filaments, thus allowing erythrocytes to migrate from the surrounding splenic cords into the sinus lumen. The lining cells rest on a fenestrated basal lamina and are supported by reticular fibers, some of which form hoop-like structures encircling the sinus at right angles to the long axis. In most domestic mammals, venules rather than venous sinuses are present. Their wide lumina are lined by a thin endothelium with a discontinuous basal lamina supported by reticular cells and fibers. Openings between endothelial cells in this wall are common (Fig. 8-17).

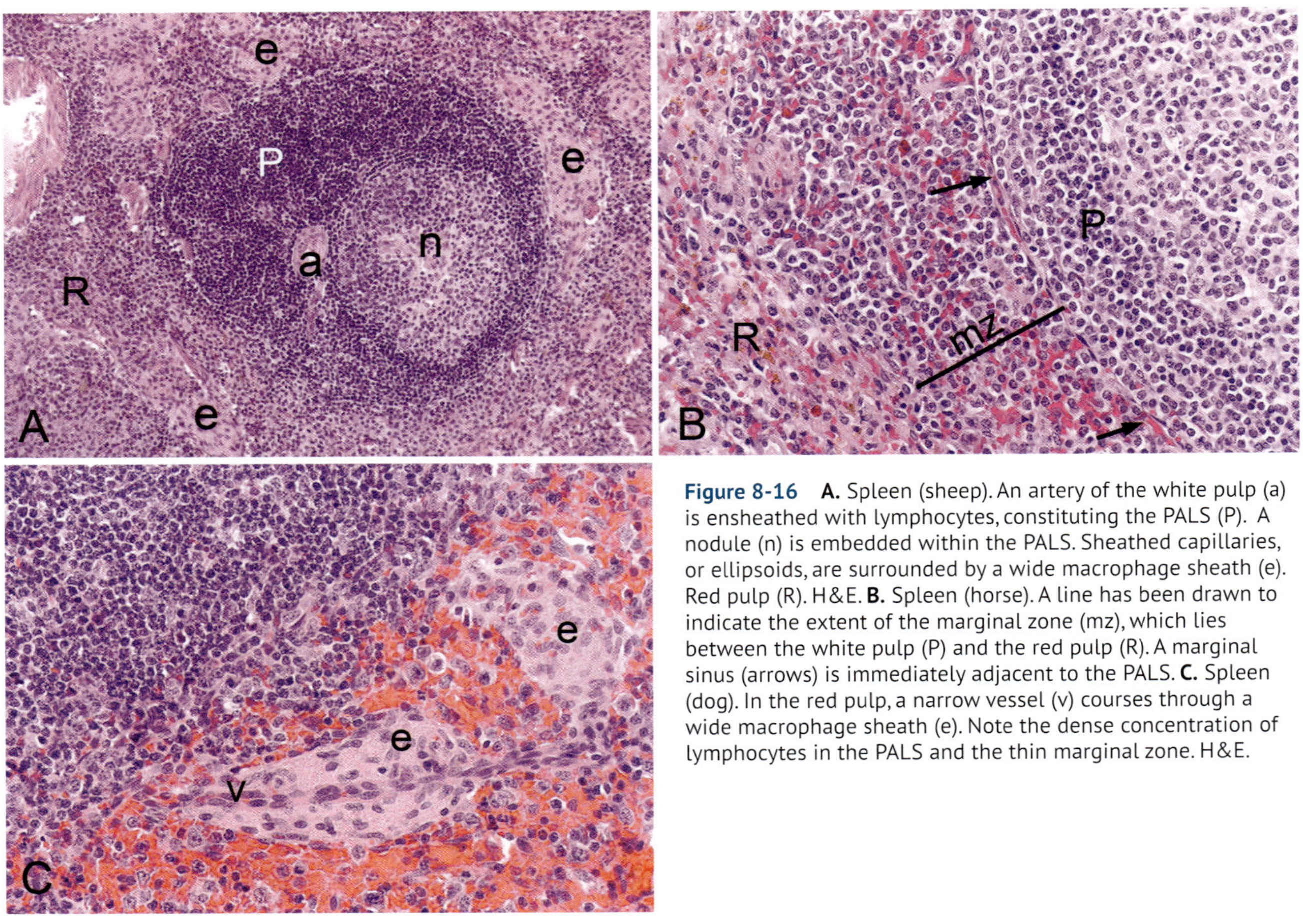

Figure 8-16 **A.** Spleen (sheep). An artery of the white pulp (a) is ensheathed with lymphocytes, constituting the PALS (P). A nodule (n) is embedded within the PALS. Sheathed capillaries, or ellipsoids, are surrounded by a wide macrophage sheath (e). Red pulp (R). H&E. **B.** Spleen (horse). A line has been drawn to indicate the extent of the marginal zone (mz), which lies between the white pulp (P) and the red pulp (R). A marginal sinus (arrows) is immediately adjacent to the PALS. **C.** Spleen (dog). In the red pulp, a narrow vessel (v) courses through a wide macrophage sheath (e). Note the dense concentration of lymphocytes in the PALS and the thin marginal zone. H&E.

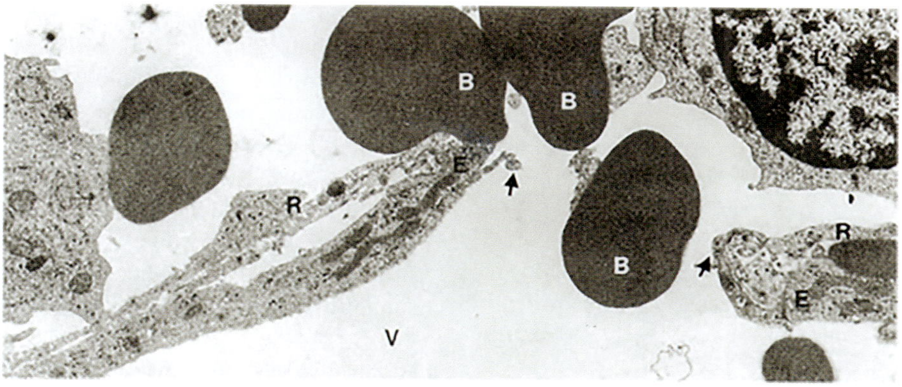

Figure 8-17 Spleen (sheep). Electron micrograph of a venule with erythrocytes (B) passing through an opening in the wall. Lumen (V), endothelium (E), reticular cells (R), and lymphocyte (L). Arrows indicate the edges of the endothelial opening (×8000).

The narrow splenic cords, situated between the sinuses, form a vast three-dimensional network comprised of reticular fibers with enmeshed reticular cells, erythrocytes, macrophages, lymphocytes, plasma cells, and other leukocytes. The membranous processes of the reticular cells tend to form channel-like structures that may function to guide blood toward the endothelial slits in the sinus walls. In nonsinusal spleens, the splenic cords are wider than in sinusal spleens. The red pulp of ruminant and porcine spleens contains numerous smooth muscle cells, whereas that of horses and dogs has myofibroblasts, cells resembling fibroblasts but possessing some features of smooth muscle (e.g., actin filaments and dense bodies).

White Pulp

White pulp is lymphatic tissue that is distributed throughout the spleen and consists of lymphatic nodules and diffuse lymphatic tissue called periarterial lymphatic sheaths (PALS) (Figs. 8-16 and 8-18). Nodules of the white pulp are B-cell

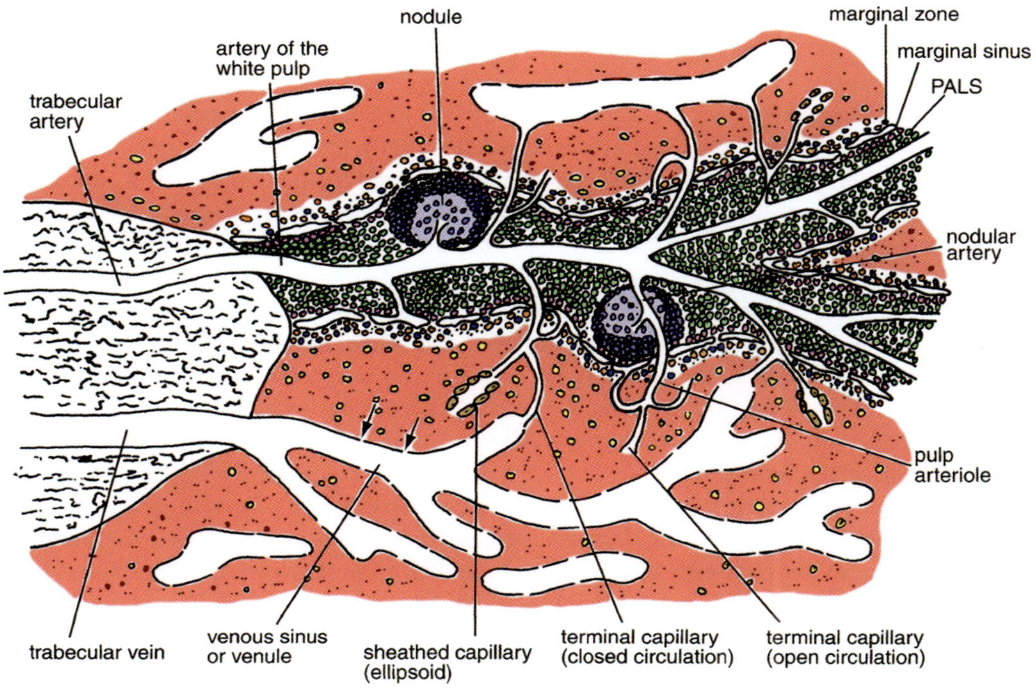

Figure 8-18 Schematic drawing of the splenic parenchyma with emphasis on the vasculature. Trabecular artery, artery of the white pulp with lymphatic sheath, nodular artery, pulp arteriole, sheathed capillary (ellipsoid), terminal capillaries emptying into reticular mesh (open circulation), terminal capillaries emptying into venous sinus or venule (closed circulation), venous sinus or venule, and trabecular vein. Arrows indicate openings in the wall of sinuses or venules. Periarterial lymphatic sheath (PALS).

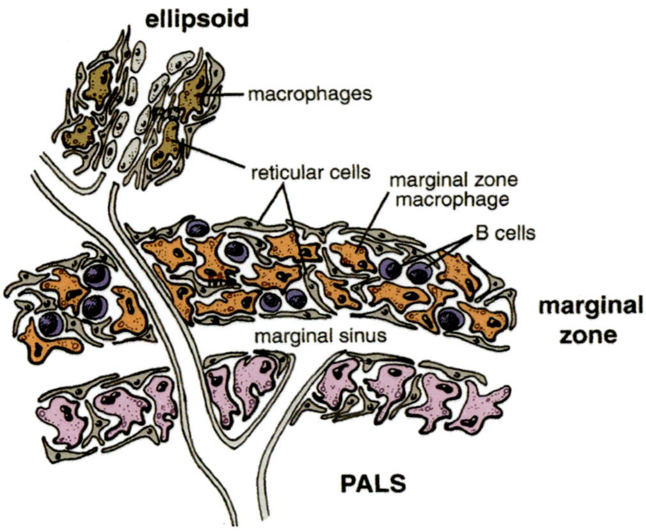

Figure 8-19 Schematic drawing of the marginal zone and an ellipsoid. Blood vessels leave the PALS to pass through a rim of macrophages and empty into the marginal sinus, marking the inner limit of the marginal zone. The marginal zone is composed of reticular cells, B cells, and marginal zone macrophages. Some blood vessels traverse the marginal zone and terminate in the red pulp as sheathed capillaries or ellipsoids, surrounded by a meshwork of reticular cells and macrophages.

areas and may or may not have germinal centers, depending on their functional state. The PALS are organized along the artery of the white pulp. Within the PALS, T cells are concentrated adjacent to the tunica media of the artery, whereas the peripheral region of the sheaths contains a more diverse mixture of T and B cells, macrophages, and DCs. Throughout the white pulp, reticular cells and associated reticular fibers form a three-dimensional stroma containing lymphocytes, macrophages, and DCs similar to those seen in lymph nodes.

Marginal Zone

The marginal zone lies between the white pulp and the red pulp. The periphery of the white pulp is bounded by a circumferential reticulum, the reticular cells of which branch into the marginal zone. The marginal zone blends into the splenic cords of the red pulp (Figs. 8-16 and 8-18). The reticular network of the marginal zone receives capillaries from the white pulp and some terminal capillaries of the red pulp. The capillaries empty into a marginal sinus, which is a series of anastomosing channels, not equally apparent in all species (Fig. 8-18). From here, the blood is drained slowly toward the venous sinuses or venules of the red pulp. Many macrophages and B cells are in the marginal zone. All elements of the blood, as well as antigens and particles, come into contact with the local macrophages and lymphocytes, facilitating phagocytosis and the initiation of an immune response. Bloodborne antigens trapped within the marginal zone are transported by marginal zone macrophages to the PALS, an environment rich in recirculating lymphocytes and DCs.

Blood Vessels

The circulation of blood through the spleen has important functional implications, particularly with respect to antigenic stimulation and the extraction of hemoglobin and iron from red blood cells. Branches of the splenic artery enter the hilus and extend into the large trabeculae as trabecular arteries. As the artery leaves the trabecula, it is called the artery of the white pulp (Fig. 8-18). As the artery of the white pulp becomes smaller, the PALS and marginal zone attenuate and eventually the surrounding reticulum disappears. Strands of white pulp extend across the attenuated marginal zone into the red pulp, forming bridging channels. Meanwhile, branches of the white pulp artery continue to supply capillary beds within nodules and terminate in the marginal zone or enter the red pulp, forming penicillar arteries (brushlike tufts). Each branch of the penicillar artery extends into the red pulp as a pulp arteriole, which then transitions into a distinctive structure called a sheathed capillary or ellipsoid (Fig. 8-19). Here, the vessel lumen narrows, and the endothelium becomes cuboidal, with permeable junctions and a discontinuous basal lamina. The vessel is surrounded by a sheath of macrophages enclosed within a meshwork of reticular cells and fibers, called a pericapillary macrophage sheath. This sheathed capillary eventually transitions into an unsheathed terminal capillary.

Most terminal capillaries open into the spaces between the fibroblastic reticular cells of the red pulp, allowing blood to enter the venous circulation through slits in the sinus walls (referred to as "open circulation"). Terminal capillaries may expand, forming an ampulla, and open directly into the splenic sinuses or venules, forming a continuous tubular structure ("closed circulation"). The blood within the red pulp venules eventually drains into the trabecular veins and exits through the splenic vein.

Lymph Vessels and Nerves

The spleen lacks afferent lymph vessels. Instead, efferent capsular and trabecular lymph vessels originate in the white pulp, serving as exit routes for certain lymphocytes. These efferent lymph vessels ultimately drain into the splenic lymph nodes.

Species Differences

The spleens of horses, dogs, and pigs have abundant lymphatic nodules and periarterial lymphatic sheaths. Conversely, in the cat and ruminant spleens, lymphatic tissue is less abundant and occurs mainly as lymphatic nodules with shorter periarterial lymphatic sheaths.

The size and number of the sheathed capillaries also vary considerably among the domestic animals. In pigs and cats, pericapillary macrophage sheaths are large, abundant, and often particularly numerous near the white pulp. Comparatively, in horses and dogs, these sheaths are smaller than in other domestic animals, and in ruminants, they are small and narrow. Sheathed capillaries are absent in mice, rats, guinea pigs, and rabbits.

The ability to mobilize rapidly the reservoir of erythrocytes stored in the spleen differs between and within species. This is evidenced by the significant increases in hematocrit following physical activity in thoroughbred horses and greyhounds, while only moderate or small changes in hematocrit occur in other domestic animal species such as sheep.

Mucosa-Associated Lymphatic Tissue

Cells of the immune system are present either within or adjoining the mucosa of the respiratory, alimentary, and urogenital tracts, as well as the mammary gland. These lymphatic tissues function as a mucosal immune system to augment the mechanical and chemical barriers of surface mucosal epithelia. The various tissue compartments of the mucosal immune system can be divided into inductive sites where antigens are sampled from mucosal surfaces to stimulate naive T and B lymphocytes, and effector sites where immune system effector cells perform their protective functions. The inductive sites of the mucosal immune system are the organized mucosa-associated lymphoid tissue (MALT) and the regional draining lymph nodes. The effector sites consist of distinctly different histological compartments, including the lamina propria of various mucosae, the stroma of exocrine glands, and surface epithelia. MALT structures serve as the origin of lymphocyte trafficking to mucosal effector sites. They are secondary lymphatic tissues resembling lymph nodes, possessing areas of diffuse lymphatic tissue rich in T lymphocytes (T cell zones) between B-cell nodules, and populated with antigen-presenting cells, including DCs and macrophages. MALT may occur as solitary (isolated) lymphoid nodules or as larger aggregates of lymphoid nodules. Unlike lymph nodes, MALT lacks afferent lymphatics, as these structures sample exogenous antigens directly from the mucosal surfaces through a characteristic epithelium overlaying each nodule and an elevated subepithelial dome region. This epithelium contains morphologically distinct cells specialized in antigen uptake termed M cells, which typically envelop intraepithelial lymphocytes. Accordingly, the epithelium has been termed a lymphoepithelium and is also described as a nodule-associated epithelium. Recirculating lymphocytes enter MALT through high endothelial venules in the T-cell zones between B-cell nodules. The compartmental organization of MALT distinguishes it from focal lymphocytic infiltrates of the mucosa.

MALT is subdivided according to anatomical location, and the distribution and composition of these structures vary among species. Also, MALT structures vary with age and tissue state, particularly regarding the extent and duration of exposure to exogenous stimuli. Solitary lymphatic nodules are commonly found in the subepithelial CT of most mucous membranes. Aggregates of lymphatic nodules of MALT can be constitutively present at defined mucosal sites, or constitutively present but with variable locations, or induced by antigen exposure. Characterized MALT structures include conjunctiva-associated lymphoid tissue, lacrimal duct-associated lymphoid tissue, salivary gland-associated lymphoid tissue, nasopharynx-associated lymphoid tissue (NALT), larynx-associated lymphoid tissue, bronchus-associated lymphoid tissue (BALT), and gut-associated lymphoid tissue (GALT). Aggregated lymphatic nodules in the pharynx are referred to as tonsils.

Tonsils

The tonsils are aggregates of lymphatic tissues located in the nasal, oral, and auditory passages leading into the pharynx. In the oropharynx, three types of tonsils are present: the lingual tonsil, the palatine tonsil, and the tonsil of the soft palate. In the nasopharynx, the pharyngeal and tubal tonsils are present. Collectively, these lymphatic tissues are referred to as Waldeyer's ring. The tonsils serve as an early encounter site for infectious agents and other antigens. Local production of antibodies by tonsillar cells is important in initiating a rapid immune response and subsequently a more generalized response.

The tonsils are located adjacent to the lumen of the host organ and are covered by either a stratified squamous epithelium (in the oropharynx) or pseudostratified columnar epithelium (in the nasopharynx). The tonsillar surface may appear relatively smooth (e.g., palatine tonsil of dogs and cats) (Fig. 8-20A), or it may have surface invaginations, referred to as

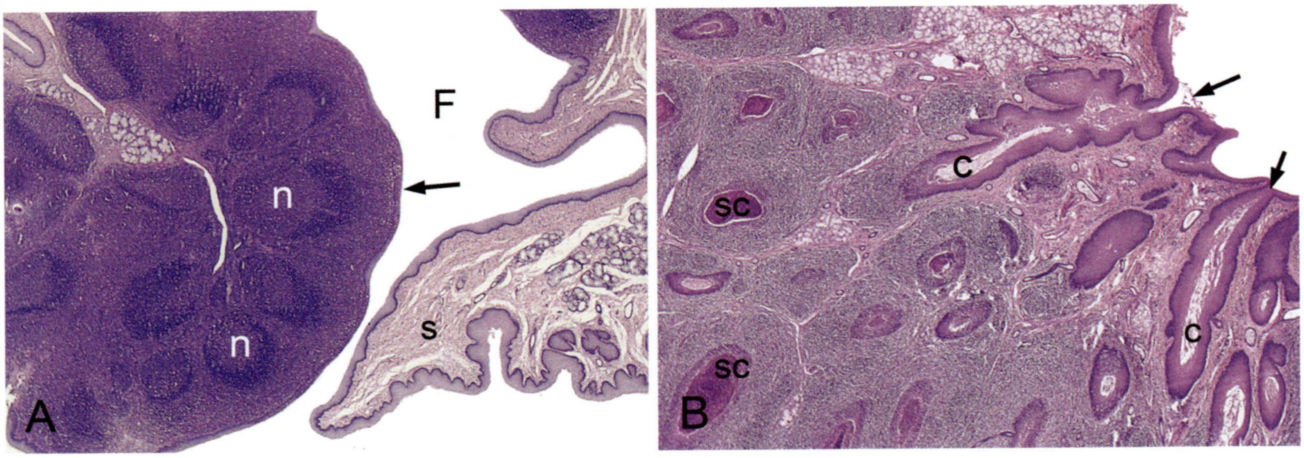

Figure 8-20 Palatine tonsil. **A.** Dog. The lymphatic tissue is embedded in a fossa (F) and is partly covered by a semilunar fold (s). The smooth tonsillar surface (arrow) is a stratified squamous epithelium and overlies many lymphatic nodules (n). **B.** Calf. The stratified squamous epithelium invaginates, forming tonsillar fossulae (arrows) that continue as blind epithelial tubes or crypts (c) surrounded by lymphatic tissue. Salivary corpuscles (sc). H&E.

tonsillar fossulae, which extend as deep, penetrating crypts (e.g., lingual tonsil in horses and palatine tonsil in horses and ruminants) (Fig. 8-20B). These invaginations allow for a high concentration of lymphatic tissue in a given area.

The epithelium is usually infiltrated to a variable degree with lymphocytes, neutrophils, and macrophages. Epithelial regions of immune cell infiltration are referred to as reticular epithelium. This infiltration is particularly pronounced in the tonsils of the oropharynx. Leukocytes that reach the lumen form salivary corpuscles (Fig. 8-20B). When they are not washed out of the fossulae by secretions from the surrounding salivary glands, these cells, along with microorganisms, may obstruct the fossulae and cause inflammation.

Beneath the epithelium, diffuse lymphatic tissue with plasma cells surrounds lymphatic nodules, which frequently have a germinal center and a cap (mantle) of small lymphocytes adjacent to the epithelium. The tonsil is separated from the surrounding tissue by a distinct CT capsule, facilitating its "enucleation" (e.g., palatine tonsil of the dog). Tonsillar blood vessels have essentially the same distribution and character as those of lymph nodes (see the "Lymph Nodes" section above). Afferent lymph vessels are absent. A plexus of lymph capillaries is present in the deep layers of the tonsil, draining into larger efferent lymph vessels within the tonsillar capsule.

Species Differences In cattle, there is a moderate amount of tonsillar tissue, whereas the lymphoid tissues of Waldeyer's ring are less well developed in sheep and goats. The lymphatic tissues of the pharynx in pigs are well developed, and particularly so in horses. Rats and mice lack tonsils, although well-developed NALT is present. A palatine tonsil is present in rabbits.

Gut-Associated Lymphatic Tissue

The GALT includes solitary and aggregated lymphatic nodules, intraepithelial lymphocytes, subepithelial lymphocytes, plasma cells, and macrophages. Peyer's patches, which are aggregated lymphatic nodules found in the small intestine, are visible as elevations in the mucosa (Figs. 8-7 and 8-21). The most conspicuous aggregate of lymphatic nodules appears as a single large patch in the ileum and distal jejunum of ruminants, pigs, horses, and carnivores (see the "Ileal Peyer's Patch of Ruminants" section above). Also, the small intestine contains numerous discrete smaller Peyer's patches. These smaller aggregates of lymphatic nodules, along with the scattered aggregated or solitary nodules of the colon and rectum, are secondary lymphatic tissues. They function to maintain immunological tolerance to food proteins and commensal bacteria, as well as in inducing active immune responses to pathogenic microorganisms. The secondary lymphatic tissues of GALT persist in the adult while the primary lymphatic tissues of GALT (such as the ileal Peyer's patch in sheep and cattle or the cloacal bursa in birds) undergo involution at around sexual maturity.

The aggregated lymphatic tissue of the intestine (Fig. 8-22) contains several components: (a) submucosal lymphatic nodules with high mitotic activity, (b) a zone of small lymphocytes forming a cap over the submucosal lymphatic nodule (the mantle), (c) an internodular region rich in T cells and postcapillary venules through which lymphocytes recirculate, (d) an elevated region overlying lymphatic nodules (the dome), and (e) nodule-associated epithelium. The domes are located between typical small intestinal villi and crypts. The nodule-associated epithelium covering the dome lacks goblet cells but includes M cells with numerous microfolds on their luminal surface (Fig. 8-21). These M cells typically envelop groups of lymphocytes and occasionally enclose macrophages and DCs.

There are regional differences in GALT across different segments of the intestine. Peyer's patches found in the jejunum have small pear-shaped lymphatic nodules, along with large domes and extensive submucosal internodular areas. In contrast, the elongated continuous ileal Peyer's patch has long oval lymphatic nodules, smaller domes, and reduced submucosal internodular areas.

Species Differences In the large intestine of cattle, lymphatic nodules are found either in the lamina propria or as part of lymphoglandular complexes. These complexes are characterized by one or more lymphatic nodules in the submucosa, accompanied by one or more epithelial crypts extending from the mucosal surface into the lymphatic tissue. GALT structures in rats and mice resemble jejunal Peyer's patches.

Bronchus-Associated Lymphatic Tissue

BALT is the acronym for bronchus-associated lymphatic tissue, which includes clusters of lymphocytes present in the walls of bronchi and bronchioles, primarily situated near bifurcations in the respiratory airways. Both T and B cells are present, usually located between an arteriole and bronchial epithelium, though they are not organized into nodules like intestinal aggregated lymphatic nodules. The development of BALT is antigen-dependent, and it is not a constitutive structure across all species. The presence of BALT varies widely: it is present in 100% of rabbits and rats, 50% in guinea pigs, and 33% in pigs, while it is absent in normal cat and human lungs. BALT is not well developed in sheep and cattle.

Hemal Nodes and "Milk Spots"

Hemal nodes are described in various mammalian species, especially in ruminants, rats, horses, pigs, and humans. In ruminants, they are prevalent in the sublumbar area along the vena cava and abdominal aorta. These organs

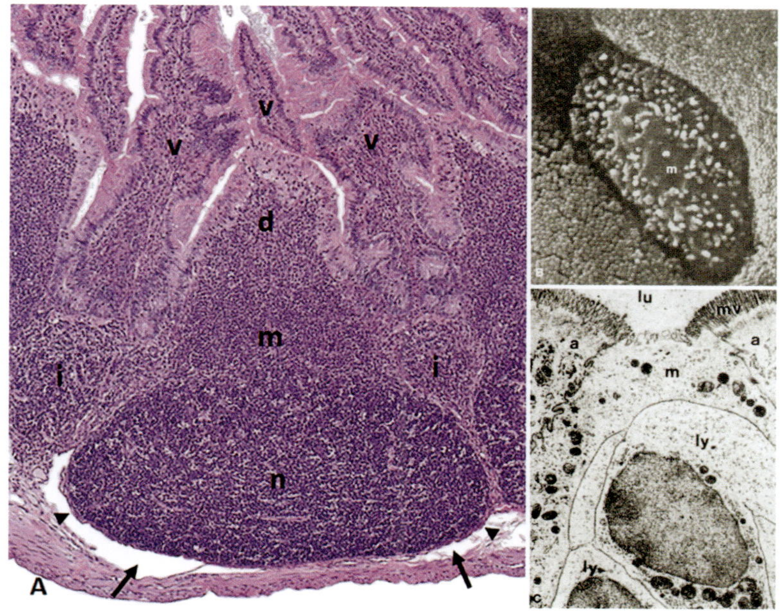

Figure 8-21 **A.** Jejunal aggregated lymphatic nodules (lamb). A large, saclike lymphatic nodule (n) is separated from other nodules in the submucosa by wide internodular (T-cell) regions (i). A prominent mantle (m) is interposed between the nodule and a broad dome region (d) that extends into the gut lumen. Villus (v), lymphatic sinuses (arrows), and capsule of nodule (arrowheads). H&E. **B.** Jejunal Peyer's patch (3-week-old calf). Short microfolds are present on an M cell (m) at the surface of the dome; adjacent absorptive cells have densely packed microvilli (×10,000). **C.** Jejunal Peyer's patch (3-week-old calf). An M cell (m) with microfolds is wedged between two microvilli-bearing (mv) absorptive cells (a) and envelops lymphocytes (ly). Lumen (lu) (×7500).

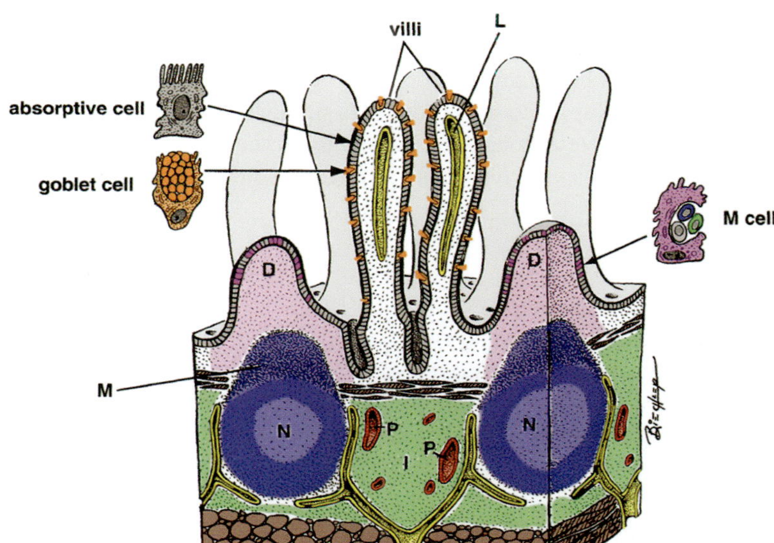

Figure 8-22 Schematic drawing of a portion of the small intestine showing aggregated lymphatic nodules. Submucosal lymphatic nodules (N) are capped by a mantle (M) and situated beneath the dome (D). The nodule-associated epithelium overlying the dome contains many M cells interspersed among absorptive cells but lacks goblet cells. Postcapillary venules (P) and T lymphocytes are present in the internodular region (I), which, along with the lamina propria of the villi, is drained by lymphatic vessels (L).

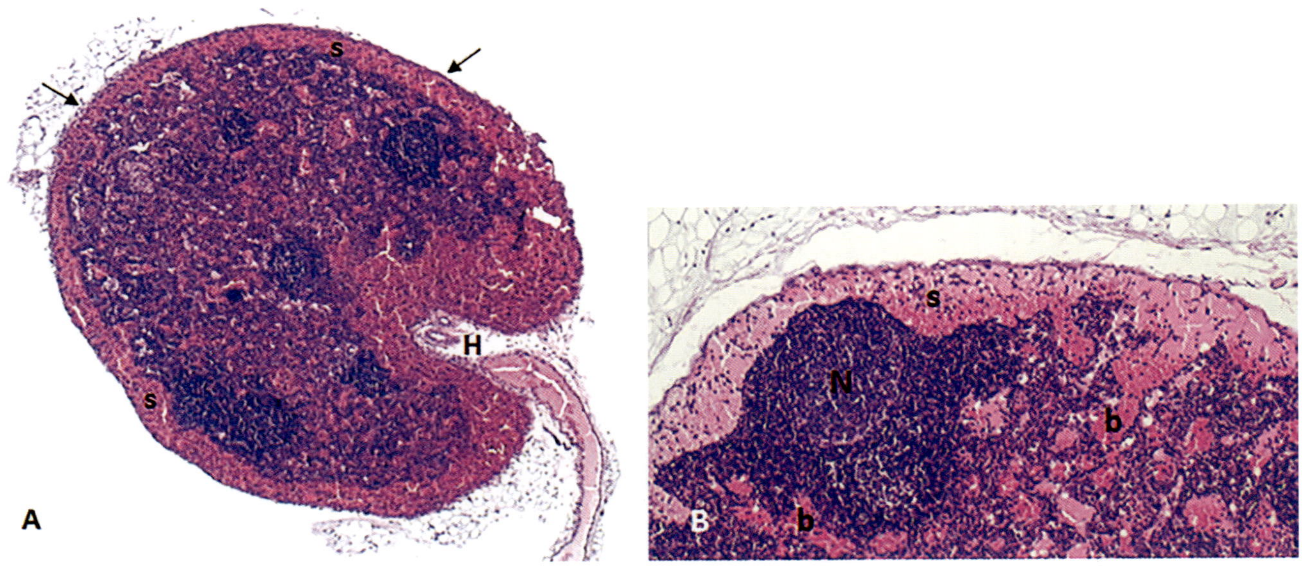

Figure 8-23 Hemal node (lamb). **A.** A wide subcapsular sinus (s) filled with blood is present beneath a thin CT capsule (arrows). Blood vessels enter and exit the hemal node at a hilus (H). **B.** A lymphatic nodule (N) is situated adjacent to the subcapsular sinus (s). Cords of diffuse lymphatic tissue are separated by blood sinuses (b). H&E.

are typically small, ranging from brown to dark red, with wide variations in size, number, and histologic characteristics. Hemal nodes develop during fetal life from lymph node primordia that lose their lymph vessels, thus receiving all cells and antigens from the blood. Although the functional significance of hemal nodes is unclear, it is likely that they respond to bloodborne antigens.

Each hemal node is covered by a thin CT capsule containing a hilus with blood vessels. Below the capsule, a subcapsular blood sinus and lymphatic nodules are present. In young animals, lymphocytes accumulate in a distinct region resembling the deep cortex of a lymph node, although with few nodules (Fig. 8-23). In healthy adults, the node is generally filled with red blood cells. Upon antigenic stimulation, many nodules may form, accompanied by a decrease in red blood cell presence. The sinuses are wide, with few macrophages and lymphocytes. The diffuse lymphatic tissue contains relatively few lymphocytes but has many macrophages that digest erythrocytes and granulocytes. A typical medulla is lacking.

The vascular supply to hemal nodes is similar to that of lymph nodes, but all venules have a thin endothelium. Many lymphocytes and erythrocytes pass through this endothelium.

So-called "milk spots" refer to small aggregations of lymphocytes and macrophages found along the blood vessels of the omentum.

Clinical Correlations

Follicular hyperplasia is the most common type of reactive lymphoid proliferation, which can occur as a reaction to infection with bacteria, viruses, or other microbes. It is characterized by an increased number and size of lymphoid nodules, resulting from a stimulation of the B-cell compartment (Fig. 8-24A). Lymphoma is one of the most common types of cancer found in dogs, affecting lymphocytes. While it often manifests in lymph nodes, other organs can also be involved, such as the liver, spleen, and gastrointestinal tract. In the "diffuse" form, the neoplastic infiltrate effaces most or all of the lymph node architecture (Fig. 8-24B).

Additionally, diseases connected to the complex immune system can manifest as immunodeficiencies, hypersensitivity, or autoimmune diseases. Immunodeficiency diseases related to phagocytes (Chapter 6) are often viral in nature (i.e., feline panleukopenia and leukemia viruses). Excess inflammatory responses also involve immune cells (monocytes, macrophages, and neutrophils). The production of proinflammatory cytokines such as tumor necrosis factor, interleukin (IL)-1, and IL-6 from phagocytes can lead to septic shock. Similarly, blood leukocytes and tissue cells (i.e., mast cells) participate in type I hypersensitivity reactions through the production of histamine, leukotrienes, and eosinophil chemotactic factors, to name a few. Type II hypersensitivity is autoimmune in nature where antibodies attack normal cells, most commonly blood cells. Erythrocytes (hemolytic anemias), white blood cells (leukopenias), and platelets (thrombocytopenia) can be the target of this autoimmune reaction.

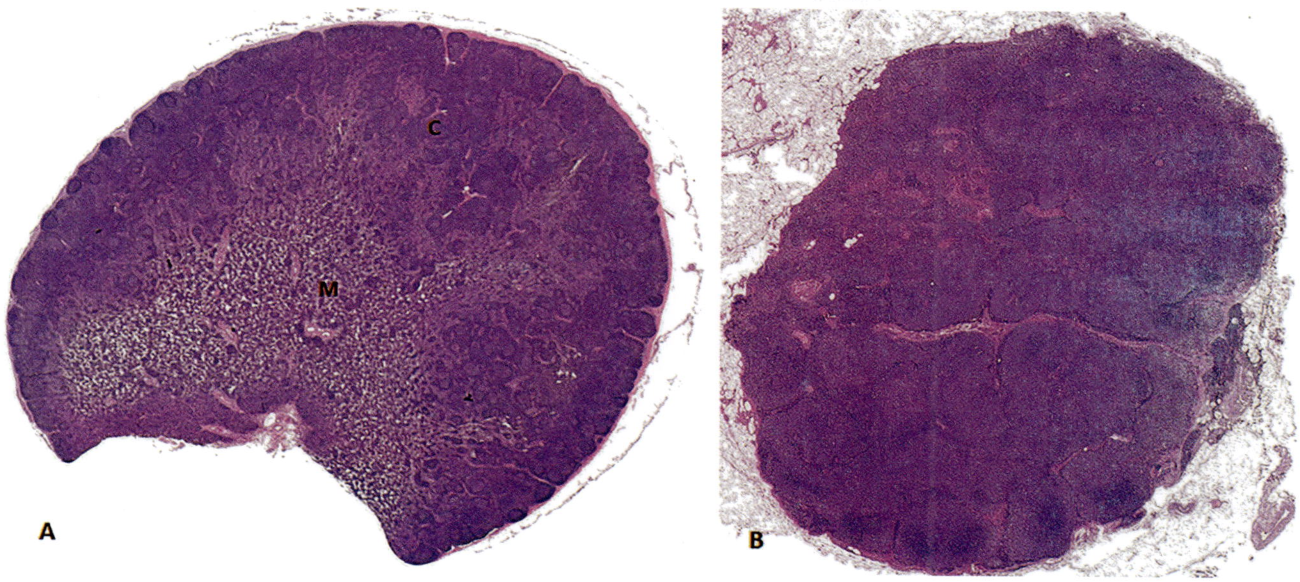

Figure 8-24 **A.** Lymph node (cow). Follicular hyperplasia. The lymph node appears enlarged, with numerous nodules, many exhibiting germinal centers, present throughout the cortex (C). Expansion of nodules into the medulla (M) is observed. H&E. **B.** Lymph node (dog). Lymphoma. The lymph node is enlarged, but unlike follicular hyperplasia, the parenchyma is filled with lymphoblastic cells, obscuring the normal architecture of the node, including a distinct cortex and medulla. H&E. (Courtesy of G. Gunnes.)

Essentials

1) The **immune system** comprises organs, aggregated lymphatic tissues, and cells that work to maintain the integrity of the body. A rapid *innate immune response* recognizes and responds to broad threats to the host. An *adaptive immune response* develops more slowly and responds specifically to a threat.
2) **Cells of the immune system:** Lymphocytes recognize foreign antigens, which are crucial for adaptive immunity. B lymphocytes produce antibodies and are responsible for humoral immunity; T lymphocytes are responsible for cell-mediated immunity. Lymphatic tissues contain organized compartments rich in B lymphocytes (nodules) and adjacent areas rich in T lymphocytes. Phagocytic cells respond to threats by phagocytosing and destroying harmful microbes and substances. Some phagocytic cells can phagocytose, process, and present antigens to lymphocytes. Stromal cells help structure lymphatic tissues and regulate immune responses.
3) Primary lymphatic organs produce large numbers of naive lymphocytes that populate lymphatic tissues, collectively recognizing diverse pathogens.
4) The **thymus**, a primary lymphatic organ, produces T lymphocytes. Its capsule sends septa that divide the parenchyma into lobules with a peripheral cortex and a central medulla. Thymic epithelial cells and interdigitating cells act to select lymphocytes to leave the thymus. Tingible body macrophages remove apoptotic lymphocytes not selected for survival. Hassall's corpuscles are characteristic of the thymic medulla.
5) The **bone marrow** is a primary lymphatic organ responsible for producing B lymphocytes. In some species, tissues associated with the gut mucosa, such as the ileal Peyer's patch of sheep and cattle and the cloacal bursa of birds, also contribute to naive B lymphocyte production.
6) Secondary lymphatic tissues can trap foreign organisms and substances and induce immune protection.
7) The **lymph node**, a secondary lymphatic organ, receives lymph via afferent lymph vessels, which penetrate a capsule to empty lymph into a subcapsular sinus. Trabeculae traverse the cortex and medulla, followed by sinuses. Drained lymph is collected in efferent lymph vessels exiting the node at a hilus with blood vessels. The outer cortex contains B lymphocyte nodules that may contain germinal centers, while the deep cortex and internodular tissue are rich in T lymphocytes and high endothelial venules important for lymphocyte recirculation. The medulla consists of medullary cords of immune cells separated by a network of sinuses and trabeculae. The parenchyma of the node is supported by a network of fibroblastic reticular cells.

8) The **spleen**, a major secondary lymphatic organ, filters blood. Blood vessels enter and exit at the hilus in the capsule, continuing into trabeculae. The parenchyma is divided into red pulp (venous sinuses and splenic cords filled with red blood cells) and white pulp (mostly T lymphocytes in PALS surrounding arteries, with B lymphocyte nodules). Blood vessels empty into the marginal zone between the red pulp and the white pulp, an area rich in macrophages and specialized B cells. Other blood vessels pass through sheathed capillaries (ellipsoids) and empty into splenic cords.
9) Mucosa-associated lymphatic tissues (**MALTs**) are secondary lymphatic tissues situated within or adjacent to the mucosa of the respiratory, alimentary, and urogenital tracts, as well as the mammary gland. These tissues lack afferent lymph vessels and sample antigens directly from mucosal surfaces. MALTs maintain immunological tolerance and induce active responses to pathogenic microbes.
10) **Tonsils** are aggregates of lymphatic tissues in the pharynx. The tonsillar surface may be adjacent to the lumen or adjacent to deep, penetrating crypts. Reticular epithelium may be infiltrated with lymphocytes. Tonsils are separated from surrounding tissue by a capsule.
11) Gut-associated lymphatic tissues include **Peyer's patches**, which are aggregates of lymphatic nodules in the small intestine. Submucosal B cell nodules are separated by internodular T cell areas containing high endothelial venules. A dome covers the nodule, extending across the mucosa to a specialized epithelium containing M cells that sample exogenous antigens from mucosal surfaces.
12) **Hemal nodes** lack lymph vessels and filter blood only. Hemal nodes are prominent in ruminants.

Suggested Readings

Abramson J, Anderson G. Thymic epithelial cells. *Annu Rev Immunol* 2017;35:85–118.

Alexandre YO, Mueller SN. Splenic stromal niches in homeostasis and immunity. *Nat Rev Immunol* 2023;23:705–719.

Brandtzaeg P, Kiyono H, Pabst R, et al. Terminology: nomenclature of mucosa-associated lymphoid tissue. *Mucosal Immunol* 2008;1:31–37.

den Hann JMM, Kraal G. Innate immune functions of macrophage subpopulations in the spleen. *J Innate Immun* 2012;4:437–445.

Fletcher AL, Acton SE, Knoblich K. Lymph node fibroblastic reticular cells in health and disease. *Nat Rev Immunol* 2015;15:350–361. doi: 10.1038/nri3846.

Heesters BA, Myers RC, Carroll MC. Follicular dendritic cells: dynamic antigen libraries. *Nat Rev Immunol* 2014;14:495–504. doi: 10.1038/nri3689.

Huang JY, Lyons-Cohen MR, Gerner MY. Information flow in the spatiotemporal organization of immune responses. *Immunol Rev* 2022;306:93–107.

Jalkanen S, Salmi M. Lymphatic endothelial cells of the lymph node. *Nat Rev Immunol* 2020:20. doi: 10.1038/s41577-020-0281-x.

Kondo K, Ohigashi I, Takahama Y. Thymus machinery for T-cell selection. *Int Immunol* 2018;31:119–125.

Lanning D, Zhu X, Zhai S-K, et al. Development of the antibody repertoire in rabbit: gut-associated lymphoid tissue, microbes, and selection. *Immunol Rev* 2000;175:214–228.

Liebler-Tenorio EM, Pabst R. MALT structure and function in farm animals. *Vet Res* 2006;37:257–280.

Nagy N, Oláh I, Vervelde L. Structure of the avian lymphoid system. In: Kaspers B, Schat KA, Göbel TW, et al., eds. Avian Immunology. 3rd Ed. London, UK: Academic Press, 2021: 11–44.

Qi H, Kastenmüller W, Germain RN. Spatiotemporal basis of innate and adaptive immunity in secondary lymphoid tissue. *Annu Rev Cell Dev Biol* 2014;30:141–167.

Roozendaal R, Mebius RE, Kraal G. The conduit system of the lymph node. *Int Immunol* 2008;20:1483–1487.

Thapa P, Farber DL. The role of the thymus in the immune response. *Thorasic Surg Clin* 2019;29:123–131.

Tizard IR. Veterinary Immunology. 10th Ed. St. Louis, MO: Elsevier, 2018.

Watanabe N, Wang YH, Lee HK, et al. Hassall's corpuscles instruct dendritic cells to induce CD4+CD25+ regulatory T cells in human thymus. *Nature* 2005;436:1181–1185.

Weill J-C, Weller S, Reynaud C-A. B cell diversification in gut-associated lymphoid tissues: from birds to humans. *J Exp Med* 2023;220:e20231501. doi: 10.1084/jem.20231501.

Zidan M, Pabst R. Histology of hemal nodes of the water buffalo (*Bos bubalus*). *Cell Tissue Res* 2010;340:491–496.

9

Respiratory System

Charles G. Plopper

CHAPTER MENU

The primary function of the respiratory system is to provide for the exchange of the respiratory gases (oxygen and carbon dioxide) between the organism and the environment. The conducting airways provide a series of air passages for moving air to and from the gas exchange area in the lungs. The conducting airways also serve as a protective function by conditioning incoming (inhaled) air. This conditioning includes heating the air to body temperature, saturating it to 100% relative humidity, and filtering out noxious gases and particulates. The conducting airways also conserve body heat and water by extracting them from the air during expiration. The mucociliary blanket, which covers the mucosal surface of conducting airways, serves to trap inhaled particles and conveys them and cellular debris out of the system. Other structures, such as the nasolacrimal duct, vomeronasal organ, paranasal recesses and sinuses, auditory tube, and equine guttural pouch, connect to the conducting airways.

The distal, smallest conducting airways connect to the gas exchange area, which includes the respiratory bronchioles, alveolar ducts, and alveolar sacs. Gas exchange occurs in alveoli, where only a thin blood–air barrier is present between pulmonary capillary blood and respired air. An extensive pulmonary capillary bed receives the entire output of the right ventricle of the heart.

Dellmann's Textbook of Veterinary Histology, Seventh Edition. Edited by Marxa L. Figueiredo and John J. Turek.

Companion website: www.wiley.com/go/figueiredo/vethistology7e

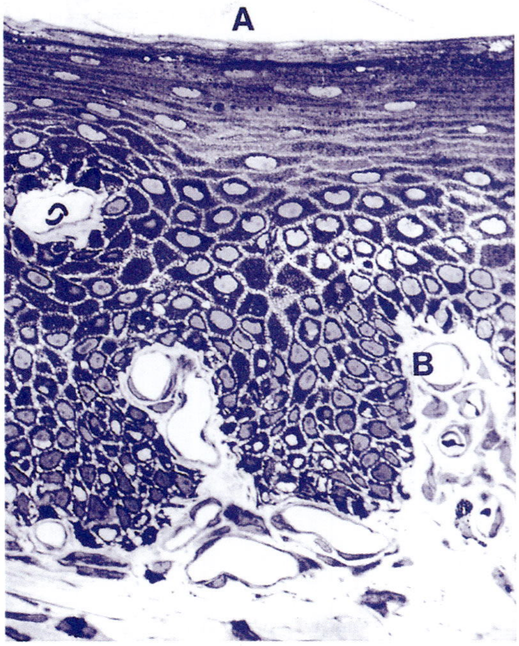

Figure 9-1 Stratified squamous epithelium in the cutaneous region of the canine nasal cavity. Airway lumen (A) and dermal papilla (B). 1 µm. Azure II (×385). (With permission from Adams DR, Hotchkiss DK. The canine nasal mucosa. *Zentralbl Veterinarmed C Anat Histol Embryol* 1983; 12:111).

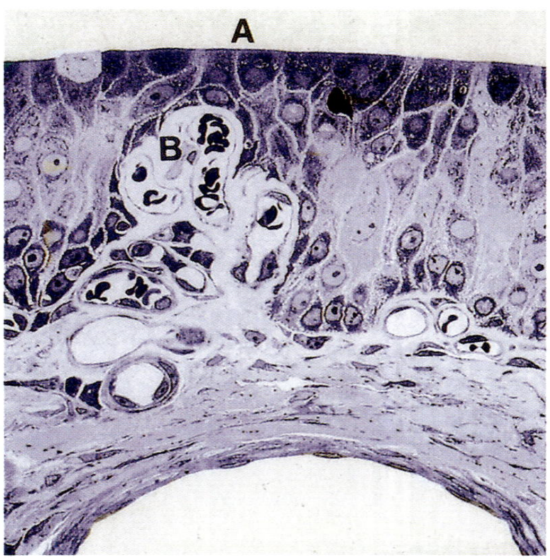

Figure 9-2 Stratified cuboidal epithelium in the transitional zone of the canine nasal cavity. Airway lumen (A) and connective tissue (CT) papilla (B). 1 µm. Azure II (×385). (With permission from Adams DR, Hotchkiss DK. The canine nasal mucosa. *Zentralbl Veterinarmed C Anat Histol Embryol* 1983; 12:113).

Nasal Cavity, Vomeronasal Organ, and Paranasal Sinuses

Nasal Cavity

Each nasal cavity is divided into a cutaneous region, a respiratory region, and an olfactory region. The skin of the nasal apex is continuous through a tissue gradient with the mucous membrane of the caudal part of the nasal cavity proper.

Cutaneous Region

Rostrally, the **cutaneous region** (nasal vestibule) is lined by a relatively thick keratinized stratified squamous epithelium (Fig. 9-1). At midvestibule, the epithelium is thinner and nonkeratinized. Superficial cells have microridges on their free surface. The caudal portion of the cutaneous region and the rostral third of the nasal cavity proper are a **transitional zone** lined by an epithelium that varies from stratified cuboidal to nonciliated pseudostratified columnar. Surface epithelial cells in the transitional zone contain multilobated nuclei, have microvilli on their free surface, and are frequently spherical (Fig. 9-2).

The propria-submucosa of the cutaneous region interdigitates via papillae with the epithelium. The papillae contain small vessels, nerves, and numerous migratory cells, including mast cells, plasma cells, lymphocytes, macrophages, and granulocytes. Lymphocytes and other migratory cells are also frequently observed in the basal portion of the epithelium. Bundles of collagen fibers, larger blood vessels and nerves, and serous glands are located deep in the propria-submucosa.

In horses, a nasal diverticulum lined with skin opens into the cutaneous region of the nasal vestibule; this region is lined by an integument containing vibrissae, sebaceous glands, and sweat glands. In dogs, the papillary layer of the vestibular propria-submucosa has particularly numerous papillae and capillary loops.

Respiratory Region

The epithelium lining the caudal two-thirds of the nasal cavity proper, excluding the olfactory region, is classified as **respiratory epithelium** (ciliated pseudostratified columnar). In contrast, the epithelium lining the middle nasal meatus is thinner and contains fewer ciliated and goblet cells. The ciliated pseudostratified epithelium of the nasal cavity contains several cell types, including ciliated, secretory, brush, and basal cells (Figs. 9-3 to 9-5).

Individual **ciliated cells** are columnar and have 200 to 300 motile cilia and numerous microvilli projecting into the nasal lumen. The supranuclear portion of the cell contains basal bodies, a Golgi complex, and numerous mitochondria; small strands of rough endoplasmic reticulum (rER) are scattered throughout the cell. Defects in the fine structure of cilia may result in ineffective ciliary beat or immotility. Immotile cilia syndrome is a condition associated with congenital ciliary abnormality, resulting in respiratory tract infections.

Secretory cells of the respiratory epithelium extend from the basal lamina to the epithelial surface. Their luminal surface bears microvilli. The morphologic and histochemical appearance of these cells is both species and regionally variable. Their description as mucous or serous is based on their glycoprotein content.

Granules of **mucous epithelial cells** are relatively electron-lucent and contain sialylated or sulfated acid glycoproteins. The supranuclear portion of mucous epithelial cells varies in appearance with the secretory phase from tall and slender with few granules to wide and globular with numerous mucous granules. Globular mucous cells, known as **goblet cells**, have nuclei pressed to the base of the cell by the supranuclear mass of large mucous granules. Organelles usually present in the perinuclear region of the goblet cell include a Golgi complex, rER, and mitochondria. Goblet cells of most species primarily secrete sulfated glycoprotein as a major component of mucus.

Granules of **serous epithelial cells** have electron-dense cores, contain neutral glycoproteins, and are smaller than those of mucous cells.

Brush cells have long, thick microvilli and a cytoplasm containing mitochondria and many filaments. These cells may be sensory receptors associated with endings of the trigeminal nerve.

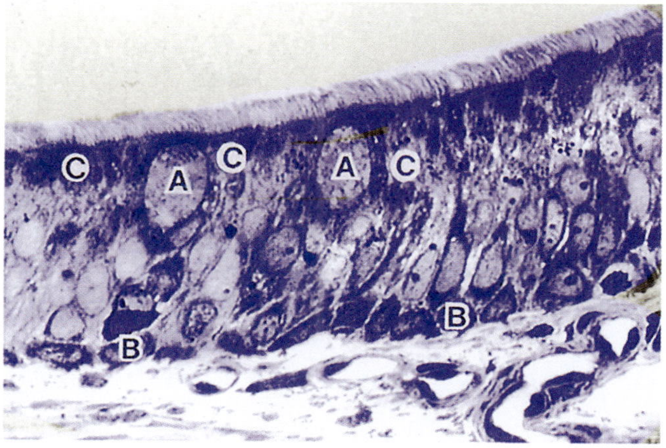

Figure 9-3 Ciliated pseudostratified columnar epithelium with goblet cells lining the respiratory region of the nasal cavity. Goblet cells (A), basal cells (B), and ciliated cells (C). 1 μm. Azure II (×590).

Basal cells are small polyhedral cells located along the basal lamina. The cytoplasm of basal cells contains numerous bundles of tonofilaments and free ribosomes. Basal cells are characterized by anchoring attachments (desmosomes) to other cell types and to the basal lamina (hemidesmosomes). While basal cells appear to have some role in replacing other cell types, the rate of cell proliferation is very low and most of the replacement cells are derived from the other cell types in the epithelium.

Another unnamed cell in the nasal mucosa has surface microvilli and contains a significant amount of smooth endoplasmic reticulum (sER) but little secretory material. This cell type is believed to function in the metabolism of xenobiotic compounds (see below).

The respiratory mucosa (respiratory epithelium plus underlying propria-submucosa) of the nasal cavity is more vascular than the mucosae of the cutaneous, transitional, or olfactory regions. The highly vascular propria-submucosa, containing arteries and large thin-walled veins oriented, rostro-caudally, is called the **cavernous stratum** (Fig. 9-6). The veins profusely anastomose and are referred to as **capacitance vessels** because they determine the degree of mucosal congestion and, inversely, nasal patency. Constriction of nasal blood vessels is affected by α-adrenergic stimulation via the sympathetic nervous system. Periods of vascular engorgement varying from 30 minutes to 4 hours followed by periods of decongestion normally occur in the cavernous stratum of mammals; during this nasal cycle, the vascular activity in one side of the nose alternates with that in the other side.

Serous or mixed nasal glands are present between the numerous veins of this stratum (Fig. 9-7). Acini of nasal glands also secrete secretory immunoglobulin A, lysozyme, and odorant-binding protein.

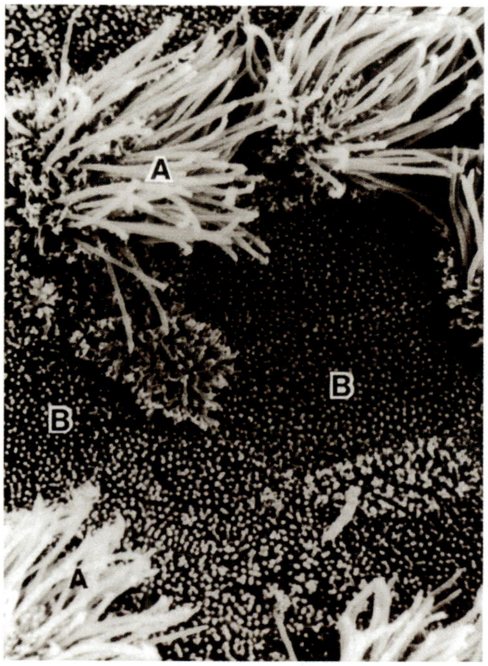

Figure 9-4 Scanning electron micrograph of respiratory epithelium (ciliated pseudostratified columnar epithelium). Ciliated cells with cilia and microvilli (A) and secretory cells with apical microvilli (B) (×3500).

Nerves in the nasal mucosa include sensory fibers arising from the terminal, olfactory, vomeronasal, and maxillary division of the trigeminal nerves and efferent fibers of the autonomic nervous system. Nerves are distributed throughout all compartments of the nasal mucosa including within epithelium.

Lymphatic nodules are commonly present in the caudal part of the nasal cavity, adjacent to the choana, which is the opening between the nasal cavity and the nasopharynx.

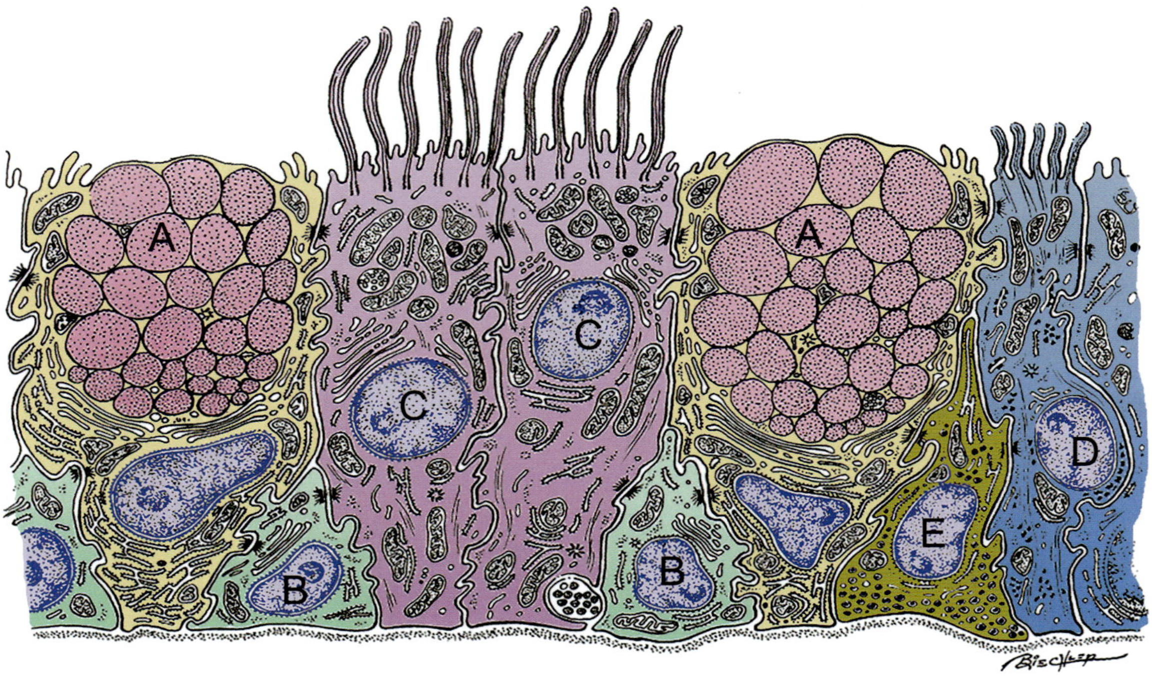

Figure 9-5 Drawing of the fine-structural characteristics of respiratory epithelial cells. Goblet cells (A), basal cells (B), ciliated cells (C), brush cell (D), and small granule cell (E).

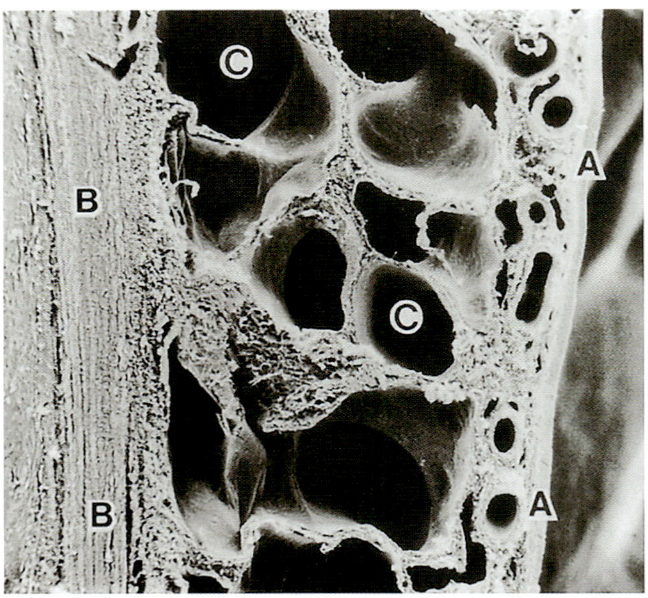

Figure 9-6 Scanning electron micrograph of a section of the respiratory mucosa of the bovine nasal cavity. Epithelium (A), perichondrium (B), and lumina of blood vessels (C) in the cavernous stratum (×40).

Metabolically active exogenous compounds (xenobiotics) that reach nasal tissues via air or blood pathways may remain firmly bound to tissue elements unless degraded. Cytochrome P-450-dependent monooxygenase enzymes in surface epithelium and in acinar cells of the lateral nasal gland (see below) actively metabolize endogenous compounds (e.g., progesterone and testosterone) and exogenous compounds. These enzymes convert lipid-soluble exogenous compounds, some of which are highly toxic (e.g., formaldehyde and acetaldehyde), into water-soluble metabolites.

Olfactory Region

The olfactory region comprises the dorsocaudal portion of the nasal cavity, including some of the surfaces of the ethmoid conchae, dorsal nasal meatus, and nasal septum. Olfactory mucosa may be discerned from adjacent respiratory mucosa because it has a thicker epithelium, numerous tubular glands, and many bundles of nonmyelinated nerve fibers in the lamina propria.

The olfactory mucosa is lined by a ciliated pseudostratified columnar epithelium, the **olfactory epithelium**, consisting of three primary cell types: neurosensory, sustentacular, and basal (Fig. 9-8).

Neurosensory olfactory cells are bipolar neurons with perikarya (cell bodies) in a wide basal zone of the epithelium, dendrites extending to the lumen, and axons reaching the olfactory bulb of the brain. A club-shaped apex, the **dendritic bulb**, protrudes from each dendrite into the lumen (Fig. 9-9). Ten to thirty cilia emanate from each dendritic bulb. Each cilium is 50 to 80 μm long and consists of a wide, short basal portion and a long, thin, tapering distal portion. The number of microtubules decreases from the typical nine peripheral doublets (fused pairs of microtubules) plus two single central microtubules in the basal portion to singlets of one to four microtubules distally. The perikaryon has typical neuronal structural characteristics. Individual axons converge as they pass into the lamina propria, forming bundles of nonmyelinated nerve fibers. Neurosensory cells are continuously replaced during the life of the animal by cells derived from basal cells.

Sustentacular cells are columnar cells with a narrow base and a wide apical portion. Their oval nuclei form the most superficial nuclear layer in the epithelium. Microvilli, often branched, cover the luminal surface of sustentacular cells. Juxtaluminal junctional complexes occur between sustentacular cells and the adjacent dendrites of neurosensory cells. Pigment granules are present in the infranuclear cytoplasm. Sustentacular cells are also replaced by basal cells.

Basal cells of the olfactory mucosa are similar in structure to those of the nonolfactory epithelium.

Olfactory glands, the cells of which contain pigment granules, are located in the propria-submucosa. The intraepithelial portion of their ducts is lined by squamous cells. The glands secrete a watery product, which may serve to enhance the solubility of airborne odorants and cleanse the cilia, facilitating access to new odorants.

The olfactory mucosa also exhibits very high levels of cytochrome P-450 monooxygenase activity and is the primary site for chemically induced nasal tumors.

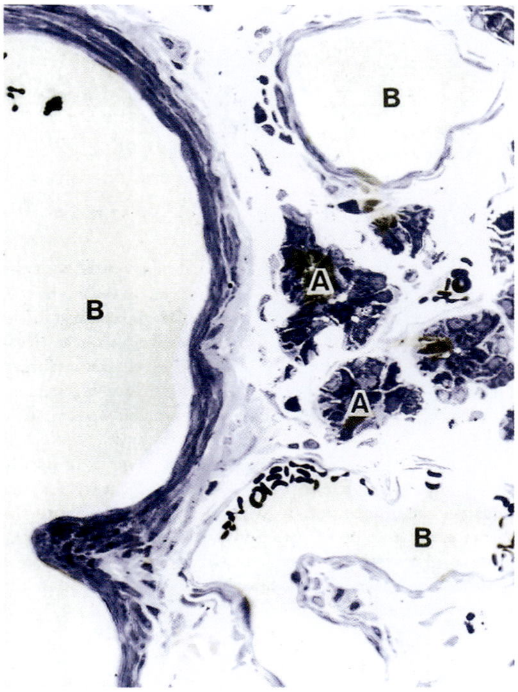

Figure 9-7 Nasal gland acini (A) occupy the CT between the veins of the cavernous stratum (B) of the respiratory mucosa. 1 μm. Azure II (×425).

Vomeronasal Organ

Located in the mucosa of the ventral portion of the nasal septum, the tubular, blind-ended bilateral **vomeronasal organ** consists of an internal epithelial duct (vomeronasal duct), a middle propria-submucosa, and an external cartilaginous support. Rostrally, the vomeronasal duct joins the **incisive duct**, which connects the nasal cavity with the oral cavity, except in horses, where the ventral end of the incisive duct is blind.

In transverse section, the vomeronasal duct is crescent-shaped, with a convex lateral wall and a concave medial mucosal wall. The epithelial lining transitions from a stratified cuboidal lining rostrally, near the incisive duct, to a ciliated pseudostratified columnar epithelium over much of the caudal portion of the vomeronasal duct. The medial pseudostratified columnar epithelium has neurosensory, sustentacular, and basal cells (Fig. 9-10). The dendritic portions of vomeronasal neurosensory cells lack dendritic bulbs and, with the exception of those in dogs, have microvilli instead of cilia on their apical surfaces. Neurosensory cells are periodically replaced in the adult mammal. The lateral pseudostratified columnar epithelium has ciliated and nonciliated columnar, goblet, and basal cells.

Vomeronasal glands, located in the highly vascular propria-submucosa, secrete into the vomeronasal duct most commonly through the commissures between lateral and medial mucosal walls. Secretory

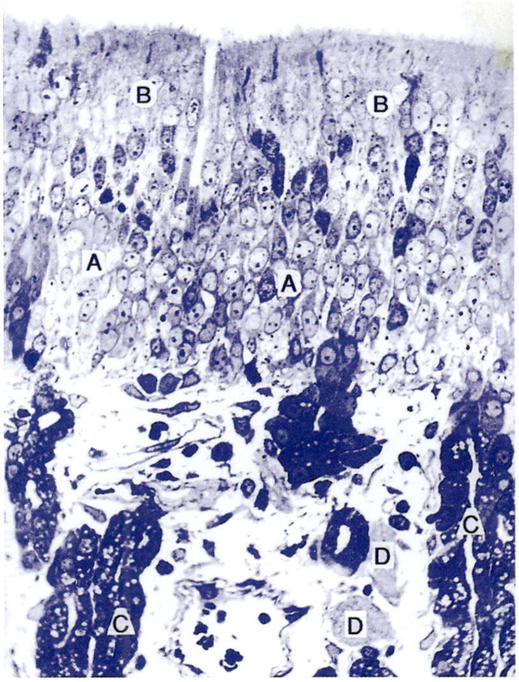

Figure 9-8 Mucosa of the canine olfactory region. Nuclei of neurosensory cells (A), nuclei of sustentacular cells (B), olfactory glands (C), and olfactory nerves (D). 1 μm. Azure II (×410).

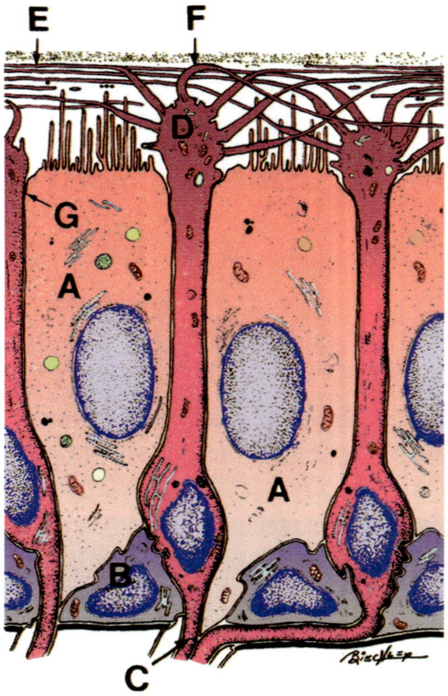

Figure 9-9 Schematic drawing of the olfactory epithelium. Sustentacular cells (A), basal cell (B), axon of the receptor cell (C), dendritic bulb (D), thin distal portion of cilium (E), thick proximal portion of cilium (F), and junctional complex between receptor and sustentacular cells (G).

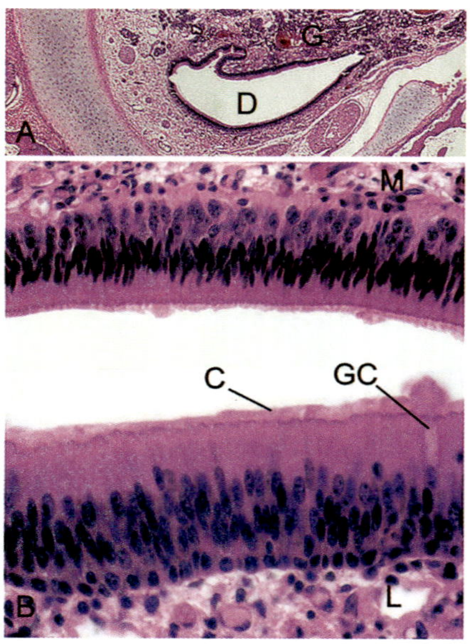

Figure 9-10 **A.** Canine vomeronasal gland (G) and duct (D) (×25). **B.** The lateral epithelium (L) includes ciliated (C), nonciliated, and goblet cells (GC), whereas the medial epithelium (M) contains neurosensory and sustentacular epithelial cells (×400). Hematoxylin and eosin (H&E) (Image by W. E. Haensly).

granules of the acinar cells contain neutral glycoproteins. The hyaline **vomeronasal cartilage** is J-shaped, enclosing all but the dorsolateral portion of the organ.

The vomeronasal organ functions in the chemoreception of liquid-soluble compounds of low volatility. Sensing of these compounds is believed to function in sexual behavior of both the female and the male, in maternal behavior, and in the interaction of the fetus with its amniotic environment. In several mammals, vomeronasal detection of the odor of a female results in an elevation of plasma testosterone in the male. The vomeronasal organ is associated with the lip-curl type of facial grimace (flehmen response) action used by some male mammals to sample substances in the urine of the female; odorant particles may reach the incisive duct with inhaled air, through contact with the tongue, or during passage through the mouth with food or water. These substances, dissolved in fluid in the incisive duct, are sucked into the vomeronasal duct by constriction of blood vessels within the propria-submucosa of the vomeronasal organ. When these vessels dilate, the dissolved substances are expelled from the vomeronasal lumen.

Paranasal Sinuses

The mucosae of the paranasal sinuses are thinner than those of the respiratory region of the nasal cavity with which they are continuous. Glands and blood vessels in the propria-submucosa are scant. The epithelium is ciliated pseudostratified columnar, containing a few goblet cells. The ciliary beat carries mucus toward openings that connect the sinuses with the nasal cavity.

The **lateral nasal gland** (Fig. 9-11) is a relatively large compound gland that secretes neutral glycoproteins via a long duct into the nasal vestibule. It is present in the maxillary recess of carnivores, in the maxillary sinus of pigs, and at the nasomaxillary aperture in horses and small ruminants, but it is absent in cattle. In addition, separate maxillary recess glands are present in carnivores.

Nasopharynx

The **nasopharynx** is the portion of the pharynx located dorsal to the soft palate, extending from the nasal cavity to the laryngopharynx. Its lining consists mostly of respiratory epithelium, but stratified squamous epithelium covers the caudodorsal portion of the soft palate, making contact either with the dorsal wall of the nasopharynx during deglutition or with the epiglottis. The propria-submucosa is loose connective tissue (CT) containing mixed glands, and lymphatic nodules are prominent in the dorsal portion of the nasopharynx, where they aggregate as the pharyngeal tonsil.

Larynx

The **larynx** opens rostrally into the laryngopharynx and is continuous caudally with the trachea (Fig. 9-12). It is lined by mucosa and supported by cartilage.

The epithelium lining the epiglottis, laryngeal vestibule, and vocal folds is nonkeratinized stratified squamous; caudal to the vocal fold, the laryngeal epithelium gradually changes into respiratory epithelium (Fig. 9-3). Respiratory epithelium also lines the equine laryngeal ventricle. The epithelium on the laryngeal surface of the epiglottis, aryepiglottic folds, and arytenoid cartilages may contain taste buds in all species except horses. Sensory receptors of the cranial laryngeal nerve in the epithelium respond to the presence of fluids, such as water, milk, gastric fluid, and saliva; stimulation of these receptors results in reflex apnea.

The propria-submucosa beneath the stratified squamous epithelium is a dense, irregular CT, while the propria-submucosa beneath the respiratory epithelium is a loose CT rich in elastic fibers, leukocytes, plasma cells, and mast cells. Diffuse lymphatic tissue or solitary lymphatic nodules are frequently observed. In pigs and small ruminants, a paraepiglottic tonsil is present on either side of the base of the epiglottis; this tonsil occurs occasionally in cats. Mixed glands (Fig. 9-13) occur in the propria-submucosa but are absent in the vestibular and vocal folds. Numerous elastic fibers are present in the vocal ligament and, to a lesser extent, in the vestibular ligament.

The laryngeal cartilages are connected to each other, to the trachea, and to the hyoid apparatus by ligaments. Extrinsic skeletal muscles move the larynx during swallowing, while intrinsic skeletal muscles move individual laryngeal cartilages during respiration and phonation. Most of the laryngeal cartilages are of the hyaline type. The epiglottis, the cuneiform and corniculate cartilages or processes, and the vocal process of the arytenoid cartilage contain elastic cartilage. In carnivores, the epiglottis often consists of a peripheral cartilaginous wall enclosing white adipose tissue, strands of elastic fibers, and small areas of elastic cartilage. A loose CT forms the tunica adventitia surrounding the laryngeal cartilages and muscles.

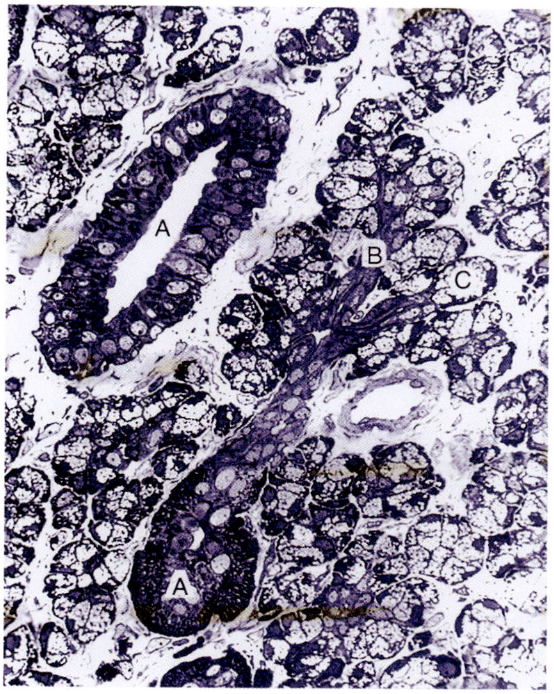

Figure 9-11 Two striated ducts (A), an intercalated duct (B), and acinar cells (C) in the canine lateral nasal gland. 1 μm. Azure II (×425).

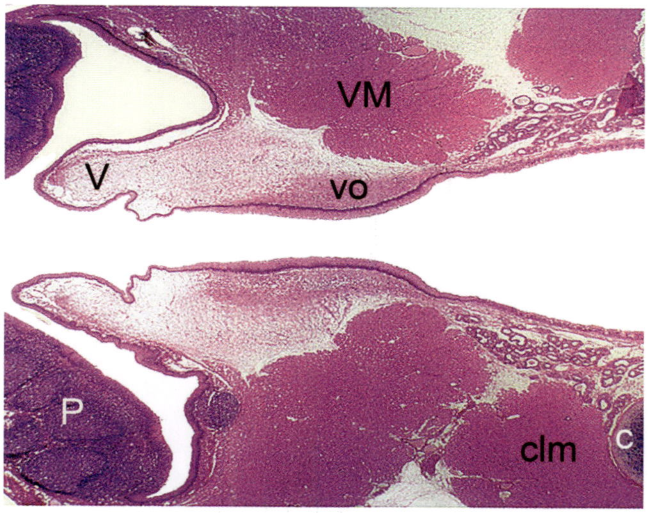

Figure 9-12 Horizontal section through a feline larynx. Ventricular ligaments (V) and vocal ligaments (vo) protrude into the lumen. This region is lined by nonkeratinized stratified squamous epithelium, which changes to respiratory epithelium. Skeletal muscles include the vocalis (VM) and cricoarytenoideus lateralis muscle (clm). A paraepiglottic tonsil (P) is present at the base of the epiglottis. A portion of the cricoid cartilage (c) is present. Larynx, cat, H&E (x16). (Image by W.E. Haensly).

Trachea and Extrapulmonary Bronchi

Distal to the larynx, the respiratory system consists of a series of branching tubes (Fig. 9-14), the tracheobronchial airways, which open into the extensive alveolar gas exchange, approximately 25 times the body surface. The **trachea**, the largest in diameter and length among these tubes, serves as the air passageway connecting the larynx to the bronchi. It is a semiflexible, semicollapsible tube that extends from the larynx into the thoracic cavity.

The lining epithelium of the tracheobronchial tree is respiratory epithelium (Fig. 9-15), containing ciliated cells, brush cells, secretory cells, bronchiolar exocrine cells, basal cells, and neuroendocrine cells. Ciliated cells, brush cells, and secretory cells of the trachea are similar to those of the upper respiratory system (see the *Respiratory Region* section). **Goblet cells** are the predominant secretory cell type in domestic mammals. Bronchiolar exocrine cells are relatively scarce or even absent in the larger airways, which are described later in the chapter. **Neuroendocrine cells** are APUD cells, i.e., they are characterized by *a*mine *p*recursor *u*ptake and *d*ecarboxylation and are identifiable through histochemical methods. Structurally, they are typically pyramid shaped with their bases on the

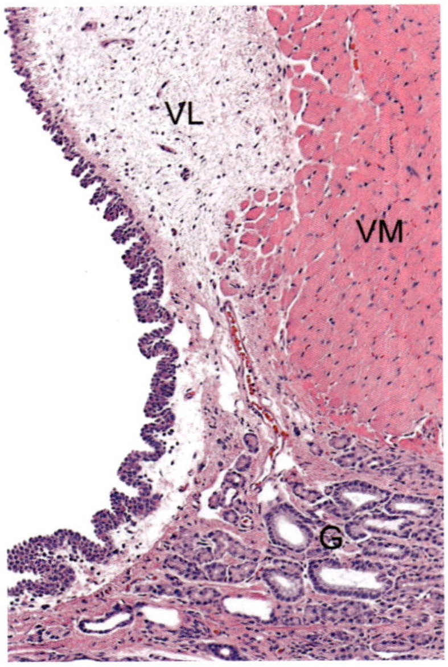

Figure 9-13 Section through the caudal portion of a rat vocal fold. Mixed glands (G), vocal ligament (VL), and vocalis muscle (VM). H&E (×200). (Courtesy of Purdue Veterinary Medicine).

basal lamina and contain dense-cored, argyrophilic granules, abundant ER, Golgi complex, ribosomes, and many filaments at the fine-structural level. These cells are most abundant in young animals and are sometimes associated with nerves.

A variety of **migratory cells** also are observed in the epithelium. These include lymphocytes, globule leukocytes, and mast cells. **Globule leukocytes** are cells of unknown function that contain relatively large acidophilic, metachromatic granules.

The tracheal propria-submucosa consists of loose CT and a subepithelial layer of longitudinally oriented elastic fibers. Cell types present include fibrocytes, lymphocytes, plasma cells, globule leukocytes, and mast cells. The propria-submucosa contains tubuloacinar seromucous glands that open into the tracheal lumen via ducts that are lined with ciliated cells, mucus-secreting cells, and various intermediate cells. The tubular portions of the **tracheal glands** are lined by mucus-secreting cells, while their acinar portions are lined primarily by serous secretory cells. The mucus-secreting cells generally secrete sulfated acid glycoproteins. Serous cells are the major secretory cells of the glands in most species, and their secretory product is a neutral glycoprotein that is sometimes sulfated. Tracheal glands provide most of the secretory material that covers the ciliated surface in the trachea. These glands are abundant in the proximal portions of the trachea of virtually all domestic mammalian species.

The most distinctive feature of the trachea is hyaline cartilage (Fig. 9-15), which in most species occurs as roughly C- or U-shaped separate pieces. In some individuals, however, the cartilage is fused in places to form a continuum. The dorsal free ends of the cartilages are bridged by the **trachealis muscle**, a band of smooth muscle. In most species, the muscle attaches to the perichondrium on the internal side of the cartilage. In carnivores, this attachment is on the external surface of the cartilage. Nerves and large blood vessels are generally associated with the smooth muscle band. The external perichondrium is surrounded by the loose CT of the adventitia.

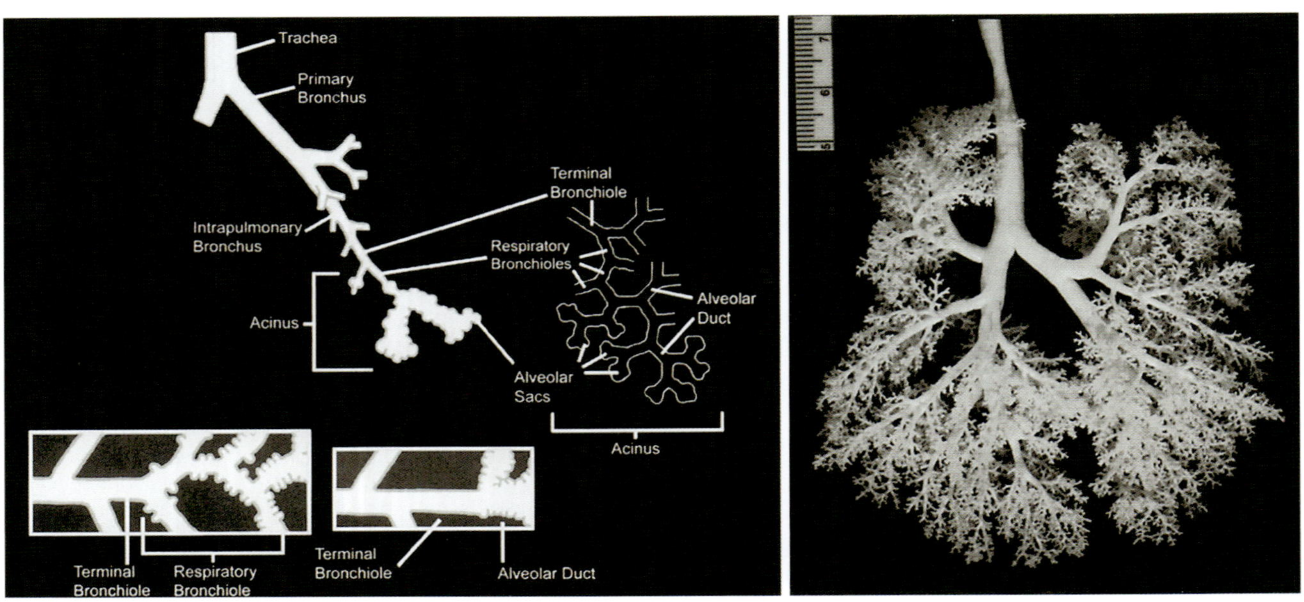

Figure 9-14 Comparison of a schematic drawing of the organization of the tracheobronchial airways and gas exchange area (left) and a cast of the air space in the tracheobronchial airways (right). In many species, terminal bronchioles have a very short transition to alveolar ducts (inset, lower right), while in other species the transition is extensive with many generations of bronchioles containing alveolar outpocketings and are called respiratory bronchioles (inset, lower left).

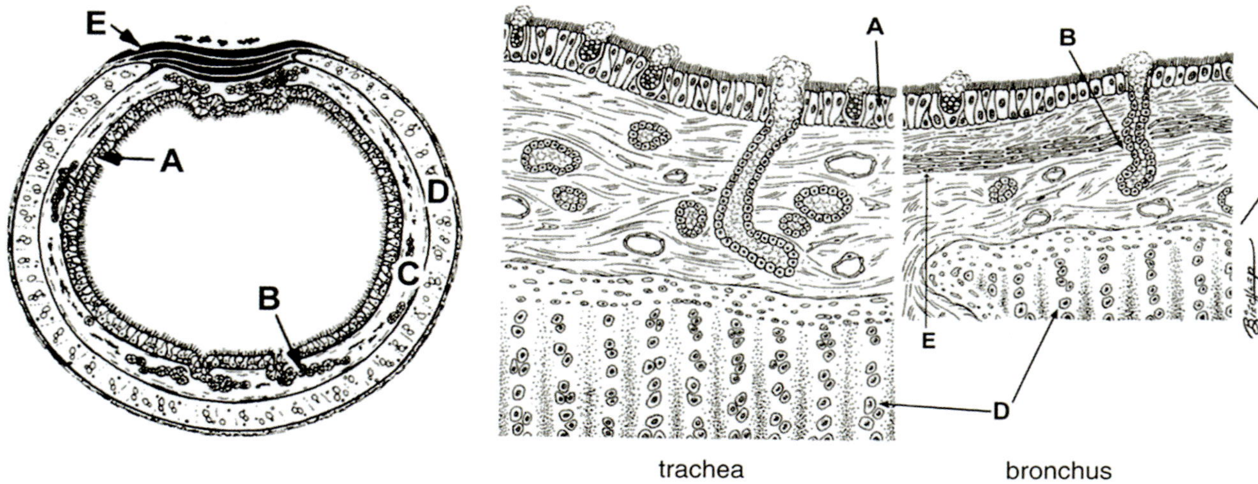

Figure 9-15 Schematic drawing of a cross-section of the trachea and detailed sections through parts of the wall of the trachea and a bronchus. Note the differences in the height of the epithelium (A), the glandular density (B), the thickness of the soft tissue in the propria-submucosa (C), the presence of hyaline cartilage as rings in the trachea versus plates in the bronchus (D), and the location of smooth muscle (E).

Within the thoracic cavity, the trachea terminates by bifurcating into two **primary bronchi**. Distal to the bifurcation, the primary bronchi provide branches that enter the lungs. The structural characteristics of primary bronchi are the same as those of the trachea, except that cartilage is in the form of irregular plates.

Lung

Most of the thoracic cavity is occupied by right and left lungs. The lungs of mammals may be divided into intrapulmonary conducting airways, gas exchange area (parenchyma), and pleura (Fig. 9-14). The intrapulmonary conducting airways (bronchi and bronchioles) compose approximately 6% of the lung. The gas exchange area, consisting of respiratory bronchioles (also referred to as the transition zone), alveolar ducts, alveolar sacs, and alveoli, comprises approximately 85% of the lung. The lung is encapsulated by a layer of CT covered by mesothelial cells termed the **visceral (pulmonary) pleura**. Along with the pleura, the intrapulmonary nervous and vascular tissue (pulmonary arteries, pulmonary veins, and bronchial arteries) comprise the remaining 9 to 10% of the lung.

Intrapulmonary Conducting Airways

Bronchi

The bronchial tree is formed by a primary bronchus and the various orders of airways that it supplies (Fig. 9-14). The largest segments of the intrapulmonary conducting airways are called **lobar bronchi**, each of which enters a lobe of the lung at its hilum. The lobar bronchi divide into two smaller branches, which then divide again, and this process continues until the gas exchange area is reached. The first two or three generations of branching from a lobar bronchus supply portions of the lung lobe called **bronchopulmonary segments**. Each succeeding generation of branching consists of a greater number of airways and has a larger total cross-sectional area than the generation before it.

The histologic appearance of a bronchus is generally similar to that of the trachea, except that the various layers are thinner (Fig. 9-15). Bronchi are lined by a respiratory epithelium composed primarily of ciliated cells, secretory cells, and basal cells. Proximodistally (from the proximal to the distal parts of the bronchial tree), the composition of the epithelium changes. Mucous cells and basal cells decrease in number, while ciliated cells remain at about the same density, and bronchiolar exocrine cells increase. At the same time, both the epithelial height and the thickness of the propria-submucosa progressively decrease.

The propria-submucosa is loose CT containing mixed glands (**bronchial glands**) in all species except goats; bronchial glands are less abundant in distal bronchi. The hyaline cartilage of the proximal bronchi is in the form of irregular plates, and the smooth muscle is interspersed either between or on the luminal side of the plates. The muscle cells are generally arranged in a circular fashion, perpendicular to the long axis of the airway. The amount of cartilage decreases proximodistally, whereas smooth muscle becomes relatively more abundant. The adventitial CT is primarily loose, with many collagen fibers and variable numbers of elastic fibers. Many of the fibers are oriented longitudinally, whereas others are oriented perpendicularly to the long axis of the airway. Adventitial and submucosal nerve plexuses and intraepithelial nerve endings are present. In most domestic species, the extensive vascular supply is derived from the systemic circulation via the bronchial artery.

Bronchioles

Bronchioles arise from bronchi, branch into several generations, and terminate as terminal bronchioles (Fig. 9-14). Several generations of **bronchioles** are present in horses, cattle, and sheep, whereas generally only one or two generations are present in carnivores.

Bronchioles have roughly circular cross-sectional profiles and are lined with simple columnar or cuboidal epithelium (Fig. 9-16), composed of ciliated cells and **bronchiolar exocrine cells** (also known as club cells). These cells have characteristics of both secretory cells and cells capable of metabolizing xenobiotic compounds. The secretory granules contain either neutral glycoprotein or low-molecular-weight protein. sER is abundant in cells from horses and sheep but is minimally present in those from carnivores, cattle, and pigs. Glycogen is the predominant feature of bronchiolar exocrine cells in carnivores and cattle and is rarely observed in most other species. In carnivores, the epithelium of terminal bronchioles primarily consists of bronchiolar exocrine cells.

The propria-submucosa is sparse loose CT; glands and cartilage are absent. The smooth muscle is arranged in separate circular and oblique fascicles. Numerous nerve fibers occur in the area immediately below the epithelium and interspersed between muscle fascicles.

The adventitia is loose CT, including elastic fibers oriented circularly or obliquely. The outer border of the adventitia is attached to the alveolar gas exchange area and is lined by alveolar epithelial cells and a pulmonary capillary bed.

Gas Exchange Area

The **gas exchange area**, also referred to as parenchyma, can be organized into either functional or structural units. The functional unit of the gas exchange area is called the **acinus** or terminal respiratory unit (Figs. 9-14 and 9-17). The acinus includes all air spaces distal to a single terminal bronchiole, including branching respiratory bronchioles, alveolar ducts, alveolar sacs, and alveoli.

The **lobule** is a structural unit rather than a functional unit. It comprises a cluster of acini that is separated from adjacent clusters by CT septa. These CT septa are termed **interlobular septa** and are composed of collagen, elastic fibers, and blood vessels. Both bronchial arteries and pulmonary veins are located within interlobular septa. The lungs of cattle, sheep, and pigs are highly lobulated and have complete septa. The lungs of horses have incomplete septa and are considered poorly lobulated. Carnivores do not have interlobular septa.

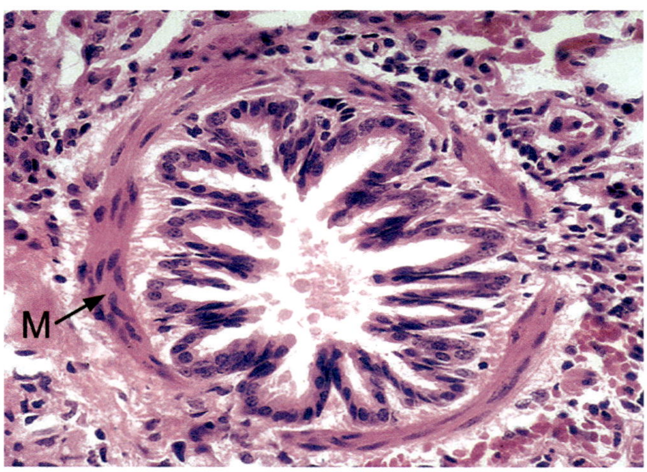

Figure 9-16 Cross-section of a bronchiole. The bronchiolar epithelium is simple cuboidal to simple columnar and includes ciliated cells and bronchiolar exocrine or club cells. Cartilage and glands are lacking in the propria-submucosa, and smooth muscle (M) is a prominent feature of the bronchiolar wall. A thin adventitia of CT lies outside the muscle. Lung, horse. H&E (×400). (Image by W. E. Haensly).

Respiratory Bronchioles

Bronchioles in which the walls possess outpocketings of gas exchange tissue, i.e., alveoli, are termed **respiratory bronchioles**. They are also called the **transition zone**, which is the focus of most lung disorders. The histologic appearance of respiratory bronchioles is similar to that of terminal bronchioles, with the exception that the epithelium is interrupted by alveoli (Figs. 9-17 and 9-18). The smooth muscle is arranged in fascicles that underlie the simple columnar or cuboidal epithelium. The alveoli open between these muscle bundles.

In respiratory bronchioles of carnivores, extensive alveolarization occurs (Fig. 9-18); generally, there are fewer alveoli in the proximal generation of branching. The epithelium consists almost entirely of bronchiolar exocrine cells. In horses, cattle, sheep, and pigs, respiratory bronchioles are short or absent. In carnivores, a minimum of three to four generations of branching of respiratory bronchioles are present (Fig. 9-19).

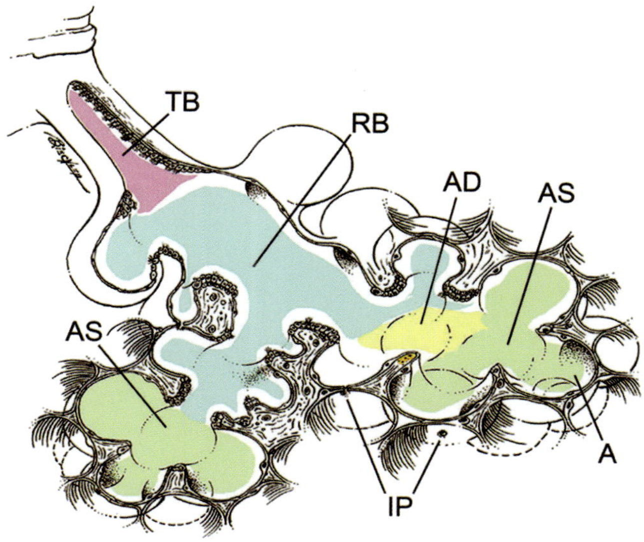

Figure 9-17 Schematic illustration of the gas exchange area originating from a terminal bronchiole (TB). Respiratory bronchiole (RB), alveolar duct (AD), alveolar sac (AS), alveolus (A), and interalveolar pore (IP).

Alveolar Ducts and Alveolar Sacs

Respiratory bronchioles branch into tubular structures termed **alveolar ducts** (Figs. 9-14 and 9-17 to 9-19). The ducts are comparable to hallways lined by doorless rooms on all sides. Each of these doorless rooms is an alveolus. Between one and five generations of alveolar ducts are supplied by a single respiratory bronchiole. The walls of an alveolar duct are composed of the open sides of alveolar air spaces and the terminations of the interalveolar septa that separate these alveoli. Spiraling bands of smooth muscle and elastic fibers are oriented perpendicular to the long axis of the alveolar ducts. They lie underneath the epithelium at the terminations of the interalveolar septa.

The alveolar ducts terminate in clusters of alveoli called **alveolar sacs** (Figs. 9-14 and 9-17). A shared space into which several alveolar sacs open is called an **atrium**.

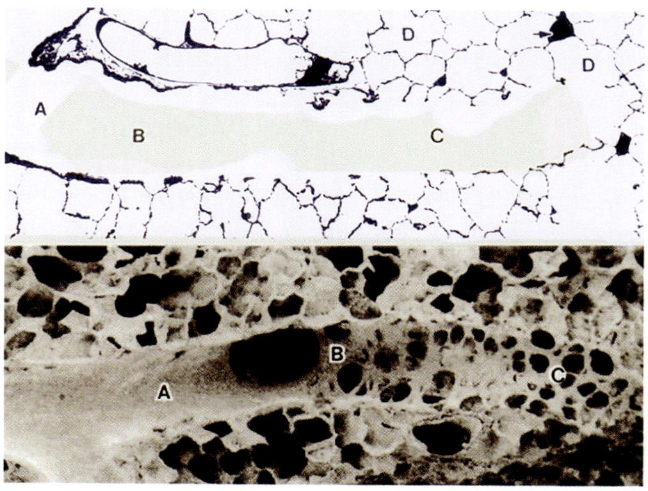

Figure 9-18 Light microscopic and scanning electron microscopic appearance of a terminal bronchiole and gas exchange area in the feline lung. Terminal bronchiole (A), respiratory bronchiole into which a few alveoli open (B), alveolar duct completely surrounded by alveoli (C), and alveoli sacs/alveoli (D). Methylene blue–Azure II (top: ×55; bottom: ×70).

Alveoli

The basic unit for gas exchange in the pulmonary parenchyma is the **alveolus** (Figs. 9-14, 9-20, and 9-21). Alveoli are spheroid air spaces lined with epithelium, which open into an alveolar sac, alveolar duct, or respiratory bronchiole; they are separated by interalveolar septa.

The alveolar epithelial lining, located adjacent to the air space, comprises two types of epithelial cells: type I and type II alveolar epithelial cells. The **type I** or **squamous alveolar epithelial cell** (respiratory epithelial cell) is flat with a central nucleus and rests on a continuous basal lamina (Fig. 9-20). Its thin cytoplasm has few mitochondria, minimal amounts of rER, and a moderate number of endocytotic vesicles. This cell type covers approximately 97% of the interalveolar septal surface in all the species studied thus far. The average surface area of a type I cell ranges from 5000 to 7000 μm^2.

The **type II** or **granular (great) alveolar epithelial cell** (Fig. 9-22) is a cuboidal cell with a central nucleus. This cell type covers the remainder of the interalveolar septal surface area (approximately 3%). Its alveolar surface bears microvilli and ranges from 100 to 280 μm^2 per cell. This cell contains mitochondria, rER, microvesicles, a Golgi complex, and multiple characteristic osmiophilic vesicles called **lamellar bodies**. These lamellar bodies are believed to be primarily phospholipid and are the source of phospholipids in pulmonary surfactant that lines the air spaces. The type II alveolar cell is the progenitor cell for both type I and type II cells.

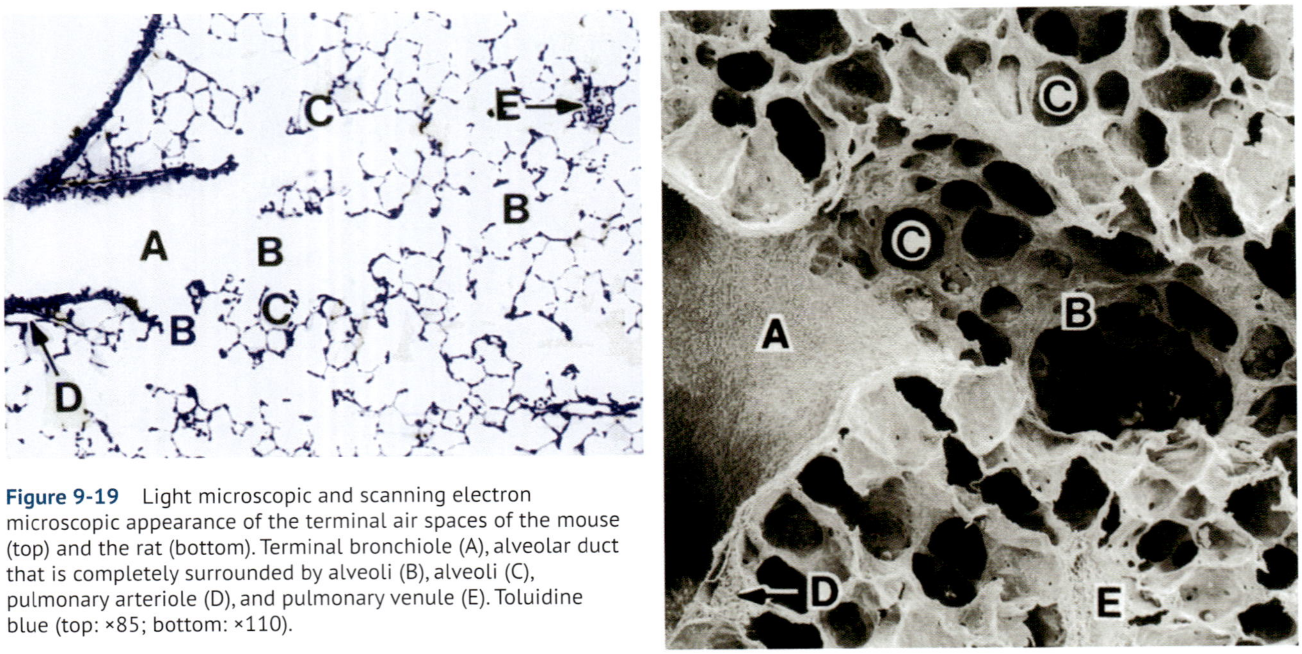

Figure 9-19 Light microscopic and scanning electron microscopic appearance of the terminal air spaces of the mouse (top) and the rat (bottom). Terminal bronchiole (A), alveolar duct that is completely surrounded by alveoli (B), alveoli (C), pulmonary arteriole (D), and pulmonary venule (E). Toluidine blue (top: ×85; bottom: ×110).

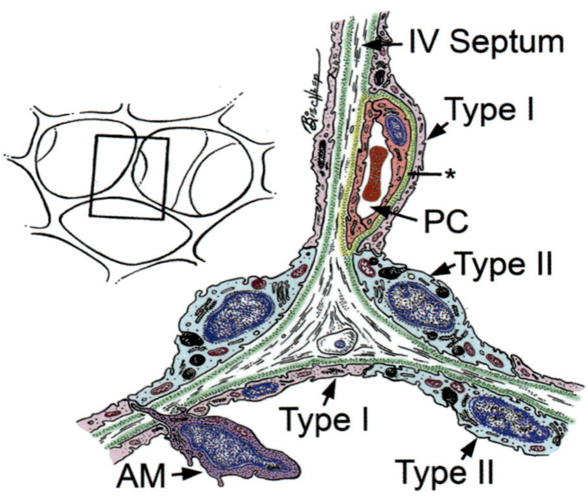

Figure 9-20 Schematic illustration of parts of three adjacent alveoli, as outlined in the rectangle (inset): type I alveolar epithelial cell, type II alveolar epithelial cell, interalveolar (IV) septum, pulmonary capillary (PC), and alveolar macrophage (AM). Note the merger of the basal laminae of the pulmonary capillary and adjacent alveolus (*).

Pulmonary **alveolar macrophages** are likewise present on the air side of the interalveolar septa (Fig. 9-23). As active phagocytic cells, they are part of the mononuclear phagocyte system distributed throughout the body.

Interalveolar septa are thin sheets of CT containing a capillary plexus (Fig. 9-20). The interalveolar **interstitial CT** contains collagen and elastic fibers, as well as fibrocytes. Additionally, pericytes, macrophages, lymphocytes, and plasma cells may also be present.

The capillary bed of the interalveolar septa is an intermeshed network of short, branching vessels. Individual capillary beds traverse the walls of three to seven alveoli when passing from a pulmonary arteriole to a pulmonary venule. Most endothelial cells have attenuated cytoplasm in the region adjacent to type I alveolar epithelial cells. In these attenuated areas, the basal laminae of alveolar epithelial cells and endothelial cells fuse. Capillary endothelial cells (Fig. 9-20) are characterized by few organelles and relatively numerous endocytotic vesicles. The intercellular junctions tend to be loose or leaky, and the tight junctions have few anastomosing ridges. The surface area of the gas exchange capillary bed is between 66 and 75% of the surface area of the air side of the interalveolar septa.

The alveoli contain a small amount of fluid, consisting of a biphasic layer of plasma filtrates overlaid by a thin layer of phospholipids. This phospholipid layer or **pulmonary surfactant** reduces the intraalveolar surface tension, preventing alveolar collapse.

The **blood–air barrier** consists of the surface-lining layer of pulmonary surfactant and fluid, the alveolar type I cell, fused basal laminae of the alveolar epithelial cell and the underlying capillary endothelial cell, the capillary endothelial cell, and the plasmalemma of a red blood cell (Fig. 9-20). The average thickness of this barrier is 1.5 μm in most species, with the thinnest areas ranging from 0.2 to 0.7 μm. At its thickest, this barrier consists of the above-mentioned layers and interstitial CT and cells between the basal laminae of epithelial and endothelial cells. The blood–air barrier prevents the massive release of fluid filtrate from capillaries into the air space while permitting diffusion of oxygen and carbon dioxide between blood capillaries and alveoli (Figs. 9-20 and 9-23).

Openings in the interalveolar septa interconnect adjacent alveoli. These openings, called **septal pores** (alveolar pores) (Figs. 9-21 and 9-23), are lined by epithelial cells and permit air and alveolar macrophages to pass from one alveolus to another.

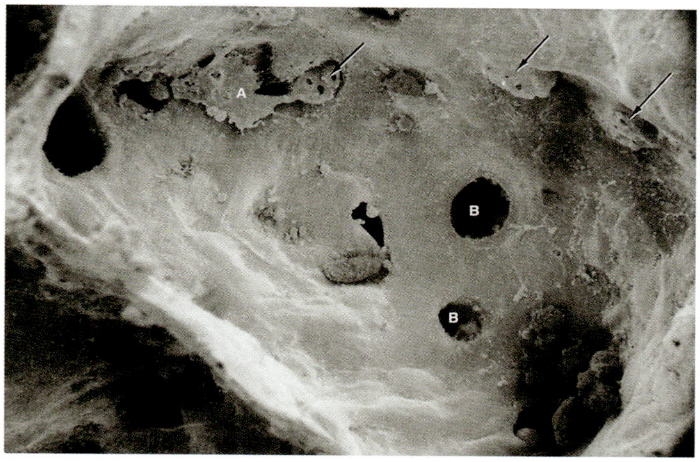

Figure 9-21 Scanning electron micrograph of a portion of an alveolus in the equine lung. Type II (granular) alveolar epithelial cells bulge into the lumen (arrows). On the left is a pulmonary alveolar macrophage (A). Note the pores in the interalveolar septum (B) (×1232). (Courtesy of W. S. Tyler).

Pleura

The visceral, or pulmonary, pleura is a serous membrane that completely covers both lungs, except at the hilum and pulmonary ligament. This covering layer consists of squamous to cuboidal mesothelial cells overlaying varying amounts of elastic fibers and dense irregular CT. Pleural mesothelial cells contain large amounts of rER and mitochondria; their free surfaces are covered by microvilli. At its thickest, the CT elements of the pleura consist of two or more layers of elastic laminae, many dense irregular bundles of collagen fibers, pulmonary capillaries, and two additional sets of vessels. These two sets of vessels include capillaries and small arterioles from the bronchial circulatory system and lymph vessels. The pulmonary capillaries supply the superficial portion of the gas exchange area. The CT of the pulmonary pleura is continuous with that of the interalveolar septa. The thickness of the pulmonary pleura varies from species to species and within different regions of the same species. The pleura is thinnest in the dog and cat, where the submesothelial CT is minimal, and the only blood supply is derived from the pulmonary artery. Conversely, the pleura is thick in large domestic mammals.

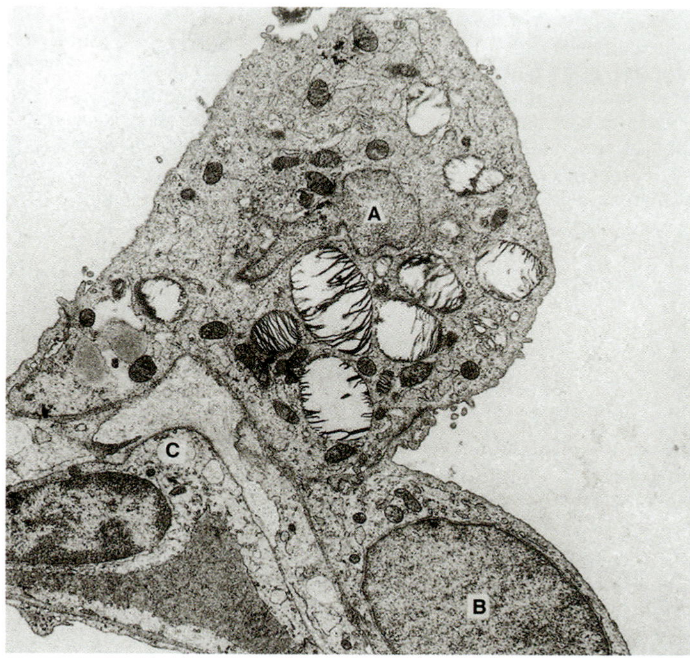

Figure 9-22 Electron micrograph of a type II (granular) alveolar epithelial cell (A) containing numerous characteristic lamellar bodies and a type I (squamous) alveolar epithelial cell (B). Capillary endothelial cell (C) (×8200). (From Tyler WS, Gillespie JR, Nowell JA. Modern functional morphology of the equine lung. *Equine Vet J* 1971).

Blood Vessels and Lymphatics

Blood is supplied to the lungs through two different circulatory systems: **pulmonary** and **bronchial**. **Pulmonary arteries** carry the entire output of unoxygenated blood from the right ventricle. These arteries and their branches operate under low pressure; thus, their walls have fewer elastic and collagen fibers and fewer smooth muscle cells than vessels of comparable size in the systemic circulatory system. Pulmonary arteries and the tracheobronchial tree have a common adventitia.

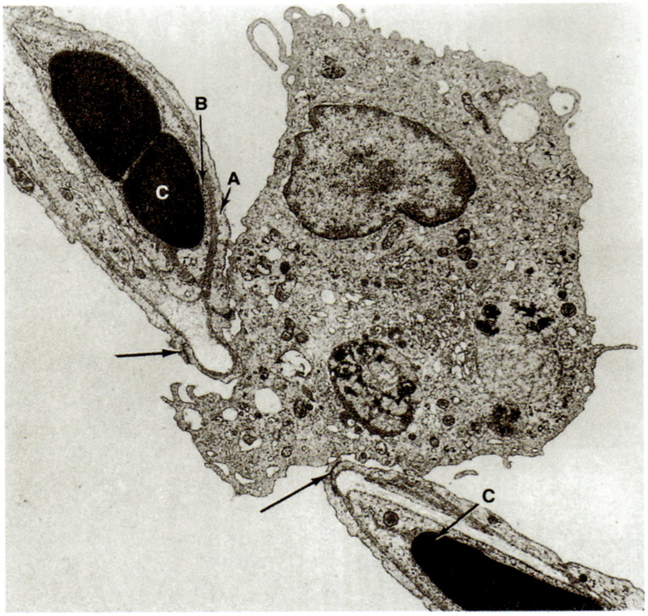

Figure 9-23 Electron micrograph of an alveolar macrophage projecting through a septal pore. The macrophage has numerous filopodia, phagosomes, and phagolysosomes. The thin layer of cytoplasm of the type I (squamous) alveolar epithelial cells (A) is separated by a basal lamina from the capillary endothelium (B). Erythrocytes (C) are in the capillary lumen. The dark lines (arrows) are tight junctions between adjacent squamous alveolar epithelial cells (×8100). (From Tyler W. S., Gillespie J.R., Nowell J.A. Modern functional morphology of the equine lung. *Equine Vet J* 1971;3:84–94.)

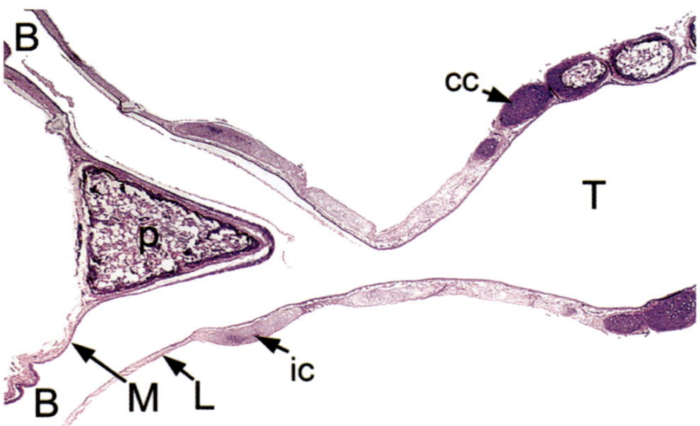

Figure 9-24 The avian syrinx is located at the junction between the trachea (T) and bronchi (B). Medial (m) and lateral (l) tympanic membranes vibrate to produce sound. The syrinx has three cranial cartilages (cc) in the female or four in the male. Four intermediate cartilages (ic), a pessulus (p), and three caudal cartilages (not shown) form the balance of the syrinx. Syrinx, chicken. H&E (×25). (Image by W.E. Haensly.)

The **bronchial arteries** are under high pressure as a part of the systemic arterial circulatory system. The blood vessels in this system have the same wall structure as those of other systemic arteries of the same size. In all species, the bronchial artery supplies blood to the large bronchi, the major pulmonary vessels, and the pulmonary lymph nodes. Anastomoses between the bronchial and pulmonary arterial circulatory systems have been identified in the walls of medium-sized bronchi and bronchioles of horses, cattle, and sheep.

All blood from the lungs is carried back to the heart by the **pulmonary veins**, constituting a low-pressure system. The pulmonary veins have thin walls with little smooth muscle in dogs, cats, horses, and goats. Conversely, pulmonary veins with large muscle bundles are present in cattle and pigs. In most species, the pulmonary veins are located at the periphery of lobules and course toward the hilum within interlobular septa. However, in cattle, horses, pigs, and sheep, the pulmonary veins accompany the bronchial tree on the side opposite that of pulmonary arteries.

The **pulmonary lymphatics** begin as lymph capillaries distributed throughout the interstitium, except for the interstitium of interalveolar septa. Collecting lymph vessels are found throughout the CT of the lung, except for areas surrounding alveoli, alveolar sacs and ducts, and respiratory bronchioles.

Innervation

Innervation of the lungs originates from two sources: the parasympathetic system (via the vagus nerve) and the sympathetic system (via the middle cervical and cervicothoracic ganglia). Additionally, general visceral afferent sensory fibers from pulmonary tissue are also conveyed through the vagus nerve. Fibers from the vagus nerves intermingle to form a plexus along the walls of the airway tree and the pulmonary vasculature, with ganglia present in the adventitia of large airways. Individual nerve fibers are distributed irregularly over the wall of arteries, veins, and airways. Free nerve endings are present near glands, within smooth muscle bundles, and in the interalveolar septa.

Avian Respiratory System

In contrast to the mammalian respiratory system, the respiratory system of birds contains a simpler larynx, a syrinx, and only four orders or generations of conducting airways, a compact spongy lung, and air sacs. The highly efficient avian respiratory system comprises lung tissue positioned between conducting airways and air sacs. During inspiration, air is drawn into the nasal cavity and through the lung tissue to the air sacs; during expiration, the reverse process occurs. Birds breathe more slowly and deeply than mammals, and unlike in mammals, the lung volume of birds remains relatively constant while the volume of their air sacs changes during ventilation.

The nasal cavity is lined by epithelia similar to those of mammals, with stratified squamous epithelium rostrally, olfactory epithelium dorsocaudally, and respiratory epithelium lining most of the remaining areas. In the respiratory epithelium, groups of goblet cells form intraepithelial glands. Large air spaces, the paired infraorbital sinuses, are often clinically involved in respiratory infections. These sinuses drain into the nasal cavity and are lined by respiratory epithelium.

The larynx, devoid of vocal folds, produces minimal sound. The trachea is similar in structure to that in mammals, except that the tracheal cartilages form complete rings encircling the airway; the cartilage rings overlap and interlock with adjacent rings. The trachealis muscle is absent, and intraepithelial mucous glands are numerous (Fig. 9-24). As a result of differences in cartilage structure and smooth muscle content, the trachea of birds, unlike that of mammals, does not undergo phasic changes in diameter during breathing.

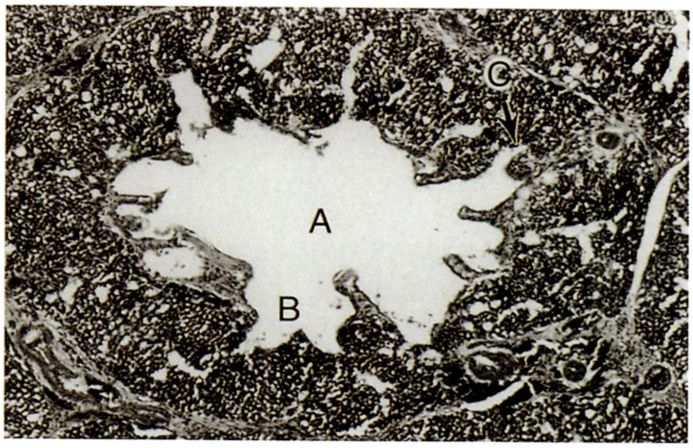

Figure 9-25 Tertiary bronchus (parabronchus) of a chicken lung. An atrium (B) opens into the lumen (A) of the tertiary bronchus. Air capillaries (C) open into the atria. H&E (×110).

Vocalization occurs in the avian **syrinx**, a specialized region at the tracheobronchial junction with considerable species-dependent structural variation. The intrasyringeal (tympaniform) membranes, which vibrate during the production of sound, are lined by stratified squamous epithelium.

The avian lungs consist of primary, secondary, and tertiary bronchi, as well as atria and air capillaries. Extrapulmonary primary bronchi continue as intrapulmonary **primary bronchi** or **mesobronchi**, each of which terminates by opening into an abdominal air sac. The epithelium of the primary bronchi resembles that of the trachea. Bronchial cartilages are incomplete along the medial aspect of the proximal bronchi and become patch-like distally. **Secondary bronchi** branch off from each intrapulmonary primary bronchus, with many connecting to other air sacs. **Tertiary bronchi**, or **parabronchi**, approximately 100 to 150 μm in diameter, interconnect the secondary bronchi. The epithelium varies from respiratory epithelium in the secondary bronchi to simple cuboidal or squamous epithelium in the tertiary bronchi. A network of spiraling bundles of smooth muscle is present in the lamina propria of the secondary and tertiary bronchi. Numerous small air spaces, or **atria**, open into the tertiary bronchi, with the projecting tips of the **interatrial septa** containing smooth muscle and lined by squamous cells (Fig. 9-25).

Gas exchange in the avian lung occurs between blood and **air capillaries**. These capillaries, 5 to 15 μm in diameter, open into the atria. Simple squamous epithelium lines the majority of the atria and air capillaries. The epithelial portion of the gas exchange area consists of both type I and type II cells, similar to those of mammals; a biphasic fluid lining layer, similar to surfactant of mammals, is also observed in birds.

The terminal **air sacs** are lined by a simple squamous to cuboidal epithelium. Epithelial surfaces adjacent to the ostia of bronchi are ciliated.

Clinical Correlations

The respiratory tract is constantly exposed to potentially harmful agents such as microorganisms or toxic substances in inspired air or through the blood supply. Respiratory disease in mammals and avian species spans an extensive array of agents that includes viral, bacterial, fungal, and parasitic pathogens. All levels of the respiratory system are subject to disease and inflammation of the larynx, trachea, and bronchi is common as well as various pneumonia types of the deeper airways (lobar, focal, and interstitial pneumonia). The structure and function of the respiratory system dictate the patterns of disease observed within it. Bronchi often contain bronchus-associated lymphoid tissue, which becomes activated and proliferates during lung infections. In Figure 9-26, a bronchiole is shown that is surrounded by small cells with dark nuclei

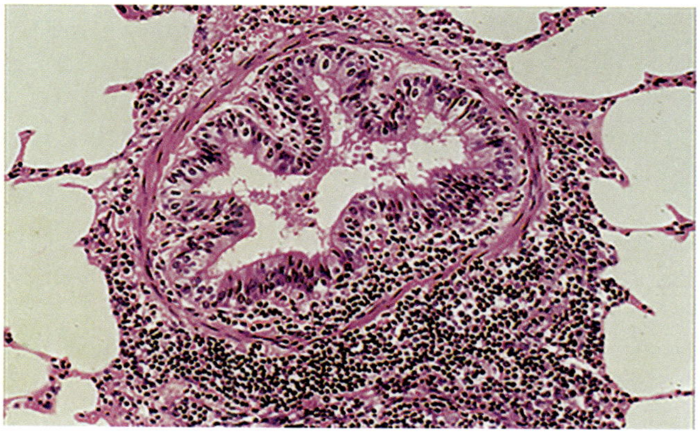

Figure 9-26 Lung, Bronchiole (calf). H&E (Reprinted with permission from Salguero Bodes FJ, Pallares Martinez FJ. Aughey and Frye's Comparative Veterinary Histology with Clinical Correlates. 2nd ed. Boca Raton: CRC Press, 2023.)

and scant cytoplasm (lymphocytes). This invasion of lymphoid cells into the bronchiolar wall, termed "cuffing" pneumonia due to their arrangement, is an example of a chronic, nonsuppurative pneumonia commonly seen in calves. Mycoplasma infections are often implicated in these cases.

Essentials

A cross-section through the trachea will reveal the mucosa, submucosa with submucosal glands, and the perichondrium on the surface of the tracheal hyaline cartilage. On one side of the trachea can be found the trachealis muscle. The ***trachea*** has a thick basement membrane underneath the trachea epithelium. The ***extrapulmonary primary bronchi*** have more complete cartilage rings than the trachea, and they have spiral bands of smooth muscle that completely encircle the bronchi. The ***intrapulmonary bronchi*** have irregular cartilage plates and a smooth muscle muscularis. As the ***bronchus*** becomes smaller, the epithelium may transition from pseudostratified ciliated columnar to simple ciliated columnar. ***Bronchioles*** lack cartilage plates but have smooth muscle. At the ***terminal bronchiole***, there are few to no goblet cells, with bronchiolar exocrine cells (club cells) being the predominant cell type. The terminal bronchiole transitions to the respiratory bronchiole with club cells and some ciliated cells proximally and primarily club cells distally. The walls of ***respiratory bronchioles*** are interrupted by alveoli. Respiratory bronchioles lead into alveolar ducts. While ***alveolar ducts*** contain smooth muscle, their epithelium is composed of simple squamous Type I pneumocytes. The alveolar ducts lead into ***alveolar sacs*** and ***alveoli***. Surfactant producing Type II pneumocytes are located at the intersection points of the alveoli. Alveolar macrophages may be present in the alveolar lumen. The blood-gas or ***blood-air barrier*** in the lungs is thin, facilitating efficient gas exchange, and consists of Type I pneumocytes, endothelial cells, and a shared basement membrane. The visceral pleura of the lung is covered by a thin mesothelial layer attached to the lung that acts as a seal. Under the mesothelium lies a CT layer with blood vessels, lymphatics, and nerves.

Suggested Readings

Adams DR, Hotchkiss DK. The canine nasal mucosa. Zentralbl Veterinärmed C Anat Histol Embryol 1983;12:109.

Bodes FJS, Martínez FPM. Respiratory System. In: Aughey and Frye's Comparative Veterinary Histology with Clinical Correlates, 2nd Ed., CRC Press, 2023: 69.

Farrington JE, Sannes PL. Basement membranes and the extracellular matrix. In: Parent RA, ed. Comparative Biology of the Normal Lung. San Diego: Elsevier, Inc, 2015: 119.

Harkema JR. Comparative anatomy and epithelial cell biology of the nose. In: Parent RA, ed. Comparative Biology of the Normal Lung. San Diego: Elsevier, Inc, 2015: 7.

Lascola KM. Overview of respiratory diseases of horses. In: The Merck Veterinary Manual, 2023. Retrieved [May 5, 2024].

Mercer RR, Crapo JD. Architecture of the gas exchange region of the lungs. In: Parent RA, ed. Comparative Biology of the Normal Lung. San Diego: Elsevier, Inc, 2015: 93.

Peake JL, Pinkerton KE. Gross and subgross anatomy of lungs, connective tissue septa, distal airways and structural units. In: Parent RA, ed. Comparative Biology of the Normal Lung. San Diego: Elsevier, Inc, 2015: 21.

Pinkerton KE, Gehr P. Architecture and cellular composition of the air-blood tissue barrier. In: Parent RA, ed. Comparative Biology of the Normal Lung. San Diego: Elsevier, Inc, 2015: 105.

Pinkerton KE, Van Winkle LS, Plopper CG, et al. Architecture of the tracheobronchial tree. In: Parent RA, ed. Comparative Biology of the Normal Lung. San Diego: Elsevier, Inc, 2015: 33.

Plopper CG, Hyde DM. Epithelial cells of the bronchiole. In: Parent RA, ed. Comparative Biology of the Normal Lung. San Diego: Elsevier, Inc, 2015: 83.

Reynolds SD, Pinkerton KE, Mariassy AT. Epithelial cells of trachea and bronchi. In: Parent RA, ed. Comparative Biology of the Normal Lung. San Diego: Elsevier, Inc, 2015: 61.

Salguero Bodes FJ, Pallares Martinez FJ. Aughey and Frye's Comparative Veterinary Histology with Clinical Correlates. 2nd ed. Boca Raton: CRC Press, 2023.

St George JA. Secretory glycoproteins of the trachea and bronchi. In: Parent RA, ed. Comparative Biology of the Normal Lung. San Diego: Elsevier, Inc, 2015: 53.

Tyler WS, Gillespie JR, Nowell JA. Modern functional morphology of the equine lung. *Equine Vet* J 1971;3:84.

10

Digestive System

Ji-Ming Feng

CHAPTER MENU

Dellmann's Textbook of Veterinary Histology, Seventh Edition. Edited by Marxa L. Figueiredo and John J. Turek.

Companion website: www.wiley.com/go/figueiredo/vethistology7e

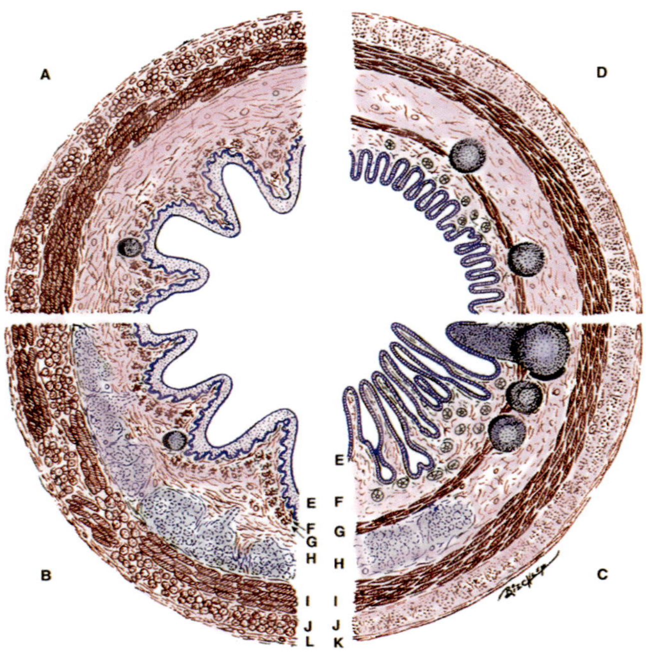

Figure 10-1 Schematic drawing of cross-sections through various portions of the digestive tract. Esophagus without submucosal glands (A). Esophagus with submucosal glands (B). Small intestine with and without submucosal glands and with aggregated lymphatic nodules (C). Large intestine (D). Tunica mucosa: Epithelium (E), lamina propria (F), and lamina muscularis (G). Tela submucosa (H). Tunica muscularis: Circular layer (I) and longitudinal layer (J). Tunica serosa (K) and tunica adventitia (L).

The digestive system, consisting of a series of tubular organs and associated glands, primarily functions to break down ingested food into smaller units that can be absorbed into the circulation and used for the maintenance of the organism.

Morphologic adaptations for specialized functions are characteristic of the digestive systems of the domestic species. Considerable variations in the teeth, stomachs, and large intestines mainly result from the variety of food consumed. For example, the teeth of carnivores are adapted for tearing flesh, whereas those of herbivores are specialized for grinding roughage. The forestomach of ruminants and the cecum and colon of horses reflect structural variations that facilitate the microbial digestion of rough, fibrous food.

Although the large accessory digestive glands—salivary glands, liver, and pancreas—are located outside the tubular portion of the digestive system, they originate as epithelial evaginations from the digestive tube. Their ducts penetrate the walls of the tubular organs to discharge secretory products into the lumina.

General Structure of Tubular Organs

A general structural pattern exists for all tubular organs of the digestive, respiratory, urinary, and reproductive systems (Fig. 10-1). Familiarity with this general pattern is helpful in understanding the specific characteristics of each organ. The wall of a typical tubular organ is composed of four coats or layers, each called either a **tunic** or a **tela**. A tela has a delicate weblike structure, while a tunic is comprised of denser tissue.

Tunica Mucosa

The tunic adjacent to the lumen is the **tunica mucosa**, also referred to as a mucous membrane or simply the mucosa. A mucosa lines all organs that communicate with the outside of the body and is protected by a layer of **mucus**, a viscous material containing cast-off epithelial cells, leukocytes, and **mucin**, a product of specialized glands. Structures within or associated with the oral cavity, such as the lips, cheeks, and tongue, have a mucosa, even though they are not typical tubular organs. The mucosa is composed of three layers or laminae: an epithelium, a lamina propria, and a lamina muscularis.

The mucosal **epithelium** rests on a basement membrane and may consist of any type of surface epithelium, depending on the specific function of the organ.

The **lamina propria** is a layer of connective tissue (CT) located immediately beneath the epithelium. In most organs, this is a loose CT containing fine collagen, elastic, and reticular fibers, as well as the typical cells found in loose CT (see Chapter 3). The lamina propria also is classified as diffuse lymphatic tissue because it contains many immunocompetent T and B lymphocytes. These lymphocytes initiate the immune response against injurious agents that have breached the epithelium. Blood vessels essential for the nourishment of the epithelium, along with lymph capillaries and nerves, are present also in the lamina propria. In some organs, the lamina propria contains glands that are referred to as **mucosal glands** because they are confined to the mucosa.

The **lamina muscularis**, also called **muscularis mucosae**, is variably present. It consists of one to three layers of smooth muscle. The lamina muscularis allows independent movement of the mucosa, possibly to facilitate the movement of luminal contents or to assist in the expression of secretions from mucosal glands.

Tela Submucosa

The **tela submucosa**, or simply **submucosa**, is a CT layer that may contain glands (**submucosal glands**). In most organs, the submucosa CT is denser than that of the lamina propria. Also present are blood vessels, lymph vessels, and the **submucosal (Meissner) plexus**, a ganglionic nerve plexus of the autonomic nervous system. In organs lacking a lamina muscularis, the lamina propria and submucosa blend without a clear line of demarcation, forming a **propria-submucosa**.

Tunica Muscularis

The **tunica muscularis**, or **muscularis externa**, consists of smooth muscle or skeletal muscle responsible for moving the ingesta through the digestive tract and mixing it with glandular secretions. Usually, two layers of muscle are present in the tunica muscularis of the tubular organs of the digestive system. The muscle fibers of the inner layer are oriented circularly or in a tightly coiled pattern, whereas those of the outer layer are arranged longitudinally or in a loosely coiled pattern. Between these layers is a ganglionic nerve plexus of the autonomic nervous system, the **myenteric (Auerbach) plexus**.

Tunica Serosa/Adventitia

The outermost layer of the digestive tract may be either a tunica serosa or a tunica adventitia. The **tunica serosa** (serosa or serous membrane) is composed of a CT layer with a covering of mesothelium. Organs that border the pleural, pericardial, and peritoneal cavities are covered by a serosa. In each of these locations, the serosa is given a special name: pleura, epicardium, and peritoneum, respectively. All organs not bordering these cavities, such as the cervical part of the esophagus, lack a mesothelium. Instead, they have a CT layer called a **tunica adventitia**, or simply **adventitia**, which blends with the surrounding fascia (Fig. 10-1).

Oral Cavity

Lips

The transition from the integument to the digestive system occurs at the lips, where the outer surface is covered by skin and the inner surface is covered by a mucosa. Near the **mucocutaneous junction**, the skin lacks hair follicles and the epidermis is thicker, with a more elaborate interdigitation with the underlying CT (Fig. 10-2). The mucosa of the lips is covered by strati-

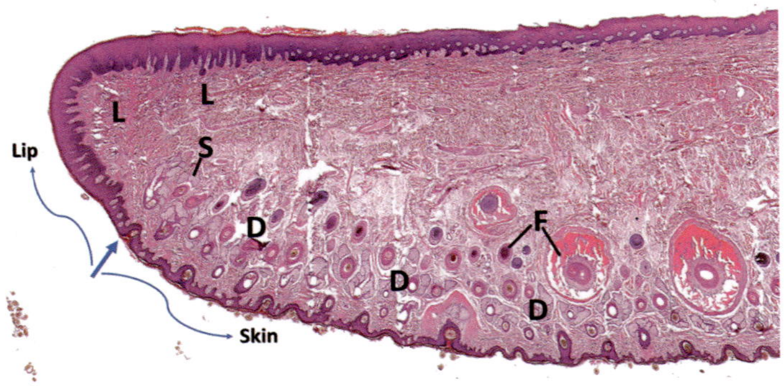

Figure 10-2 Lip (sheep). Transitional junction (arrow) of keratinized stratified squamous epithelium of skin and mucosa. Note that the dermis (D) of the skin contains many hair follicles (F) and their associated sebaceous glands (S), while the lamina propria (L) of the lip lacks any. Hematoxylin and eosin (H&E) (×20). (Image by J. Feng.)

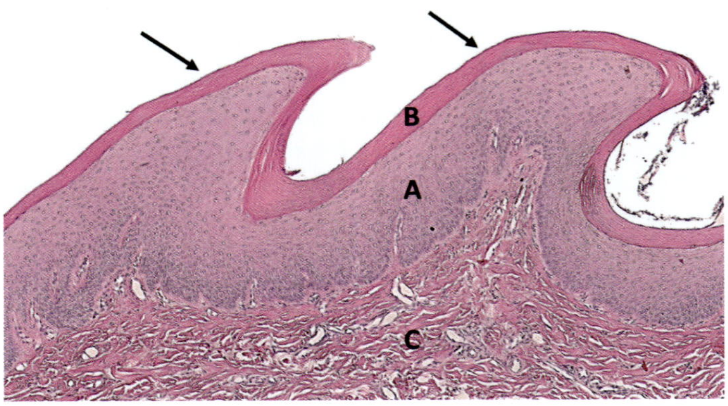

Figure 10-3 Cheek (large ruminant). Caudally oriented conical buccal papillae (arrows) covered by stratified squamous epithelium (A) with keratinized surface layers (B); lamina propria (C). H&E (×100). (Image by J. Feng.)

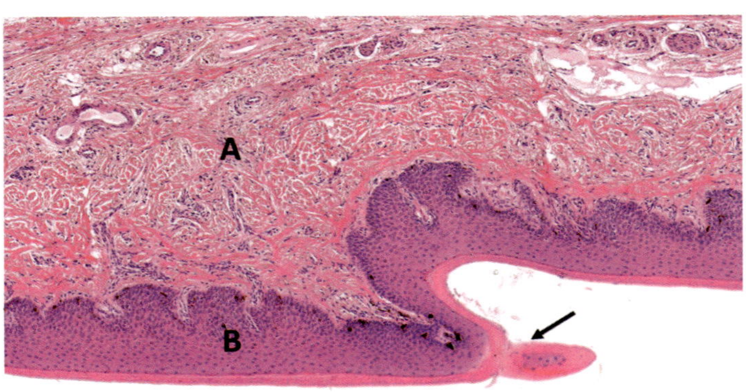

Figure 10-4 Hard palate mucosa (large ruminant). Propria-submucosa (A), keratinized stratified squamous epithelium (B), and caudal surface of ruga (arrow). H&E (×100). (Image by J. Feng.)

fied squamous epithelium that is keratinized in ruminants and horses but nonkeratinized in carnivores and pigs. The lamina propria and submucosa blend without a clear line of demarcation. Aggregates of serous or seromucous minor salivary glands, referred to as **labial glands**, are distributed throughout the propria-submucosa. The tunica muscularis consists of skeletal muscle fibers from the orbicularis oris muscle.

Cheeks

The cheeks, like the lips, are composed of an external covering of skin, a middle muscular layer (the buccinator muscle), and an internal mucosa lined by stratified squamous epithelium that may or may not be keratinized, depending on the specific area or species. In ruminants, the mucosa is studded with macroscopic, caudally directed, conical **buccal papillae** that facilitate the grasping and mastication of food (Fig. 10-3). The **buccal glands** are minor salivary glands located in the propria-submucosa and among the skeletal muscle bundles of the cheek, with some secretory units extending into the dermis. The glands are compound tubuloacinar glands and may be serous, mucous, or seromucous, depending on their location and the species.

Hard Palate

The bones of the hard palate are covered by a mucosa that exhibits a series of transverse ridges called **rugae**. This mucosa is covered by a keratinized stratified squamous epithelium, which is particularly thick in ruminants (Fig. 10-4). The lamina propria has a well-developed papillary layer that blends with the submucosa without an intervening lamina muscularis, forming a propria-submucosa. The propria-submucosa is composed of a dense network of collagen and reticular fibers and blends with the adjacent periosteum. In horses, the propria-submucosa has a rich network of capillaries and veins. Branched tubuloacinar mucous and seromucous minor salivary glands (**palatine glands**) are located in the caudal part of the hard palate in all domestic mammals except pigs. The rostral portion of the mucosa of the hard palate is especially thick in ruminants and forms the dental pad (**pulvinus dentalis**). The dental pad consists of a heavily keratinized stratified squamous epithelium overlying a thick layer of dense irregular CT (Fig. 10-5). During grazing, the lower (inferior) incisor teeth firmly press against the pad, facilitating effective grasping of forage.

Soft Palate

The soft palate consists of a core of skeletal muscle fibers with mucosa covering both surfaces. The oropharyngeal (ventral) surface is covered by a stratified squamous epithelium. The nasopharyngeal (dorsal) surface is covered caudally by stratified squamous epithelium and rostrally covered by ciliated, pseudostratified columnar epithelium. Between these epithelial types, a narrow transition zone of transitional epithelium is present. The propria-submucosa contains branched tubuloacinar mucous and seromucous **palatine glands**. Lymphatic tissue occurs in the mucosa of both the oropharyngeal and the nasopharyngeal surfaces; in pigs and horses, a macroscopically visible **tonsil** is present on the oropharyngeal surface. Longitudinally oriented skeletal muscle fibers (the palatinus muscle) and CT are located between the two mucous membranes.

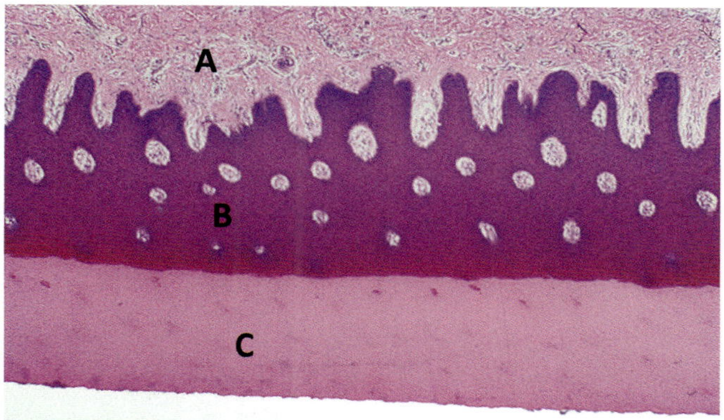

Figure 10-5 Dental pad (sheep). Propria-submucosa (A) with papillae interdigitating with stratified squamous epithelium (B) and a very thick stratum corneum (C). H&E (×48).

Tongue

The tongue is a muscular organ covered by a mucosa. It is important in the prehension, mastication, and deglutition of food.

The epithelium covering the tongue is stratified squamous. It is keratinized and thick on the dorsum, and nonkeratinized and thin on the ventral surface. The dorsum bears numerous macroscopic **lingual papillae**. These papillae differ somewhat in shape, are named according to their morphologic characteristics, and serve either a mechanical or a gustatory function. The filiform, conical, and lenticular papillae are purely mechanical; they facilitate the movement of ingesta within the oral cavity. The fungiform, vallate, and foliate papillae are gustatory; that is, they contain the taste buds that are responsible for the perception of taste.

The **filiform papillae** are the most numerous type. They are slender, threadlike structures that project above the surface of the tongue and are covered by a keratinized stratified squamous epithelium with a thick stratum corneum. They are supported by a highly vascularized CT core. In equines, filiform papillae consist of very fine keratinized threads projecting above the surface (Fig. 10-6). The CT core terminates at the base of each thread. In ruminants, a keratinized cone projects above the surface, and the CT core has several secondary papillae. Cats have large papillae with two prominences of unequal size (Fig. 10-7). The caudal prominence is especially large and gives rise to a caudally directed keratinized spine, supported by a more rounded rostral papilla with a thinner stratum corneum. The filiform papillae of dogs may have two or more apices; the caudal apex is the largest and has a thicker stratum corneum than the other(s) (Fig. 10-8).

The **conical papillae** occur on the root of the tongue in dogs, cats, and pigs, and on the **torus linguae** of ruminants (see the "Special Lingual Structures" section below). They are larger than the filiform papillae and typically have lower levels of keratinization. They contain both primary and secondary CT papillae. In pigs, these papillae are more accurately referred to as **tonsillar papillae** because they contain a core of lymphatic tissue, collectively constituting the **lingual tonsil**.

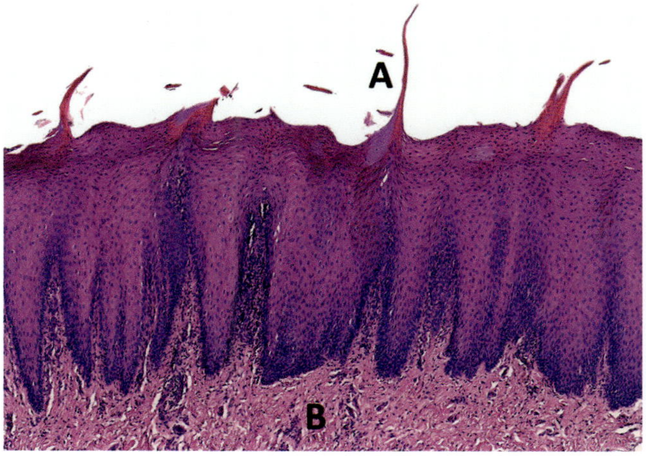

Figure 10-6 Tongue (horse). Filiform papillae are keratinized threads extending from the surface of the stratified squamous epithelium on the dorsum of the tongue (A); submucosa propria (B). H&E (×80). (Image by J. Feng.)

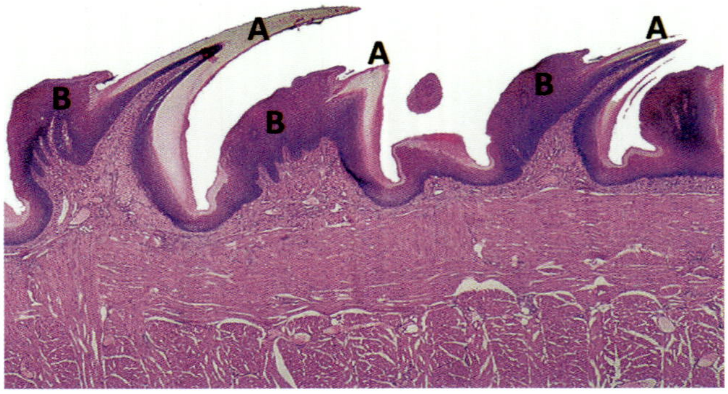

Figure 10-7 Tongue (cat). Three filiform papillae of cat, each with a caudally directed keratinized spine arising from the caudal prominence (A) and supporting rostral papilla (B). H&E (×80). (Image by J. Feng.)

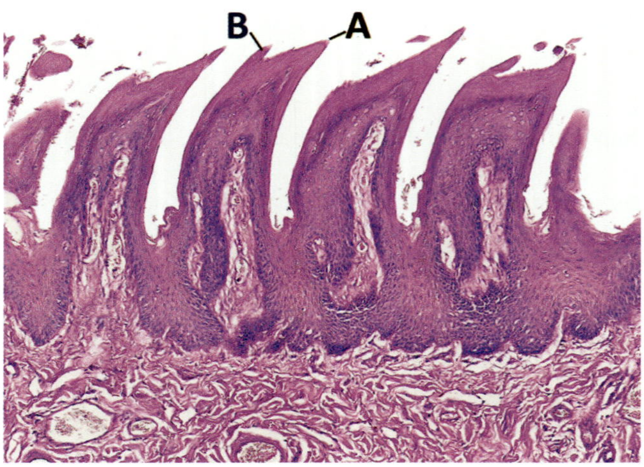

Figure 10-8 Tongue (dog). Filiform papillae of dog with two (A and B) or more caudally directed apices. H&E (×120). (Image by J. Feng.)

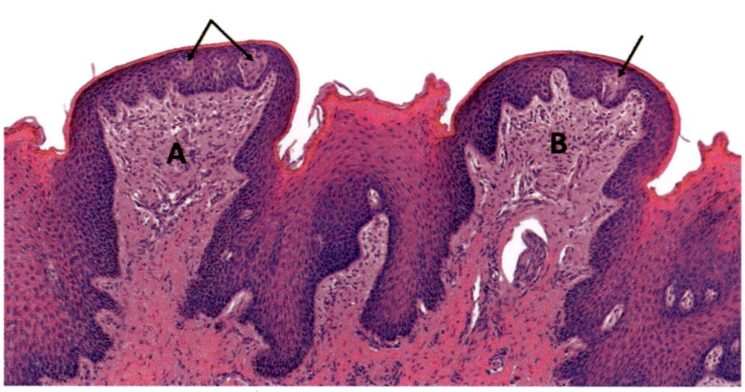

Figure 10-9 Tongue (goat). Two fungiform papillae (A and B) with taste buds (arrows). H&E (×130). (Image by J. Feng.)

The **lenticular papillae** are flattened, lens-shaped projections found on the torus linguae of ruminants. They are covered by keratinized stratified squamous epithelium and have a core of dense irregular CT.

The **fungiform papillae** are scattered among the filiform papillae and have a dome-shaped upper surface in horses and pigs (Fig. 10-9). The shape is suggestive of a mushroom, hence the name "fungiform." These papillae are covered by a nonkeratinized stratified squamous epithelium containing one or more taste buds on the upper surface. Taste buds are sparse in these papillae in the tongues of horses and cattle, more numerous in those of sheep and pigs, and abundant in those of carnivores and goats. The CT core is rich in blood vessels and nerves.

The circumvallate or **vallate papillae** are located on the dorsum of the tongue, just rostral to the root. They are large, flattened structures completely surrounded by an epithelium-lined sulcus (Fig. 10-10). These papillae extend only slightly, if at all, above the lingual surface and are covered by a stratified squamous epithelium. The epithelium on the papillary side of the sulcus contains many taste buds. Groups of serous **gustatory glands** are located deep to the sulcus and have ducts that open into the sulcus at various levels (Fig. 10-10). Mucous glands may also be found beneath the papillae, but their secretory products are emptied directly onto the lingual surface. The CT core is rich in blood vessels and nerves. The number of vallate papillae varies with the species; horses and pigs typically have one pair, carnivores have 4 to 6 pairs, and ruminants have 8 to 24 pairs.

The **foliate papillae** are parallel folds of the lingual mucosa located on the margin of the tongue, just rostral to the palatoglossal arch. Taste buds reside in the epithelium lining the sides of these folds. Gustatory sulci separate the folds (Fig. 10-11A). Deep to the sulci lie serous gustatory glands, whose ducts empty into the sulci. Foliate papillae are absent in ruminants; in cats, they are rudimentary and lack taste buds.

The **taste buds** are ellipsoid clusters of specialized epithelial cells embedded in the stratified squamous epithelium of the fungiform, vallate, and foliate papillae of the tongue (not found in filliform papillae). They also occur widely dispersed in the soft palate, epiglottis, or other areas of the oral cavity and pharynx. Each taste bud consists of a cluster of spindle-shaped epithelial cells that extend from the basement membrane to a small opening, the **taste pore**, at the epithelial surface

(Fig. 10-11B). In most mammalian species, three cell types have been identified: type I, type II, and type III cells. Type I and type II cells have apical microvilli that project into the taste pore, while type III cells have a club-shaped apex that also projects into the taste pore. The type III cell is characterized by clusters of cytoplasmic vesicles, resembling synaptic vesicles, adjacent to intraepithelial nonmyelinated afferent nerve fibers. Therefore, the type III cell is considered to be the **chemoreceptor (taste) cell**, whereas the type I and type II cells are believed to serve a **sustentacular** (**supportive**) role. The average lifespan of these cells is approximately 10 days, with new cells continuously recruited from mitotically dividing cells in the perigemmal region (Latin *gemma*, meaning "bud").

The proper (intrinsic) lingual muscles consist of longitudinally, transversely, and perpendicularly arranged bundles of skeletal muscle (Fig. 10-12). Because of the diverse arrangement of these muscle fibers, the tongue has extensive mobility, facilitating the movement of food into and within the oral cavity.

The ventral surface of the tongue is covered by nonkeratinized stratified squamous epithelium. The mucosa contains an abundance of capillaries, arteriovenous (AV) anastomoses, and branches of the lingual artery and vein, which participate in thermoregulation.

Scattered among the muscle fibers and in the propria-submucosa of the tongue are clusters of seromucous minor salivary glands, collectively referred to as the **lingual glands**.

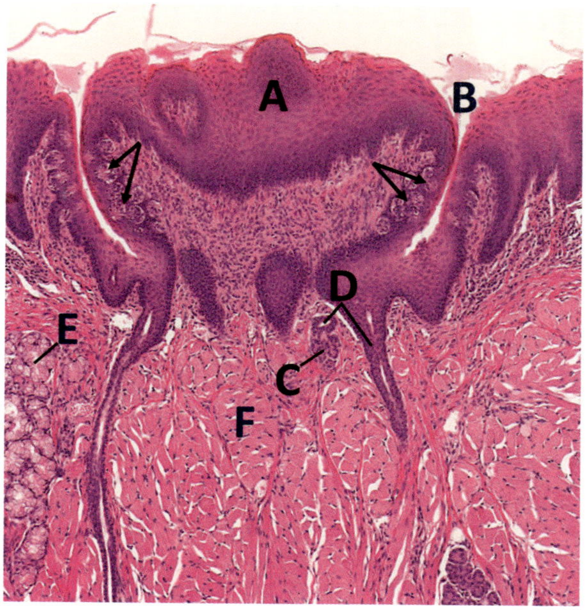

Figure 10-10 Tongue (mammal). A vallate papilla (A) with a surrounding sulcus (B), taste buds in the epithelium (arrows), serous gustatory glands (C) and their ducts (D) opening into the sulcus, mucous glands (E), and striated muscle fibers (F). H&E (×100). (Image by J. Feng.)

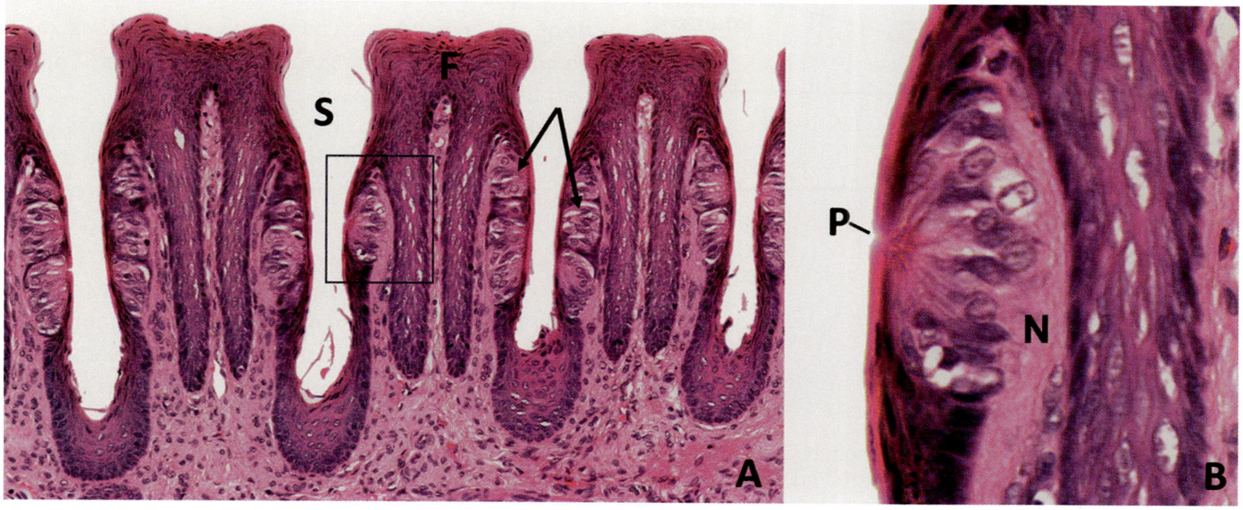

Figure 10-11 Tongue (rabbit). Foliate papillae (F) with prominent taste buds (arrows) and a deep gustatory sulcus (S) in the left panel (**A**, ×100). The right panel (**B**, ×600) magnifies a taste bud (from the boxed region of panel **A**) to show the taste pore (P) and nonmyelinated nerve fibers (N). H&E. (Image by J. Feng.)

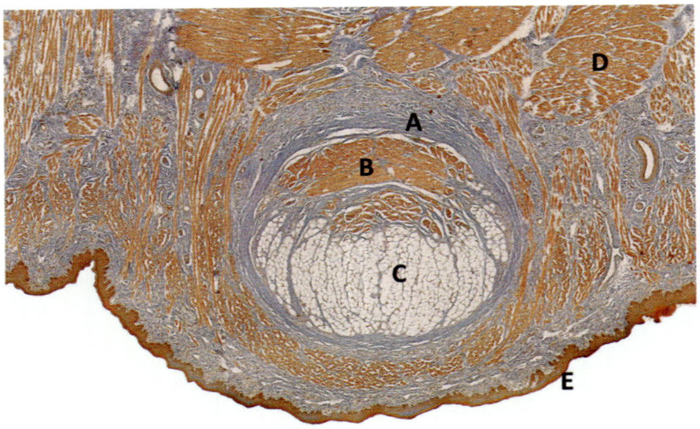

Figure 10-12 Lyssa (dog). The lyssa has a dense irregular CT capsule (A) enclosing skeletal muscle (B) dorsally and white adipose tissue (C) ventrally. Intrinsic lingual muscles (D) and the ventral surface of tongue (E) are visible. Trichrome staining (×30). (Image by J. Feng.)

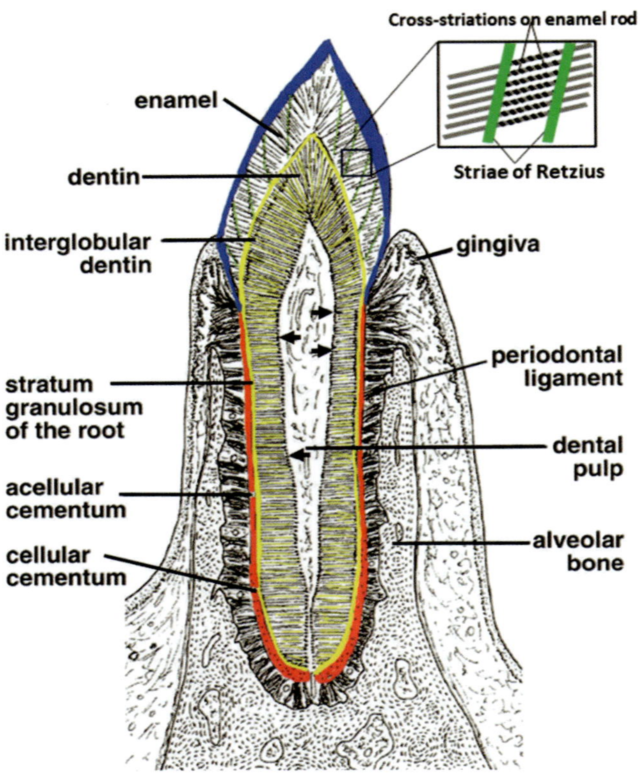

Figure 10-13 Schematic drawing of a longitudinal section through a brachydont tooth in situ. The dental pulp fills the pulp cavity of the tooth. The location of the odontoblasts, at the periphery of the dental pulp, is indicated by arrows. Their processes pass through the dentinal tubules and project outward. (From Dellmann HD. Veterinary Histology: An Outline Text–Atlas. Philadelphia: Lea & Febiger, 1971.; Modified by J. Feng).

Special Lingual Structures

The **lyssa** of the tongue in carnivores is a cordlike structure enclosed in a dense irregular CT capsule. It extends longitudinally in the midline near the ventral surface of the apex of the tongue. In dogs, the lyssa is filled with white adipose tissue, skeletal muscle, blood vessels, and nerves, whereas in cats it mainly contains white adipose tissue (Fig. 10-12). The tongue of pigs contains a similar structure. Horses have a middorsal fibroelastic cord known as the **dorsal lingual cartilage**, which includes hyaline cartilage, skeletal muscle, and white adipose.

The ruminant tongue has a large prominence, the **torus linguae**, covering the caudal portion of the dorsum and is characterized by a thickened mucosa. CT papillae extend almost to the surface of the epithelium, which is thicker than that in other regions of the tongue. Lenticular papillae and conical papillae are scattered over the surface of this area.

Teeth

Teeth are highly mineralized structures in the oral cavity that serve domestic mammals in procuring, cutting, and crushing food, as well as in offense and defense. Each tooth consists of a highly mineralized outer part surrounding the **pulp cavity**. This cavity contains the **dental pulp**, which contains a core of CT, blood vessels, lymph vessels, and nerves (Fig. 10-13).

Brachydont and Hypsodont Teeth

Two types of teeth occur in domestic mammals: **brachydont** and **hypsodont**. These teeth differ in their rates of growth and in the arrangement of their layers of mineralized tissue.

Brachydont teeth are short and stop growing after eruption is completed (Fig. 10-13). They have a **crown** (the portion above the gingiva), a **neck** (the constricted region just below the gingival line), and one or more **roots** embedded in a bony socket called the **alveolus**. The crown is covered by a cap of enamel that extends down to the neck. The root is covered by a layer of cementum that may slightly overlap the enamel at the neck. Beneath both the enamel and the cementum lies a thick layer of dentin. Brachydont teeth include those of carnivores (and humans), the incisor teeth of ruminants, and the teeth of pigs, except for the canine teeth.

Hypsodont teeth are much longer than brachydont teeth, characterized by an elongated crown (often called the "body") that extends below the gingival line. In some species, their roots form very late (equine teeth) or are even absent altogether (as seen in boar tusks and rodent incisors), allowing them to continue to grow throughout much, if not all, of the adult life of the animal (Fig. 10-14). Unlike brachydont teeth, hypsodont teeth have cementum covering the entire crown (both above and below the gingival line).

Beneath the cementum is a layer of enamel extending throughout the length of the body and nearly to the apex of the root. This enamel invaginates into the dentin, creating **infundibula**, funnel- or cup-like invaginations visible from the occlusal surface (Fig. 10-14). Along the peripheral sides, these infoldings form the **enamel plicae**, characteristic of the cheek teeth (premolars and molars) in horses and ruminants. The occlusal surface of each cheek tooth is corrugated because of the irregular wearing of the mineralized tissues. Because enamel is the hardest of the mineralized tissues, it is most resistant to wear and forms sharp **enamel crests** (**ridges or lophs**) projecting above the occlusal surface. Dentin and cementum are less resistant and wear away more readily. These uneven enamel crests make the occlusal surface highly effective for grinding food. Hypsodont teeth include all teeth of horses, the cheek teeth of ruminants, the canine teeth of pigs, and the incisor teeth of rodents.

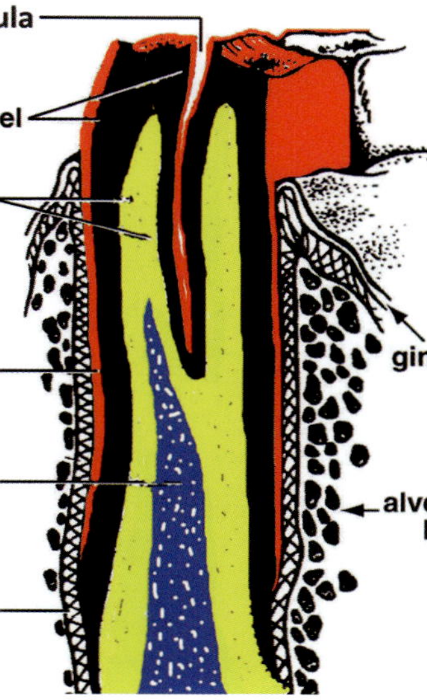

Figure 10-14 Schematic drawing of a longitudinal section through a hypsodont tooth in situ. (Modified by J. Feng.)

Structure

The mineralized tissues of the teeth are enamel, dentin, and cementum. Each of these has a separate origin and differs morphologically and in degree of mineralization.

Enamel covers the external surface of the crown in brachydont teeth and lies beneath a layer of cementum in hypsodont teeth. It is the hardest substance in the body, composed of 99% mineral (**hydroxyapatite**) and 1% organic matrix by weight. Histologically, enamel is composed of long, slender rods called **enamel prisms**, held together by **inter-rod enamel**. The enamel rods extend to the enamel surface in an almost perpendicular trajectory from the dentin–enamel junction. Each enamel rod exhibits inconspicuous **cross-striations** (Figs. 10-13 and 10-15), representing the daily enamel deposition during odontogenesis. The more visible lines or bands that obliquely cross the enamel rods are the **incremental lines (or striae) of Retzius**, indicating a longer (weekly) periodic deposition of enamel (Fig. 10-13). Enamel is produced by **ameloblasts** that differentiate from the inner enamel epithelium of the enamel organ (see the "Development" section below). Ameloblasts disappear from the fully developed brachydont tooth, but a small population of columnar cells remains at the base of the hypsodont tooth to continue enamel production.

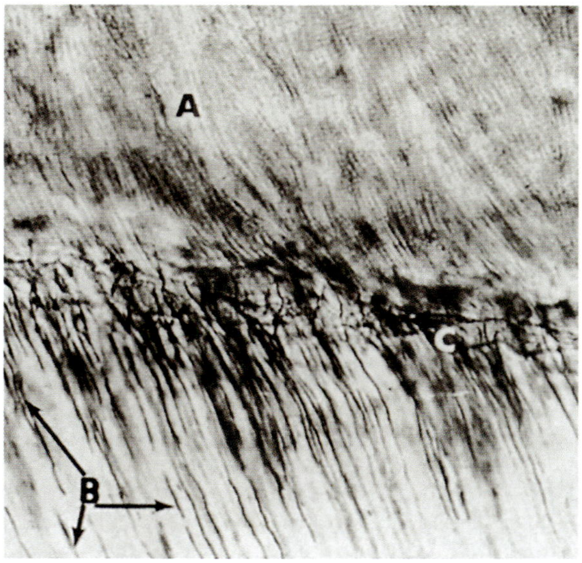

Figure 10-15 Ground section of a human tooth. The junction of enamel (A) and dentin (B). Numerous enamel rods with inconspicuous cross-striations are visible in the enamel. Straight dentinal tubules (dark lines), indicated by arrows in dentin, facilitate penetration of odontoblastic processes into live dentin tissue. At the junction area (C), the dentinal tubules change direction and become torturously intertwined, with the spaces between them forming interglobular dentin. Unstained (×235).

Cementum resembles bone in all its structural features. **Acellular cementum** is composed of lamellae oriented parallel to the tooth surface (Figs. 10-13 and 10-16). **Cellular cementum** has cementocytes, which occupy lacunae and canaliculi like those of bone (Figs. 10-13 and 10-16). Bundles of collagen fibers, called **cementoalveolar (Sharpey's) fibers**, extend from the alveolar bone into the cementum of the tooth (Fig. 10-16). Collectively, these fibers form the **periodontal ligament**, which anchors the tooth in the alveolus. **Cementoblasts** located at the junction of the cementum and the periodontal ligament produce the fibrous matrix of the cementum, and then later mineralize the cementum by depositing hydroxyapatite crystals within this matrix. Once surrounded by matrix, the cementoblasts are termed **cementocytes**. In brachydont teeth, the roots are covered by a layer of cementum that may slightly overlap the enamel

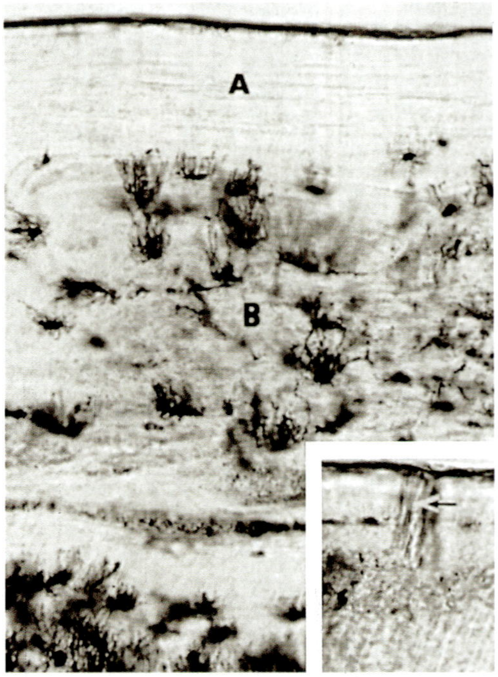

Figure 10-16 Ground section of a human tooth. Lamellae of acellular cementum (A) oriented parallel to the surface of the root. Cellular cementum with cementocytes (B) (×185). Inset: Cementoalveolar (Sharpey's) fibers (arrow) embedded in the cementum. Unstained (×185).

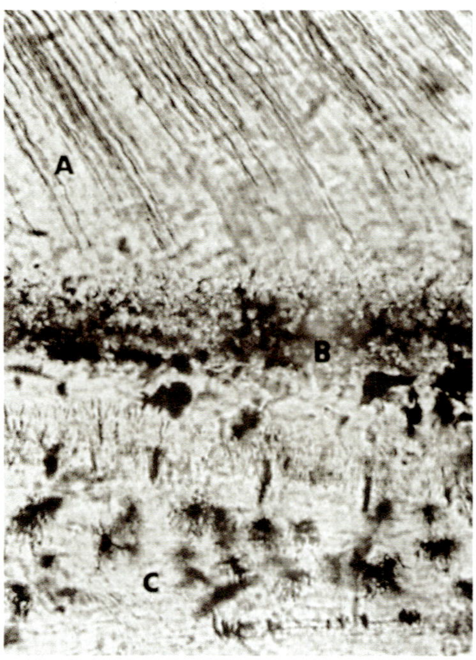

Figure 10-17 Ground section of a human tooth. Dentin–cementum junction. Dentin (A) containing dentinal tubules (the dark lines), incompletely mineralized Tomes' granular layer of the root (B), and cementum (C) with lacunae. Unstained (×185).

at the neck of the tooth. Cementum covers the outside surface of equine and ruminant hypsodont teeth, both above and below the gingiva. It begins just above the region where the ameloblasts produce enamel, at the base of the tooth. Equine cementum differs in that it has cementocytes throughout and lacks the acellular form seen in brachydont teeth. Equine cementum is also unique in that it is vascular and innervated.

Dentin is a highly mineralized tissue that constitutes a major part of the tooth. It underlies the enamel of the crown and the cementum of the root in brachydont teeth and also underlies the enamel of the body in hypsodont teeth. Dentin also forms the wall of the pulp cavity. It consists of a matrix of organic material, primarily randomly oriented collagen fibrils and glycoproteins, upon which minerals are deposited, primarily hydroxyapatite along with carbonate, magnesium, and fluoride. The composition is approximately 70% mineral and 30% organic matter. Dentin is produced by a layer of columnar cells called **odontoblasts**, located adjacent to the interior surface of the dentin in the outer layer of the dental pulp. **Odontoblast processes** extend through channels known as **dentinal tubules** (Fig. 10-15), which run roughly parallel from the inner to the outer surface of the dentin. **Peritubular dentin** immediately surrounds the odontoblast processes and is more highly mineralized than **intertubular dentin**, which constitutes the remainder of the dentin. Unmineralized organic material, termed **predentin**, lies between the apex of the odontoblast cell body and the mineralized dentin. Mineralization of predentin begins with the small spherules that are globular in appearance, surrounded by **interglobular dentin** composed of small, unmineralized or incompletely mineralized areas at the dentin–enamel junction (Fig. 10-15). These poorly mineralized dentin areas are also numerous in the root adjacent to the cementum, forming the **stratum granulosum** known as the **Tomes' granular layer** (Figs. 10-13 and 10-17). Odontoblasts continue to produce dentin throughout the life of the tooth, although at a slower rate after the tooth erupts. Two main types of incremental growth lines present in dentin are **Andresen's** lines, which are long-period weekly depositional lines, and **von Ebner lines**, which are short-period daily depositional lines.

The **dental pulp** occupies the pulp cavity of the tooth. It is composed of CT cells and fibers, amorphous ground substance, numerous blood and lymph vessels, and nerves. Its texture resembles embryonic CT, with delicate collagen fibers coursing through the amorphous ground substance. The most peripheral part of the pulp is the layer of odontoblasts, from which the odontoblast processes extend into the dentinal tubules. Basal processes from the odontoblasts extend into the amorphous ground substance or unite with similar processes from neighboring cells. Because dentin is continuously deposited on the inside of the tooth, the size of the pulp cavity gradually reduces as the animal ages.

Development

In the embryo, an invagination of the oral ectoderm into the underlying mesenchyme forms the **dental lamina** (Fig. 10-18), a continuous, arch-shaped sheet of epithelial cells extending along the future site of the gingiva in both the upper and lower jaws. Isolated thickenings arise on the labial side of the dental lamina, where each deciduous and permanent tooth develops. These thickenings are the primordia of the **enamel organ**, which eventually gives rise to the enamel. As the enamel organ develops, it adopts the appearance of an inverted cup, attached to the dental lamina by a thin stem (Figs. 10-18 and 10-19). The epithelial cells lining the inner surface of the cup form the **inner enamel epithelium**, while those covering the outer surface form the **outer enamel epithelium**. The epithelial cells between these two layers become stellate and take on the appearance of CT, thus forming the **stellate reticulum** of the enamel organ. The mesenchyme, derived from neural crest ectoderm and enclosed by the cup of the enamel organ, condenses to form the **dental papilla**, which will develop into the future dental pulp. The internal contour of the cup is a replica of the shape of the tooth crown to be produced (Fig. 10-20).

As the enamel organ enlarges, another layer of cells develops from the stellate reticulum and overlays the inner enamel epithelium. This new layer, called the **stratum intermedium**, induces the transformation of the simple squamous inner enamel epithelial cells into enamel-producing columnar **ameloblasts**. Meanwhile, the neural crest-derived mesenchymal cells of the dental papilla adjacent to the ameloblasts differentiate into **odontoblasts**, which produce **dentin**. Dentin is deposited around the odontoblast processes in mineralized sheaths anchored to the basement membrane of the inner enamel epithelium. As more dentin is produced, the cell bodies of the odontoblasts recede toward the developing pulp cavity. Shortly after dentin deposition begins, the ameloblasts begin to

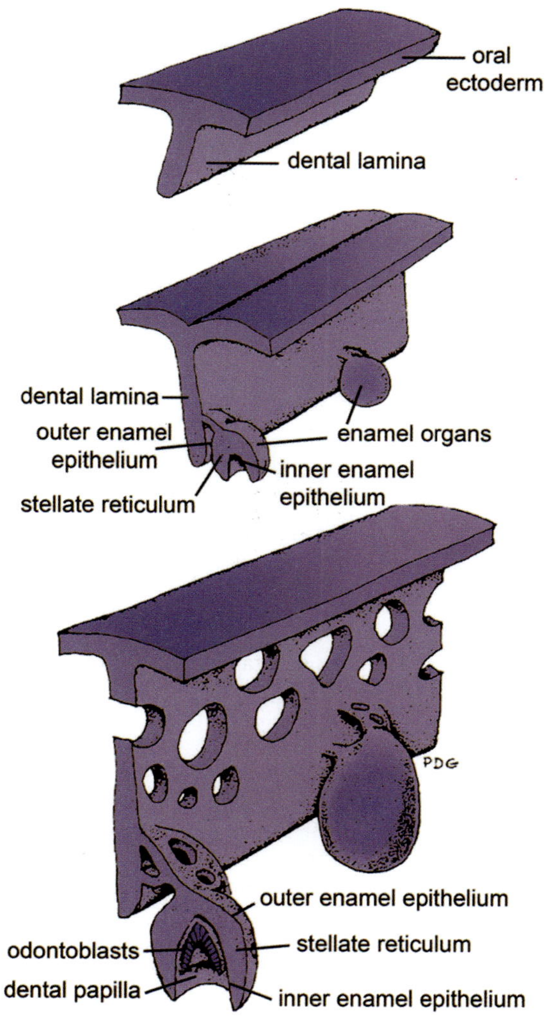

Figure 10-18 Stages in the development of the tooth. The dental lamina degenerates (appears as holes) as the teeth mature.

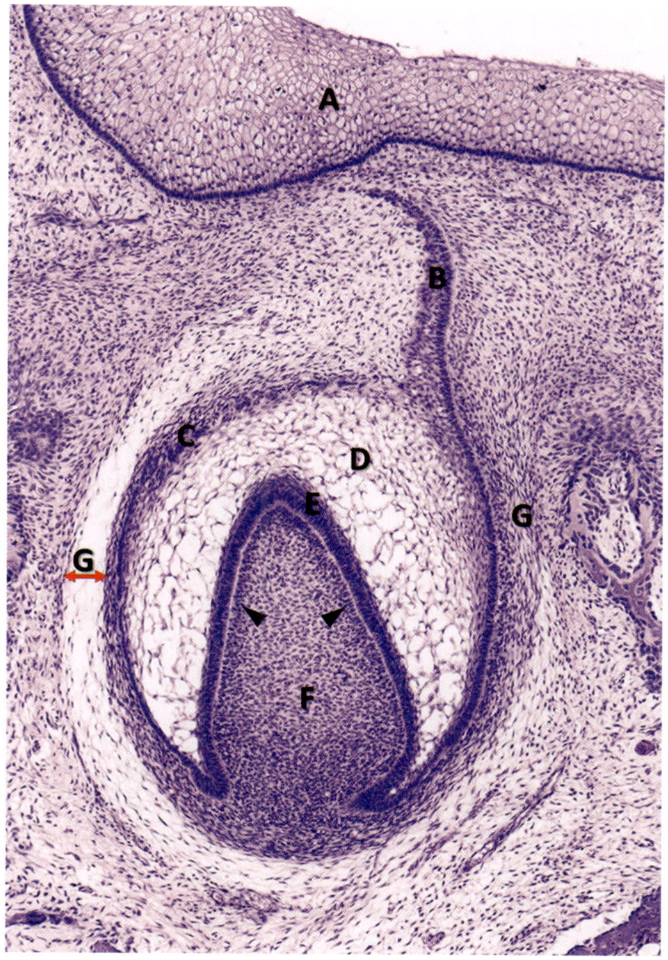

Figure 10-19 Developing tooth (pig). Oral ectoderm (A), dental lamina (B), outer enamel epithelium of enamel organ (C), stellate reticulum of enamel organ (D), inner enamel epithelium of enamel organ (E), dental papilla (F) with peripheral odontoblasts (arrowheads), and developing dental sac (G). H&E (×60). (Image by J. Feng.)

produce the enamel matrix (Figs. 10-20 and 10-21). Deposition of dentin and enamel begins at the crown apex and continues down the crown sides toward the tooth neck.

The formation of the root of the tooth begins shortly before eruption. The root is formed by a downward growth of a sheet of cells originating from the enamel organ at the junction of the inner and outer enamel epithelia. This downward-growing sheet of cells, called the **Hertwig's epithelial root sheath** (HERS) (Fig. 10-20), surrounds the CT of the dental papilla and induces the formation of odontoblasts that produce the dentin of the root.

The entire enamel organ and developing tooth are enclosed by the **dental sac (or dental follicle)**, a thickened CT layer that completely surrounds the developing tooth (Fig. 10-19). In brachydont teeth, after the crown erupts through the dental sac, **dental mesenchymal stem cells** from the collapsed dental sac penetrate the disintegrated HERS to contact the dentin of the root. They then differentiate into **cementoblasts**, which deposit **cementum** over the roots. In hypsodont teeth, the differentiation of cementoblasts from the collapsed dental sac occurs before the tooth erupts, and therefore, cementum covers the entire tooth.

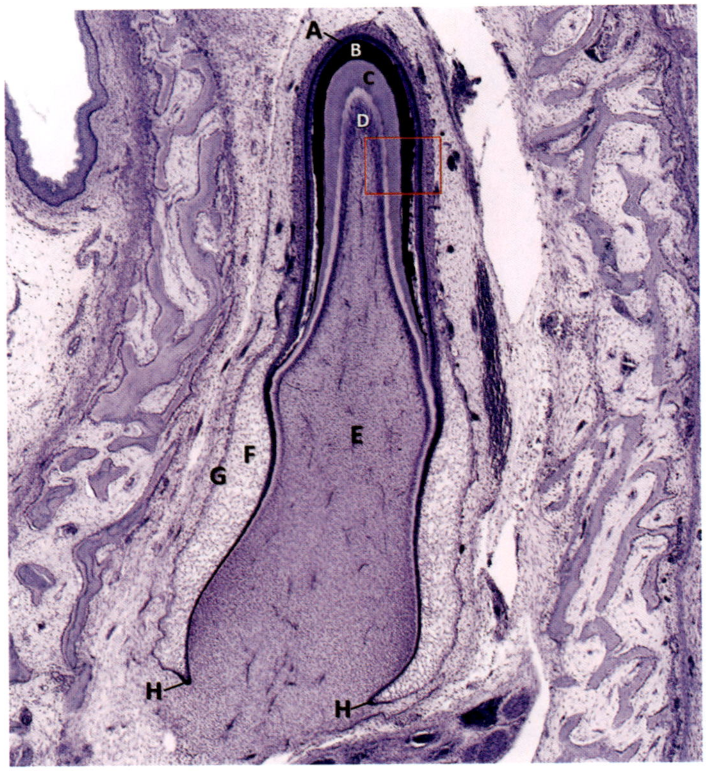

Figure 10-20 Developing permanent tooth (cat). Ameloblasts (A), enamel (B), dentin (C), odontoblasts (D), dental pulp (E), stellate reticulum (F), outer enamel epithelium (G), and Hertwig's epithelial root sheath (H). H&E (×43). (Image by J. Feng.) (Boxed region is magnified in Fig. 10–21).

Salivary Glands

General Characteristics

The salivary glands comprise a series of secretory units (glandular epithelium) that originate from the oral ectoderm and grow into the underlying mesoderm as compound glands (see Chapter 2). The **major salivary glands** include the parotid, mandibular, and sublingual glands. The **minor salivary glands** are named according to their location, for example, labial, lingual, buccal, palatine, molar (in cats), and zygomatic (in carnivores).

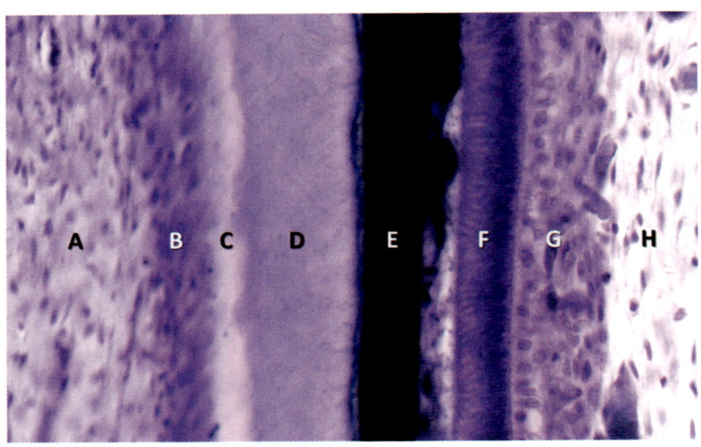

Figure 10-21 The boxed region from Figure 10-20 is enlarged and relabeled to show the detailed structures of the developing tooth (cat). Dental pulp (A), odontoblasts (B), predentin (C), dentin (D), enamel (E), ameloblasts (F), stratum intermedium and stellate reticulum (G), and dental sac (H). H&E (×400). (Image by J. Feng.)

Saliva is a mixture of both serous and mucous secretory products from salivary glands. It is important in the moistening of the ingested food and the lubrication of the surface of the upper digestive organs, aiding in the flow of ingesta into the stomach. Saliva also dissolves water-soluble components of food, thereby facilitating access to the taste buds and influencing the sense of taste. In domestic mammals, saliva has a minor role in food digestion before it reaches the stomach. Ruminants, however, produce large volumes of saliva, which is an important source of fluids in the rumen.

Parotid Salivary Gland

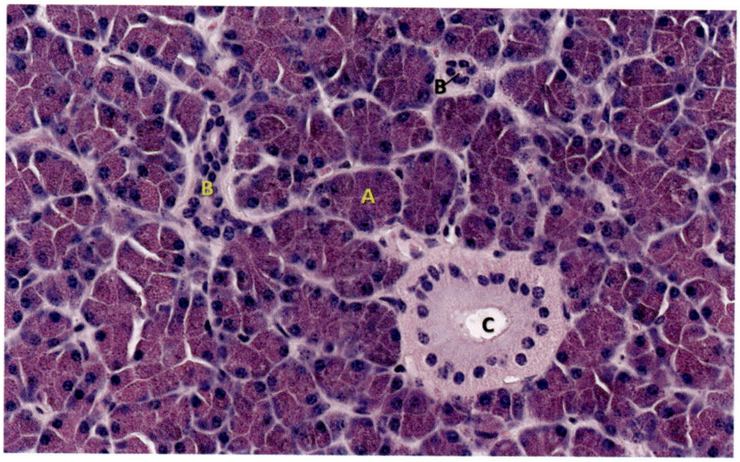

Figure 10-22 Parotid salivary gland (horse). Serous acini (A), intercalated ducts (B), and striated duct (C). H&E (×530). (Image by J. Feng.)

The parotid salivary gland in domestic mammals is predominantly serous, although isolated mucous secretory units may occur in dogs and cats. Structurally, it is a compound acinar gland composed of numerous lobules separated by thin CT septa. Each lobule consists of acini formed by pyramid-shaped cells with basally located nuclei, filled with eosinophilic secretory granules (Fig. 10-22), referred to as **zymogen granules**, containing inactive digestive enzyme precursors. Myoepithelial cells are located between the secretory cells and the basement membrane.

The narrow lumen of the acinus opens into a short **intercalated duct** lined by low cuboidal epithelium (see Fig. 2-18). The intercalated duct then connects to a larger **striated or salivary duct** lined by simple columnar epithelium and characterized by striations in the basal portion of the cells (see Figs. 2-18 and 10-22). These striations result from perpendicularly oriented mitochondria within numerous cytoplasmic compartments formed by deep infoldings of the basal cell membrane. This structure increases the basal membrane surface area containing energy-requiring ion pumps located near mitochondria, facilitating active transport between cells and the underlying tissue. The striated ducts are easily recognized as the largest structures within the lobule and participate in the secretory process. They extend to the edge of the lobule, where they join **interlobular ducts** located in the CT septa between lobules (see Fig. 2-18).

Interlobular ducts are lined by simple columnar epithelium, which changes to stratified columnar epithelium as the ducts become larger and fuse with similar ducts draining other lobules. These interlobular ducts converge to form the parotid duct. The epithelium changes from stratified columnar to stratified squamous where the parotid duct opens into the vestibule of the oral cavity.

Mandibular Salivary Gland

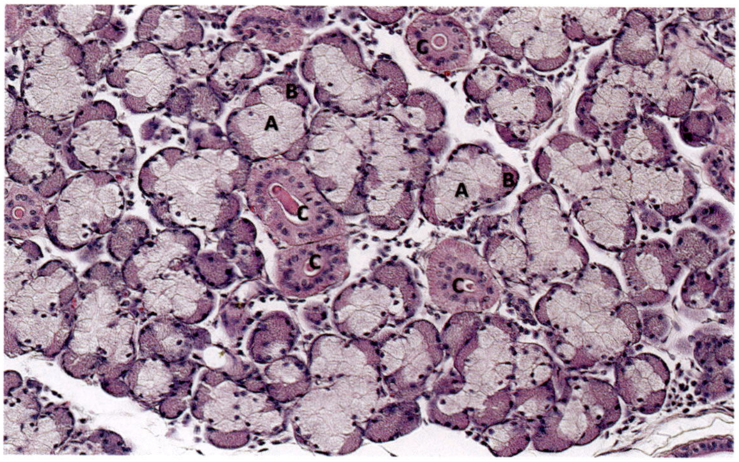

Figure 10-23 Mandibular salivary gland (horse). Mucous acinus (A) with peripheral serous demilunes (B) and striated ducts (C). H&E (×280). (Image by J. Feng.)

The mandibular salivary gland is a seromucous (mixed) compound tubuloacinar gland. The morphological structure of its secretory unit varies somewhat between species but generally consists of a tubular unit ending in an enlarged terminal acinus. Mucus-secreting cells line the lumens of both the tubule and acinus, with serous demilunes occurring at the periphery (Fig. 10-23); their alignment and positioning can be influenced by tissue fixation and histological preparation methods. The serous secretory product reaches the lumen through intercellular canaliculi between the mucous cells. Variations in this basic pattern may include separate serous and mucous acini or mucous tubular units with enlarged, serous acinar end pieces. In dogs and cats, the mucous elements predominate. **Myoepithelial cells** surround the secretory units (see Fig. 2-19). The duct system resembles that of the parotid salivary gland. In the epithelium of the main duct, goblet cells may occur.

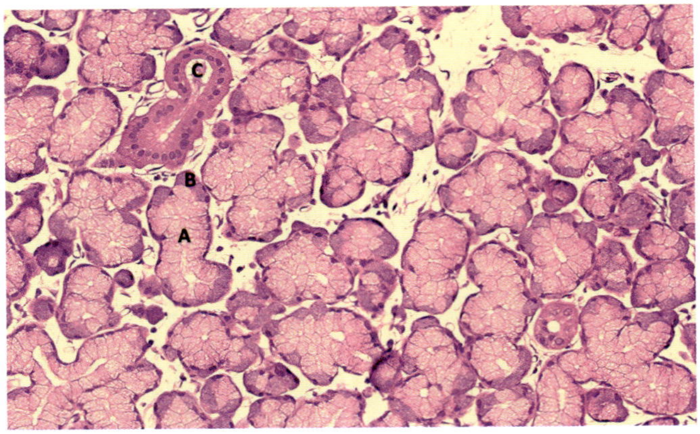

Figure 10-24 Sublingual salivary gland (dog). Mucous acini (A) with serous demilunes (B) and striated ducts (C). H&E (×320). (Image by J. Feng.)

Sublingual Salivary Gland

Like the mandibular salivary gland, the sublingual salivary gland is a seromucous (mixed) compound tubuloacinar gland (Fig. 10-24). The number of mucous acini and serous demilunes, and the seromucous nature of their secretory products, vary among species. In cattle, sheep, and pigs, sublingual glands are almost entirely mucous, with few serous demilunes. In dogs and cats, in addition to mucous acini and demilunes, there are clusters of serous acini. The mucous cells form tubular secretory units that connect serous acini with intercalated ducts. Striated and intercalated ducts are less prominent in cats and dogs but well developed in horses, ruminants, and pigs. The interlobular ducts originate with a low simple columnar epithelium that increases in height and becomes two-layered in larger ducts. The main duct is lined with stratified cuboidal epithelium, with goblet cells present in cattle and pigs.

Minor Salivary Glands

Clusters of minor salivary glands, composed of serous, seromucous, or mucous types, are distributed throughout the oral cavity and are generally named based on their location. The **lingual glands** are located in the propria-submucosa and among the intrinsic muscle bundles of the tongue. The **gustatory glands**, associated with the vallate and foliate papillae (Fig. 10-10), are entirely serous, with ducts opening into the sulcus at the base of the papillae. The **labial, buccal, palatine**, and **pharyngeal glands** contribute both mucous and serous secretory products to the saliva. Histologically, these glands exhibit diverse forms such as acinar, tubuloacinar, or tubular structures. Mucous tubules and acini frequently have serous demilunes associated with them; however, striated ducts are not typical in minor salivary glands. The duct system within lobules is lined with simple cuboidal epithelium, transitioning to two-layered cuboidal epithelium in larger interlobular ducts. The stratification of the duct epithelium increases toward the oral cavity, where it transitions to a stratified squamous type.

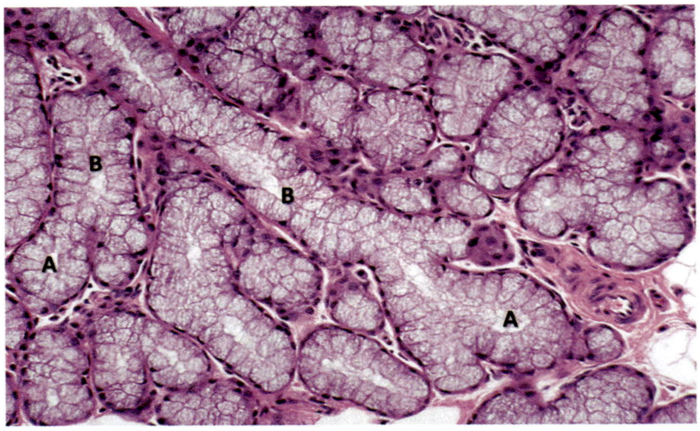

Figure 10-25 Zygomatic salivary gland (dog). Mucous acini (A) and mucous tubules (B). H&E (×300).

Among the domestic species, the **zygomatic salivary gland** is present only in carnivores. Its parenchyma is composed of long, branched tubuloacinar secretory units that primarily secrete mucus (Fig. 10-25). Intercalated and striated ducts are almost nonexistent. The interlobular and main ducts are similar to those of the other glands.

The **molar salivary gland** of cats is histologically similar to the zygomatic salivary gland. It is a compound tubuloacinar gland primarily secreting mucus. Intercalated and striated ducts are absent, and interlobular ducts are lined with a two-layered cuboidal epithelium. Several main ducts empty into the vestibule of the oral cavity opposite the molar teeth.

Pharynx

The pharynx connects the oral cavity to the esophagus and the nasal cavity to the larynx. It contains openings to the oral cavity (oropharynx), nasal cavity and auditory tubes (nasopharynx), and the larynx and esophagus (laryngopharynx). The pharynx wall is composed of a mucosa, a tunica muscularis (skeletal muscle), and an adventitia. The mucosa is lined with stratified squamous epithelium throughout, except for a portion of the nasopharynx, where it is lined by a ciliated, pseudostratified columnar epithelium. Unlike many other mucosal layers, a lamina muscularis is absent here. The propria-submucosa contains collagen and elastic fibers intermingled with lymphatic tissue and mucous glands. The tunica muscularis consists entirely of skeletal muscle. The adventitia is dense irregular CT that attaches the pharynx to the surrounding tissues.

Esophagus

The esophagus connects the laryngopharynx with the stomach and contains all the layers typical of a tubular organ of the digestive system (Figs. 10-1 and 10-26), although with some variations among different species (Table 10-1). An internal annular fold, the **pharyngoesophageal limen**, marks the junction of the laryngopharynx and esophagus in carnivores.

The mucosa is composed of three layers: a stratified squamous epithelium, a lamina propria, and a lamina muscularis. The degree of keratinization of the stratified squamous epithelium varies by species: carnivores typically have nonkeratinized epithelium, pigs have slightly keratinized epithelium, horses show more keratinization, and ruminants have highly keratinized epithelium. The lamina propria consists largely of a dense meshwork of fine collagen fibers interspersed with abundant and evenly distributed elastic fibers. The lamina muscularis contains only longitudinally oriented smooth muscle bundles. In some species, such as pigs and dogs at the cranial end of the esophagus, this layer may be absent. Cats, horses, and ruminants have isolated smooth muscle bundles near the pharynx that increase in number and become confluent toward the stomach. In pigs, the lamina muscularis is especially well developed in the caudal end, where it is as thick as the outer layer of the tunica muscularis.

The submucosa is loose CT containing large, longitudinally oriented arteries, veins, large lymph vessels, and nerves. Seromucous glands containing mucous acini with serous demilunes are present in this layer in pigs and dogs (Fig. 10-26). In pigs, these glands are abundant in the cranial half of the esophagus but do not extend into the caudal half. In contrast, in dogs, these glands are present throughout the esophagus, extending into the cardiac gland region of the stomach. Near the stomach (caudally), the density of these glands may be up to four times greater than at the beginning of the esophagus (cranially). Glands are present only at the pharyngoesophageal junction in horses, cats, and ruminants. Mixed acini with serous demilunes occur in cattle. The loose structure of the submucosa allows the mucosa of the relaxed esophagus to form longitudinal folds.

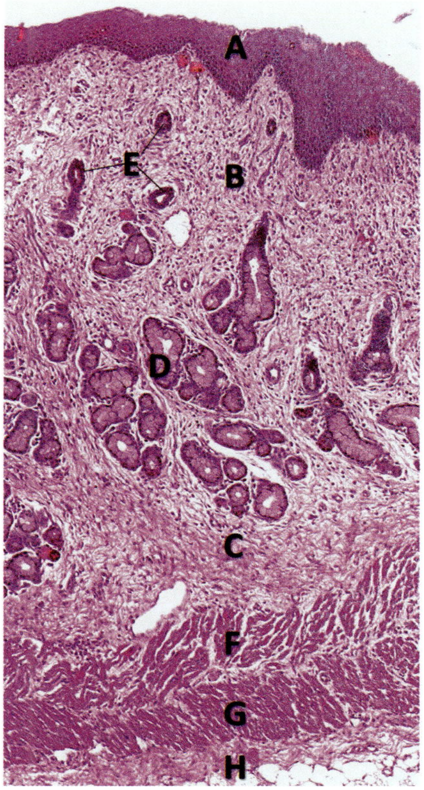

Figure 10-26 Esophagus, midcervical region (dog). Nonkeratinized stratified squamous epithelium of the tunica mucosa (A), lamina propria of the tunica mucosa (B), submucosa (C), submucosal glands (D), submucosal gland duct (E), inner circular layer of the tunica muscularis (F), outer longitudinal layer of the tunica muscularis (G), and adventitia (H). Note that a lamina muscularis is absent in this region of the canine esophagus. H&E (×73). (Image by J. Feng.)

The tunica muscularis of the esophagus consists of two layers of muscle. In ruminants and dogs, it consists entirely of skeletal muscle (Fig. 10-26). In horses, skeletal muscle comprises the cranial two-thirds of the tunica muscularis but gradually transitions to smooth muscle in the caudal third. Pigs have a similar arrangement to horses but with a middle third containing mixed smooth and skeletal muscle. In cats, the skeletal muscle may extend four-fifths of the length of the esophagus before transitioning to smooth muscle. Near the cranial end of the esophagus, the muscle layers interdigitate and spiral, but more caudally, they become organized into inner circular and outer longitudinal layers. The inner circular muscle layer thickens at the cardiac ostium of the stomach in all domestic mammals, forming the **cardiac sphincter muscle**. This muscle is especially prominent in horses, measuring 10 to 15 mm. In ruminants, the skeletal muscle of the esophagus extends into the wall of the **reticular sulcus** (**groove**).

In the cervical part of the esophagus, the tunica muscularis is surrounded by an adventitia, a loose CT containing blood vessels, lymph vessels, nerves, and fat (Fig. 10-26). In most species, the thoracic part of the esophagus is largely covered by a serosa, specifically the mediastinal pleura. In horses, the abdominal part of the esophagus is approximately 2.5 cm in

Table 10-1 Characteristics of the Esophagus

	Horses	Pigs	Cattle	Goats	Sheep	Dogs	Cats
Stratified squamous epithelium[a]	Keratinized	Keratinized	Keratinized	Keratinized	Keratinized	Nonkeratinized	Nonkeratinized
Lamina muscularis	[b]	Absent in cranial part Highly developed in caudal part	[b]	[b]	[b]	Absent in cranial part Interrupted in middle part	[b]
Submucosal glands	[c]	Present only in cranial half	[c]	[c]	[c]	Present throughout and extend into stomach	[c]
Tunica muscularis[d]	Cranial two-thirds striated Caudal one-third smooth	Cranial part striated Middle part mixed Caudal part smooth	Striated throughout and extends into the reticular sulcus			Striated throughout	Cranial part striated Caudal one-third to one-fifth smooth
Tunica adventitia	Loose CT cells and fibers with blood and lymph vessels and nerves surround the esophagus. A tunica serosa may be present in the thoracic cavity (mediastinal pleura) or near the stomach (visceral peritoneum).						

[a] Epithelial adaptation to food texture: Coarse food ingestion leads to highly keratinized epithelia; soft food results in slightly keratinized to nonkeratinized epithelia.
[b] Isolated bundles of smooth muscle near pharynx, increases in thickness near stomach.
[c] Present only at the pharyngoesophageal junction.
[d] Inner circular muscle layer becomes thicker at the cardiac ostium of the stomach (forming the cardiac sphincter muscle), especially in horses.

length and is also covered by a serosa (visceral peritoneum). In carnivores, the abdominal part is not only shorter but also covered by visceral peritoneum. In other species, the esophagus–stomach junction is at or near the diaphragm and lacks a mesothelial covering.

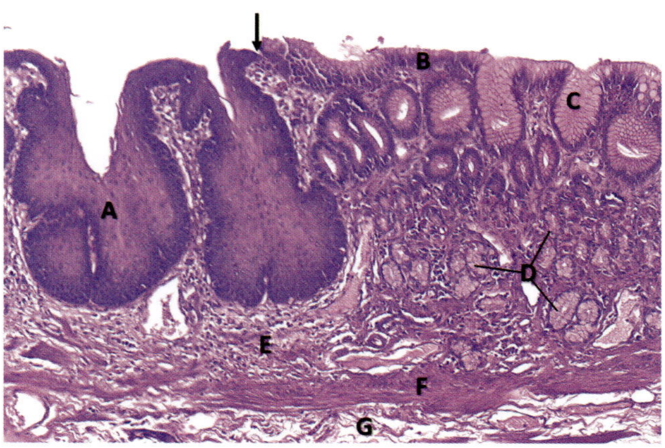

Figure 10-27 Esophagus–stomach junction (cat). Epithelium of esophagus (A), epithelium of stomach (B), junction of nonkeratinized stratified squamous epithelium with simple columnar epithelium (arrow), gastric pits (C), cardiac glands (D), lamina propria (E), lamina muscularis (F), and submucosa (G). H&E (×180). (Image by J. Feng.)

Esophagus–Stomach Junction

The morphologic characteristics of this junction vary considerably among species. In carnivores, there is an abrupt transition from the stratified squamous epithelium of the esophagus to the simple columnar epithelium of the cardiac gland region (Fig. 10-27). In cats, this junction is 3 to 5 mm cranial to the cardia (cardiac part) of the stomach, whereas in dogs, it is 1 to 2 cm cranial to the cardia. In horses and pigs, the stratified squamous epithelium extends throughout the nonglandular portion of the stomach mucosa, whereas in ruminants, it lines the entire forestomach. In species where the esophageal glands extend along the entire length of the esophagus, they may briefly continue into the submucosa of the stomach. In species with skeletal muscle extending into the stomach (carnivores and ruminants), there is a gradual transition from skeletal to smooth muscle.

Stomach

The stomach is an enlarged part of the digestive tube specialized for initiating the enzymatic and hydrolytic breakdown of food into digestible nutrients. The tunica muscularis aids in mixing the ingesta with gastric secretions. In carnivores, the stomach is entirely lined with glandular mucosa. In contrast, herbivores have both a glandular and a nonglandular region of the mucosa, the latter of which is lined with stratified squamous epithelium.

The stomach wall has all the layers of a typical tubular organ (Fig. 10-28 [1]). The mucosa is composed of an epithelial layer, a lamina propria (of loose CT), and a lamina muscularis. The submucosa contains collagen fibers, white adipose tissue, blood vessels, and the Meissner (submucosal) nerve plexus (Fig. 10-28 [2]). The tunica muscularis has three layers: inner oblique, middle circular, and outer longitudinal. The Auerbach (myenteric) nerve plexus (Fig. 10-28 [3]) is located between the middle and outer muscle layers. The serosa is composed of mesothelium overlying a layer of loose CT.

Nonglandular Region of the Tunica Mucosa

The nonglandular region of the stomach mucosa is absent in carnivores and small in pigs. In horses, the nonglandular region extends a considerable distance from the esophagus and ends at the **margo plicatus**. Its greatest development occurs in ruminants, lining the entire **forestomach** (rumen, reticulum, and omasum) (Fig. 10-29), detailed later in this chapter.

The epithelium lining the nonglandular region of the mucosa is stratified squamous, potentially keratinized depending on species and diet. The lamina propria is of typical loose CT, and the lamina muscularis is distinct. The junction between the nonglandular and glandular regions of the mucosa is abrupt, where stratified squamous epithelium meets simple columnar epithelium.

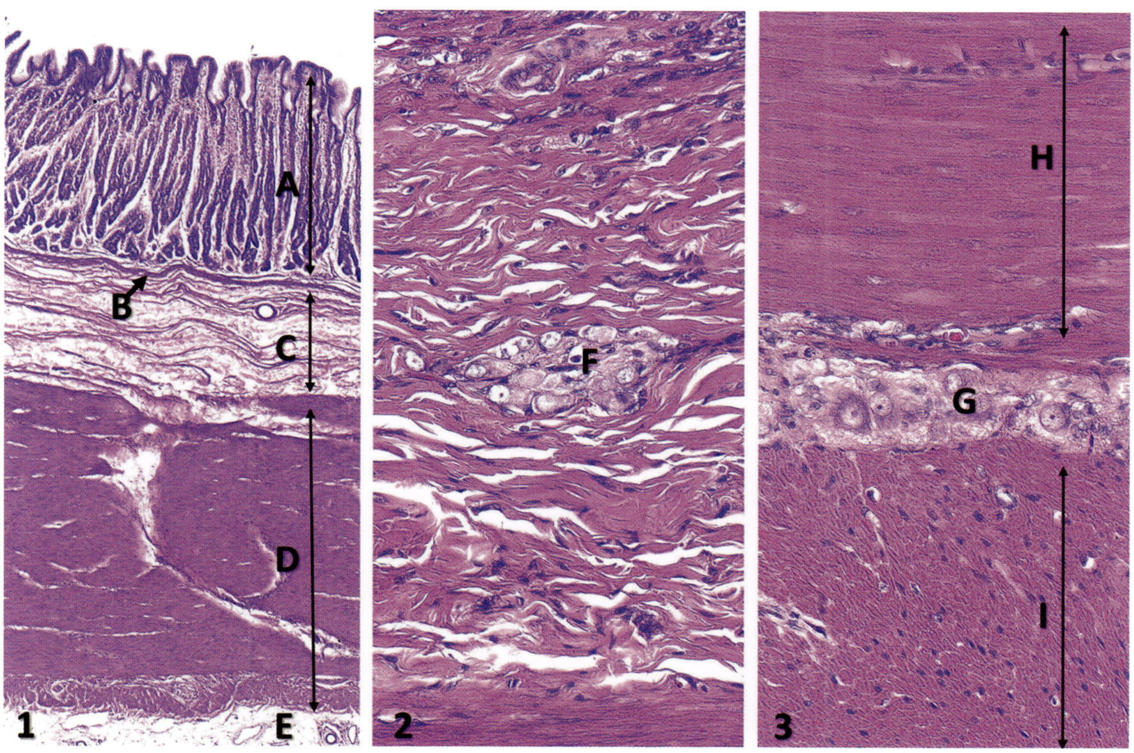

Figure 10-28 Proper gastric (fundic) gland region of the stomach mucosa in dogs. 1. Section through the proper gastric gland region: Tunica mucosa (A), lamina muscularis (B), tela submucosa (C), tunica muscularis (D), and tunica serosa (E). H&E (×50). 2. Meissner (submucosal) nerve plexus (F) within the submucosa. H&E (×200). 3. Auerbach (myenteric) nerve plexus (G) located between the circular (H) and longitudinal (I) layers of the tunica muscularis. H&E (×200). (Image by J. Feng.)

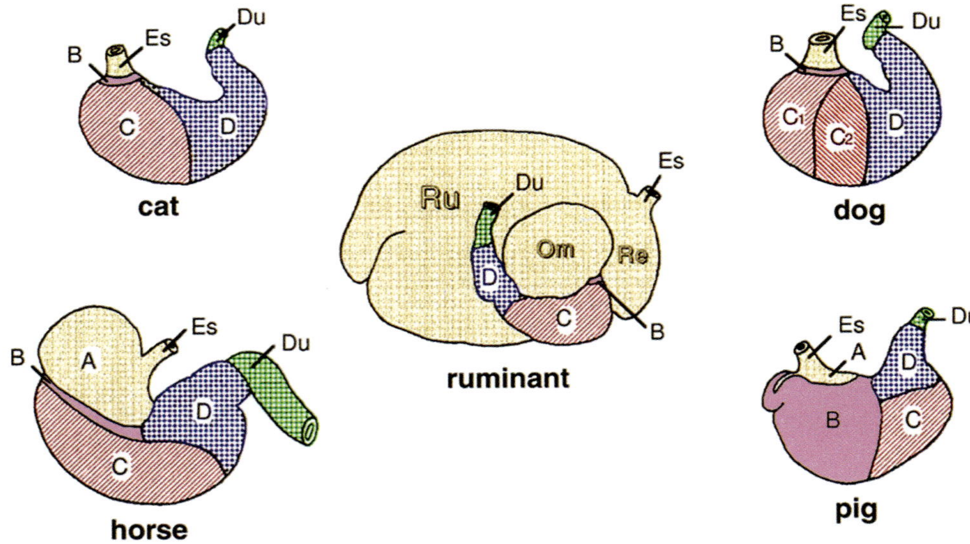

Figure 10-29 Schematic drawing illustrating the regions of the gastric tunica mucosa. A: Nonglandular region of the mucosa lined by stratified squamous epithelium, including the rumen (Ru), reticulum (Re), and omasum (Om); B: cardiac gland region; C: fundic gland region, showing light (C1) and dark (C2) zones in the dog; D: pyloric gland region, esophagus (Es), and duodenum (Du).

Glandular Region of the Tunica Mucosa

The structure of the glandular region of the mucosa follows the general pattern described earlier. The mucosa forms extensive folds (**gastric folds**), which flatten as the stomach fills. The surface is covered with small invaginations called **gastric pits**, which are continuous with the **gastric glands** and receive their secretory products (Fig. 10-30). The mucosal

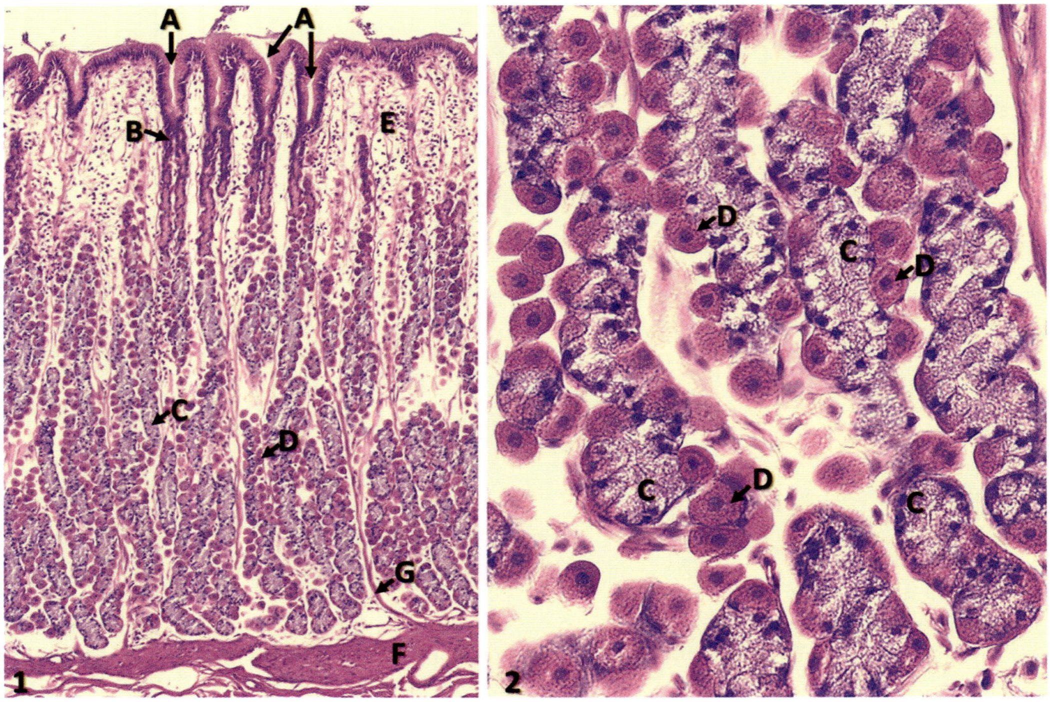

Figure 10-30 Proper gastric gland region of tunica mucosa, stomach (dog). 1. Under lower magnification (×80). 2. Fundic glands under higher magnification (×400). Gastric pits (A), mucous neck cells (B), chief cells (C), parietal cells (D), lamina propria (E), lamina muscularis (F), and its branch (G) penetrating the lamina propria. H&E. (Image by J. Feng.)

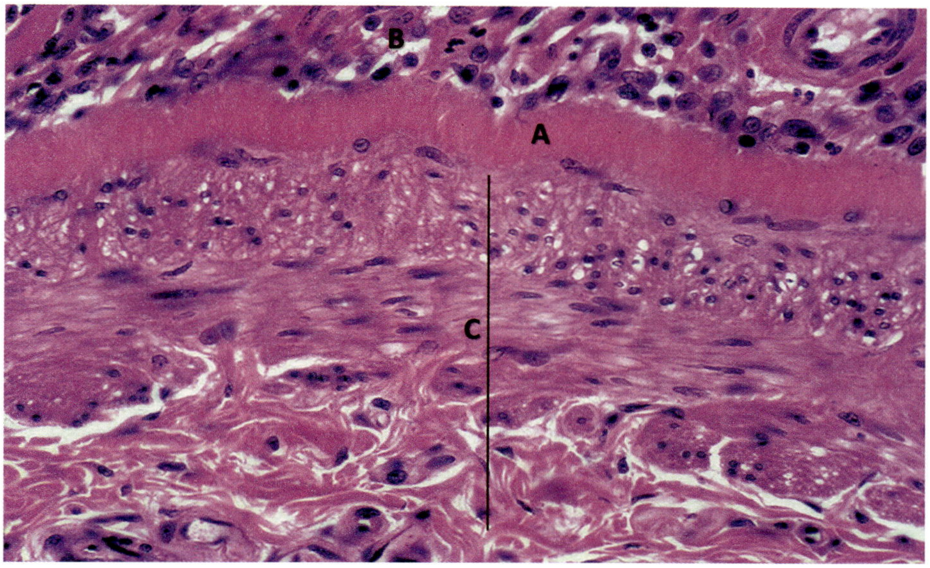

Figure 10-31 Proper gastric gland region of tunica mucosa, stomach (cat). Stratum compactum of lamina propria (A), fundus of proper gastric gland (B), and lamina muscularis comprising three layers with different orientations (C). H&E (×300).

surface, including the gastric pits, is lined with tall simple columnar epithelial cells that continuously secrete mucus, forming a protective coat that prevents digestion of the mucosa. These surface epithelial cells have a rapid turnover rate; new cells originating from mitosis in the gastric pits replace them approximately every 3 to 4 days. The gastric glands are densely packed within the lamina propria (Fig. 10-30). The loose CT in this area is often difficult to visualize because of the large amount of glandular epithelium. In carnivores, there may be a layer of densely packed collagen fibers called the **stratum compactum** between the bases of the gastric glands and the lamina muscularis (Fig. 10-31). The function of this layer may be to limit penetration of the stomach wall by sharp bones in the gastric contents.

The lamina muscularis is relatively thick, usually comprising three layers (Fig. 10-31). Small bundles of smooth muscle cells extend into the lamina propria, coursing between the gastric glands (Fig. 10-30 [1]).

The glandular region of the stomach mucosa is subdivided into three distinct regions according to the various glandular types present: **cardiac, proper gastric** (**fundic**), and **pyloric**. The distribution of these glandular regions in domestic mammals is illustrated in Fig. 10-29.

Cardiac Gland Region

The cardiac gland region of the mucosa occupies a narrow strip at the junction of the glandular and nonglandular mucosae in all domestic mammals except pigs, where it covers nearly half the stomach, including most of the **diverticulum ventriculi** (Fig. 10-29). The **cardiac glands** are relatively short, simple, branched, coiled tubular glands that secrete a mucous product (Fig. 10-32). The cells of these glands are cuboidal, with nuclei located in the basal portion of the cells. The cardiac glands empty into relatively shallow gastric pits (Fig. 10-32). Parietal cells (described below) may occur at the junction of the cardiac and proper gastric (fundic) gland regions.

Proper Gastric (Fundic) Gland Region

The proper gastric (fundic) gland region of the mucosa is well developed in all domestic mammals (Fig. 10-29). In carnivores, it occupies more than half of the stomach mucosa; in horses, more than one-third; and in pigs, approximately one-fourth. In ruminants, two-thirds of the abomasum mucosa is occupied by proper gastric glands. Also note in Fig. 10-29 that this gland region actually occupies the fundus of the stomach only in dogs, cats, and humans; therefore, the term "**proper gastric**" is used to clarify its location within the stomach.

Proper gastric glands are simple, branched, straight tubular glands that extend to the lamina muscularis (Fig. 10-30 [1]). The gland consists of a short **neck**, a long **body**, and a slightly dilated blind end known as the **fundus**. Four structurally and functionally distinct cell types comprise the secretory epithelium of the proper gastric gland: mucous neck cells, chief cells, parietal cells, and endocrine cells.

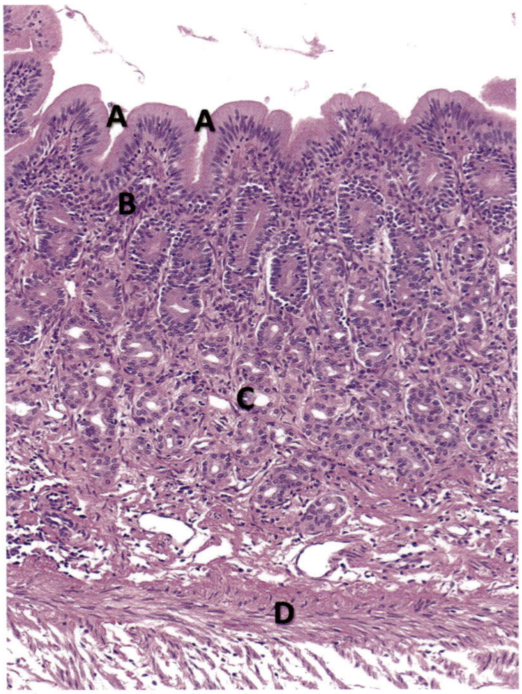

Figure 10-32 Cardiac gland region of tunica mucosa, stomach (dog). Shallow gastric pits (A), lamina propria (B), cardiac glands (C), and lamina muscularis (D). H&E (×130). (Photo by J. Feng.)

The **mucous neck cells** occupy the neck of the proper gastric gland (Fig. 10-30 [1]). They are typical mucous cells with a flat nucleus situated toward the base of the cell. While they appear similar to the mucus-producing surface epithelial cells, their cytoplasm is more basophilic. In addition, when treated with Periodic Acid-Schiff (PAS), the mucous neck cells are intensely positive throughout, whereas the surface cells only have PAS-positive material in the upper two-thirds of the cell.

The **chief cells** are the most numerous cells in the gastric glands (Fig. 10-30 [1] and [2]). They are cuboidal or pyramidal, with a spherical nucleus located near the base of the cell. The region between the nucleus and the free surface appears lacy due to clear spaces that remain after fixation. In their living state, these vacuoles contain zymogen granules that can be demonstrated with special fixation and staining. Thus, chief cells are also referred to as zymogen cells. The basal area of the chief cell has abundant rough endoplasmic reticulum (rER), resulting in a basophilic staining reaction. Chief cells secrete **pepsinogen**, which is converted into pepsin by hydrochloric acid (HCl).

The **parietal cells** (or **oxyntic cells**) are larger and less numerous than the chief cells. They have a tendency to occur singly and are peripheral to the chief cells (Fig. 10-30 [1] and [2]). Usually, only a narrow apex of the cell borders the gland lumen, while the base of the cell often bulges outward from the gland's external surface. Parietal cells have a spherical nucleus and their cytoplasm stains deeply with eosin, appearing granular due to the presence of numerous mitochondria. At the apex, the cell membrane invaginates to form a branching **intracellular canaliculus** that extends toward the center of the cell and communicates with the lumen of the gastric gland. Numerous microvilli of varying lengths project into the canaliculus, providing an extensive surface area necessary for the active transport system involved in producing free HCl. Parietal cells form carbonic acid through the action of the enzyme carbonic anhydrase. Carbonic acid dissociates into bicarbonate ions, which remain in the cell, and hydrogen ions, which are transported across the cell membrane into the intracellular canaliculus. There, hydrogen ions combine with chloride ions to form free HCl within the canaliculus and lumen of the gastric gland.

Throughout the glandular regions of the gastric mucosa and continuing into the small and large intestines are **endocrine cells** (**enteroendocrine cells**) responsible for producing gastrointestinal hormones such as gastrin, secretin, cholecystokinin, and gastric inhibitory polypeptide. These hormones are released either into the blood or lymphatic systems, where they circulate throughout the body or diffuse locally to target cells (i.e., a paracrine mode of secretion). These cells are difficult to identify in routine hematoxylin and eosin (H&E) sections and generally appear clear or poorly stained. Many of these cells demonstrate an affinity for silver stains and therefore have been referred to as **argentaffin cells** or **argyrophilic cells** (see Fig. 10-49). Some of these cells also can be demonstrated with potassium dichromate solutions just like the **enterochromaffin cells** in the small intestine and are therefore referred to as **enterochromaffin-like cells**. The difference between them is that the enterochromaffin cells secrete serotonin, whereas the enterochromaffin-like cells secrete histamine, a potent stimulator of gastric acid production in parietal cells. Most frequently, endocrine cells are wedged between the basement membrane and the chief cells and do not reach the epithelial surface. However, some extend to the lumen and are believed to monitor luminal contents and respond by releasing hormones. At least 12 different endocrine cell types have been identified by electron microscopy in the gastrointestinal tract. They all have numerous small membrane-bounded granules, mostly within the basal cytoplasm, along with relatively sparse rER and small Golgi complexes. The endocrine cells of the gastrointestinal tract are part of the **diffuse neuroendocrine system**, as discussed in Chapter 12.

Pyloric Gland Region

The pyloric gland region occupies approximately half of the gastric mucosa in carnivores but only about one-third in horses and in the abomasal mucosa in ruminants. In pigs, the pyloric gland region is smaller, representing approximately one-fourth of the mucosa (Fig. 10-29).

The gastric pits are considerably deeper than those in the cardiac and fundic (proper gastric) gland regions (Fig. 10-33). **Pyloric glands** are simple, branched, coiled tubular glands that are relatively short compared to the other gastric glands. The cells of the pyloric glands have the appearance of typical mucus-secreting cells, with flat nuclei located at the base of the cell and a lightly stained apical cytoplasm.

At the pylorus–duodenum junction, **submucosal intestinal glands** extend into the submucosa of the pyloric gland region from the duodenum. The middle circular layer of the tunica muscularis thickens at the pylorus to form the **pyloric sphincter** muscle, which causes the submucosa and mucosa to bulge into the lumen. In ruminants and pigs, this protuberance, called the **torus pyloricus**, is especially prominent.

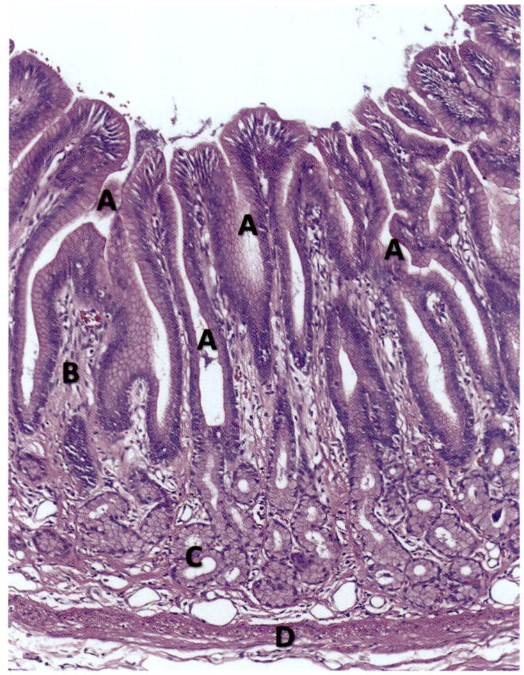

Figure 10-33 Pyloric gland region of tunica mucosa, stomach (dog). Deep gastric pits (A), lamina propria (B), short pyloric glands (C), and lamina muscularis (D). H&E (×80). (Image by J. Feng.)

Species Differences

In carnivores, the cardiac gland region is relatively narrow, with the proper gastric and pyloric gland regions occupying the remainder of the stomach. In dogs, the proper gastric gland region is divided into two zones. The light zone has a thinner mucosa with deep gastric pits and short, tortuous glands that appear in groups and do not reach the lamina muscularis. The dark zone, adjacent to the pyloric gland region, has a thicker mucosa, shallow gastric pits, and proper gastric glands that more closely resemble those of other species (Fig. 10-29).

The stomach of the pig has a very large cardiac gland region that contains numerous lymphatic nodules in the lamina propria. Parietal cells in the proper gastric gland region tend to occur in clusters.

The stomach of the horse has an extensive nonglandular region of the mucosa that terminates abruptly, forming the **margo plicatus** (Fig. 10-34). The cardiac gland region is almost nonexistent, whereas the proper gastric and pyloric gland regions follow the normal pattern.

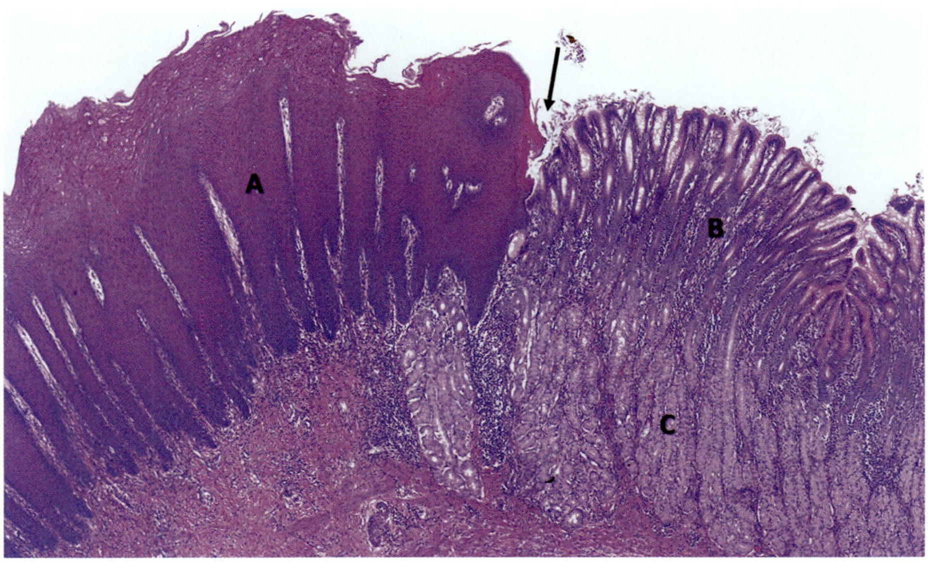

Figure 10-34 Junction of nonglandular and glandular horse stomach (margo plicatus). Nonglandular and nonkeratinized stratified squamous epithelium (A), simple columnar glandular epithelium with gastric pits (B), junction of stratified squamous epithelium and glandular epithelium (arrow), and gastric glands (C). H&E (×60). (Image by J. Feng.)

Ruminant Stomach

The stomach of ruminants is composed of four structurally distinct parts. The first three parts (the rumen, reticulum, and omasum) are collectively called the **forestomach** or **proventriculus** (Fig. 10-29). The forestomach is lined entirely by a nonglandular mucosa with a keratinized stratified squamous epithelium. The fourth part of the ruminant stomach (the **abomasum**) is lined by a glandular mucosa similar to that of other species.

The forestomach effectively breaks down coarse, fibrous ingesta into absorbable nutrients through both mechanical and chemical actions. The rumen functions as a fermentation vat where a large population of bacteria and protozoa act on the ingesta, producing short-chain, volatile fatty acids that are absorbed through the mucosa into the blood. Meanwhile, the reticulum and omasum exert a mechanical action on the ingesta, reducing the mass to fine particles. The wall of the omasum is especially well adapted for this function. In addition to fermentation and mechanical activities, significant absorption occurs across the keratinized stratified squamous epithelium of all three portions of the forestomach. The enzymatic digestive processes in the abomasum further degrade the ingesta, along with accompanying microorganisms, into substances such as glucose and amino acids in a manner similar to that of the stomach of nonruminants.

Rumen

The mucosa of the rumen is characterized by small tongue-shaped **papillae** (Figs. 10-35 and 10-36), which vary considerably in size and shape across different regions of the rumen. These papillae develop prenatally and remain small as long as the animal is on a milk diet. However, when roughage is introduced into the diet and fermentation begins in the rumen, the papillae rapidly increase in size (Fig. 10-36).

The ruminal epithelium is keratinized stratified squamous and performs at least three important functions: protection, metabolism, and absorption (Figs. 10-37 and 10-38). The stratum corneum forms a protective shield against the rough, fibrous ingesta. The deeper layers metabolize short-chain, volatile fatty acids, particularly butyric, acetic, and propionic acids, which are the chief products of fermentation. Additionally, sodium, potassium, ammonia, urea, and many other products are absorbed from the ruminal contents.

The **stratum corneum** varies in thickness from one to two cells up to as many as 10 to 20 cells. Stainable nuclei may or may not be present. The **stratum granulosum** is usually one to three cells thick, characterized by flattened cells containing keratohyalin granules in the cytoplasm. Cells of the stratum granulosum near the stratum corneum are frequently swollen and have a pyknotic nucleus surrounded by clear, electron-lucent cytoplasm. The peripheral cytoplasm of these cells contains keratohyalin granules, tonofilaments, and numerous membrane-bounded, electron-dense granules (Fig. 10-38). The **stratum spinosum** consists of polyhedral cells that are slightly larger than the basal cells (Fig. 10-38). The thickness of this layer varies from 1 to 10 cells. Cytologic features of these cells include numerous mitochondria and ribosomes distributed throughout the cytoplasm. Adjacent cells are interconnected through numerous desmosomes (Fig. 10-38). The cells of the **stratum basale** are columnar and extend numerous processes to the basement membrane, significantly increasing the basal cell membrane surface area. The cytologic features of the basal cells are similar to those of the stratum spinosum.

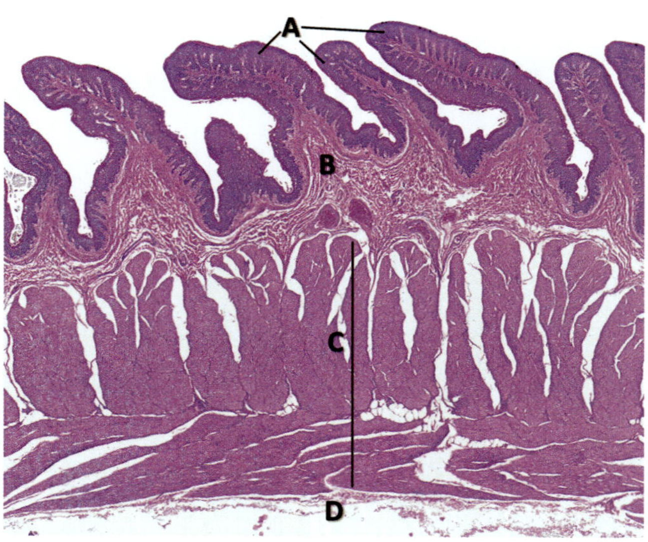

Figure 10-35 Rumen (goat). Papillae (A), propria-submucosa (B), tunica muscularis (C), tunica serosa (D). H&E (×30). (Image by J. Feng.)

The intercellular spaces throughout the entire epithelium are distended to varying degrees. These spaces may appear wide, containing flocculent material passing through the epithelium (Fig. 10-38), or, in other areas, they may be collapsed without flocculent material, indicating periods of little or no movement of material across the epithelium.

A lamina muscularis is *absent*, allowing the lamina propria to blend directly with the submucosa, forming a combined propria-submucosa. Each papilla has a core (an extension of the propria-submucosa) with a dense

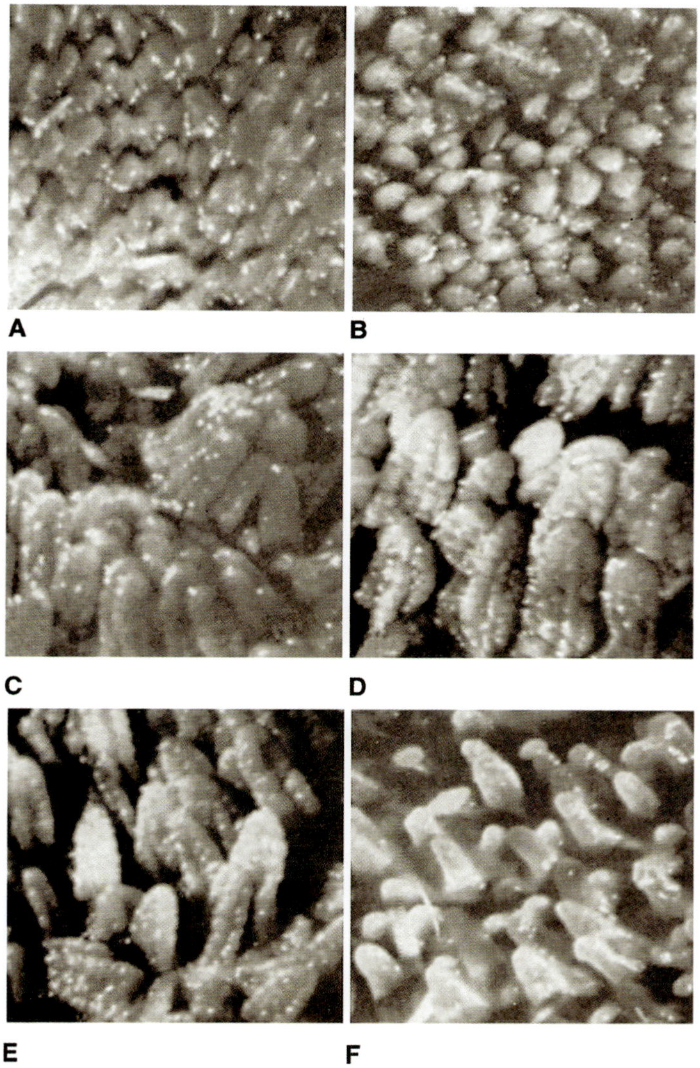

Figure 10-36 Changes in ruminal papillae caused by age and diet (same steer) (×2). **A.** Six months of age and on a milk diet since birth. Papillae are rudimentary. **B.** Hay and grain diet for 3 weeks. Papillae are enlarged. **C.** Hay and grain diet for 2 months. **D.** Hay and grain diet for 3 months. Papillae have reached maximal length. **E.** After returning to a milk diet for 3 days. Papillae are smaller. **F.** After returning to a milk diet for 10 days. Papillae are strikingly reduced. (From Stinson AW, Brown EM. Veterinary Histology Slide Sets. East Lansing, MI: Michigan State University, Instructional Media Center, 1970.)

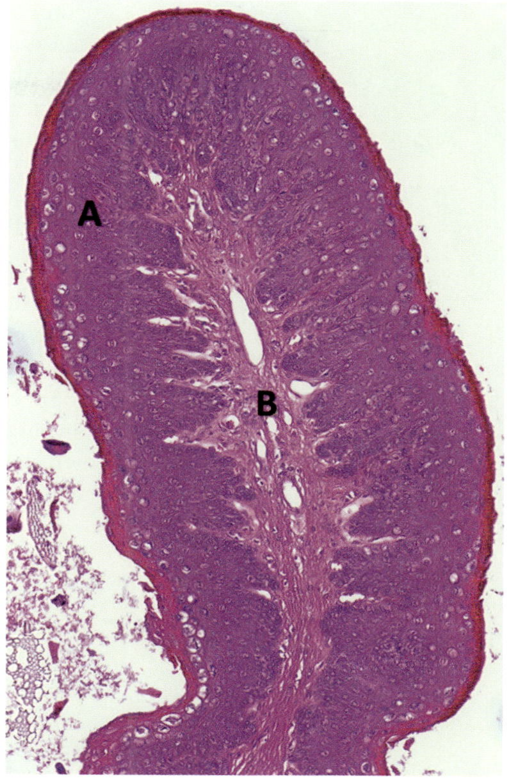

Figure 10-37 Tip of ruminal papilla (goat). Keratinized stratified squamous epithelium (A) and lamina propria (B). H&E (×150). (Image by J. Feng.)

feltwork of collagen, elastic, and reticular fibers. A dense network of fenestrated capillaries lies just beneath the basement membrane of the epithelium. Closer to the tunica muscularis, the CT of the propria-submucosa is more loosely arranged. Within this layer lies a network of blood vessels and the submucosal nerve plexus.

The tunica muscularis is composed of inner circular and outer longitudinal layers of smooth muscle. The myenteric plexus is located between these layers.

The serosa of the rumen is a loose CT covered by a mesothelium. It contains varying amounts of white adipose tissue, as well as blood vessels, lymph vessels, and nerves distributed within the loose CT.

Reticulum

The reticulum has a mucosa with permanent interconnecting folds, the **reticular crests**, which give it the appearance of a honeycomb (Fig. 10-39). These crests are of two different heights: the taller (primary) crests separate the mucosal surface into shallow compartments called **reticular cells**, which are further subdivided by shorter (secondary) crests into smaller areas. The sides of the crests have vertical ridges, and the mucosa between the crests is covered by conical **reticular papillae** that project into the lumen.

The keratinized stratified squamous epithelium resembles that of the rumen. The propria-submucosa consists predominantly of a feltwork of collagen and elastic fibers. A lamina muscularis is located only in the upper part of the larger reticular crests, causing the lamina propria and submucosa to blend imperceptibly (Fig. 10-40). This lamina muscularis is

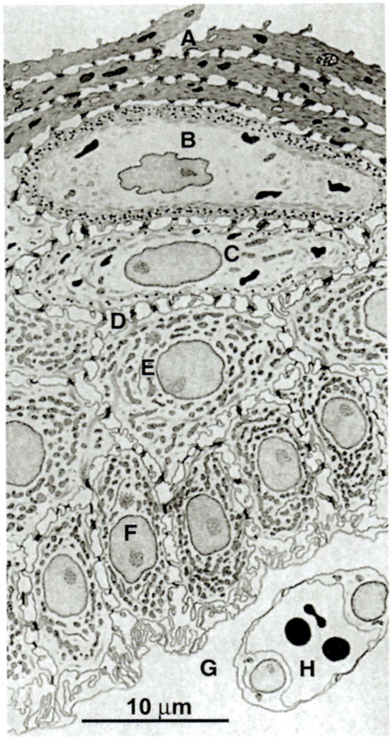

Figure 10-38 Drawing from an electron micrograph of ruminal epithelium. Stratum corneum (A), swollen cells of the stratum granulosum (B), flat cells of the stratum granulosum (C), intercellular canaliculi (D), stratum spinosum with desmosomes (E), stratum basale (F), lamina propria (G), and capillary in lamina propria (H). (From Stinson AW, Brown EM. Veterinary Histology Slide Sets. East Lansing, MI: Michigan State University, Instructional Media Center, 1970).

continuous with that of the esophagus. Smooth muscle bundles extend from one crest to another, creating a continuous network of smooth muscle throughout the reticular mucosa where the crests intersect.

The tunica muscularis consists of two layers of smooth muscle cells that follow an oblique course and cross at right angles. The serosa is similar to that of the rumen.

Omasum

The omasum is nearly filled with approximately 100 longitudinal folds, known as **laminae**, which originate from the internal surface of the greater curvature and sides of the organ (Fig. 10-41). Among these, the largest laminae, about 12 in number, feature a thick, concave-free edge that extends close to the lesser curvature.

Successive orders of shorter laminae (second, third, fourth, and fifth) progressively decrease in length. The omasal contents are compressed into thin layers within the narrow spaces between the laminae (**interlaminar recesses**). These contents are further broken down into a fine pulp by numerous rounded, horny **omasal papillae** that stud the surface of the mucosa (Fig. 10-42). The papillae are oriented to facilitate the movement of solid contents from the reticulo-omasal ostium into the interlaminar recesses, where the laminae work to move the contents out through the omaso-abomasal ostium.

The lining is keratinized stratified squamous epithelium, and the glandular lamina propria contains a dense subepithelial capillary network. A lamina muscularis forms a thick layer just beneath the lamina propria on both sides of the laminae (Fig. 10-42). The submucosa is very thin.

The tunica muscularis is composed of a thin outer longitudinal layer and a thicker inner circular layer of smooth muscle. The innermost fibers of the circular layer extend into the large omasal laminae (first through third orders) as the intermediate muscle sheet (Fig. 10-42).

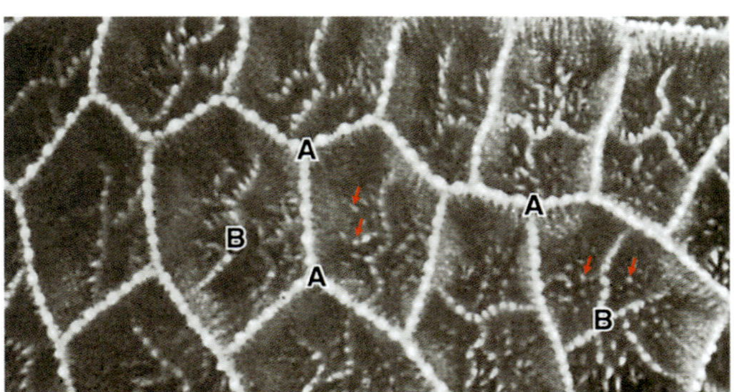

Figure 10-39 Surface view of the reticulum mucosa. Primary crests (A) delineating the large reticular cells, secondary crests (B) subdividing the large reticular cells into smaller reticular cells, and conical papillae (arrows). (Courtesy of A. Hansen.)

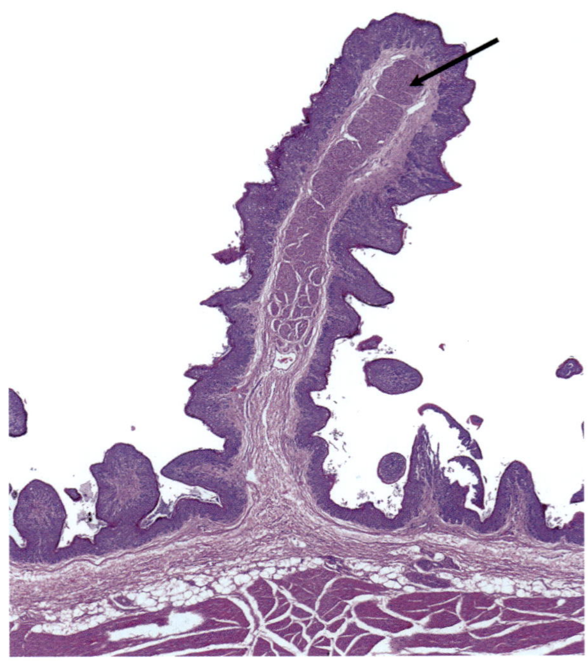

Figure 10-40 Reticulum (goat). Cross-section through a primary crest with condensed lamina muscularis (arrow) in the upper portion. H&E (×30). (Image by J. Feng.)

Abomasum

The omaso-abomasal ostium is demarcated by two mucosal folds called the **vela abomasica**. Here, the epithelium changes abruptly from keratinized stratified squamous to simple columnar. In cattle, this transition occurs at the apex of the folds, whereas in small ruminants, it occurs on the omasal side. On the abomasal side of the folds, the lamina propria becomes less dense and often contains a lymphatic nodule beneath the epithelial junction. The mucosa of the abomasum has all the characteristic glandular regions of the stomach described previously (Fig. 10-29).

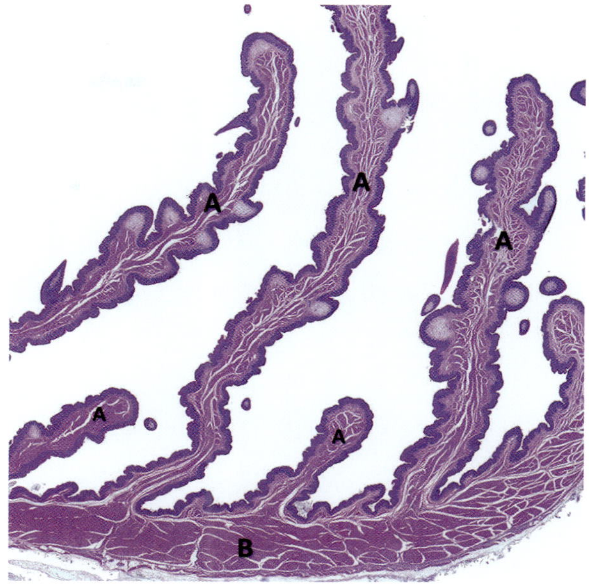

Figure 10-41 Omasum (sheep). Portion of the wall including laminae of different sizes (A) and tunica muscularis (B). H&E (×9). (Image by J. Feng.)

Small Intestine

The small intestine is divided into three parts: the **duodenum, jejunum**, and **ileum**. Intestinal digestion, or reduction of food to an absorbable form, begins when the contents from the stomach are acted upon by pancreatic secretions, bile, and intestinal fluids, continuing throughout the length of the small intestine.

The digestive and absorptive functions of the small intestine are facilitated by several specialized structures. Digestive functions require voluminous amounts of digestive enzymes in addition to a copious supply of mucus to protect the lining cells from mechanical injury and irritating compounds. The enzymes originate from the columnar absorptive cells and the pancreas. The enzymes produced by the columnar absorptive cells are membrane-bound at the microvillous luminal surface, while those produced by the pancreas mix freely with luminal contents. Mucus is produced by **submucosal glands** (**Brunner's glands**) in the duodenum (Figs. 10-43 and 10-44) and by **goblet cells**, which are intermingled with the columnar absorptive cells throughout the entire intestine (Figs. 10-46 and 10-47).

The efficiency of the absorptive function is enhanced by three structural features that increase the surface area exposed to intestinal contents: (a) the upper two-thirds of the small intestine has circularly disposed mucosal folds (**plicae circulares**) extending approximately two-thirds of the way around the lumen (Fig. 10-43). In ruminants, these folds are permanent, but in all other domestic mammals, they disappear when the organ is distended; (b) the surface of the mucosa is covered with finger-like projections called intestinal **villi** (Figs. 10-45 and 10-46). Villi vary in length depending on the small intestine region and species, appearing long and slender in carnivores and short and wide in cattle; and (c) microvilli are present on the free surface of the simple columnar epithelial cells of the villi (Fig. 10-47).

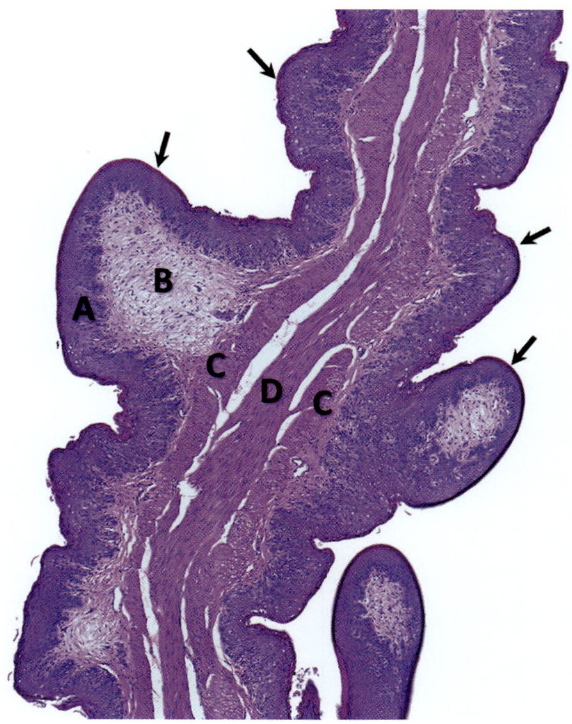

Figure 10-42 Omasum (sheep). Portion of a large lamina containing omasal papillae (arrows). Keratinized stratified squamous epithelium (A), lamina propria (B), lamina muscularis (C), and extension of inner circular layer of tunica muscularis (D). H&E (×50). (Image by J. Feng.)

Tunica Mucosa

The mucosa includes the lining epithelium, a lamina propria with glands, and a lamina muscularis. The villi are mucosal projections and are the most characteristic feature of the small intestine. The **intestinal glands** (**crypts of Lieberkühn**), which open between the bases of the villi, penetrate the

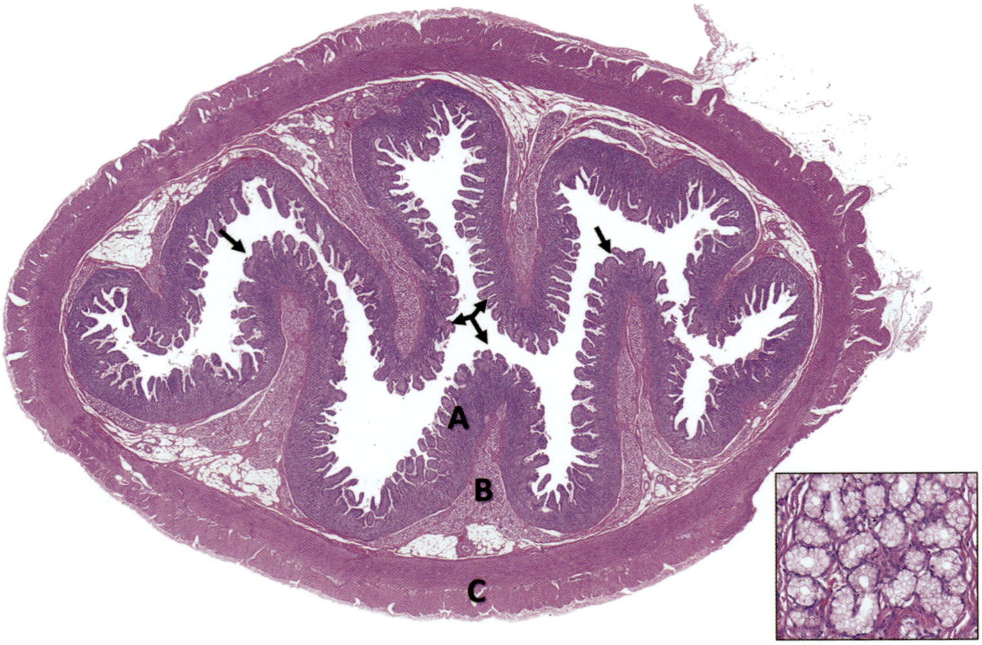

Figure 10-43 Oblique section of the duodenum (dog). Circular folds (plicae circulares) (arrows). Mucosa (A), submucosal glands (B), and tunica muscularis (C). H&E (×10). Inset: Magnified submucosal glands. H&E (400×). (Image by J. Feng.)

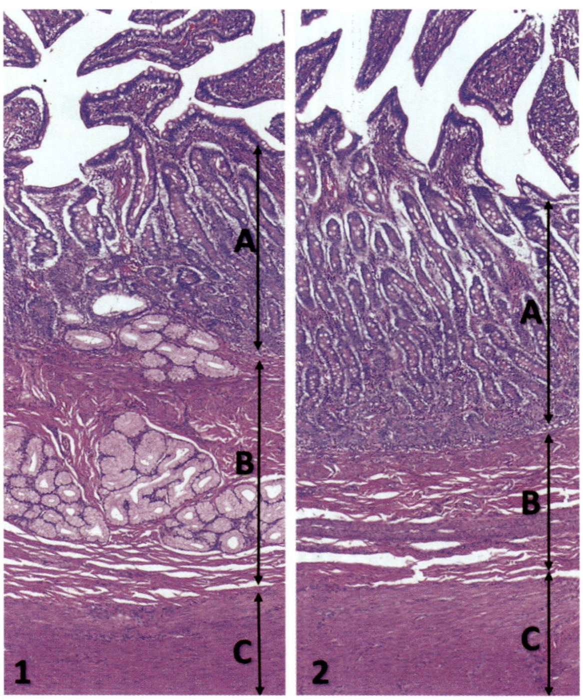

Figure 10-44 Duodenum (dog). 1. Area near pylorus with submucosal glands. 2. A more caudal area lacking submucosal glands. Tunica mucosa with villi and intestinal (mucosal) glands (A), tela submucosa (B), and tunica muscularis (C). H&E (×50). (Image by J. Feng.)

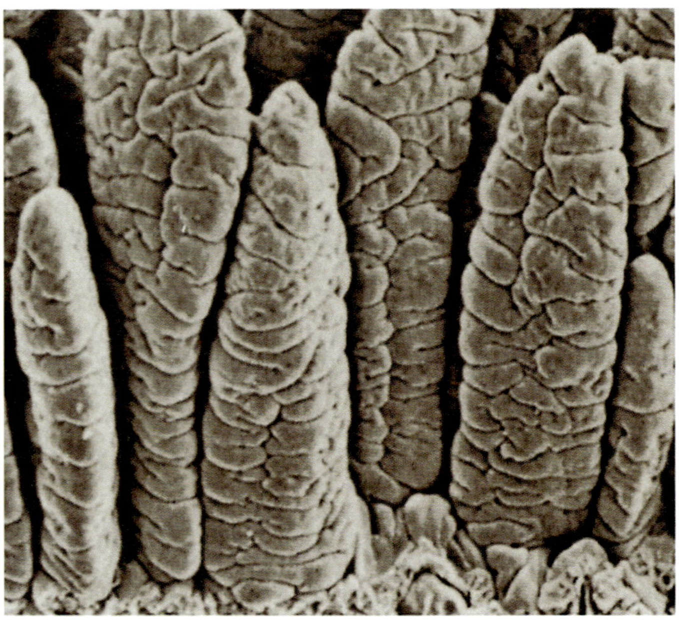

Figure 10-45 Scanning electron micrograph of intestinal villi, ileum (calf). These villi are in a contracted state (×85). (Courtesy of J. F. Pohlenz.)

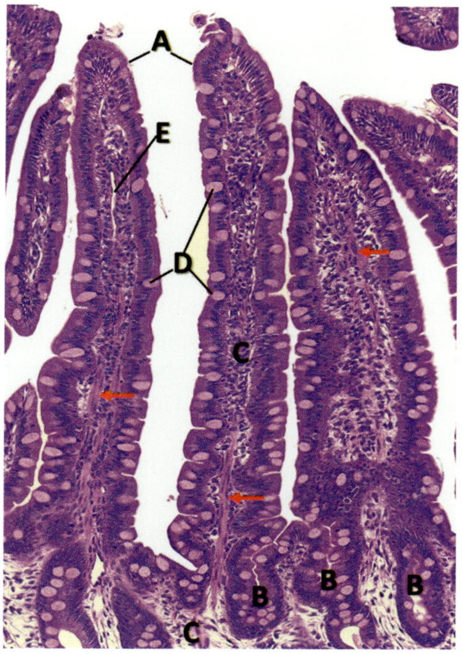

Figure 10-46 Villi and intestinal glands of the small intestine (dog). Finger-like villi (A) project into the lumen, while the intestinal glands (B) invaginate into the lamina propria (C). Simple columnar epithelium with many goblet cells (D), lymphatic capillary (lacteal) (E), and smooth muscle (arrows). H&E (×140). (Image by J. Feng.)

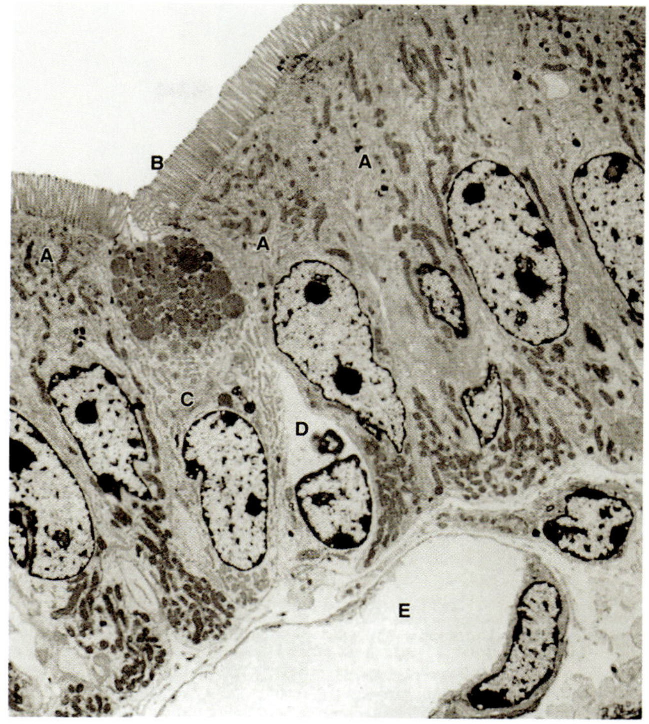

Figure 10-47 Transmission electron micrograph of jejunum surface epithelium (calf). Simple columnar epithelial cells (A) with microvilli (B). A goblet cell (C) and a migrating lymphocyte (D) are also present. Immediately below the epithelium is a capillary (E) (×5000). (Courtesy of J. F. Pohlenz.)

mucosa as far as the lamina muscularis. These simple tubular glands are sometimes referred to simply as mucosal glands (Figs. 10-44 and 10-46).

The lumen of the small intestine is lined by a simple columnar epithelium containing numerous goblet cells interspersed among columnar absorptive cells (Fig. 10-47). Junctional complexes, located between the epithelial cells at the luminal surface, prevent the fluid of the intestinal contents from diffusing into the lamina propria without going through the cells. The columnar **absorptive cells** have ovoid nuclei situated near the cell base and prominent microvilli that form a striated border. In electron micrographs, mitochondria are seen near the nucleus and in the basal region (Fig. 10-47). The apical cytoplasm contains a terminal web and extensive smooth endoplasmic reticulum (sER) necessary for the synthesis of triglycerides. A prominent supranuclear Golgi complex functions in digestive enzyme secretion as well as in the transformation of emulsified fats into chylomicrons, small fat droplets transported by the blood. Free ribosomes and rER are located in the basal part of the cell.

Goblet cells are dispersed among the columnar absorptive cells (Figs. 10-46 and 10-47). As **mucinogen** is produced within the cell, the apical portion of the cell becomes distended, mucinogen droplets accumulate, and the nucleus and remaining cytoplasm are pushed toward the narrow cell base resting on the basement membrane (Fig. 10-47) (for more details, see Chapter 2). The number of goblet cells decreases at the tips of the villi; however, the density of goblet cells is two to three times greater in the ileum than in the duodenum.

The simple tubular **intestinal glands** (**crypts of Lieberkühn**) are lined by a variety of cell types. The principal cell type within these glands is the **undifferentiated columnar cell**. These cells multiply, differentiate, and migrate onto the villus, where they differentiate into columnar absorptive cells and goblet cells. As they progress toward the villus tip, they eventually slough off into the lumen. Because of this continuous cell renewal process, many mitotic figures are observed among the glandular cells. This mitotic activity is constant and bears no relation to the amount of ingesta or enzyme activity. The epithelium is renewed approximately every 2 to 3 days.

Near the base of the intestinal glands, **acidophilic granular cells** (**of Paneth**) are present in ruminants and horses (Fig. 10-48). They are pyramid-shaped cells with prominent spherical, acidophilic granules located between the nucleus and the cell apex. The acidophilic granular cells have all the characteristics of enzyme-producing cells, and substantial evidence

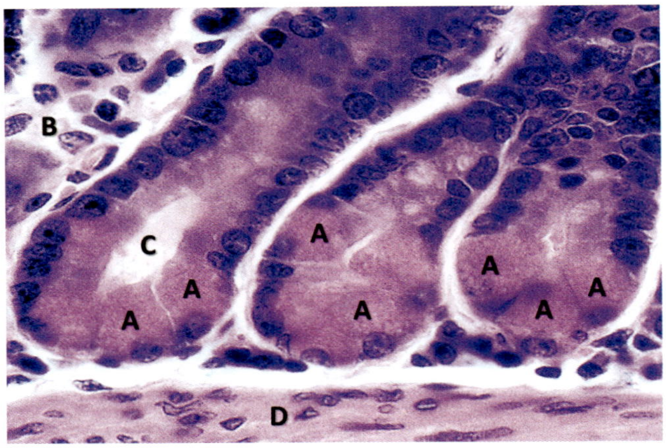

Figure 10-48 Mucosal glands, small intestine (horse). Acidophilic granular cells (of Paneth) (A) in the base of three intestinal glands, lamina propria (B), lumen of one intestinal gland (C), and lamina muscularis (D). H&E (×400).

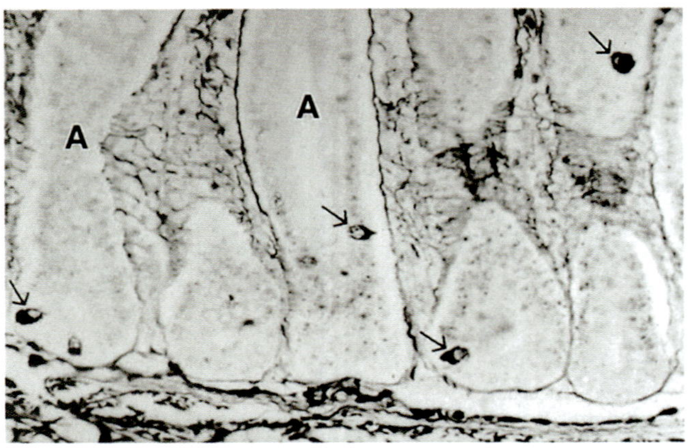

Figure 10-49 Mucosal glands, small intestine (cat). Lumen of an intestinal mucosal gland (A) and enteroendocrine cells (arrows). Silver stain (×320).

shows that they produce **peptidases**, which hydrolyze peptide bonds, and **lysozyme**, an antibacterial compound. These cells also contain zinc, which has been reported to be important in the activation of peptidases. **Enteroendocrine cells** are also present in the intestinal glands, as described earlier in the "Proper Gastric (Fundic) Gland Region" section (Fig. 10-49).

The lamina propria forms the cores of the villi and surrounds the intestinal glands. It is composed of loose CT with a prominent reticular fiber framework. Within this extensive fiber network are blood and lymph vessels, leukocytes, fibrocytes, smooth muscle cells, plasma cells, and mast cells. **Globule leukocytes** are found in the intestinal mucosa of most domestic species. They contain large eosinophilic globular material surrounding a small nucleus. Recent studies suggest they are derived from mast cells and participate in the immune response. Diffuse lymphatic tissue and solitary lymphatic nodules are present throughout the lamina propria of the small intestine, with their numbers increasing toward the ileum. A **stratum compactum** similar to that found in the stomach may be present between the bases of the intestinal glands and the lamina muscularis of carnivores.

A single lymphatic capillary, the **lacteal**, is located in the center of the lamina propria within the villus (Fig. 10-46). This vessel has a blind terminal end at the tip of the villus and serves as the origin of the lymph vessels that form a plexus at the bases of the villi. This basal plexus gives rise to a larger plexus surrounding the intestinal glands and the lymphatic nodules. Longitudinally oriented smooth muscle cells that originate from the lamina muscularis extend to the tip of the villus (Fig. 10-46). Contraction of these muscle cells causes the villus to shorten and likely contributes to lateral movements. Muscle contraction also aids in pumping the lymph out of the lacteal into the plexus below. A single arteriole from an arterial plexus in the submucosa penetrates the lamina muscularis and courses into the villus, where it forms an arteriovenular loop and a capillary network immediately beneath the surface epithelium. During digestive activity, this vascular network becomes engorged with blood, causing the villus to lengthen. In contrast, during muscular contraction, blood is expelled as the villus shortens. Thus, the villi act as pumping stations for moving both blood and lymph into the general circulation.

The lamina muscularis is composed of inner circular and outer longitudinal layers of smooth muscle that tend to be thin and incomplete, except in dogs. The thickness and completeness of the lamina muscularis may vary depending on the species, the individual animal, and the specific intestinal region.

Tela Submucosa

The submucosa is a layer of CT denser than that of the lamina propria. Tubuloalveolar **submucosal glands** (**Brunner's glands**), located within this CT, open into the base of the intestinal mucosal glands (Figs. 10-43 and 10-44). The submucosal glands are mucous in dogs and ruminants, serous in pigs and horses, and seromucous in cats. The serous (proteinaceous) or mucous secretory product of these glands lubricates the surface epithelium and provides protection from the acidic gastric chyme. The glands are present in all domestic mammals, but their distribution varies with the species. For example, they are confined to the proximal portion of the duodenum in dogs, whereas in horses, they extend well into the jejunum.

Solitary (isolated) lymphatic nodules are present in the submucosa throughout the small intestine. Large **aggregated lymphatic nodules** (**Peyer's patches**) occur in all three segments of the small intestine, but they are usually considered more characteristic of the ileum (Fig. 10-50). These masses of lymphatic tissue can be identified grossly, except in cats, as they create well-delineated elevations on the mucosal surface. Aggregated lymphatic nodules are largest in cattle and most numerous in horses. The intestinal glands may extend into the submucosa in areas of the small intestine where the lamina muscularis is disrupted by the aggregated lymphatic nodules. (See Chapter 8 for details on this gut-associated lymphatic tissue.)

The submucosa also contains the submucosal (Meissner's) nerve plexus, from which nerve fibers extend into the villi.

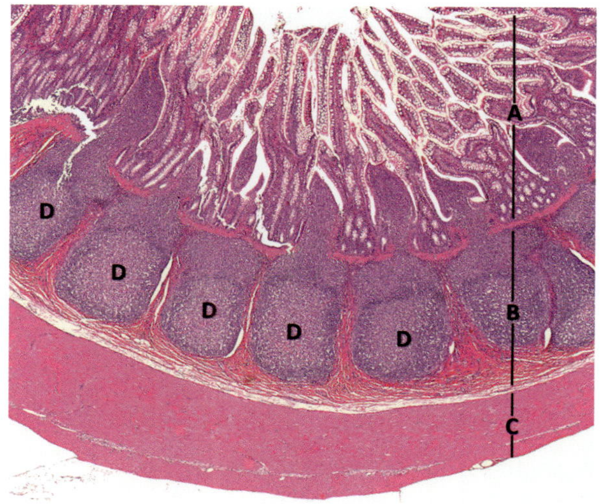

Figure 10-50 Ileum (cat). Tunica mucosa (A), submucosa (B), tunica muscularis (C), and Peyer's patches—the aggregated lymphatic nodules (D). H&E (×25). (Image by J. Feng.)

Tunica Muscularis

In all species, the tunica muscularis of the small intestine consists of inner circular and outer longitudinal smooth muscle layers. The tunica muscularis is thickest in horses, where the two layers are nearly equal in thickness. The CT between the two muscle layers contains the myenteric plexus.

Tunica Serosa

A serosa covers the entire small intestine. It consists of a layer of loose CT covered by mesothelium.

Blood Supply

Branches of the celiac and cranial mesenteric arteries travel through the mesoduodenum and mesentery (mesojejunum and mesoileum) and penetrate the tunica muscularis at the mesenteric attachment line. These arteries then branch out to supply the tunica muscularis and continue into the submucosa, where they form a submucosal arterial plexus. The plexus gives rise to short arterioles, which supply capillary beds around the lamina muscularis and intestinal (mucosal) glands, and long arterioles that reach the villi tips. Within the villi, a single arteriole supplies a capillary network and extends to the tip of the villus, where it joins a venule, forming an arteriovenular loop. Venules from the villi and the periglandular capillary bed converge to form a submucosal venous plexus. This network gives rise to veins that traverse the tunica muscularis in parallel to the arterial supply and drain into the portal vein. The circulatory system in the small intestine of horses, carnivores, and pigs differs from the previously described pattern. These animals lack arteriovenular loops in the villi. Instead, they have arteriovenous (AV) anastomoses in the submucosa, which precede the villous circulation. During digestion, circularly arranged smooth muscle cells in the AV anastomoses contract, diverting blood flow to the villi. When the digestive process is inactive, these AV anastomoses remain open, allowing for a partial bypass of the villus circulation.

General Identifying Features

The various regions of the small intestine in domestic mammals are not as clearly defined microscopically as they are in humans. For example, the submucosal glands do not extend the full length of the duodenum in sheep, goats, and carnivores. In contrast, in horses, cattle, and pigs, these glands reach into the jejunum. Likewise, the aggregated lymphatic nodules (**Peyer's patches**), often considered an identifying feature of the ileum, can be found anywhere along the small intestine of domestic mammals.

Because the length of the villi varies with physiologic activities and among species, it is not a reliable characteristic for the identification of the various segments.

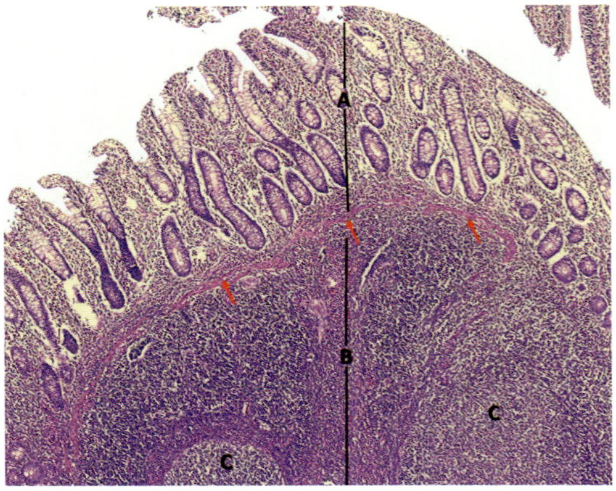

Figure 10-51 Cecum (pig). Tunica mucosa (A), submucosa (B), lymphatic nodules (C), and lamina muscularis (arrows). H&E (×26). (Image by J. Feng.)

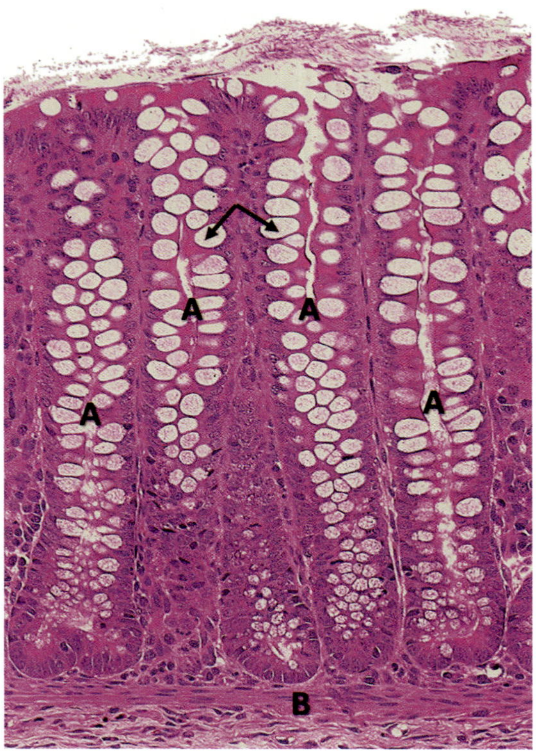

Figure 10-52 Colon (dog). Tunica mucosa with intestinal glands (A) containing numerous goblet cells (arrows) and lamina muscularis (B). H&E (×180). (Image by J. Feng.)

Large Intestine

The large intestine is composed of the cecum, colon, rectum, and anal canal. It is a site for microbial action on the ingesta, absorption of water, vitamins, and electrolytes, and secretion of mucus. Many gross anatomical and functional variations in the large intestine relate to the breakdown of cellulose-containing material consumed by herbivores. However, despite these differences, the cecum, colon, and rectum are difficult to differentiate in histologic sections. Characteristics common to these three segments of the large intestine are the absence of villi, longer and less coiled simple tubular intestinal glands with many goblet cells (Fig. 10-51), the lack of acidophilic granular (**Paneth**) cells, and an increased number of lymphatic nodules. Plicae circulares are absent in the large intestine, but longitudinal folds are present. Animals raised for food production tend to accumulate white adipose tissue in the submucosa.

Cecum

The cecum varies in size among different species. In herbivores with simple stomachs (e.g., horses), the cecum is large and is an important bacterial fermentation reservoir. In contrast, in carnivores, the cecum is small. Across all domestic mammals, the cecum has a substantial number of lymphatic nodules scattered throughout its length (Fig. 10-51). Lymphatic nodules are especially numerous around the ileal ostium (the opening from the ileum into the cecum or colon) in pigs, ruminants, and dogs. However, in horses and cats, lymphatic nodules are concentrated near the apex of the cecum.

Colon

The mucosa of the colon is substantially thicker than that of the small intestine because of the increased length of the intestinal glands. Since villi are absent, the mucosal surface is smooth (Fig. 10-52). The number of goblet cells is increased compared to the small intestine (Fig. 10-52). The submucosa is often distended by lymphatic tissue, which can disrupt the lamina muscularis and allow intestinal glands to extend into it.

In pigs and horses, the outer longitudinal layer of the tunica muscularis in the cecum and colon forms large, flat muscle bands containing numerous elastic fibers known as the **taenia ceci** and **taenia coli**. In the cecum and ventral colon of horses, these bands have more elastic fibers than smooth muscle cells.

Rectum

Like that of the cecum and colon, the mucosa of the **rectum** is smooth, and except for the increased number of goblet cells, the basic structures are similar as well. In horses and cattle, the rectal wall is thicker than that of the colon. In carnivores, the outer longitudinal layer of the tunica muscularis is thickened. Elastic fibers are most prominent in the rectum of horses and cattle and least prominent in sheep and goats. The outer longitudinal layer of the tunica muscularis contains more elastic fibers than the inner circular layer. The cranial portion of the rectum is covered by a serosa, whereas the retroperitoneal portion is surrounded by an adventitia, which blends with the pelvic fascia.

Near its junction with the anal canal, the rectal mucosa in ruminants forms longitudinal folds known as **rectal columns** (**columnae rectales**). All domestic mammals have an extensive venous plexus in the lamina propria of this region of the rectum. In dogs, approximately 100 solitary lymphatic nodules are a prominent feature of the rectum. They are visible grossly because of pitlike depressions, **rectal pits**, in the mucosa overlying the lymphatic nodules.

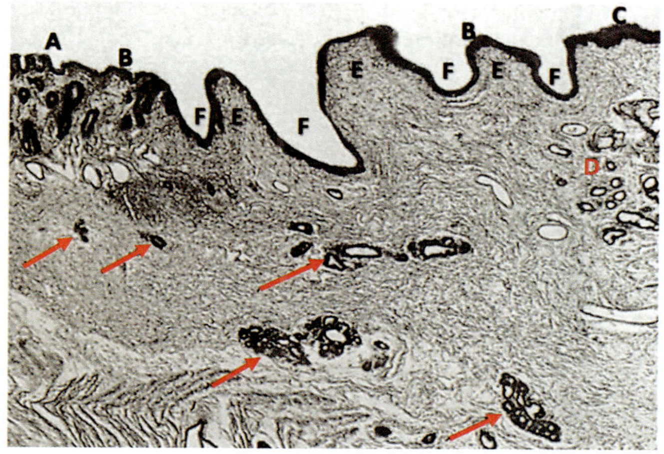

Figure 10-53 Rectum and anal canal (dog). Rectum (A), anal canal (B), skin (C) with sweat and sebaceous glands (D), columns (E), anal sinuses (F), and anal glands (arrows). H&E (×66). (Modified from Adam WS, Calhoun ML, Smith EM, et al. Microscopic Anatomy of the Dog: A Photographic Atlas. Springfield, IL: Charles C. Thomas, 1970.)

Anal Canal

The **anal canal** is the terminal segment of the digestive tract, where the simple columnar epithelium of the rectum changes abruptly to nonkeratinized stratified squamous epithelium at the **anorectal line** (Fig. 10-53). Also at the anorectal junction, the lamina muscularis of the rectum terminates.

The mucosa of the anal canal is smooth and lacks glands in ruminants and horses. In pigs and carnivores, however, the anal mucosa is divided into three distinct zones: (1) the columnar zone (zona columnaris ani), (2) the intermediate zone (zona intermedia), and (3) the cutaneous zone (zona cutanea). The **columnar zone** contains longitudinal folds, the **anal columns**, between which are grooves called **anal sinuses** (Fig. 10-53). The **intermediate zone** is a narrow strip located between the columnar zone and the cutaneous zone. Both the columnar and intermediate zones are lined with nonkeratinized stratified squamous epithelium, and modified tubuloalveolar sweat glands known as **anal glands** occupy the propria-submucosa. The anal glands produce a lipid secretion in cats and dogs (Fig. 10-53) and a mucous secretion in pigs. The **cutaneous zone** begins at the **anocutaneous line**, where the nonkeratinized stratified squamous epithelium of the intermediate zone changes abruptly to a keratinized form, marking the beginning of the cutaneous zone. This zone is lined with keratinized stratified squamous epithelium. In carnivores, the ducts from the **anal sacs** (**paranal sinuses**) open at the junction of the intermediate and cutaneous zones. These anal sacs and ducts are bilateral evaginations of the anal mucosa. In dogs, the mucosa of the outermost part of the cutaneous zone, near the junction with the skin, contains large, modified sebaceous glands known as **circumanal glands**. The anatomy and function of anal sacs, associated glands, and the circumanal glands are discussed further in Chapter 16.

At the anorectal junction, the outer longitudinal layer of the tunica muscularis of the rectum terminates. However, the inner circular layer continues into the anal canal and terminates as the internal anal sphincter muscle. The external anal sphincter muscle, which is circularly disposed skeletal muscle, surrounds the internal anal sphincter muscle.

Liver

The liver is the largest gland in the body and is characterized by multiple, complex functions: excretion (waste products), secretion (bile), storage (lipids, vitamins A and B, and glycogen), synthesis (fibrinogen, globulins, albumin, and clotting factors), phagocytosis (foreign particulate matter), detoxification (lipid-soluble drugs), conjugation (toxic substances and steroid hormones), esterification (free fatty acids to triglycerides), metabolism (proteins, carbohydrates, lipids, hemoglobin, and drugs), and hemopoiesis (in the embryo and potentially in the adult). An understanding of the structure of the liver is vital to the interpretation of these processes.

Capsule and Stroma

Each lobe of the liver is covered by a typical serosa (visceral peritoneum) overlying a thin CT capsule. CT from this capsule extends into the liver lobes as interlobular CT, surrounding individual liver lobules and supporting the vascular and bile duct systems. A fine network of reticular fibers surrounds the cells and sinusoids, with the capsule and interlobular CT possibly containing smooth muscle cells. Interlobular CT is very distinct and forms septa in pigs (Fig. 10-54), but scant and difficult to see in other species (Fig. 10-55). This difference accounts for the tougher texture of pork liver compared to that of beef liver.

Portal areas are expanded regions of interlobular CT which contain groups of vessels and ducts, including branches of the **portal vein, hepatic artery, bile duct**, and **lymph vessels**. These portal areas are present throughout any section of the liver (Figs. 10-54 and 10-55).

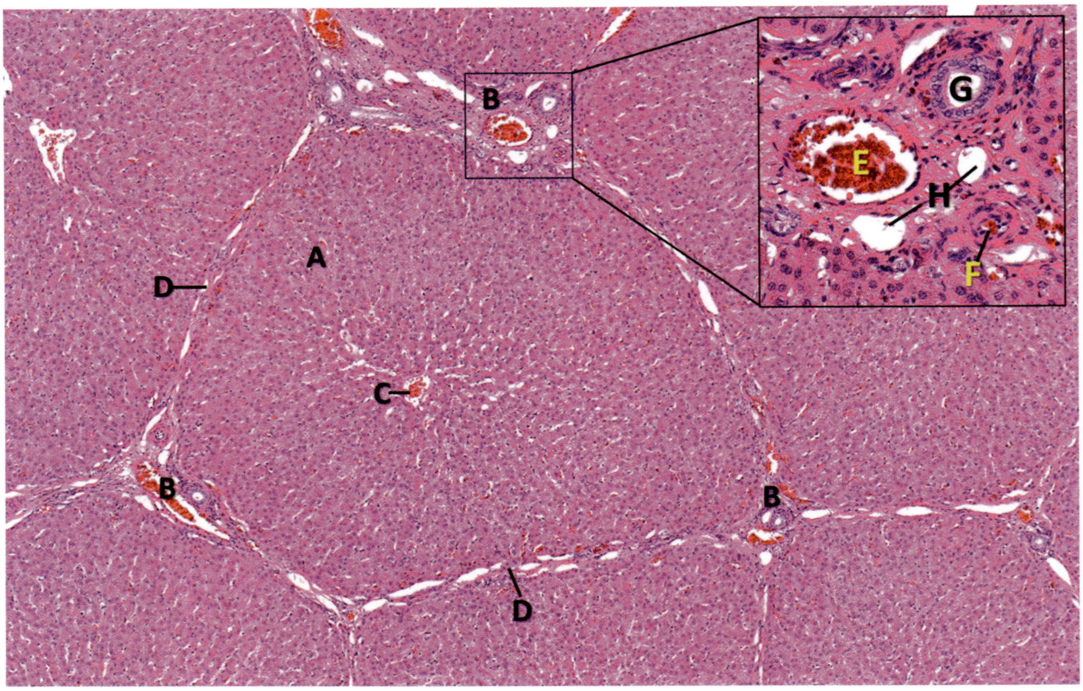

Figure 10-54 Liver (pig). Liver lobules (A), portal areas (B), central vein (C), and distinct interlobular CT (D). H&E (63×). Inset: Magnified portal area with branches of portal vein (E), hepatic artery (F), bile duct (G), and lymph capillaries (H). H&E (400×). (Image by J. Feng.)

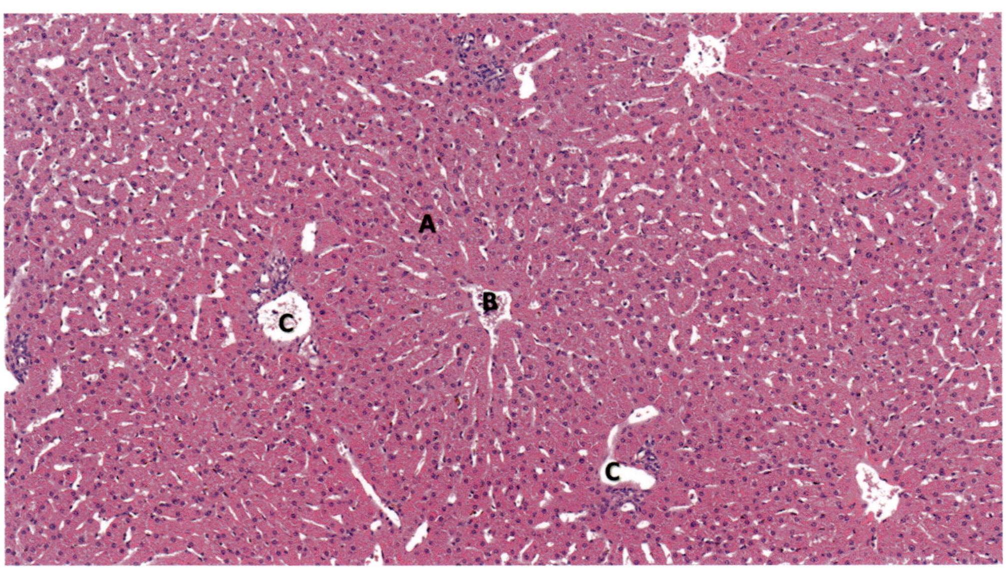

Figure 10-55 Liver (horse). Lobule (A) with central vein (B) is not separated from adjacent lobules by CT as is that of the pig in Figure 10-54. Interlobular portal venules (C) in portal areas. H&E (×124). (Image by J. Feng.)

Parenchyma

The **hepatocytes** are organized in rows or plates called **hepatic laminae**, arranged radially around the **central vein**. Each hepatocyte has six or more surfaces of three types: (a) microvillous surfaces facing the perisinusoidal space; (b) canalicular surfaces bordering the bile canaliculi; and (c) contact surfaces between adjacent hepatocytes where apposed cell membranes may have tight junctions and desmosomes (Fig. 10-56).

Hepatocytes typically have a centrally located spherical nucleus with one or more prominent nucleoli, occasionally showing binucleation. The appearance of the cytoplasm of hepatocytes varies widely, depending on nutritional and functional changes. Mitochondria are abundant, and the Golgi complex is usually near bile canaliculi but may be also juxtanuclear. There are numerous lysosomes, clusters of free ribosomes, and well-developed rER and sER that are often interconnected. At the ultrastructural level, glycogen is seen as dense granules in a rosette configuration. In routine histologic preparations, glycogen-rich areas appear grainy or as irregularly shaped empty spaces, whereas lipid-rich areas appear as round vacuoles. Bile pigments may be seen as fine yellow granules throughout the cytoplasm of normal hepatocytes. In cytology preparations stained with Wright's stain, these bile pigments appear as blue-green granules both inside and outside hepatocytes.

Considerable evidence indicates that not all hepatocytes are not functionally identical. Instead, specific enzyme patterns and metabolic systems may correlate with the position of the cell within the lobule. While hepatocyte metabolic activity is generally believed to be closely associated with blood supply, the extent of their similarity or dissimilarity in terms of metabolic systems, susceptibility to insults, and nutritional needs remains unresolved.

Bile Canaliculi and Bile Ducts

Hepatocytes absorb bilirubin (the principal bile pigment) from the blood, conjugate it, and secrete it as one component of bile. Bile salts, protein, and cholesterol are the other components. Bile is discharged into **bile canaliculi**, which are minute canals (0.5 to 1.0 μm in diameter) located between apposed hepatocytes (Figs. 10-56 and 10-57). These canaliculi are expanded intercellular spaces bordered by cell membranes with short microvilli that project into the lumen. Tight junctions prevent bile from escaping into the narrow intercellular space adjacent to the canaliculus.

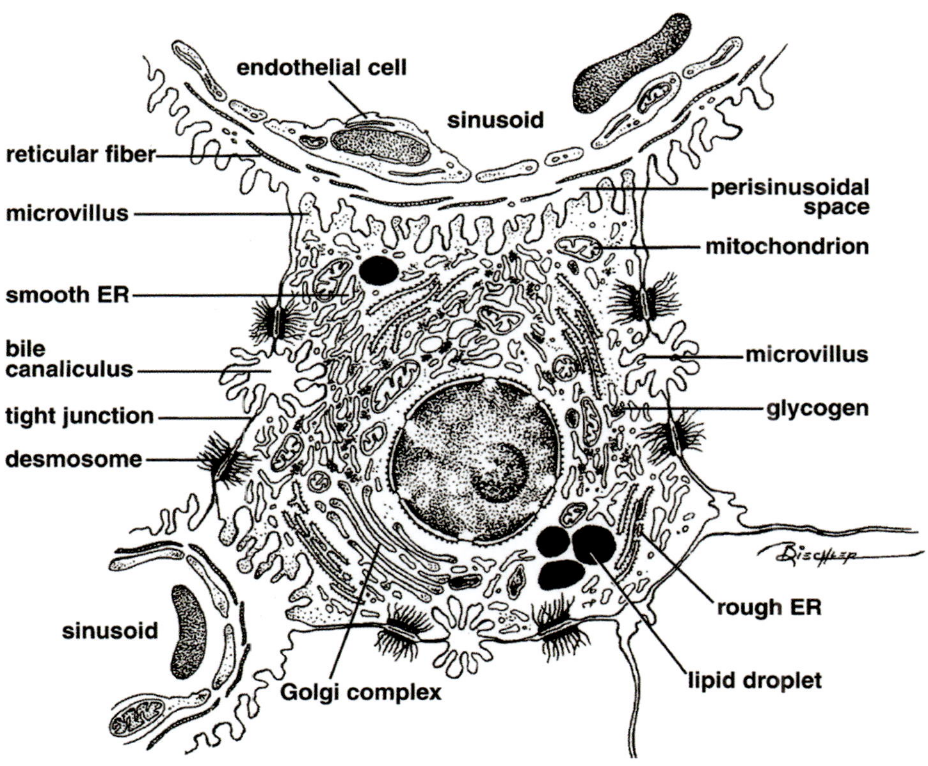

Figure 10-56 Drawing of an electron micrograph of a hepatocyte and adjacent structures.

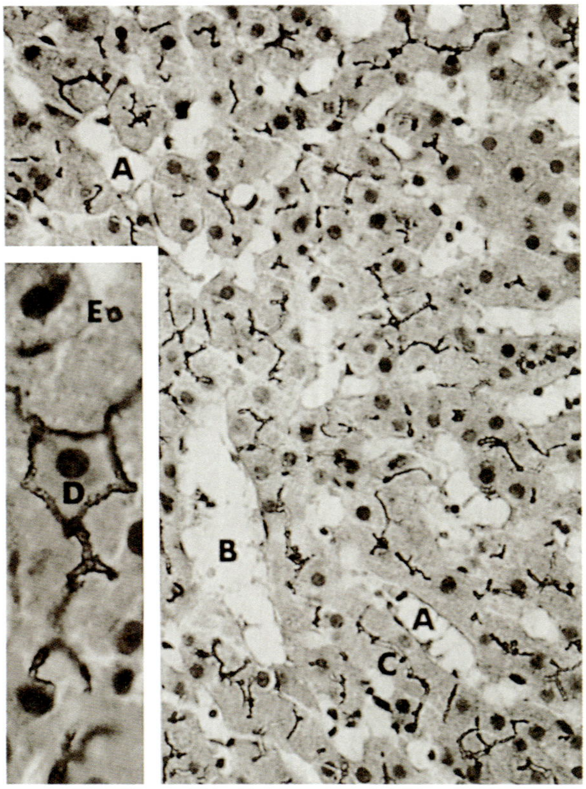

Figure 10-57 Liver (pig). Sinusoids (A), central vein (B), and liver laminae with bile canaliculi between the cells (C). Silver stain (×300). Inset: Bile canaliculi surrounding a hepatocyte (D) and a cross-section of a bile canaliculus (E). Silver stain (×768).

Bile flows through the bile canaliculi toward the periphery of the classic lobule, where it enters small **bile ductules** lined by low simple cuboidal epithelium. These ductules join **interlobular bile ducts** located in the portal canals, which are lined by simple cuboidal or simple columnar epithelium. Interlobular bile ducts converge to form progressively larger **intrahepatic ducts**, which ultimately exit the liver lobes through the **hepatic ducts**. The extrahepatic biliary passages include the hepatic ducts, the cystic duct (absent in horses), the bile duct, and the gallbladder. Hepatic ducts drain each individual liver lobe, while the **cystic duct** drains the gallbladder. The hepatic ducts and the cystic duct unite to form the **bile duct**, which empties into the duodenum. All of the extrahepatic biliary passages are lined by tall simple columnar epithelium.

Blood Supply

The vascularity of the liver is directly related to its multiple functions. The liver has a dual blood supply: the **portal vein** brings blood from the intestines and associated organs, while the **hepatic artery** supplies the liver cells with oxygenated blood. These vessels enter the liver at a hilus, called the porta, located on its visceral surface. Branches (rami) of these two vessels enter the liver lobes, where they branch out and follow the interlobular CT. The smaller branches within the portal area are termed the **interlobular portal venule** and the **interlobular hepatic arteriole** (Fig. 10-54).

The interlobular portal venules give rise to small branches, sometimes called distributing venules, which form the axis of the liver acinus. Short terminal venules arise from the distributing venules and end directly in the sinusoids. Most of the blood from the interlobular hepatic arterioles enters a capillary plexus within the portal area and interlobular CT; only a small portion of the blood reaches the sinusoids directly by way of terminal arterioles.

The **hepatic sinusoids** are blood capillaries located between hepatic laminae, that course through the lobule to transport blood from terminal branches of the interlobular hepatic arteriole and interlobular portal venule to the **central vein**. These sinusoids often communicate with each other via interruptions in the hepatic laminae. This branching arrangement ensures that hepatocytes are in proximity to at least one sinusoidal surface. Sinusoids are lined by a porous endothelium resting on a discontinuous basal lamina (Fig. 10-56). The endothelial cells contain small pores that lack diaphragms. The pores are too small to allow the passage of blood cells, but blood plasma can flow through them freely. In the liver of ruminants, the sinusoids differ in that the endothelium is nonporous and the basal lamina is continuous.

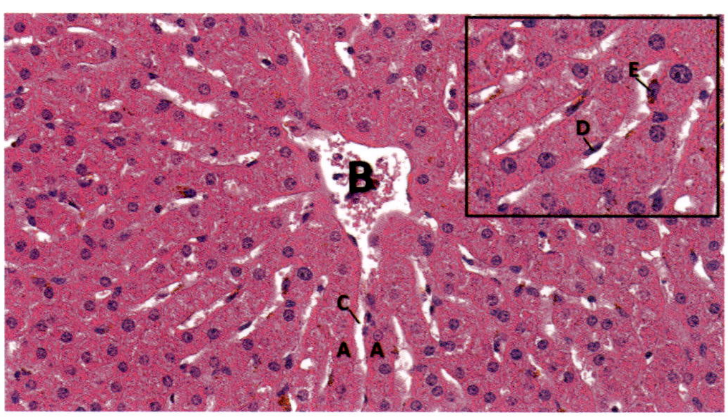

Figure 10-58 Liver laminae and sinusoids (horse). The hepatic cells are arranged in laminae (A) radially toward the central vein (B). The sinusoids (C) are the slits between the laminae. H&E (×400). Inset: Endothelial cell (D) lining the sinusoid and a Kupffer cell (E). H&E (×800). (Image by J. Feng.)

Kupffer cells, the resident **macrophages** with a stellate shape, are present within the sinusoid lumen and are attached to the luminal surface of endothelial cells (Fig. 10-58). Derived from blood monocytes, they are integral components of the monocyte-macrophage system. These cells often extend long pseudopodia through the endothelial pores or between the cells and are highly phagocytic (Fig. 10-59).

The endothelium is separated from the hepatocytes by a space called the **perisinusoidal space (or space of Disse)**. Hepatocyte microvilli project into the perisinusoidal space, which is filled with plasma, allowing a direct exchange of substances between blood and hepatocytes.

In addition to the hepatocyte microvilli, the perisinusoidal space contains reticular fibers as well as **perisinusoidal adipocytes** (**Ito cells** or **hepatic stellate cells**). These cells act as pericytes and are believed to store vitamin A and synthesize type III collagen following liver injury.

Blood within the sinusoids exits the lobule via the **central vein** (Figs. 10-54 and 10-55). Central veins are lined by endothelium resting on a thin adventitia. They connect with **sublobular veins** at the periphery of the lobules. Sublobular veins join to form progressively larger veins that eventually form the **hepatic veins**, which drain directly into the caudal vena cava.

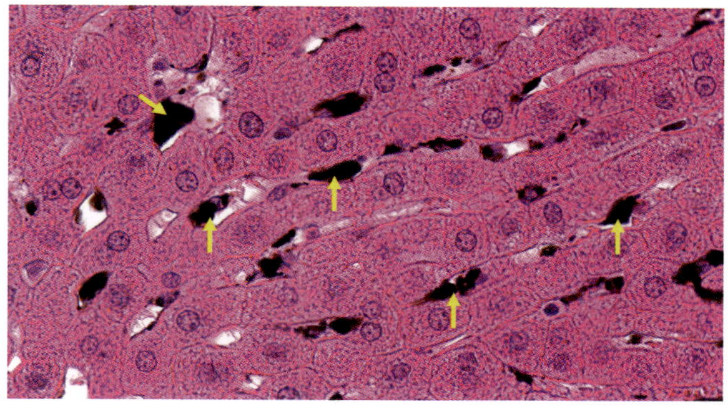

Figure 10-59 Phagocytic activity of Kupffer cells in liver (rat). The Kupffer cells taking up the intravascular injected carbon particles before sacrifice are visualized as black spots (arrows). H&E (×800). (Image by J. Feng.)

Lymph and Lymph Vessels

Lymph in the liver is formed within the perisinusoidal space. It flows toward the periphery of the lobule and enters the intercellular spaces of the portal area and interlobular CT. Here, it diffuses into lymph capillaries within the portal areas (Fig. 10-54). From there, the lymph is carried from the portal areas by larger lymph vessels that ultimately exit the liver at the porta. These lymph vessels proceed to drain to the hepatic lymph nodes.

The Classic Liver Lobule—The Anatomic Unit of the Liver

The clear delineation afforded by abundant interlobular CT in the liver of pigs has led to the recognition of **hepatic lobules** (**classic liver lobules**). This morphologic unit is organized around the central vein (Figs. 10-54, 10-55, and 10-60). Each lobule forms a polyhedral prism of hepatic tissue measuring approximately 2 mm long and approximately 1 mm wide. Cross-sectional profiles of this lobule are roughly hexagonal, with the sinusoids converging from the periphery to the central vein, where they drain. Portal areas are present at approximately three of the six angles of the lobule. The parenchyma located between the portal areas and the central vein consists of cells arranged in branching plates or laminae (Fig. 10-58). These laminae are a single cell thick, and the surfaces of the cells facing the sinusoids are exposed. Throughout the laminae, there is an interconnected network of bile canaliculi formed by the adjacent cell membranes of hepatocytes (Fig. 10-57).

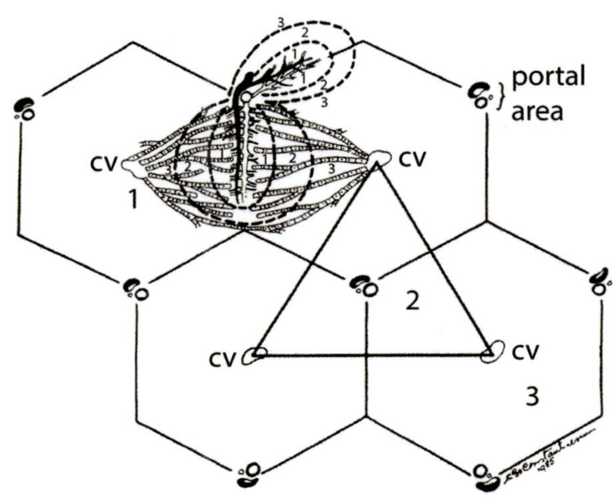

Figure 10-60 Schematic drawing of the functional units of the liver in relation to the anatomic unit (classic hepatic lobule). 1. *Liver acinus* with three zones on each side of the vascular backbone. 2. *Portal lobule* with an interlobular bile ductule (in the portal area) as the axis and one central vein (CV) at each point of the triangle. 3. *Classic hepatic lobule* (anatomical unit) with the central vein as its axis.

The Portal Lobule and the Liver Acinus—Functional Units of the Liver

The **portal lobule** is a functional unit developed to highlight the exocrine function of the liver, specifically bile secretion. It is defined as a triangular area consisting of the parenchyma of three adjacent classic lobules, drained by the bile ductule located in the portal area. Thus, the axis (center) of the portal lobule is the interlobular bile ductule in the portal area, while the peripheral angles are formed by the central veins of the three adjacent lobules (Fig. 10-60).

The **liver acinus** is a functional unit that delineates the vascular supply to the parenchyma. It forms a roughly diamond-shaped area made of parts of two classic lobules, supplied by terminal branches of the interlobular portal venule and interlobular hepatic arteriole. These blood vessels run perpendicular to a portal area between two hepatic lobules to form the axis of the acinus, and the two central veins are positioned at the opposite points of the diamond shape (Fig. 10-60). Within the liver acinus, three distinct zones have been identified. **Zone 1** is closest to the vascular axis of the acinus. In this zone, hepatocytes receive an excellent nutrient and oxygen supply and are metabolically most active. Cells in this zone also may be the first to encounter and process toxic substances entering the liver. **Zone 2** exhibits intermediate metabolic activity, receiving a moderate supply of oxygen and nutrients. **Zone 3**, which borders the central vein, experiences the lowest supply of oxygen and nutrients, making these hepatocytes less metabolically active and more susceptible to hypoxic conditions.

Gallbladder

Bile produced by the liver is *stored* in the gallbladder and *concentrated* by the reabsorption of water and inorganic salts. In its contracted (empty) state, the gallbladder mucosa forms numerous folds (**plicae**). As it fills and expands, these folds tend to flatten, resulting in a smoother mucosal surface. A tall simple columnar epithelium lines the luminal surface of the gallbladder and extends into mucosal **crypts**, which are small epithelial diverticula that can resemble glands (Fig. 10-61). Two types of columnar cells are present in the gallbladder epithelium. The most common type is the "light" cell, which has a pale cytoplasm of uniform density. The cytoplasm of the apical region contains vesicles but is devoid of organelles. Electron-dense bodies with smooth outlines occur in the subapical and supranuclear cytoplasm. The less numerous "dark" cells are scattered among the light cells. They have a narrow profile and contain a dark, dense cytoplasm with few organelles and a nucleus that is more heterochromatic than that of the light cells. The epithelial cell surface is covered with microvilli, and tight junctions (zonulae occludens) between adjacent cells prevent the passage of fluids from the lumen of the organ. Goblet cells are characteristic of the epithelium in some species, such as cattle, while globule leukocytes may be found in the epithelium of cats. Endocrine cells, possibly belonging to the APUD system (characterized by *a*mine *p*recursor *u*ptake and *d*ecarboxylation), have been described in gallbladder epithelium of cattle.

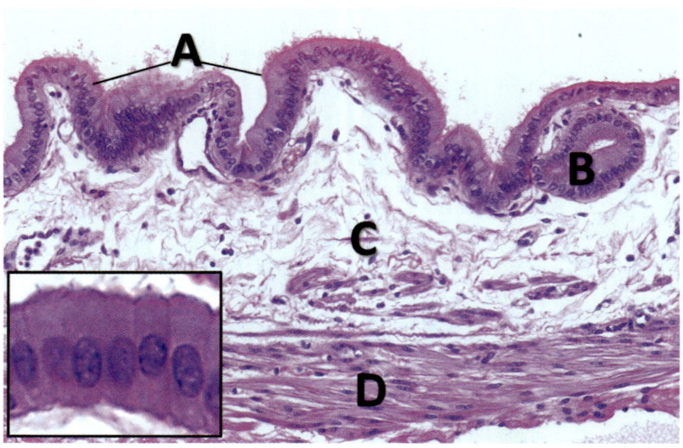

Figure 10-61 Gallbladder (dog). Mucosal plicae (A), cross-sections of a mucosal crypt (B), propria-submucosa (C), and tunica muscularis (D). H&E (×250). Inset: Simple columnar epithelial lining. H&E (×800). (Image by J. Feng.)

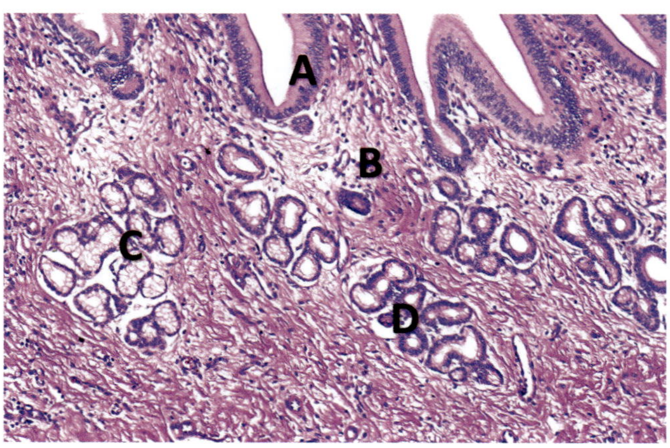

Figure 10-62 Gallbladder (large ruminant). Simple columnar epithelium (A), propria-submucosa (B), mucous glands (C), and serous glands (D). H&E (×186). (Image by J. Feng.)

The propria-submucosa (lacking a lamina muscularis) is composed of loose CT. Lymphatic tissue, which can be either diffuse or nodular, is often present. In some species, particularly ruminants, glands are present in the propria-submucosa. These glands may be serous or mucous, depending on the species, individual, or their location within the mucosa (Fig. 10-62). The tunica muscularis consists of thin bundles of smooth muscle cells that generally course in a circular direction. The muscle is supplied by both sympathetic and parasympathetic axons.

The walls of the hepatic, cystic, and bile ducts are composed of the same tunics as the gallbladder.

Pancreas

The pancreas is an encapsulated, lobulated, compound tubuloacinar gland containing both exocrine and endocrine parts (Fig. 10-63). The exocrine part functions to produce a variety of enzymes, including amylase, lipase, and trypsin, which act on the products of gastric digestion as they reach the duodenum. The endocrine part, known as pancreatic islets (or islets of Langerhans), produces mainly glucagon by A cells and insulin by B cells (Fig. 10-64). The histologic structure of the islets is discussed in Chapter 12.

The parenchyma of the pancreas is separated into distinct lobules by a CT stroma. Each lobule is composed of secretory units and intralobular ducts.

The secretory units of the pancreas are tubuloacinar, with a small lumen. The tubular portion is more prominent in ruminants. The glandular epithelial cells are generally pyramid-shaped, with a spherical nucleus located near the base of the cells (Fig. 10-65). The cytoplasm surrounding the nucleus is intensely basophilic and contains an extensive rER and

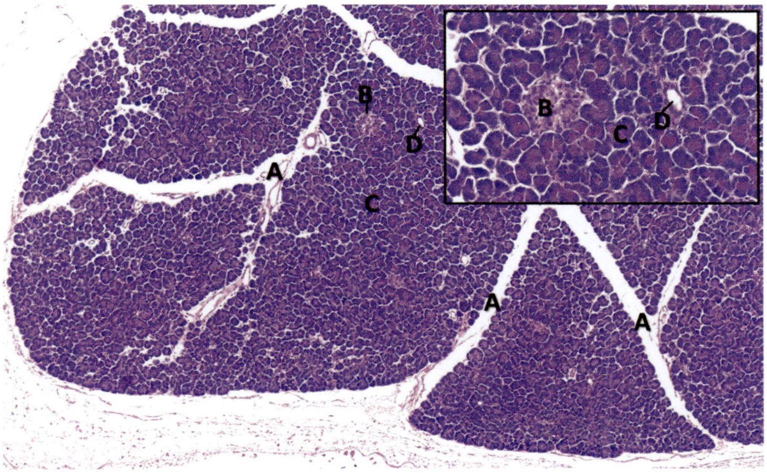

Figure 10-63 Lobulation of pancreas (dog). The lobules are divided by the interlobular CT (A). Pancreatic islet (B), pancreatic acini (C), and intralobular duct (D). H&E (×180). Inset: Magnified pancreas parenchyma. H&E (×400). (Image by J. Feng.)

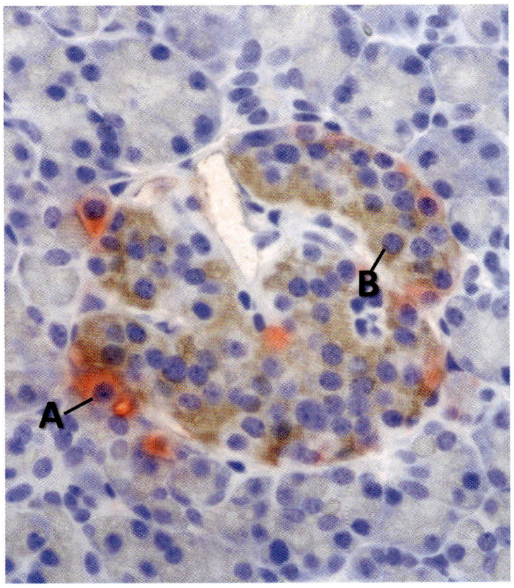

Figure 10-64 Pancreatic islet surrounded by pancreatic acini (dog). Glucagon-producing A cells are stained in red (A) and insulin-producing B cells are stained in yellow brown (B). Immunohistochemistry with hematoxylin counterstain (×400). (Image by J. Feng.)

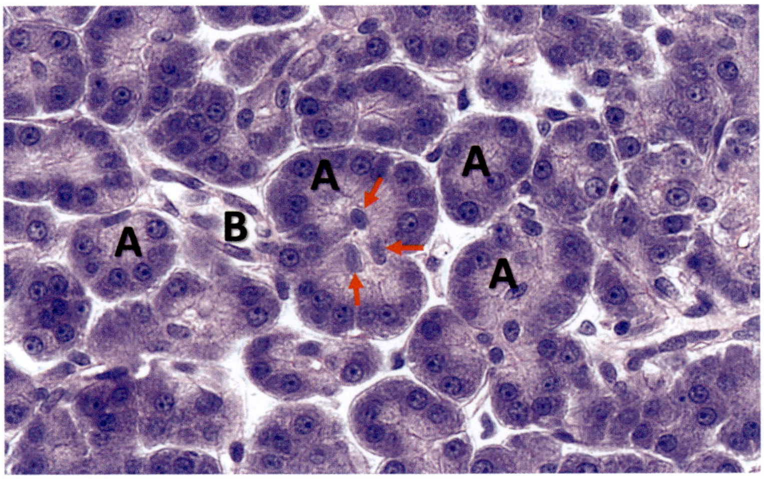

Figure 10-65 Pancreas (dog). Pancreatic acini (A), intercalated duct (B), and three centroacinar cells (arrows). H&E (×800). (Image by J. Feng.)

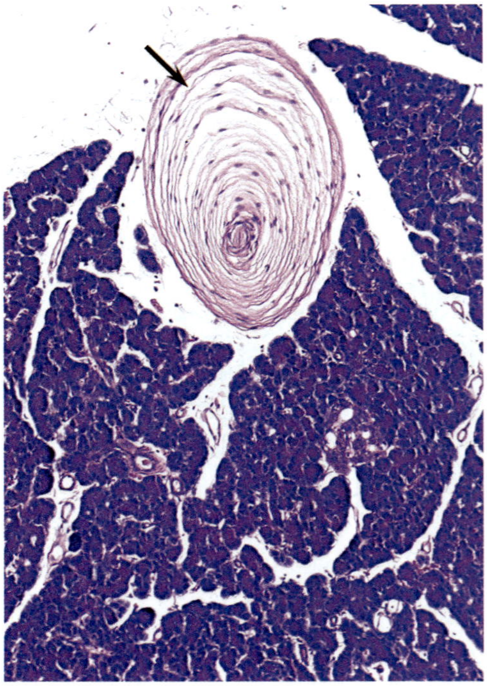

Figure 10-66 Pancreas (cat). An onion-shaped Pacinian corpuscle (arrow) in the interlobular CT. H&E (×150). (Image by J. Feng.)

numerous mitochondria. The apical region of the cells contains eosinophilic, membrane-bounded zymogen granules that are filled with the zymogens synthesized in the rER. An extensive Golgi complex is located between the nucleus and the zymogen granules. Acinar cells have receptors for **cholecystokinin**, a hormone produced by endocrine cells in the small intestine. Cholecystokinin stimulates the release of pancreatic enzymes as well as the contraction of the tunica muscularis of the gallbladder.

The tubuloacinar secretory unit is continuous with a short **intercalated duct**. This duct begins with flattened cells that extend into the lumen of the acinus; therefore, they are referred to as **centroacinar cells** (Fig. 10-65). Centroacinar cells, along with intercalated duct cells, secrete bicarbonate and water when stimulated by the polypeptide **secretin**. Bicarbonate helps raise the pH of intestinal contents, thereby facilitating the action of digestive enzymes in the intestine. Intercalated ducts join **intralobular ducts**, which are lined by low, simple cuboidal epithelium. Unlike the "striated" intralobular ducts of the parotid salivary gland, those in the pancreas lack this feature. The intralobular ducts continue into **interlobular ducts** lined by simple columnar epithelium. These interlobular ducts converge to eventually form the main **pancreatic duct** and the **accessory pancreatic duct**, both of which empty into the duodenum. Goblet cells may be present in the epithelium of larger ducts.

The stroma of the pancreas consists of a thin capsule that gives rise to delicate CT septa separating the lobules. Frequently, **lamellar (Pacinian) corpuscles** are present in the interlobular CT of the pancreas of cats (Fig. 10-66), implying a role in detecting changes in pancreatic tissue tension or pressure, potentially relevant in physiological processes such as digestion, pancreatic secretion regulation, or responses to external mechanical stimuli.

Avian Digestive System

The oral cavity is lined entirely by a keratinized stratified squamous epithelium. The propria-submucosa contains abundant diffuse lymphatic tissue and salivary glands. The tongue is also covered by a keratinized stratified squamous epithelium and contains bundles of skeletal muscle, lingual salivary glands, and the **entoglossal bone**. Taste buds are found only on the base of the tongue and the floor of the oral cavity. All salivary glands are branched tubular mucous glands with openings into a common cavity, from which an excretory duct leads to the oral cavity.

The esophagus is similar in structure both cranial and caudal to the crop. It is characterized by a thick nonkeratinized stratified squamous epithelium. The lamina propria is a loose CT containing large mucous glands. The lamina muscularis consists of longitudinally arranged smooth muscle fibers. The submucosa consists of a thin layer of loose CT. The tunica muscularis is composed of a thick inner circular layer and a thin outer longitudinal layer of smooth muscle (Fig. 10-67).

The **crop** is a sac-like diverticulum of the esophagus. It is a storage organ where the ingested food is moistened by the mucous secretions from the esophageal glands. The histologic structure of the crop is similar to that of the esophagus, but it lacks mucous glands except near its junction with the esophagus (Fig. 10-68).

Birds do not have a glandular stomach similar to that of mammals, but instead have two separate organs between the esophagus and the duodenum. The **proventriculus**, or "glandular" stomach, and the **ventriculus** (**gizzard**), or "muscular" stomach, collectively perform many of the functions of the mammalian stomach.

The mucosa of the **proventriculus** is characterized by macroscopic papillae with numerous microscopic folds (plicae) of varying height that are arranged concentrically around the single duct opening at the apex of each papilla (Fig. 10-69). Simple columnar epithelium covers these plicae and continues into three generations of ducts of the **proventricular glands** (Fig. 10-69). The glands are lined by a simple cuboidal to low columnar epithelium, where adjacent cells make direct contact only on their basal half, giving the luminal surface a serrated appearance. Only one cell type is identifiable

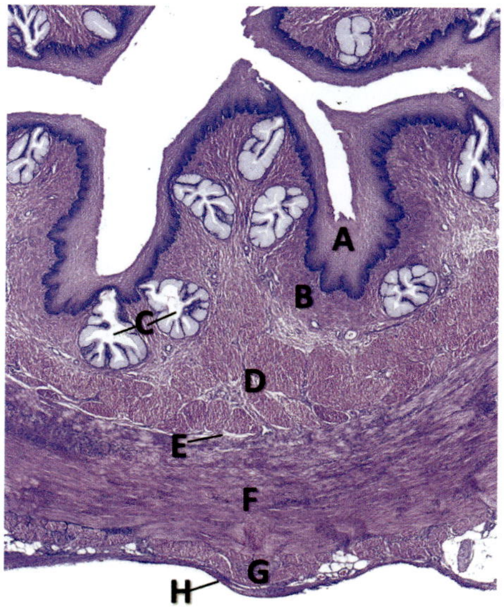

Figure 10-67 Esophagus (chicken). Nonkeratinized stratified squamous epithelium (A), lamina propria (B), mucous glands (C), longitudinal lamina muscularis (D), very thin submucosa (E), inner circular layer (F), and outer longitudinal layer (G) of tunica muscularis. H&E (×40). (Image by J. Feng.)

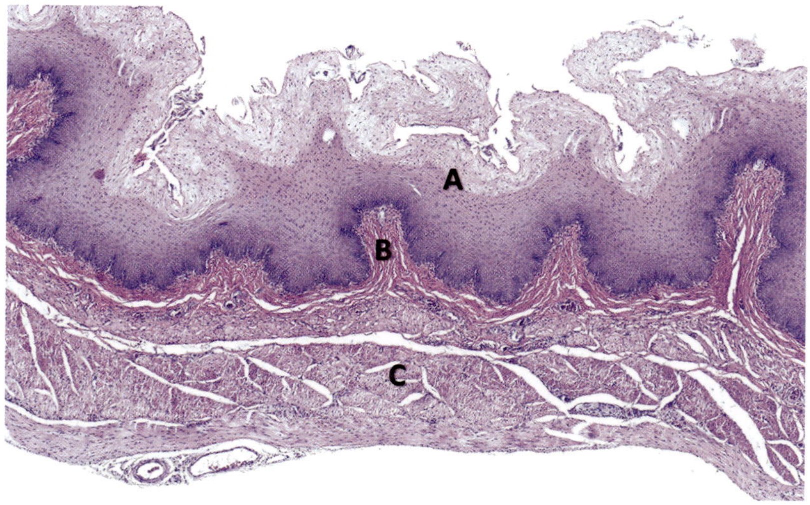

Figure 10-68 Crop (chicken). Thick nonkeratinized stratified squamous epithelium (A), lamina propria (B), and tunica muscularis (C). Note the absence of mucous glands in lamina propria. H&E (×83). (Image by J. Feng.)

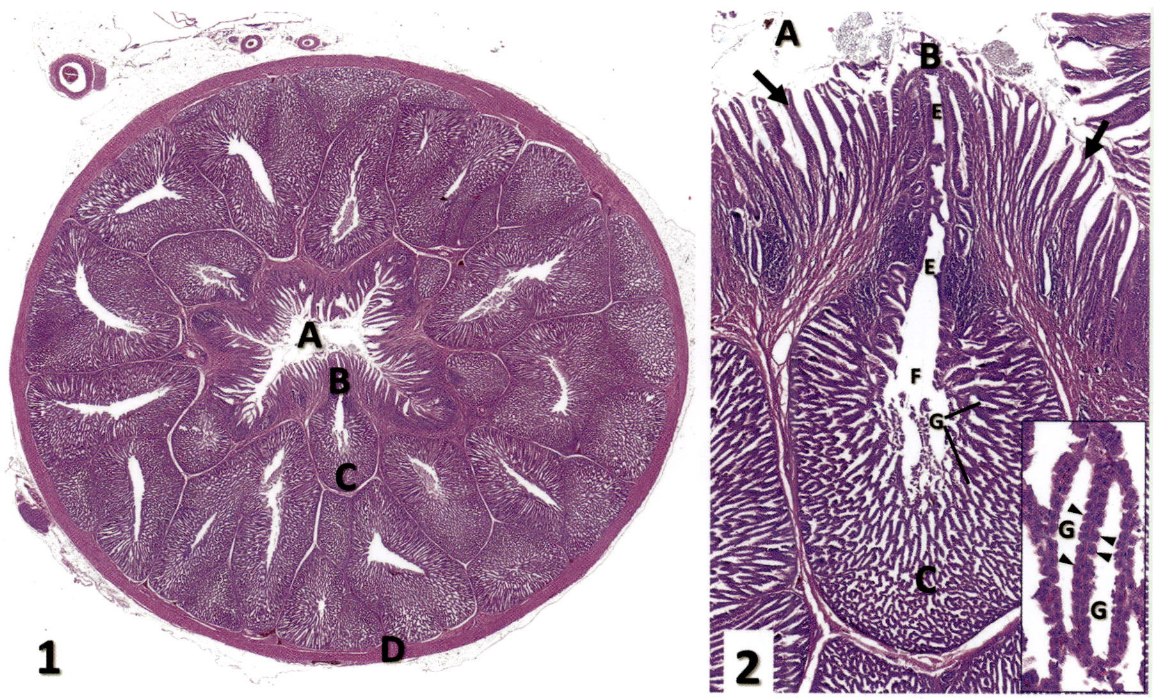

Figure 10-69 Proventriculus, glandular stomach (chicken). Lumen (A), papilla (B) with plicae (arrows), proventricular glands (C) lined with simple cuboidal oxynticopeptic cells (arrowheads in the inset), tunica muscularis (D), primary (E), secondary (F), and tertiary (G) ducts of the proventricular gland. 1. Overview under lower magnification. (x8). 2. Magnified view of papilla with plicae (×52). Inset: Two magnified glands with tertiary ducts (×400). H&E. (Image by J. Feng.)

(**oxynticopeptic cells**) that produces both pepsinogen and HCl. The secretory products are delivered into the lumen through a series of ducts (tertiary, secondary, and primary ducts). The lamina propria is typical loose CT. The lamina muscularis is split into a very thin inner layer and a thick outer layer by the proventricular glands. A typical two-layered tunica muscularis, consisting entirely of smooth muscle, underlies the loose CT of the very thin submucosa (Fig. 10-69). The proventriculus is covered by a typical **serosa**.

The **ventriculus** is a highly muscular organ responsible for grinding and macerating the ingesta (Fig. 10-70 [1]). Its lining is referred to as the **cuticle** or **koilin membrane** (Fig. 10-70 [2]), which protects the muscular walls. The membrane is not keratinous but is a polysaccharide–protein keratinoid complex (koilin) in which the cystine content is considerably less than it is in keratin; therefore, it is not a stratum corneum. The thickness of this membrane varies with the bird's diet; birds consuming grains and seeds tend to have thicker membranes than those eating softer foods such as fruits, worms, or meat. Koilin is secreted by mucosal glands (Fig. 10-70 [2]) and surface epithelial cells. The glands produce hard koilin rodlet clusters that integrate into the membrane and are separated by softer koilin produced by the surface epithelial cells. The surface epithelium is simple columnar, while the epithelium of the branched tubular mucosal glands is simple cuboidal. The gland lumens are filled with a secretory product that stains bright red with keratohyalin stains. The lamina propria and submucosa are both composed of loose CT. The lamina muscularis is discontinuous, and the tunica muscularis is a single thick layer of parallel smooth muscle cells extending from two aponeuroses at the center of the organ, crossed by bands of dense CT. The outermost layer is a typical serosa.

The histologic structure of the **small intestine** in birds is similar to that of the mammalian small intestine. The lamina propria and submucosa contain large amounts of diffuse and nodular lymphatic tissue. Submucosal glands are generally absent in the duodenum. The tunica muscularis is composed of inner circular and outer longitudinal layers of smooth muscle. The outermost tunic is a typical serosa.

Two **ceca** open into the digestive tract at the junction of the ileum and rectum. This organ has three distinct regions with slightly different histologic features. The proximal portion contains prominent villi. In adult birds, large masses of diffuse and nodular lymphatic tissue infiltrate the lamina propria and submucosa of this portion, forming grossly visible **cecal tonsils**. In the midportion, the villi are shorter and broader, and mucosal folds are present. The distal ceca are devoid of villi, with the surface epithelium of the mucosa being simple columnar with goblet cells.

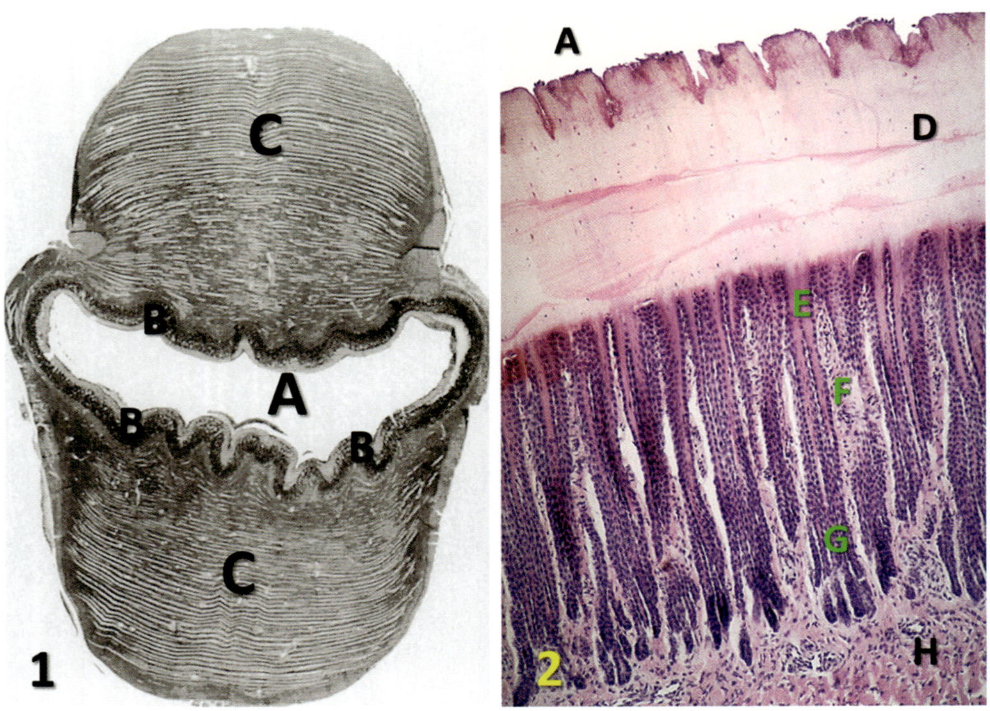

Figure 10-70 Ventriculus, gizzard, or muscular stomach (chicken). Lumen (A), mucosa layer (B), smooth muscle of tunica muscularis (C), cuticle/koilin membrane (D), gastric pit (E), lamina propria (F), mucosal glands (G), and submucosa (H). 1. Overview under lower magnification (x10). 2. A magnified view of the mucosa layer (x200). H&E.

The **rectum**, a part of the large intestine, extends from the ileum to the coprodeum of the cloaca. It resembles the small intestine in that villi are present. Scattered diffuse and nodular lymphatic tissues occur in the lamina propria and submucosa.

The **cloaca** is divided by transverse folds into three parts: the **coprodeum**, **urodeum**, and **proctodeum**. All three parts have a similar structure. Villi are present and the epithelium of the mucosa is simple columnar. The **cloacal bursa** (or **bursa of Fabricius**) is a blind sac-like dorsal diverticulum of the wall of the proctodeum of the cloaca. Masses of follicle-like lymphoid tissue accumulate in the lamina propria beneath the lining epithelium (Fig. 10-71). The bursa is considered a central (primary) lymphoid organ equivalent to mammalian bone marrow for the maturation of B lymphocytes. It regresses with age at the onset of reproductive activity (laying of eggs in females).

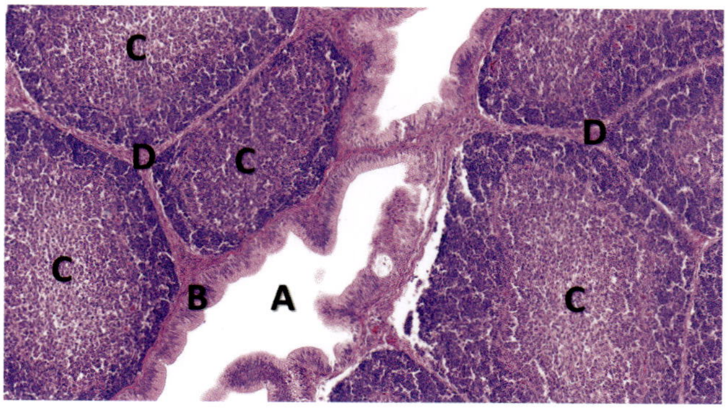

Figure 10-71 Cloacal bursa (chicken). Lumen (A) opens to the proctodeum, columnar lining epithelium (B), lymphoid tissues (C) in lamina propria, and CT septa (D). H&E (×200). (Image by J. Feng.)

Histologic features of the liver, gallbladder, and exocrine pancreas of the bird are not significantly different from those of the same organs in mammals.

Clinical Correlations

The liver plays a central role in processing material from the intestine through the portal system, exposing it to harmful factors and pathogens. Metabolic, nutritional, infectious disease, and local or metastatic neoplasms can affect the liver. Inflammation of the liver, known as hepatitis (Fig. 10-72), can occur. Hepatic lipidosis, or excess fat storage in the liver, is a clinical issue in obese animals experiencing physiological stress (e.g., dairy cattle after parturition, ewes carrying twins late in pregnancy—pregnancy toxemia). Mobilization of large amounts of triglycerides causes fatty acids to overwhelm the capacity of the liver, potentially causing rapid, fatal outcomes, with cases of sudden death not uncommon.

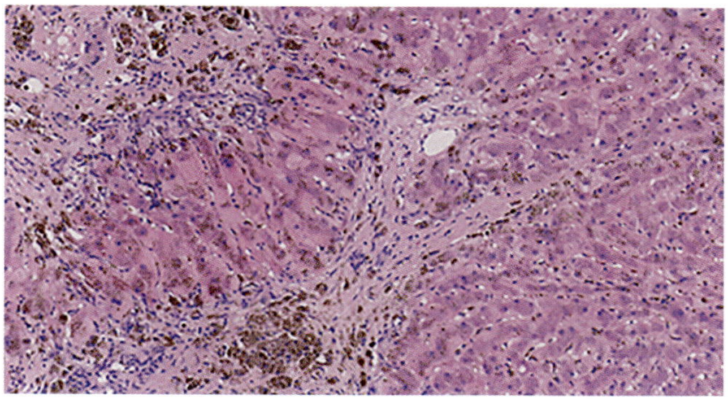

Figure 10-72 Equine liver with chronic hepatitis, showing severe fibrosis, loss of normal architecture, abundant hemosiderin (brown cells), and hepatocyte degeneration. (Reproduced with permission from Salguero Bodes FJ, Pallares Martinez FJ. Aughey and Frye's Comparative Veterinary Histology with Clinical Correlates. 2nd ed. Boca Raton: CRC Press, 2023.)

Essentials

Stomach. Mucosa has a glandular (carnivores) or a glandular and nonglandular epithelium (herbivores). Surface cells of the glandular epithelium produce mucinogen, and the gastric glands produce digestive enzymes (chief cells) and HCl (parietal cells). The nonglandular epithelium is stratified squamous epithelium with varying degrees of keratinization depending upon species.

Small Intestine (Duodenum, Jejunum, and Ileum). The mucosa is lined as a simple columnar surface epithelium over villi containing mucous-producing goblet cells and absorptive enterocytes. At the base of the villi, the epithelium extends down into crypts that can contain enteroendocrine cells and Paneth cells that produce antimicrobial peptides. The ileum contains aggregate lymphoid nodules (Peyer's patches), and surface epithelium can contain some microfolds (M cells) that transcytose macromolecules (antigens) to immune cells.

Large Intestine (Cecum Colon, Rectum, and Anal Canal). The mucosa lacks the villi of the small intestine, and it contains simple tubular intestinal glands with abundant goblet cells. The cecum often contains lymphatic nodules.

Liver. A fibrous CT capsule subdivides liver into lobes and lobules. It receives blood from the hepatic artery (20 to 30%) and the portal vein (70 to 80%). Blood flows through sinusoids lined by discontinuous endothelium that contains fixed macrophages (Kupffer cells), and blood exits the lobules via the central vein. The parenchymal cells (hepatocytes) are arranged in anastomosing and branching plates. Hepatocytes have abundant rER and sER; numerous lysosomes, peroxisomes, and mitochondria; glycogen deposits; and lipid droplets.

Liver Organization.
Classic liver lobule: It defines the flow of blood from portal areas to a central vein.
Portal lobule: It defines the flow of bile from three adjacent lobules into a bile duct.
Liver acinus: It is identified by two adjacent central veins and portal areas and defines the metabolic gradient from periportal areas to the central vein: Zone 1 (oxidative functions), Zone 2 (intermediate zone), and Zone 3 (low oxygen area; susceptible to hypoxia).

Liver Major Functions.
Gluconeogenesis: It converts amino acids, lactate, and glycerol (a component of lipids) into glucose.
Detoxification: A microsomal mixed-function oxidase enzyme system (cytochrome P450) catalyzes methylation, oxidation, or conjugation of drugs, toxins, and chemicals.
Storage: It includes glycogen, triglycerides, and vitamin A.
Plasma protein production: It includes fibrinogen, prothrombin, and albumin, as well as urea.
Acute phase proteins: They include production of bile and secretion of IgA into the bile.

Pancreas.
Structure and exocrine function: It is surrounded by a delicate capsule that subdivides the organ into lobules. Secretion of digestive enzymes occurs via a duct system (intercalated into intralobular into interlobular). Intercalated duct cells secrete HCO_3^- to inhibit enzyme activation within the duct system. Enzymes include trypsinogen, chymotrypsinogen, lipase, and amylase. The pancreas of cats has lamellar (Pacinian) corpuscles within the CT.
Endocrine function: It includes secretion of glucagon (alpha cells), insulin (beta cells), somatostatin (delta cells), ghrelin (epsilon cells), and PP cells (pancreatic polypeptide) (see Chapter 12).

Suggested Readings

Adam WS, Calhoun ML, Smith EM, et al. Microscopic Anatomy of the Dog: A Photographic Atlas. Springfield, IL: Charles C. Thomas, 1970: 102.
Boshell JL, Wilborn WH. Histology and ultrastructure of the pig parotid gland. *Am J Anat* 1978;152:447–465.
Chu RM, Glock RD, Ross RF. Gut-associated lymphoid tissue of young swine with emphasis on some epithelium of aggregated lymph nodules (Peyer's patches) of the small intestine. *Am J Vet Res* 1979;40:1720.
Costa M, Brookes SJ, Hennig GW. Anatomy and physiology of the enteric nervous system. *Gut* 2000;47(Suppl 4) :15–19; discussion iv26. doi: 10.1136/gut.47.suppl_4.iv15.iv
Dyce KM, Sack WO, Wensing CJG. Textbook of Veterinary Anatomy. 5th Ed. Philadelphia: WB Saunders Company, 2017.
Gemmell RT, Heath T. Fine structure of sinusoids and portal capillaries in the liver of adult sheep and the newborn lamb. *Anat Rec* 1972;172:57–70.
Herdt T. Regulation of gastrointestinal function. In: Cunningham JG, ed. Textbook of Veterinary Physiology. 6th Ed. Philadelphia: Elsevier, 2019.
Hyttel P, Sinowatz F, Vejlsted M, et al. Essentials of Domestic Animal Embryology. 1st Ed. Edinburgh: Elsevier, 2009.
International Committee on Veterinary Gross Anatomical Nomenclature. Nomina Anatomica Veterinaria. 6th Ed. Ithaca, NY: International Committee on Veterinary Gross Anatomical Nomenclature, 2017.
International Committee on Veterinary Histological Nomenclature. Nomina Histologica. 3rd Ed. revised Ed. Ithaca, NY: International Committee on Veterinary Histological Nomenclature, 2017.
Kadhim KK, Zuki ABZ, Noordin MM, et al. Histomorphology of the stomach, proventriculus and ventriculus of the red jungle fowl. *Anat Histol Embryol* 2011;40:226–233. doi: 10.1111/j.1439-0264.2010.01058.x.
Kmieć Z, Kmieć Z. Introduction—Morphology of the liver lobule. *Cooperation of liver cells in health and disease.* 2001:1–6.
Krstić RV. Ultrastructure of the Mammalian Cell. New York: Springer-Verlag, 1979.

Krstić RV. General Histology of the Mammal. New York: Springer-Verlag, 1985.
Nara T, Yasui T, Fujimori O, et al. Histochemical properties of sialic acids and antimicrobial substances in canine anal glands. *Eur J Histochem* 2011;55(3):e29. doi: 10.4081/ejh.2011.e29.
Salguero Bodes FJ, Pallares Martinez FJ. Aughey and Frye's Comparative Veterinary Histology with Clinical Correlates. 2nd ed. Boca Raton: CRC Press, 2023.
Titkemeyer CW, Calhoun ML. A comparative study of the structure of the small intestines of domestic animals. *Am J Vet Res* 1955;16:152–157.
Zahariev P, Sapundzhiev E, Pupaki D, et al. Morphological characteristics of the canine and feline stomach mucosa. *Anat Histol Embryol* 2010;39(5):464–471.

11

Urinary System

Marxa L. Figueiredo and John J. Turek

CHAPTER MENU

The urinary system is composed of two kidneys, two ureters, a urinary bladder, and a urethra. The kidneys excrete nitrogenous wastes and regulate the volume and composition of body fluids through the processes of blood filtration, reabsorption of filtered solutes and water, and secretion of electrolytes. The ureters conduct urine from the kidneys to the urinary bladder, which stores the urine and expels it via the urethra.

Dellmann's Textbook of Veterinary Histology, Seventh Edition. Edited by Marxa L. Figueiredo and John J. Turek.

Companion website: www.wiley.com/go/figueiredo/vethistology7e

Kidney

General Organization

Superficial Anatomic Features

In all species, both kidneys are retroperitoneal and positioned either flat against the lumbar muscles or suspended from the dorsal abdomen. The right kidney is usually slightly more cranial than the left. Within each kidney, the renal artery and vein, lymphatics, nerves, and the ureter pass through a single indentation called the hilus (or hilum).

The kidneys of domesticated animals have various shapes (Fig. 11-1). In dogs, cats, sheep, and goats, the external surface of the kidney is smooth and bean shaped. In pigs, the kidneys are smooth, elongated, and flattened. In horses, the kidneys are smooth; however, only the left kidney is bean shaped, whereas the right kidney is heart shaped. In large ruminants, the overall shape is oval, but multiple lobes are visible on the surface. The surface of the kidney is encased by a fibrous capsule primarily made up of collagen fibers (Fig. 11-2), which also may contain smooth muscle and blood vessels.

The simplest form of the mammalian kidney is the **unipapillary kidney**, which has a single renal pyramid that includes a base adjacent to the cortex and an apex known as the papilla. The unipapillary kidney is common in laboratory animals and represents the basic unit for more complex kidney structures. In species like cats, dogs, horses, sheep, and goats, the kidneys are **unilobar**, where the papillae merge or fuse to form a single renal crest, which then empties into the renal pelvis (Fig. 11-1). Pigs, large ruminants, and humans have a **multilobar** (or multipyramidal) **kidney** with numerous medullary pyramids and papillae. In these kidneys, the papillae release urine into extensions of the renal pelvis or ureter called **calyces** (both minor and major) or into the pelvis directly.

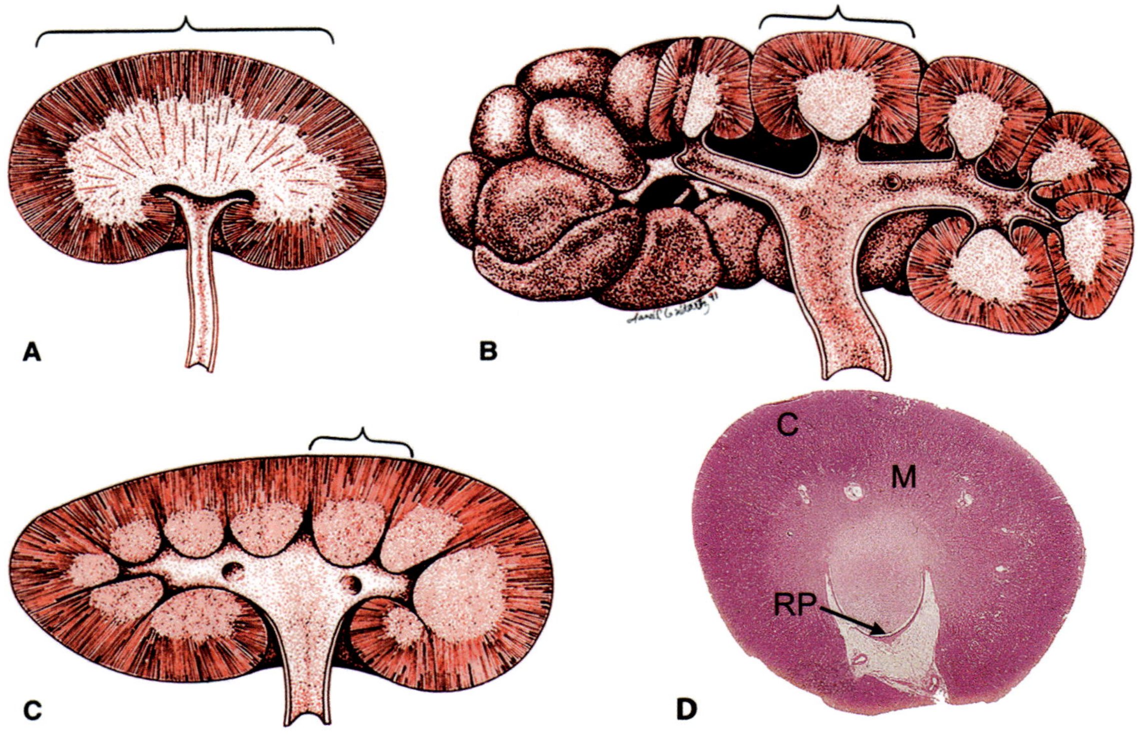

Figure 11-1 Schematic drawing of the gross structure and lobation pattern in different kidneys. **A, D.** Unilobar kidney typical of carnivores. **B.** Multilobar kidney typical of large ruminants. Each lobe is distinctly outlined by deep grooves, and this kidney lacks a renal pelvis. **C.** Multilobar kidney of the pig with a smooth surface. In the bovine kidney, the lobes are clearly demarcated (bracket in **B**), while in the porcine kidney, cortical portions of the lobes fuse (bracket in **C**). In the carnivore kidney (also equine and small ruminant kidneys), lobes fuse extensively (bracket in **A**) to give the appearance of a single lobe ("unilobar"). (Redrawn from Dellmann H-D, Brown EM. *Textbook of Veterinary Histology*. Philadelphia, PA: Lea & Febiger, 1987) **D.** Cortex (C) of cat kidney stains darker than the medulla (M). Urine from collecting tubules empties into the renal pelvis (RP). Hematoxylin and eosin (H&E) (×1). (Image by W.E. Haensly)

Cortex and Medulla

A longitudinal or transverse section through the kidney shows two regions: an outer, dark red **cortex** and an inner, lighter-colored **medulla** (Fig. 11-1D). Within the renal cortex, structures are arranged into **medullary rays** and the **cortical labyrinth** (Fig. 11-3). These terms originated from the distinct composition of the cortex relative to the medulla. Unlike the medulla, which is composed entirely of straight tubule segments, the renal cortex contains both straight and convoluted tubule segments. In a transverse section, the medulla appears striated throughout, while the straight segments within the cortex form parallel bundles that appear to radiate outward from the medulla toward the fibrous capsule, forming "medullary rays." The medullary rays contain cortical collecting ducts (CCDs), cortical thick ascending limbs (CTALs) of the loop of Henle, and proximal straight tubules (PSTs). Sections of the cortical labyrinth contain irregular profiles of convoluted tubules, including the proximal convoluted tubule (PCT), the distal convoluted tubule (DCT), and the connecting segment (CNT). In addition, the cortical labyrinth contains renal corpuscles, the distal thick ascending limb (which diverges from the medullary ray to contact the juxtaglomerular [JG] apparatus of the glomerulus), and the initial collecting tubule.

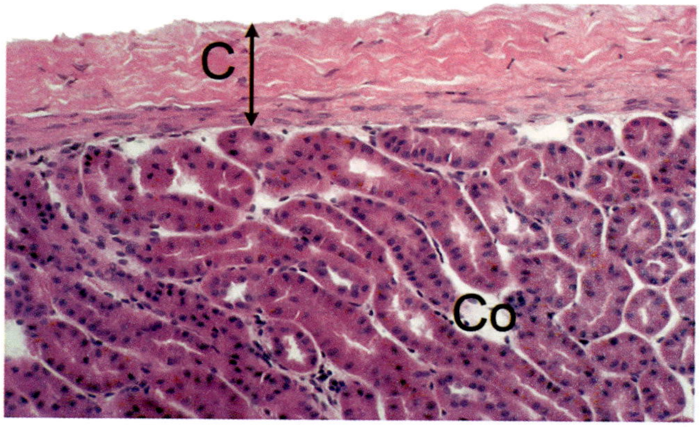

Figure 11-2 Dense irregular connective tissue (CT) forms the capsule (C) of the kidney. A portion of the renal cortex (Co) beneath the capsule shows profiles of many proximal convoluted tubules. Kidney, dog. H&E (×250). (Image by W.E. Haensly)

The **outer medulla** lies deeper than the cortex, with the arcuate blood vessels marking the border between the cortex and the outer medulla (Fig. 11-4). Within the outer medulla, there are distinct regions known as the **outer** and **inner stripes**. The outer stripe is the outermost region of the outer medulla and contains proximal straight tubules, thick ascending limbs, and collecting ducts. In contrast, the inner stripe is the inner portion of the outer medulla. Here, proximal tubules are absent, and the transition from proximal straight tubules to thin descending limbs of Henle's loop marks the boundary between the outer and inner stripes. Therefore, the inner stripe contains the collecting ducts, thick ascending limbs, and thin descending limbs of Henle's loop.

The **inner medulla** is located deeper within the kidney than the outer medulla. The transition between the thin limbs and thick ascending limbs (TAL) of Henle's loop demarcates the boundary between the inner and outer medulla. Thus, the inner medulla lacks segments of the thick ascending limb, containing only collecting ducts and descending and ascending thin limbs of Henle's loop, along with capillaries and lymphatics. Macroscopically, the inner medulla can be subdivided into the **base** and the **papilla** or **renal crest**. The base is adjacent to the outer medulla. The papilla, or renal crest, is the terminal portion of the inner medulla, which extends into the renal pelvis or calyces.

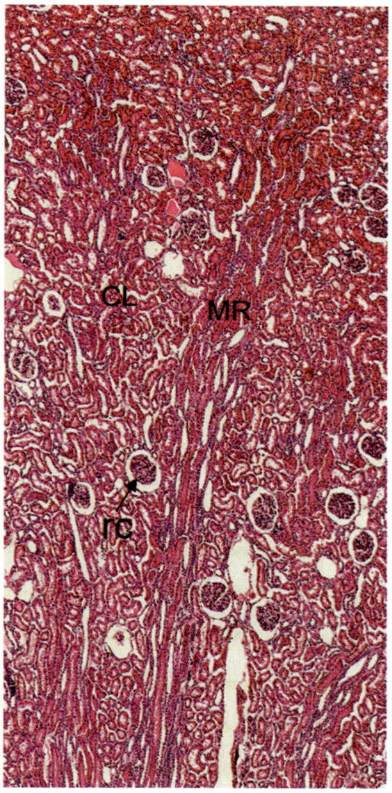

Figure 11-3 The cortex of the kidney is composed of the cortical labyrinth (CL) and medullary rays (MRs). Convoluted tubules, renal corpuscles (rc), distal thick ascending limbs, and initial collecting ducts are found in the cortical labyrinth. The medullary rays contain the cortical collecting ducts, cortical thick ascending limbs of the loop of Henle, and the proximal straight tubule. H&E (×40).

Parts of the Renal Corpuscle and the Renal Tubule

The following lists the components of the renal corpuscle and the segments of the renal tubule in sequence from where the filtrate is formed to where it is released as urine:

- I) Nephron
  - A) Renal corpuscle
    - 1) Glomerulus
      - a) Glomerular capillaries
      - b) Mesangium
    - 2) Glomerular capsule (Bowman's capsule)

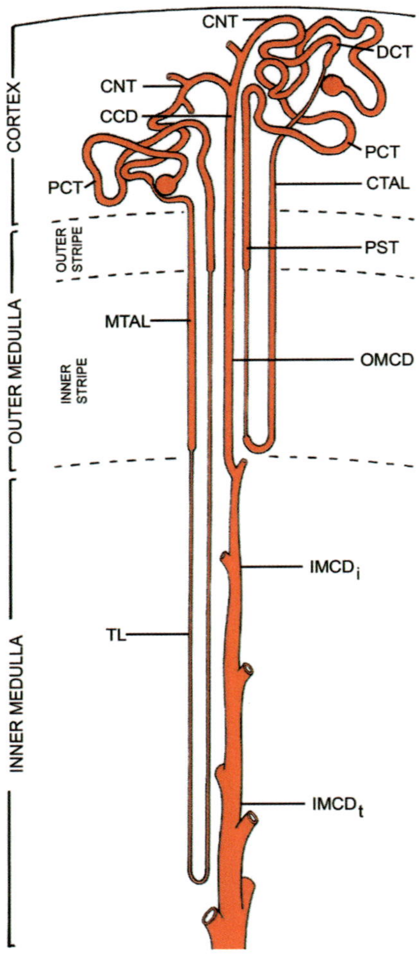

Figure 11-4 Schematic drawing of the relationships between various segments of the nephron and collecting duct and regions of the kidney. Long-looped (left) and short-looped (right) nephrons are illustrated. CCD, cortical collecting duct; CNT, connecting segment; CTAL, cortical thick ascending limb; DCT, distal convoluted tubule; IMCD, initial inner medullary collecting duct; IMCD$_t$, terminal inner medullary collecting duct; MTAL, medullary thick ascending limb; OMCD, outer medullary collecting duct; PCT, proximal convoluted tubule; PST, proximal straight tubule; TL, thin limb of the loop of Henle. Glomeruli, PCT, DCT, terminal segments of the CTAL, and CNT are located in the cortical labyrinth; PST, CTAL, and CCD are located in the medullary rays in the cortex. (From Madsen KM, Verlander JW. Renal structure in relation to function. In: Wilcox CS, Tisher CC, eds. *Handbook of Nephrology and Hypertension*. 5th Ed. Philadelphia, PA: Lippincott Williams and Wilkins, 2004.)

B) Proximal tubule
   1) Proximal convoluted tubule, including both S1 and S2 segments
   2) Proximal straight tubule, including both S2 and S3 segments
C) Thin limbs of Henle's loop
   1) Descending portion
   2) Ascending portion
D) Thick ascending limb of Henle's loop
E) Distal convoluted tubule
F) Connecting segment

II) Collecting duct
   A) Arcade—initial collecting tubule
   B) Straight portions
      1) Cortical collecting duct
      2) Outer medullary collecting duct
      3) Inner medullary collecting duct

Nephron

The **nephron** is the structural and functional unit of the kidney, consisting of the glomerulus and all segments of the renal tubule through the connecting segment. The number of nephrons varies among species. Dogs have ~400,000, whereas cats have ~200,000 per kidney. In carnivores and pigs, species where the young are relatively immature at birth, nephron formation may continue for several weeks postnatally. After renal maturity, new nephrons typically are not formed.

Nephrons can be classified either by the location of their renal corpuscles in the cortex as **superficial** (near the capsule), **midcortical**, or **juxtamedullary** (near the medulla), or by the length of their loop of Henle as **short-looped** or **long-looped** (Fig. 11-4). **Short-looped nephrons** generally have superficial or midcortical renal corpuscles and tubules that extend only into the outer medulla before returning to the cortex. In pigs, the loops turn in the medullary ray within the cortex. **Long-looped nephrons** have juxtamedullary renal corpuscles and tubules that extend deep into the inner medulla before returning to the cortex. Most species have both short- and long-looped nephrons. However, cats, dogs, and many species native to arid climates have predominantly long-looped nephrons, which are more efficient at conserving water. Conversely, beavers, which live in fresh water, have predominantly short-looped nephrons.

Renal Corpuscle

General Structure

The **renal corpuscle** is composed of the glomerular capillary tuft, the mesangium, and the glomerular capsule (Bowman's capsule) (Figs. 11-5 and 11-6). Previously, the term "**glomerulus**" referred only to the glomerular capillary tuft and mesangium, but it is now used widely to denote the entire renal corpuscle. The renal corpuscle is spherical and varies in size among species, with larger animals usually having larger corpuscles. For example, horse corpuscles average 220 µm in diameter, whereas cat corpuscles average 120 µm in diameter. Blood vessels enter and exit the glomerulus at the **vascular pole**. Opposite the vascular pole is the **urinary pole**, where the glomerular capsule opens into the proximal convoluted tubule.

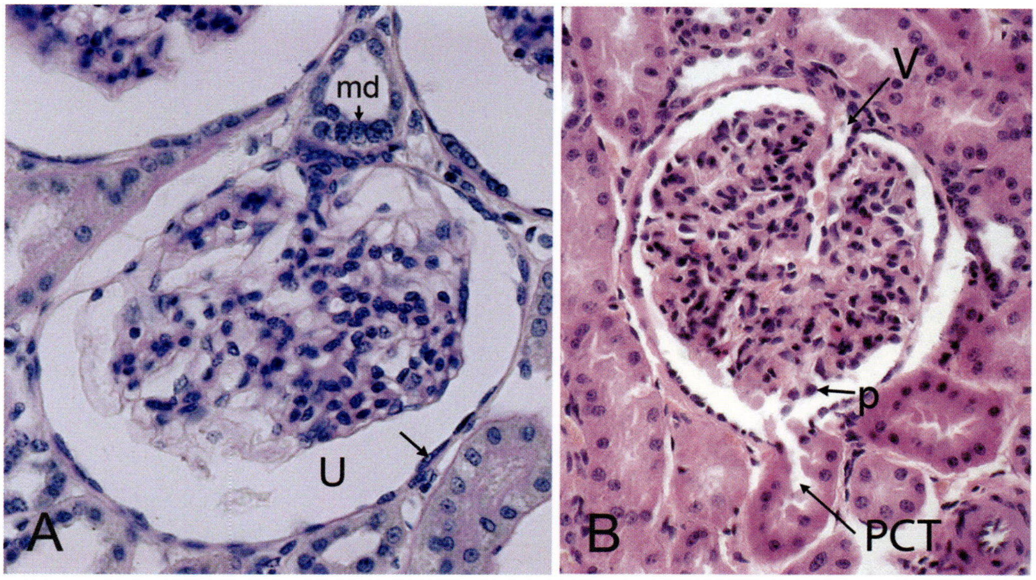

Figure 11-5 **A.** The macula densa (MD) of the juxtaglomerular apparatus is located in the thick ascending limb at the vascular pole of the renal corpuscle. The glomerular filtrate collects in the urinary space (U) of the glomerular capsule. The glomerular capsule is lined by a parietal layer of squamous cells (arrow). PAS (×200). **B.** The vascular pole (V) where afferent and efferent arterioles enter and leave the glomerulus. The glomerular capillaries are surrounded by a visceral layer of podocytes (p). The proximal convoluted tubule (PCT) begins at the urinary pole of the renal corpuscle. H&E (×200).

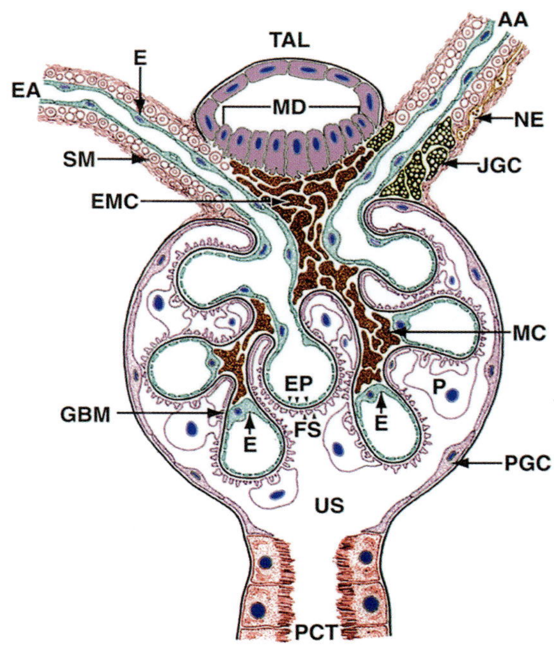

Figure 11-6 Schematic drawing of the renal corpuscle and juxtaglomerular apparatus. The afferent arteriole (AA) supplies the glomerulus, while the efferent arteriole (EA) carries blood away. Endothelial cells (E) lining the arterioles are nonporous, contrasting with glomerular endothelial cells (EP) that have pores (or fenestrations). Mesangial cells (MC) reside alongside glomerular endothelial cells on the same side of the glomerular basement membrane (GBM). The glomerular capsule surrounds the glomerulus; podocytes (P) cover the capillaries, forming the visceral layer. These podocytes reflect at the vascular pole and continue as the parietal layer of simple, squamous epithelial cells (PGC). Podocyte foot processes contact the GBM, and the spaces between these processes are the filtration slits (FS). The urinary space (US) is continuous with the lumen of the proximal convoluted tubule (PCT). The juxtaglomerular apparatus includes the macula densa (MD) in the thick ascending limb (TAL), extraglomerular mesangial cells (EMC), juxtaglomerular cells (JGC), and the afferent and efferent arterioles, both of which contain smooth muscle (SM) in the tunica media. Nerve endings (NE) are near juxtaglomerular cells. (Redrawn from Koushanpour E, Kriz W. *Renal Physiology. Principles, Structure and Function*. New York: Springer-Verlag, 1986.)

Glomerular Capillaries

The **glomerular capillary tuft** forms a network of branching and anastomosing capillaries. These capillaries are lined by a very thin layer of fenestrated endothelium; the diameter of these fenestrations or pores ranges from 50 to 150 nm (Fig. 11-7). Blood enters via the afferent arteriole and leaves through the efferent arteriole at the vascular pole (Fig. 11-6).

The **glomerular basement membrane** (GBM) serves as a barrier that separates the endothelial cells on its inner surface from the visceral epithelial cells, or podocytes, which cover its outer surface (Fig. 11-7). The GBM is composed of three

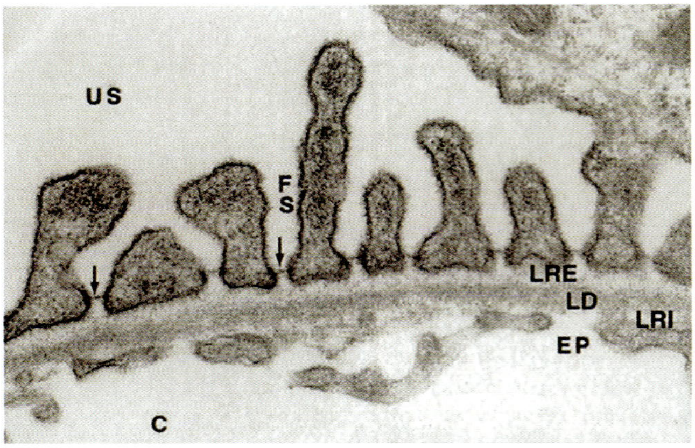

Figure 11-7 Transmission electron micrograph of the glomerular basement membrane (rat). The blood within the glomerular capillary (C) is selectively filtered as it passes through the endothelial pores (EP), the three layers of the glomerular basement membrane (lamina rara interna [LRI], lamina densa [LD], and lamina rara externa [LRE]), and the filtration slits (FS) between the podocytic foot processes, ultimately entering the urinary space (US). Note the filtration diaphragms (arrows), which bridge adjacent foot processes (×67,000).

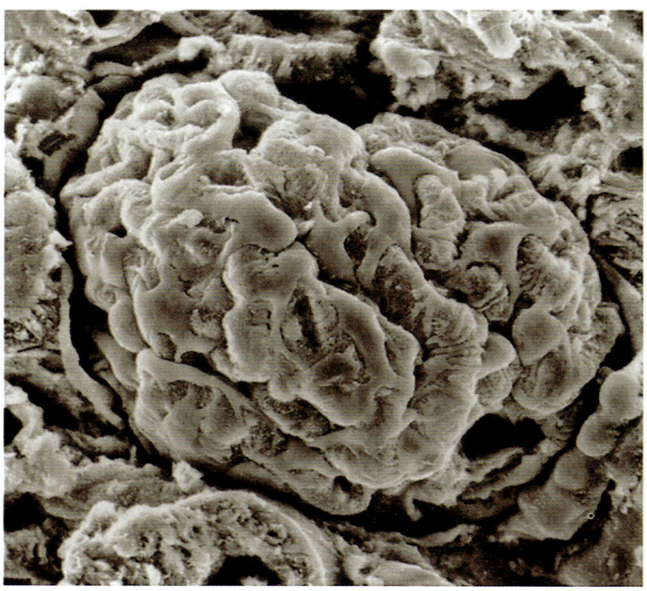

Figure 11-8 Scanning electron micrograph of the glomerulus (rat) as seen from the urinary space. The parietal layer of the glomerular capsule has been removed, revealing the visceral layer of podocytes embracing the glomerular capillaries. The large, smooth-surfaced cell bodies of the podocytes extend primary processes that branch into secondary and tertiary processes (pedicels) (×1300).

layers: the **lamina rara interna**, adjacent to the endothelium; the **lamina rara externa**, adjacent to the podocytes; and the **lamina densa**, situated between the laminae rara. These terms, lamina rara and lamina densa, refer to the electron density of the layers when viewed with a transmission electron microscope—lamina rara appears electron lucent, while lamina densa appears electron dense, and thus dark in electron micrographs. In dogs, the GBM is 100 to 250 nm thick and is largely composed of type IV collagen, heparan sulfate proteoglycans, and the glycoproteins laminin, fibronectin, and entactin. The GBM is stained by the periodic acid-Schiff (PAS) reaction, which facilitates the microscopic evaluation of the glomeruli in renal biopsies.

Mesangium

The **mesangium** forms the core of the glomerulus and is composed of specialized contractile cells embedded within an acellular matrix (Fig. 11-6). Mesangial cells have elongated, irregular cell processes and contain bundles of microfilaments made up of contractile proteins. They are interconnected to adjacent mesangial cells by gap junctions. The functions of mesangial cells include phagocytosis, production of the mesangial matrix, maintenance of capillary loop integrity, and regulation of glomerular blood flow by controlling capillary resistance. The mesangial matrix is characterized by a dense network of microfibrils surrounded by an amorphous material that is similar to the GBM.

Glomerular Capsule

The **glomerular capsule**, also known as Bowman's capsule, surrounds the glomerulus (Figs. 11-5 and 11-6). The relationship between the glomerular capillary tuft and the glomerular capsule has been compared to a fist inserted into a partially inflated balloon. In this analogy, the fist represents the glomerular capillary tuft, the part of the balloon directly covering the fist represents the visceral epithelium, and the outer layer of the balloon not in contact with the fist represents the parietal epithelium. The space between the visceral and parietal layers is called the **urinary space** or Bowman's space (Figs. 11-6 and 11-7).

The visceral epithelial cells, or **podocytes**, cover the outer surface of the glomerular capillaries (Figs. 11-8 to 11-10). Each podocyte's cell body contains the nucleus and originates several large primary processes, from which smaller secondary and tertiary processes emanate. The smallest of these extensions are called **foot processes** or **pedicels**. The secondary and tertiary foot processes of one cell interdigitate with those of adjacent cells. The narrow spaces (25 to 60 nm) between foot processes are called **filtration slits**, which are bridged by the **slit diaphragm** (Fig. 11-7). The **parietal epithelium**, consisting of a layer of simple squamous epithelium that lines the capsule, undergoes an abrupt transition at the urinary pole to the cuboidal proximal tubule epithelium (Fig. 11-11).

An additional epithelial cell in Bowman's capsule is the **peripolar cell**. Peripolar cells are located at the vascular pole of the glomerulus, situated at the junction between the parietal and visceral epithelia, and facing the urinary space. They are particularly large and prominent in sheep and goats. Peripolar cells contain dark-staining, membrane-bounded granules that contain albumin, transthyretin, immunoglobulins, neuron-specific enolase, and kallikrein but not renin. The cells also contain adseverin, a protein involved in exocytosis in secretory cells. Thus, it is believed that the peripolar cell is a secretory cell, although its specific function remains unknown.

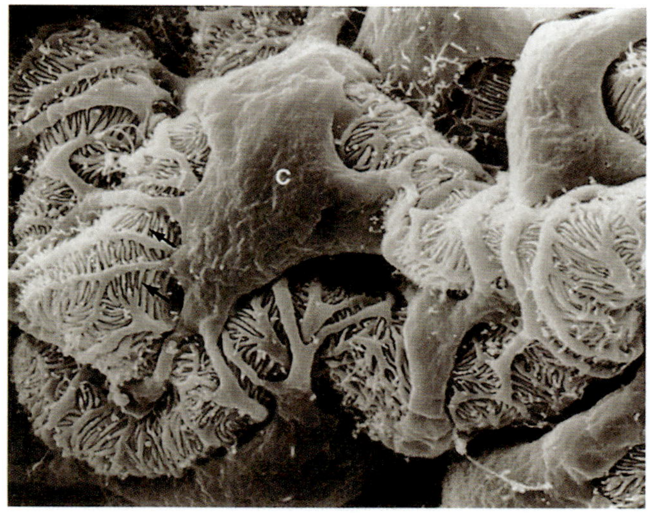

Figure 11-9 Scanning electron micrograph of podocytes (rat). The cell body (C) of one podocyte is in the center of the field. Numerous processes of varying size extend from the cell body, wrapping around the glomerular capillaries and interdigitating with secondary and tertiary processes of other podocytes (×4100).

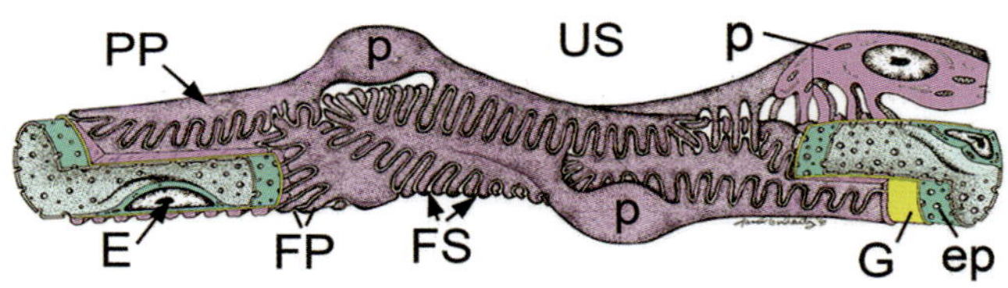

Figure 11-10 Schematic drawing of the components of the filtration barrier of the kidney. The capillaries consist of the glomerular basement membrane (G) lined by the endothelium (E), which contains numerous endothelial pores (ep) or fenestrations. Podocytes (p) cover the outer side of the GBM, with primary processes (PP) branching into secondary and tertiary processes, forming small foot processes (FP). Components of the plasma pass through the endothelial pores, the glomerular basement membrane, and the filtration slits (FS) to form the glomerular filtrate in the urinary space (US).

Renal Tubule

Proximal Tubule

The **proximal tubule** begins at the urinary pole of the renal corpuscle (Figs. 11-11 and 11-12 and Table 11-1). The proximal tubule is the longest cortical tubule segment, making proximal tubule profiles highly prevalent in histologic sections of the cortex. The initial portion of the proximal tubule is called the proximal convoluted tubule (**PCT**) because it twists and turns in the cortical labyrinth until it reaches the medullary ray. Here, it transitions into the proximal straight tubule (**PST**). The PST traverses through the medullary ray and extends into the outer stripe of the outer medulla. The proximal tubule segments are further classified as segments S_1, S_2, and S_3, based on variations in length or the abundance of features common to all proximal tubule cells. Segment S_1 corresponds to the initial portion of the PCT and is characterized by a well-developed brush border and high metabolic activity. It is responsible for the reabsorption of most filtered solutes, including glucose and amino acids. Following segment S_1, the tubule continues as segment S_2, with a gradual decrease in brush border density and metabolic activity. Segment S_3 marks the transition to the PST, where the brush border is less prominent, and reabsorptive capacity decreases further.

In general, the apical surface of the proximal tubule is covered by a brush border formed by extensive projections of the apical plasma membrane called microvilli (Figs. 11-13 and 11-14). The lateral borders of the epithelial cells are characterized by elaborate interdigitation of lateral cell processes. In addition, the basal surface of the cells has a highly folded membrane with processes from adjacent cells nestled between the folds. This arrangement resembles a cluster of tightly packed, buttressed tree stumps with their roots intertwined. The apical brush border and the basolateral plasma membrane infoldings significantly increase the surface area of the cell and thus permit the high rates of transepithelial transport within this segment.

Many long mitochondria are found between the folds of the lateral plasma membrane, creating vertical striations visible under light microscopy. This close association of mitochondria with the plasma membrane ensures that energy is readily available for the transport proteins in the basolateral plasma membrane that rely on adenosine triphosphate (ATP).

Near the apical surface, the lateral sides of the cells are joined together by tight junctions (zonulae occludens), zonulae adherens, and desmosomes (maculae adherens). Occasional gap junctions also link the cells. While tight junctions form continuous bands around the cells, those in the proximal tubule are relatively permeable to solutes and water compared to

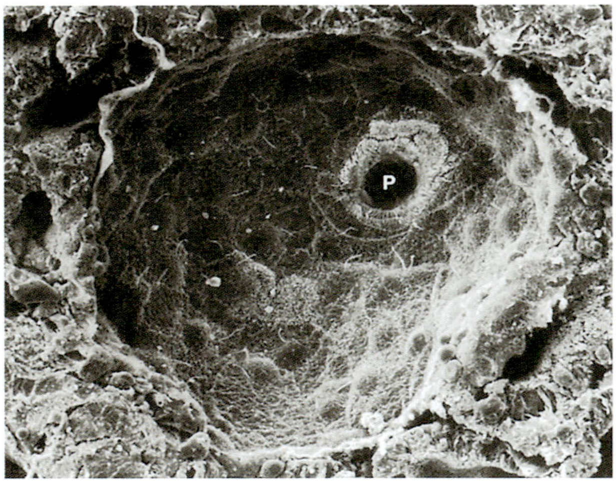

Figure 11-11 Scanning electron micrograph of the parietal layer of the glomerular capsule (rat). All the components of the renal corpuscle have been removed except the parietal layer. Each squamous cell of the parietal layer is distinctly outlined and projects a single, centrally located cilium. The opening into the proximal convoluted tubule (P) is surrounded by cells with a brush border, demonstrating the abrupt transition from the parietal epithelium to the proximal tubule epithelium (×1200).

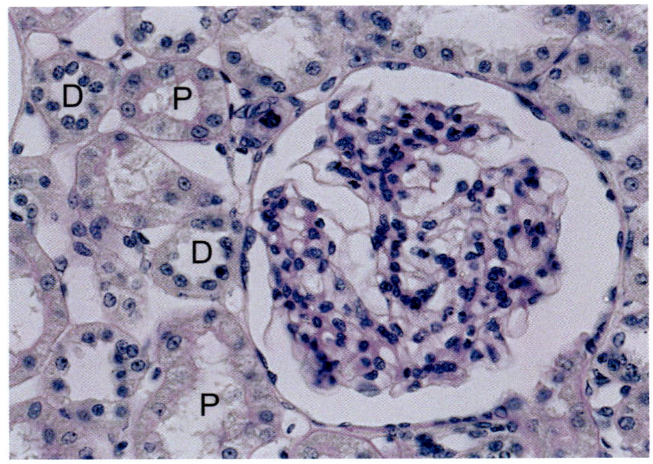

Figure 11-12 Cortical labyrinth. The cortical labyrinth contains renal corpuscles, proximal convoluted tubules (P), distal convoluted tubules (D), connecting segments, initial collecting tubules, and the terminal segment of the thick ascending limb. Nuclei of the distal convoluted tubules are located more apically than those of the proximal convoluted tubules. The periodic acid-Schiff (PAS) stain used in this section enhances the staining of the glomerular basement membrane, the basement membrane around the tubules, and the cell coat associated with the brush border of the proximal convoluted tubules (×400).

Table 11-1 Names of the Renal Tubule Segments with Corresponding Nomina Histologica Terminology

Terms in Common Use	Synonyms	Nomina Histologica Terminology
Proximal tubule		**Proximal tubule**
Proximal convoluted tubule (includes S_1 segment and first part of S_2 segment) (PCT)		Proximal convoluted tubule
Proximal straight tubule (includes latter part of S_2 segment and S_3 segment) (PST)	Thick descending limb of Henle's loop	Proximal straight tubule
Thin limbs of Henle's loop (TL)		**Thin tubules**
Thin descending limb		Thin descending tubule
Thin ascending limb		Thin ascending tubule
Distal tubule		
Thick ascending limb of Henle's loop (MTAL and CTAL)		Distal straight tubule
Distal convoluted tubule (DCT)		Distal convoluted tubule
Connecting segment (CNT)		
Collecting duct		
Initial collecting tubule		Arched collecting tubule
Cortical collecting duct (CCD)		Straight collecting tubule
Outer medullary collecting duct (OMCD)		Straight collecting tubule
Inner medullary collecting duct (IMCD)		
Initial IMCD ($IMCD_1$)		Straight collecting tubule
Terminal IMCD (includes $IMCD_2$ and $IMCD_3$)	Papillary collecting duct	Papillary duct

those in distal tubule and collecting duct segments. The single nucleus is spherical and situated in the middle to basal part of the cell. Proximal tubule cells contain an extensive endocytotic apparatus, including numerous apical vesicles, endosomes, and lysosomes. Peroxisomes, organelles containing oxidative enzymes for metabolism of toxic substances, are abundant in the PST. In cats, the PCT cells contain numerous lipid droplets (Fig. 11-15). Similarly, in dogs, PST cells contain lipid droplets, and thus the medullary rays appear lighter than the surrounding parenchyma (Fig. 11-16).

Unfortunately, the distinctive structural features of proximal tubules are not evident in many histologic sections due to interruptions in blood flow to the kidney. This interruption causes collapse of the tubules, swelling of the epithelial cells, obliteration of the tubule lumens, and disintegration of the brush border. Many of the structural features present in live animals can only be preserved with careful perfusion fixation techniques.

The PST extends into the outer medulla and typically undergoes an abrupt transition to the simple squamous epithelium of the thin descending limb (Fig. 11-17) at the border between the inner and outer stripes of the outer medulla. In dogs, this transition occurs at the corticomedullary junction; therefore, the kidney of dogs lacks an outer stripe.

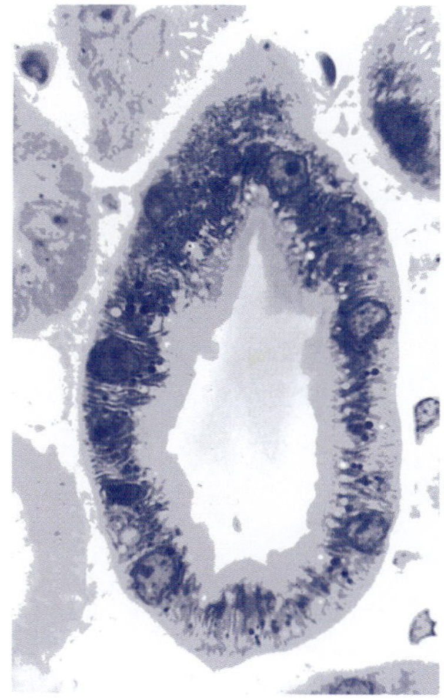

Figure 11-13 Proximal convoluted tubule (dog). The apical surface of the cells is covered by a brush border composed of microvilli. White vacuoles near the lumen and dark, round granules deeper in the cytoplasm are endocytotic vacuoles and lysosomes, respectively. The elongated dark structures oriented perpendicular to the basement membrane are mitochondria. Epon-Araldite, Azure II, methylene blue (×1320).

The Loop of Henle

The structure known as the loop of Henle includes four tubule segments: the descending thick limb, now more commonly called the **proximal straight tubule**; the **descending thin limb**; the **ascending thin limb**, predominantly found in long-looped nephrons; and the **thick ascending limb**, occasionally called the distal straight tubule.

Thin Limbs of the Loop of Henle The thin portion of the loop of Henle (TL) begins at the end of the proximal tubule (Figs. 11-4 and 11-17) and extends a variable distance into the medulla before making a hairpin turn (Fig. 11-18) and continuing toward the border between the inner and outer medulla. In long-looped nephrons, the thin epithelium extends into the inner medulla. The segment from the PST to the hairpin turn is called the **thin descending limb**, while the segment from the hairpin turn to the border of the inner/outer medulla border is called the **thin ascending limb**. Four distinct parts of the thin tubule have been identified, based on ultrastructural differences in epithelial height, amplification of the apical and basolateral cell membranes, mitochondrial count, and tight junction complexity, all of which correlate with functional differences along its length. In general, the thin limbs have a simple squamous epithelium, with transitions to low cuboidal occurring either abruptly or gradually at the two ends of the thin segments, depending on the species. The nuclei protrude into the lumen to a greater extent compared to the endothelial cells of

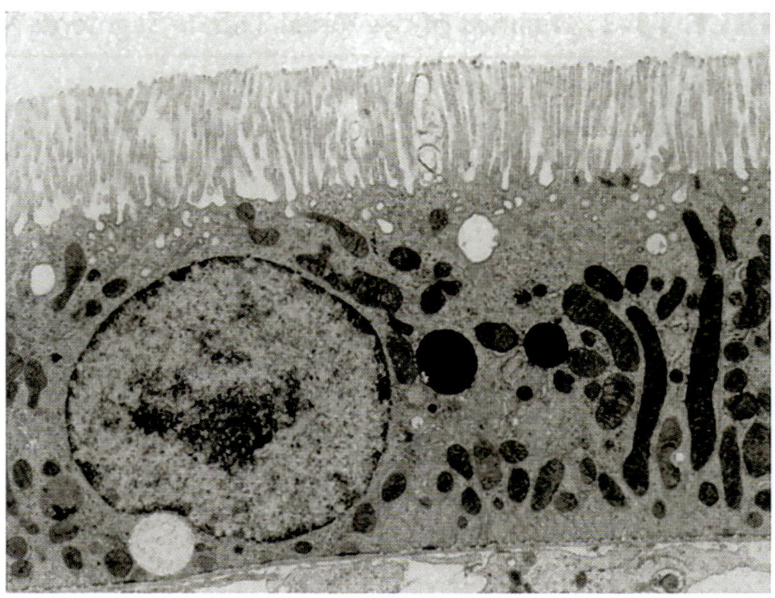

Figure 11-14 Transmission electron micrograph of a proximal straight tubule (S_3) cell (rat). Numerous microvilli cover the apical surface. Small endocytotic vesicles are present in the apical region, along with large endosomes with unstained contents and densely staining lysosomes. Numerous mitochondria also are present (×8800).

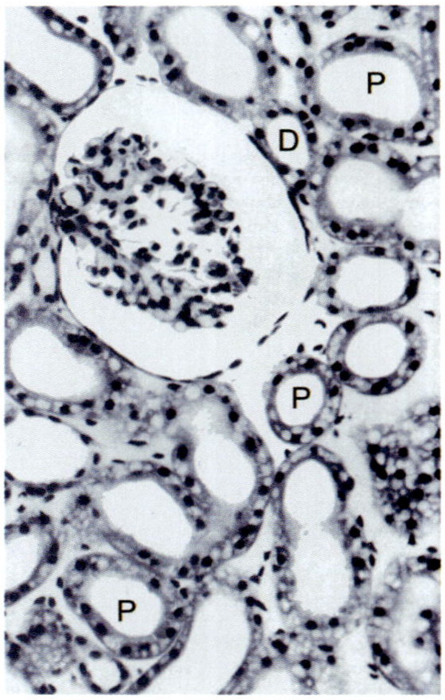

Figure 11-15 Cortical labyrinth (cat). In cats, the proximal convoluted tubules (P) contain numerous lipid droplets. Distal convoluted tubule (D) profiles are relatively rare. H&E (×335).

adjacent capillaries. In addition, the nuclei are round when viewed from the lumen, whereas endothelial nuclei are elongated along the longitudinal axis of the vessel.

Thick Ascending Limb of the Loop of Henle The **thick ascending limb** of the loop of Henle originates at the border between the inner and outer medulla and ascends into the renal cortex within the medullary ray (Fig. 11-19). The epithelium of the medullary thick ascending limb (MTAL) is taller than that of the CTAL. In short-looped nephrons, the thick ascending limb begins at the hairpin turn of Henle's loop at varying depths within the outer medulla, and the thin ascending limb extends from the turn to the transition to the TAL at the border of the inner and outer medulla. The TAL of each nephron returns to the vascular pole of its own glomerulus. At this site, the TAL contains a specialized cluster of epithelial cells called the **macula densa**, which is part of the juxtaglomerular apparatus, to be described below. The transition from the TAL to the distal convoluted tubule occurs at a variable distance beyond the macula densa.

The cells of the TAL are cuboidal with short, stubby apical micro projections, undulating cell borders, and a single central cilium on the apical surface. These cells have an impressive array of vertically oriented mitochondria and basolateral plasma membrane infoldings, necessary to accomplish the high rate of active transport characteristic of this segment. The mitochondrial density and vertical orientation are so distinctive that they appear as dark vertical striations in the tubule, even when observed by light microscopy.

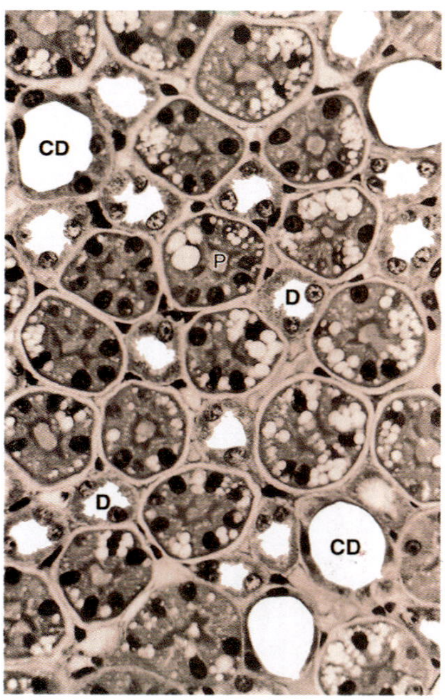

Figure 11-16 Medullary ray (dog). The three major components of the medullary ray are the proximal straight tubules (P), distal straight tubules (D), and collecting ducts (CD). In dogs, the proximal straight tubules contain numerous lipid droplets, visible here as unstained vacuoles. JB-4 plastic. H&E and phloxine (×530).

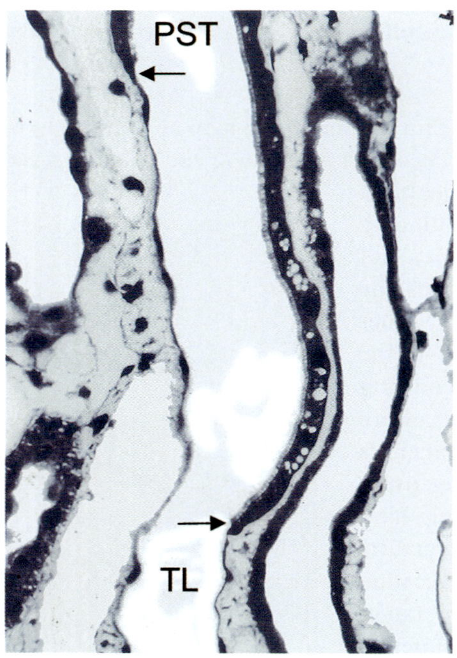

Figure 11-17 Proximal straight tubule to thin descending limb of Henle's loop (dog). The cuboidal epithelium with apical brush border of the proximal straight tubule (PST) abruptly transitions to the simple squamous epithelium with a smooth apical surface in the thin tubule (TL). Note that the transition occurs at various points (arrows) around the circumference of the tubule. JB-4 plastic. H&E and phloxine (×510).

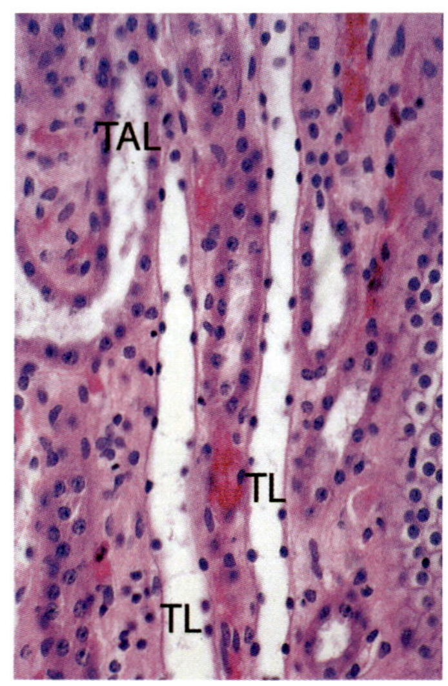

Figure 11-18 Inner stripe of outer medulla. The inner stripe of the outer medulla contains thin limbs (TL), medullary thick ascending limbs (TAL), and collecting ducts (not shown). In this tissue section, short-looped nephrons descend as thin limbs and make a hairpin turn at the junction of the outer and inner medulla to return toward the cortex as thick ascending limbs. Other thin limbs associated with long-looped nephrons continue deeper into the inner medulla without turning. Kidney, horse. H&E (×250). (Image by W.E. Haensly.)

Distal Convoluted Tubule

The **distal convoluted tubule** (DCT) is considerably shorter than the proximal convoluted tubule, resulting in its profiles being relatively rare in the cortical labyrinth. Distal convoluted tubule cells are taller than those of the cortical thick ascending limb, and their apical cell borders are simple rather than undulating. However, like the thick ascending limb, the apical surface is covered by short micro projections, and the cells have a high mitochondrial density. The nucleus is located in the apical region of the cell, whereas extensive basolateral plasma membrane infoldings containing arrays of vertically oriented mitochondria, fill the entire basal region (Fig. 11-20). Although the distal convoluted tubule is primarily composed of a uniform cell population, occasional intercalated cells are present in some species. Intercalated cells are described in detail below.

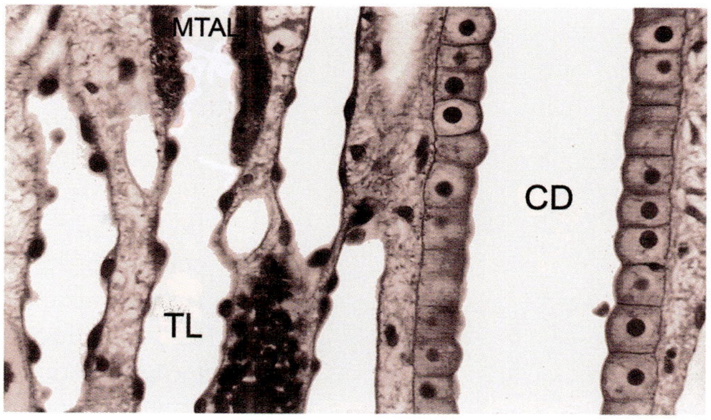

Figure 11-19 Thin ascending limb to thick ascending limb of Henle's loop (horse). The transition between the simple squamous epithelium of the thin ascending limb (TL) and the simple cuboidal epithelium of the medullary thick ascending limb of Henle's loop (MTAL) defines the border between the inner and outer medulla. The inner medullary collecting duct (CD) shown here has a tall cuboidal epithelium. JB-4 plastic. H&E and phloxine (×530).

Connecting Segment

The epithelium of the **connecting segment** is approximately the same height as the DCT. However, unlike the DCT, the connecting segment contains a variety of epithelial cell types, which may include DCT cells, connecting segment cells, intercalated cells, and principal cells. The mixture of these cell types with different cell heights, staining densities, and shapes produces an irregular appearance to the connecting segment profile under light microscopy. This appearance contrasts with the homogeneous appearance and smooth luminal surface of the DCT. Connecting segment cells are similar in morphology to DCT cells, having prominent basolateral plasma membrane infoldings, vertically oriented mitochondria, few short apical plasma membrane micro projections, and an apical nucleus. However, differences can be detected by electron microscopy between connecting segment cells and DCT cells. For example, connecting segment cells typically have fewer apical micro projections, a lower mitochondrial density, and a rounder nucleus. Definitive identification of individual profiles of these two cell types in the connecting segment may require immunocytochemical localization of cell-specific transporters. This highlights the fact that although the structure of the distal convoluted and connecting segment cells may be similar, their functions are quite distinct. Principal cells and intercalated cells are described in the section on collecting ducts.

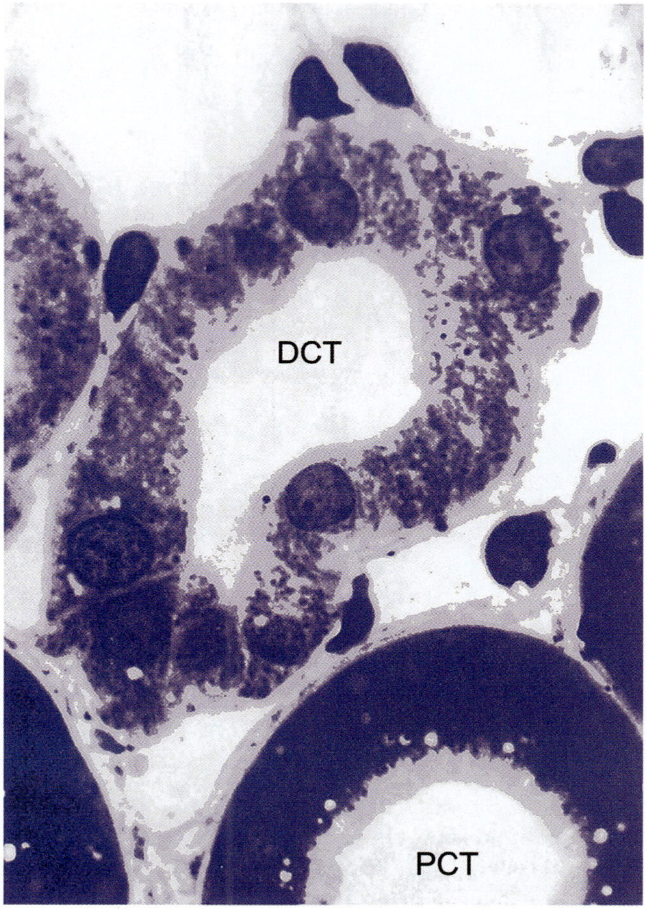

Figure 11-20 Distal convoluted tubule (dog). The cells of the distal convoluted tubule (DCT) lack a brush border, contain numerous mitochondria, and have nuclei in the apical region. Note the proximal convoluted tubule (PCT) with its distinct brush border. Epon-Araldite, Azure II, methylene blue (×1320).

Collecting Ducts

Multiple nephrons empty into a single **cortical collecting duct (CCD)**, a straight tubule segment located within the medullary ray. These collecting ducts descend through the medulla and repeatedly merge with one another. The terminal inner medullary, or papillary, collecting ducts

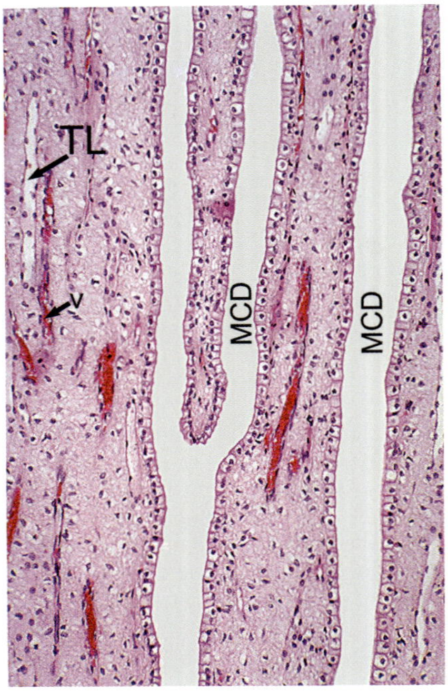

Figure 11-21 The inner medulla contains merging medullary collecting ducts (MCD) and thin limbs (TL). Thin limbs are surrounded by blood vessels that form the vasa recta (v). Kidney, horse. H&E (×160). (Image by W.E. Haensly.)

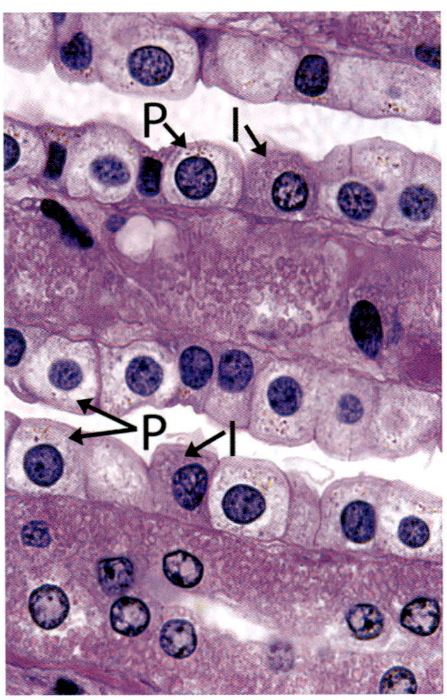

Figure 11-22 Collecting ducts. The epithelium of cortical and outer medullary collecting ducts contains both principal and intercalated cells. Principal cells (P) are low in profile with few organelles; they secrete potassium. Intercalated cells (I) secrete acid or bicarbonate; they stain darker than the principal cells. Kidney, rabbit. H&E (×1000). (Image by J. Eurell).

terminate either at the apex of the papilla or along the renal crest, forming a perforated area on the surface called the **area cribrosa**. Here, the tubule fluid, now considered urine, is released.

The collecting duct is not considered part of the nephron due to its separate origin during development. Initially, the collecting tubule and the collecting duct derive from the ureteric bud, whereas all nephron components develop from the metanephric blastema. However, during development, these two components merge to form a continuous tubule. The term **renal (uriniferous) tubule** encompasses both the nephron and the collecting duct. In the past, the collecting duct was viewed simply as a conduit for urine. However, it is now recognized that the collecting duct plays major roles in the regulation of salt, water, and acid–base excretion. Thus, while the classic definition of the nephron as the "functional unit" of the kidney is widely accepted, it should be noted that the collecting duct, although not part of the nephron, significantly contributes to overall renal function.

Connecting segments merge with the **initial collecting tubule** in the cortical labyrinth, and these then combine with the **CCD** in the medullary ray. The initial collecting tubule consists of **principal cells** and **intercalated cells**, resulting in a heterogeneous epithelium. The epithelium of the initial collecting tubule typically has a height that falls between that of the connecting segment and the cortical collecting duct.

The collecting duct descends through the medullary ray, traverses both the outer and inner medulla, and, after merging several times with other collecting ducts, terminates either at the apex of the papilla or along the edge of the renal crest. Along most of their length, the collecting ducts are lined with simple cuboidal epithelium (Figs. 11-19, 11-21, and 11-22). In carnivores, the epithelium remains low throughout, whereas in ungulates, it can transition to simple columnar or even transitional near the papillary apex.

The CCDs and **outer medullary collecting ducts (OMCDs)** contain both principal cells and intercalated cells (Fig. 11-22). **Principal cells** account for approximately two-thirds of the cell population; they are low in profile and have a smooth apical surface, with few short apical micro projections, and a single central cilium. Principal cells contain relatively few organelles, small and randomly oriented mitochondria, prominent basolateral plasma membrane infoldings, and relatively straight lateral cell membranes. These cells are involved in potassium secretion and sodium, chloride, and antidiuretic hormone (ADH)–regulated water reabsorption. **Intercalated cells** are distributed throughout most of the collecting duct. In the connecting segment, initial collecting tubule, and cortical collecting duct, at least three distinct types of intercalated cells exist: *type A*, which secretes acid; *type B*, which secretes bicarbonate; and *non-A, non-B* intercalated cells, whose function remains incompletely understood. These intercalated cell subtypes are distinguishable both by their ultrastructural characteristics and by the subcellular location of specific transporters involved in acid–base regulation. The locations of specific transporter proteins in intercalated cell subtypes are described in the section on structural–functional relationships.

Under basal conditions, type A intercalated cells contain numerous mitochondria, moderate apical plasma membrane micro projections, prominent apical cytoplasmic tubulovesicles, moderate basolateral plasma membrane infoldings, and a central nucleus. In contrast, type B intercalated cells have a denser cytoplasm and higher mitochondrial density than type A cells, along with a smooth apical surface, small cytoplasmic vesicles distributed throughout most of the cell and a vesicle-free band of cytoplasm beneath the apical plasma membrane. They also display prominent basolateral plasma membrane infoldings and an eccentric nucleus. Non-A, non-B cells are most easily identified in the connecting segment, and are characterized by a very high mitochondrial density, prominent apical plasma membrane micro projections that bulge into the tubule lumen, and relatively few cytoplasmic vesicles.

The outer medullary and initial inner medullary collecting duct (IMCD) segments contain both principal cells and acid-secreting intercalated cells, resembling type A intercalated cells. The number of intercalated cells gradually diminishes in the distal collecting duct segments, and they are essentially absent in the terminal inner medullary collecting duct.

In the terminal **IMCD**, principal cells also disappear, and the predominant cell type, called the inner medullary collecting duct cell, is a taller epithelial cell with short, apical micro projections with a prominent glycocalyx. These cells exhibit relatively little basolateral plasma membrane and contain few cytoplasmic organelles.

Vasculature of the Kidney

Each kidney is supplied by a single **renal artery** that arises from the abdominal aorta. Branching of the renal artery can occur near the hilus or within the renal sinus. These branches divide into **interlobar arteries**, which ascend in the renal parenchyma to the corticomedullary junction (Fig. 11-23). Here, the interlobar arteries form variably arched vessels called **arcuate arteries**.

The arcuate arteries give rise to **interlobular arteries**, which course within the cortical labyrinth and supply the **afferent arterioles** nourishing the glomeruli. The wall of the afferent arteriole is primarily where renin-producing juxtaglomerular cells are located. The glomerular capillary tufts are drained by **efferent arterioles**. Efferent arterioles from glomeruli located in the superficial or middle cortex distribute to **peritubular capillary networks** of fenestrated capillaries. Endothelial cells of cortical peritubular capillaries can synthesize the hormone erythropoietin (EPO), which stimulates the production of red blood cells. In unilobar kidneys, the interlobular arteries may be fewer in number and differently arranged due to the single-lobed structure, while in multilobar kidneys, they are more clearly defined, separating the renal lobes.

Efferent arterioles from juxtamedullary glomeruli supply blood to the entire medulla. These arterioles divide in the outer stripe of the outer medulla into **descending vasa recta (DVR)** (straight vessels), which supply adjacent peritubular capillary networks throughout the medulla. The capillaries then drain into **ascending vasa recta (AVR)**, which ascend in the medulla. The descending vasa recta are arterioles with a continuous endothelium, whereas the ascending vasa recta are venules with a fenestrated endothelium. Many of the descending and ascending vasa recta come together to form vascular bundles that are evenly distributed throughout the medulla (Fig. 11-24).

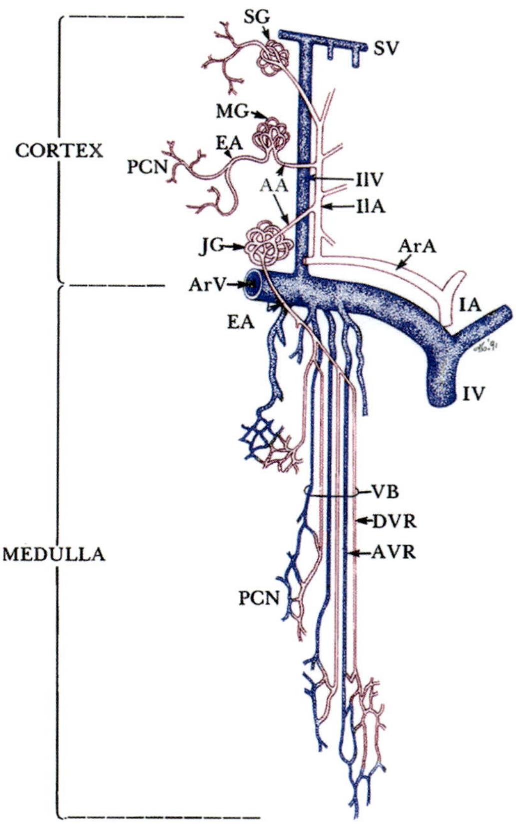

Figure 11-23 Schematic drawing of the vasculature of the kidney. Arterial blood flow starts with the renal artery, followed by interlobar arteries (IA), arcuate arteries (ArA), and interlobular arteries (IIA). Afferent arterioles (AA) supply blood to the glomeruli, from which efferent arterioles (EA) branch out. Efferent arterioles from the superficial glomeruli (SG) and midcortical glomeruli (MG) supply the peritubular capillary network (PCN) throughout the cortex. Efferent arterioles from juxtamedullary glomeruli (JG) supply the descending vasa recta (DVR) and the PCN in the medulla. Venous drainage in the cortex involves stellate veins (SV), interlobular veins (IIV), and/or arcuate veins (ArV). In the medulla, drainage primarily occurs through ascending vasa recta (AVR). Interlobular veins of the cortex and the ascending vasa recta of the medulla converge at the corticomedullary junction into arcuate veins, which drain into interlobar veins (IV), and finally into the renal vein. The descending and ascending vasa recta often form vascular bundles (VB). (Redrawn from Koushanpour E, Kriz W. *Renal Physiology. Principles, Structure and Function*. New York: Springer-Verlag, 1986.)

Veins that accompany arteries often share the same name. Venous drainage of the medulla is accomplished by the ascending vasa recta, which join either the arcuate veins or, occasionally, the interlobular veins. In contrast, venous drainage of the cortex primarily involves the peritubular capillaries, which drain into the **stellate veins**, **interlobular veins**, or **arcuate veins**. The arcuate veins subsequently empty into the **interlobar veins**, which merge to form the renal vein. This vein exits the hilus and joins the caudal vena cava. In carnivores, a network of superficial and deep cortical veins connects the capillaries to larger veins. The superficial cortical veins empty into the stellate veins near the cortical surface, whereas the deep cortical veins empty into the arcuate veins. The stellate veins are prominent in carnivores, particularly in dogs,

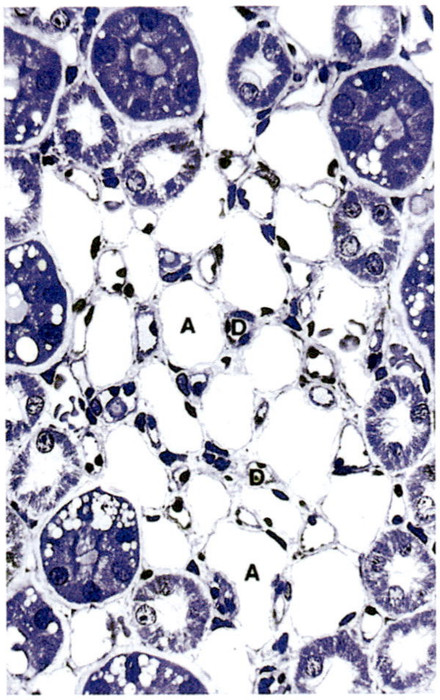

Figure 11-24 Vascular bundle in outer medulla (dog). The descending vasa recta (D) are small, round arterioles in the vascular bundle, while the ascending vasa recta (A) are large, irregularly shaped venous capillaries in the bundle. These vessels are the primary supply and drainage of the medulla. JB-4 plastic. H&E and phloxine (×530).

where they are embedded in the cortical tissue near the surface of the kidney. In cats, they are superficial and are called capsular veins. Although stellate veins in most species drain into the interlobular veins, capsular veins in cats converge toward the hilus of the kidney to join the renal vein in a direct manner rather than pass through the interlobular, arcuate, and interlobar veins.

The intrarenal arterial system lacks a robust collateral circulatory system. As a result, when a major artery is occluded, death of the tissue supplied by that artery results. For example, occlusion of an arcuate artery leads to damage to a wedge-shaped piece of the kidney, involving both cortex and medulla.

Interstitium, Lymphatics, and Nerves

The interstitium between the renal tubules and the blood vessels varies significantly across kidney regions. In the cortex, interstitial space is sparse due to the dense packing of tubules and vessels; the medulla has a more extensive matrix, particularly in its inner regions. This specialized interstitium contains interstitial cells including fibroblasts, bone marrow-derived cells, and lipid-laden interstitial cells. These lipid-laden cells produce prostaglandin E2 to influence local vascular tone and renal physiology. The kidney also serves an endocrine role through specialized cells distributed across the cortex and medulla, including peritubular capillary endothelial cells and interstitial fibroblasts, which synthesize EPO. EPO regulates erythropoiesis in response to oxygen levels, important for tissue oxygenation. In the medulla, connective tissue (CT) supports the nephron architecture, whereas pericytes and the lipid-laden interstitial cells contribute to the synthesis of medullipin I. This substance acts as a vasodilator upon conversion to medullipin II in the liver, influencing blood pressure and renal perfusion.

Lymphatics are also found in the interstitium, strategically positioned surrounding intrarenal arteries, originating either at the vascular pole of the glomerulus or more distally along the afferent arteriole, and extending toward the renal hilus. This lymphatic network supports immune surveillance and fluid balance within the kidney.

The kidney receives efferent innervation targeting the smooth muscle of arteries, afferent and efferent arterioles, and descending vasa recta; these nerves traverse the interstitium surrounding the vessels. Numerous axons and nerve terminals are also present in the vicinity of the juxtaglomerular apparatus, where they interact with the renin-producing juxtaglomerular cells of the afferent arteriole.

Juxtaglomerular Apparatus

The **juxtaglomerular apparatus** is located at the vascular pole of the glomerulus (Figs. 11-6 and 11-25). Its components include the macula densa, the extraglomerular mesangial cells, and the juxtaglomerular cells. The **macula densa** is a patch of specialized epithelial cells located in the cortical thick ascending limb as it passes between the afferent and efferent arterioles (Figs. 11-5, 11-6, and 11-25). These cells are tall and narrow relative to thick ascending limb cells, and the intercellular spaces between them appear dilated. The basal region of the macula densa is adjacent to the extraglomerular mesangial cells. The **extraglomerular mesangial cells** (lacis cells) are found between the macula densa and the two arterioles. They are continuous with the mesangial cells within the glomerulus and are arranged into several layers of flattened cells. Gap junctions connect extraglomerular mesangial cells with each other, with intraglomerular mesangial cells, and with juxtaglomerular cells, but not with macula densa cells. **Juxtaglomerular (JG or granular) cells**, primarily located in the afferent arteriole, originate from smooth muscle (Figs. 11-25 and 12-16). These cells contain membrane-bound renin granules of irregular size and shape. Sympathetic nerve endings found near the JG cells are consistent with sympathetic stimulation of renin release.

Structure–Function Relationships in the Kidney

General Function

The kidney serves several vital functions, including the excretion of metabolic wastes, regulation of body fluid volume and composition, and control of systemic blood pressure. Elimination of nitrogenous wastes, such as creatinine, urea, and uric acid, occurs largely by filtration of these substances at the glomerulus. Renal regulation of body fluid volume and composition involves adjustments in both the glomerular filtration rate and the transport processes of the various renal tubule epithelia. The kidney responds to local and systemic factors to maintain homeostasis of fluid, electrolyte, and acid–base balance.

Filtration and Regulation of Blood Pressure

Although the kidneys account for only a small percentage of the body weight in domestic animals, ranging from at most 1% in cats to 0.2% in cattle, they receive a phenomenal 20 to 25% of the cardiac output. Approximately 20% of the blood volume delivered to the kidney filters across the glomerular capillary wall to form the glomerular filtrate. However, approximately 99% of this filtrate is reabsorbed by the renal tubules, resulting in only about 1% of the filtrate volume being excreted as urine. Filtration across the glomerular capillary wall is primarily driven by the hydrostatic pressure of the intracapillary blood. Both systemic blood pressure and resistance in the afferent and efferent arterioles contribute to the intracapillary hydrostatic pressure. Filtration is primarily opposed by the osmotic pressure exerted by plasma proteins. Although the hydrostatic pressure in the urinary space also opposes filtration, its contribution is negligible under normal circumstances. The filtration barrier formed by the glomerular capillary wall is both size and charge selective. Thus, substances with a molecular weight exceeding approximately 40,000 Da are typically retained within the capillary lumen. Furthermore, smaller anionic macromolecules are retained more effectively than cationic macromolecules due to the anionic charges of the filtration barrier.

The endothelium prevents the filtration of blood cells and platelets. Water and filterable solutes pass through the endothelial pores, across the GBM, and through the filtration slits between the podocyte foot processes into the urinary space. The size selectivity of the filtration barrier is primarily created by the tightly knit proteins in the GBM lamina densa. The charge selectivity is established by the anionic molecules coating the endothelial cells and podocytes, as well as in the GBM. These elements repel and prevent the filtration of small anionic plasma proteins, even though neutral or cationic molecules of the same size and shape could be filtered. Normal filtration also requires the clearance of macromolecules trapped by the filtration barrier; mesangial cells phagocytose molecules trapped in the GBM, and podocytes phagocytose or endocytose molecules trapped at the podocyte surface and slit membrane.

Mesangial cells and podocytes maintain the structural integrity of the capillary tuft. Mesangial cells also contribute to the regulation of glomerular capillary perfusion. Largely in response to signals from the macula densa, mesangial cells contract or relax, thereby altering resistance within the capillary loops and consequently influencing glomerular blood flow. Filtration is further regulated by the resistance in the afferent and efferent arterioles.

Finally, the juxtaglomerular apparatus (Fig. 11-25) regulates not only the flow rate and perfusion pressure within individual glomeruli but also contributes to the regulation of systemic blood pressure. Juxtaglomerular cells release **renin** in response

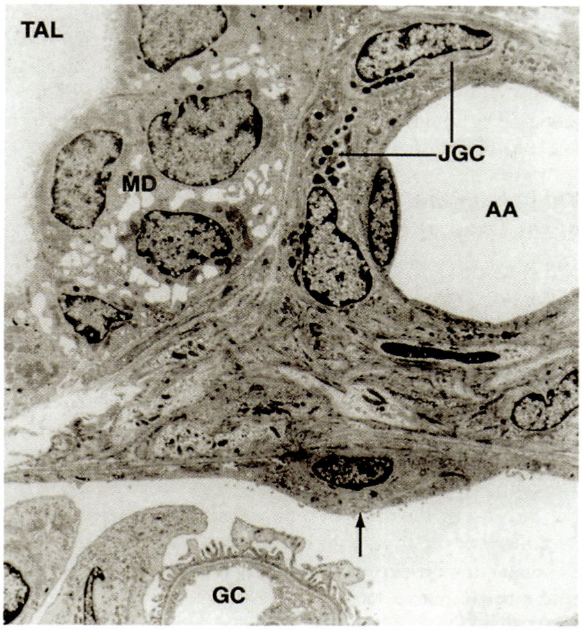

Figure 11-25 Transmission electron micrograph of a juxtaglomerular apparatus (rat). The macula densa (MD) is located in the thick ascending limb (TAL) as it passes between the afferent and efferent arterioles. Macula densa cells are typically taller and narrower than surrounding TAL cells and have dilated intercellular spaces. Two juxtaglomerular cells (JGC) containing electron-dense granules are present in the wall of the afferent arteriole (AA). Extraglomerular mesangial cells are located between the macula densa and the vascular pole of the glomerulus. A parietal epithelial cell (arrow) and a segment of a glomerular capillary (GC) are also visible (×3700).

to reduced renal perfusion pressure, sympathetic nerve stimulation, or signaling from the macula densa. Renin catalyzes the conversion of plasma angiotensinogen to angiotensin I, which is converted to **angiotensin II** in various tissues. Angiotensin II increases systemic blood pressure through vasoconstriction and by increasing intravascular volume. It increases intravascular fluid volume by stimulating sodium (and thus water) reabsorption in the proximal tubule and by triggering adrenal aldosterone secretion, which enhances sodium uptake in the collecting duct.

Tubule Function

The glomerular filtrate flows through the renal tubules, undergoing solute and water reabsorption while excess solutes are secreted. Solute and water reabsorption across the renal tubular epithelium into the peritubular capillaries occurs through transcellular and paracellular pathways.

The **transcellular pathway** uses active and passive processes to transport substances through the plasma membranes and cytoplasm. Active transport requires plasma membrane **transport proteins** and energy from ATP to move specific ions across the membrane, often against an electrochemical gradient. Plasma membranes also contain **channel proteins** and **carrier proteins** that do not require ATP; these facilitate ion or water movement across the lipid membranes, often driven by gradients generated by active transporters.

The **paracellular pathway** involves the passive movement of water and solute from the tubule lumen to the interstitium through epithelial cell junctions and lateral intercellular spaces. Movement through the paracellular pathway is also driven by gradients produced by active transporters but is limited by the permeability of the tight junctions between cells. Proximal tubules have permeable tight junctions, allowing significant paracellular transport, but the epithelium cannot maintain large gradients. In the thick ascending limb, distal convoluted tubule, and collecting duct, the tight junctions are relatively impermeable; thus, little paracellular transport occurs, but high salt and water gradients can be sustained.

The structure of renal tubule epithelial cells reflects their function. For example, transmembrane transport relies on the surface area of the plasma membrane and the generation of mitochondrial ATP. The proximal tubule's high capacity for transcellular transport is enabled by the amplification of both the apical and basolateral plasma membranes, as well as a high mitochondrial density. At the other extreme, only limited transcellular transport occurs in the thin limbs of Henle's loop, which have relatively simple plasma membranes and few mitochondria.

Proximal Tubule

The proximal tubule (Figs. 11-13 and 11-14) normally reabsorbs approximately 85% of the water and salts from the glomerular filtrate, along with 100% of filtered glucose, amino acids, peptides, and low-molecular-weight proteins. Solute and water uptake are facilitated by the sodium gradient from the lumen to the blood, generated by active sodium transport across the basolateral plasma membrane. The extensive surface area of the apical plasma membrane, characterized by the brush border, contains numerous specific **transport proteins** that couple sodium uptake with other transport processes, such as bicarbonate and glucose uptake. Water reabsorption follows the chemical gradient established by active sodium reabsorption, with membrane proteins that function as water channels (**aquaporins [AQP]**) allowing water to pass through the hydrophobic lipid membrane. Since the proximal tubule lacks a tight epithelium and cannot generate significant electrochemical gradients, the tubule fluid entering the thin descending limb remains essentially isotonic despite the majority of filtered water and solutes being reabsorbed in the proximal tubule.

Low-molecular-weight proteins and peptides are filtered but normally are entirely reabsorbed in the proximal tubule. These molecules are internalized from the lumen by receptor-mediated endocytosis into endocytic vesicles and metabolized in endosomes and lysosomes. A hallmark of glomerular disease is an increase in the amount and size of filtered proteins, along with a concurrent increase in the proximal tubule lysosomal system that is visible by light microscopy. When the capacity of the lysosomal system is exceeded, protein appears in the urine; this is often the earliest sign of renal disease.

The proximal tubule also secretes organic ions, which include many drugs and toxins. Uptake of such substances from the blood and their subsequent secretion into the lumen can lead to the concentration of organic ions in the proximal tubule, sometimes reaching toxic levels. Proximal tubule damage is often the first sign of toxic injury and may progress to renal failure. An example in clinical settings is renal failure resulting from the administration of the antibiotic gentamicin, which is secreted by the proximal tubule.

Thin Limbs and Thick Ascending Limb of the Loop of Henle

The physical arrangement and transport characteristics of the thin limbs (Figs. 11-4, 11-17 to 11-19) and thick ascending limb of Henle's loop (Fig. 11-19) enable the kidney to produce concentrated urine with minimal energy expenditure. This is achieved through the creation of a **countercurrent system** by the proximity of the descending and ascending thin limbs, along with the opposite direction of tubule fluid flow in these segments. A similar countercurrent arrangement is observed in the descending and ascending vasa recta. The countercurrent mechanism, along with the active reabsorption of NaCl by the thick ascending limb and the selective permeabilities of the thin limbs to water, salt, and urea, generates and maintains a hypertonic medullary interstitium, facilitating the production of concentrated urine.

The tubule fluid exits the proximal straight tubule, passes through the thin descending limb deep into the medulla, makes a hairpin turn, and ascends through the thin ascending limb and thick ascending limb in long-looped nephrons, or solely through the thick ascending limb in short-looped nephrons. Although structurally similar, the descending and ascending thin limbs have distinct permeabilities crucial for the countercurrent concentrating mechanism. Also fundamental to this process are the progressively increasing interstitial osmolarity in the medulla and the countercurrent arrangement of the descending and ascending vasa recta. These components function together as follows. The thin descending limb of long-looped nephrons is permeable to water but impermeable to sodium and urea. As isosmotic tubule fluid enters, it encounters increasing osmolarity in the medulla, leading to passive water reabsorption. By the time it reaches the hairpin turn, luminal fluid tonicity is high. The subsequent ascent through progressively lower interstitial osmolarity renders the thin ascending limb permeable to sodium but relatively impermeable to water. Thus, sodium moves down its concentration gradient to be reabsorbed without water, resulting in nearly isotonic fluid upon reaching the thick ascending limb. These processes occur almost entirely by passive mechanisms. The low level of active transport and the selective permeabilities of the thin limbs correlate with their structure, including uncomplicated plasma membranes, few mitochondria, and complex tight junctions that prevent leaks.

The vasa recta (Figs. 11-23 and 11-24) follow a similar pattern to the thin limbs, with descending and ascending portions connected by a hairpin turn. The DVR encounter progressively higher interstitial concentrations of NaCl and urea as they traverse the medulla. DVR are not fenestrated, but they permit paracellular diffusion of NaCl and transcellular movement of urea and water into the medullary interstitium via specific proteins. On the other hand, AVR are fenestrated and thus permeable to water, NaCl, and urea, allowing equilibration to nearly isotonicity upon leaving the hypertonic medulla. This system ensures adequate blood supply to the inner medulla without compromising interstitial hypertonicity.

The thick ascending limb also contributes to medullary hypertonicity through salt reabsorption without water. Its epithelium has extensive basolateral plasma membrane infoldings containing abundant **Na^+–K^+ ATPase** (adenosine triphosphatase), which actively pumps sodium from the cell into the interstitium. The numerous mitochondria interspersed among the plasma membrane infoldings produce the necessary energy. The electrochemical gradients created by the basolateral Na^+–K^+ ATPase facilitate ion uptake from the lumen via the **Na^+–K^+–$2Cl^-$ cotransporter** in the apical plasma membrane. Exclusive to the thick ascending limb, this transporter is inactivated by the drugs furosemide and bumetanide, which are known as "loop diuretics," because they enhance salt and water excretion in Henle's loop. The thick ascending limb is impermeable to water; thus, the avid ion uptake decreases tubular fluid tonicity and increases the medullary interstitial tonicity.

Distal Convoluted Tubule

In the distal convoluted tubule (Fig. 11-20), active transport drives sodium and chloride reabsorption. Because the DCT is impermeable to water, the osmolarity of tubule fluid falls to approximately 100 mOsm/kg, earning the DCT its designation as the "diluting segment." Basolateral Na^+–K^+ ATPase moves sodium into the interstitium, while a **Na^+–Cl^- cotransporter** in the apical plasma membrane—the site of action of thiazide diuretics—facilitates sodium and chloride uptake from the lumen. Calcium is reabsorbed via active transport by basolateral **Ca-ATPase** and secondary active transport through apical calcium channels and a basolateral sodium/calcium exchanger. The complex basolateral plasma membrane infoldings accommodate numerous ion transport proteins, and the abundant mitochondria produce the energy required for high rates of active transport.

Collecting Duct

The collecting duct (Figs. 11-19, 11-21, and 11-22) regulates the final composition of urine and maintains systemic acid–base balance, as well as sodium, potassium, and water homeostasis. The various epithelial cell types in the collecting duct perform these specific physiologic functions.

Intercalated cells are primarily involved in acid–base regulation. In the CCD, different subtypes of intercalated cells facilitate acid secretion and bicarbonate resorption. Type A intercalated cells actively secrete acid via apical **H^+-ATPase** and **H^+, K^+-ATPase** pumps, while bicarbonate is reabsorbed by the basolateral Cl^-/HCO_3^- **anion exchanger**, AE1. Type B intercalated cells secrete bicarbonate via a distinct apical anion exchanger, pendrin, while protons are transported to the interstitium by basolateral proton pumps. The function of non-A, non-B intercalated cells remains unclear; however, their possession of apical **pendrin** suggests they may secrete bicarbonate, while the presence of apical H^+-ATPase suggests they may secrete protons. Medullary collecting ducts can secrete acid but not bicarbonate, containing only acid-secreting intercalated cells similar to type A intercalated cells found in the CCD.

Intercalated cells responsible for acid secretion undergo structural changes to enhance this process. Proton pumps are contained within apical cytoplasmic tubulovesicles. During acidosis, these vesicles fuse with the apical plasma membrane, thereby increasing its surface area and relocating proton pumps to effectively pump acid into the tubule fluid. Activation of bicarbonate secretion prompts similar structural changes in type B intercalated cells, where vesicles containing the anion exchanger pendrin are inserted into the apical plasma membrane.

Principal cells and IMCD cells regulate sodium and water excretion. Principal cells reabsorb sodium via Na^+–K^+ ATPase on the basolateral plasma membrane and sodium channels on the apical plasma membrane. Both pathways of sodium uptake are enhanced by the adrenal hormone **aldosterone**.

Principal cells and IMCD cells regulate renal water excretion, a process dependent on a hypertonic medullary interstitium and ADH (or vasopressin). Principal cells contain both apical and basolateral water channels known as aquaporins (AQP). Key AQP in the principal cells of the collecting duct and IMCD include AQP2, located in the apical membrane to facilitate water reabsorption in response to ADH, and AQP3 and AQP4 in the basolateral membrane. These AQPs enable precise adjustment of water reabsorption according to hydration needs. The apical water channel AQP2 is tightly regulated by ADH. During times when water conservation is necessary, ADH released from the pituitary activates AQP2, allowing water to move from the tubule fluid into the interstitium through the apical water channels, driven by the osmotic gradient created by the hypertonic medullary interstitium. In contrast, when excess water must be excreted, the absence of ADH leads to the inactivity of apical water channels, resulting in water retention within the tubule lumen.

In the IMCD, both principal and IMCD cells contain urea transporters. Urea transporters located in the apical plasma membrane (UT-A1 and UT-A3) facilitate urea uptake. Basolateral facilitated urea transport is also present, but the specific transporters are not yet known. Urea uptake via these transporters is stimulated by ADH and contributes to the maintenance of the hypertonic medullary interstitium, thereby aiding in water conservation.

Both intercalated cells and principal cells participate in regulation of potassium excretion. Principal cells secrete potassium via the basolateral Na^+–K^+ ATPase and apical potassium channels. Intercalated cells, on the other hand, are capable of potassium reabsorption via apical H^+,K^+-ATPase and basolateral potassium channels.

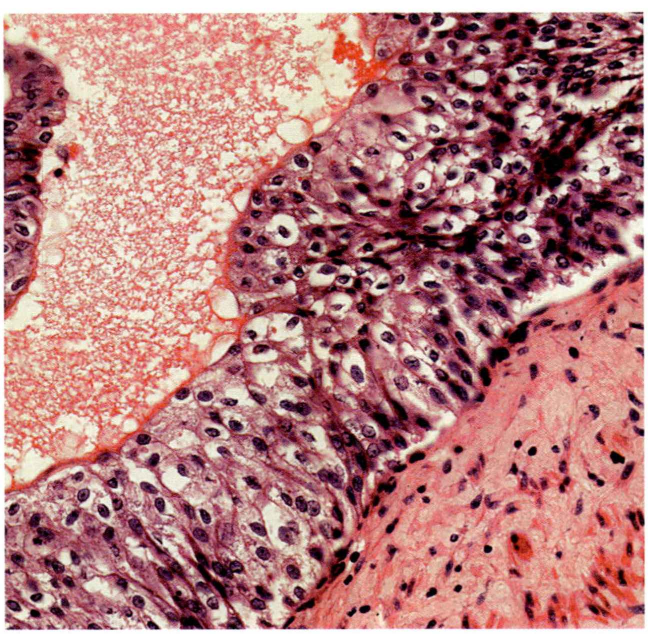

Figure 11-26 Renal calyx. Urothelium lines the inner surface of the calyx. H&E (×400).

Urinary Passages

The urinary passages include the calyces (found in large ruminant and pigs [Fig. 11-26]), renal pelvis (observed in horses [Fig. 11-27], carnivores, small ruminants, and pigs), ureters (Fig. 11-28), urinary bladder (Fig. 11-29), and urethra (Fig. 11-30). These structures have a similar histologic organization, consisting of a tunica mucosa composed of transitional epithelium (urothelium) up to eight cells deep; an underlying layer of loose CT (propria-submucosa); a tunica muscularis composed of smooth muscle forming inner longitudinal, middle circular, and

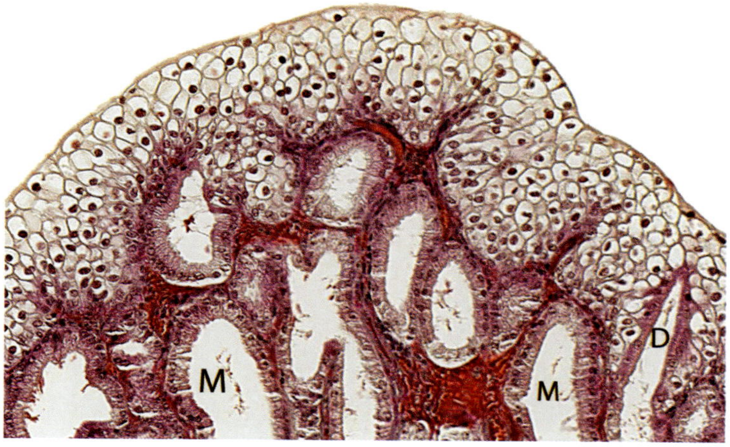

Figure 11-27 Renal pelvis (horse). Mucous glands (M) are found in the mucosa just beneath the urothelium of the renal pelvis and the proximal ureter in horses, mules, and donkeys. Ducts (D) penetrate the overlying epithelium and carry the secretion to the lumen. H&E (×200). (Courtesy of Purdue University College of Veterinary Medicine.)

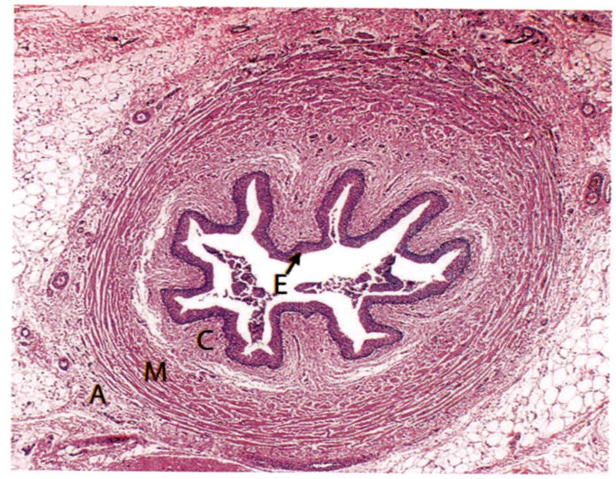

Figure 11-28 The ureter conducts urine from the kidney to the urinary bladder. The mucosa forms longitudinal folds, giving the lumen a stellate shape. A lining of urothelium (E) overlies a propria-submucosa of CT (C). The tunica muscularis (M) of the ureter is smooth muscle. CT forms the tunica adventitia (A) which blends with surrounding adipose tissue. Ureter, pig. H&E (×40). (Image by W.E. Haensly).

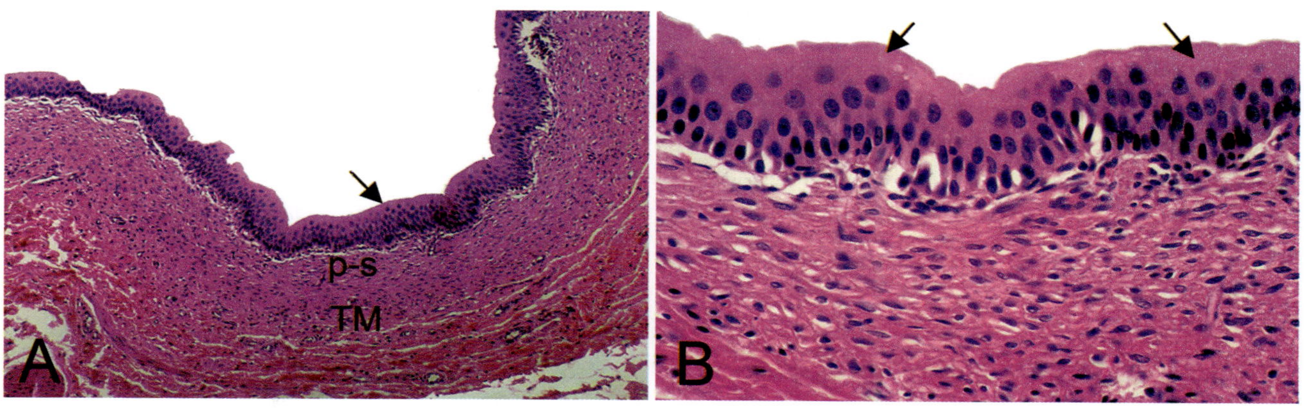

Figure 11-29 **A**. Urothelium (transitional epithelium) lines the urinary bladder (arrow). A lamina muscularis is absent in the feline bladder but present in other species. The propria-submucosa (p-s) consists of typical CT. Poorly defined layers of smooth muscle form the tunica muscularis (TM). Urinary bladder, cat. H&E (×100). **B**. Superficial cells (arrow) are large urothelial cells that line the lumen of the bladder. These cells contain intracytoplasmic membrane vesicles in the relaxed state, which are thought to integrate into the cell membrane when the bladder distends. Extensive basolateral plasma membrane infoldings interdigitate with the plasma membrane of underlying cells and help maintain epithelial integrity when the tissue is stretched. Urinary bladder, cat. H&E (×400). (Images by W.E. Haensly).

outer longitudinal layers; and a tunica adventitia made of loose CT or a tunica serosa of mesothelium and CT when a visceral peritoneal covering is present. Variations of this general pattern include the following:

1) **Renal pelvis:** In horses, mucous glands (simple branched tubuloalveolar glands) in the mucosa contribute to the viscous, stringy nature of equine urine (Fig. 11-27). The transitional epithelium is only a few cells deep.
2) **Ureter:** The ureter has a narrow lumen. When the ureter is not distended, the mucosa folds longitudinally, giving the lumen a stellate appearance in cross section (Fig. 11-28). Mucous glands are present in the proximal ureter of horses.
3) **Urinary bladder: Superficial cells** lining the lumen are large transitional epithelial cells. When the urinary bladder is relaxed, the superficial cells contain extensive intracytoplasmic membrane tubulovesicles that are believed to be inserted into the plasma membrane when the bladder is distended (Fig. 11-29). The superficial transitional cells have extensive basolateral plasma membrane infoldings that interdigitate with the plasma membrane of underlying transitional cells. Adjacent

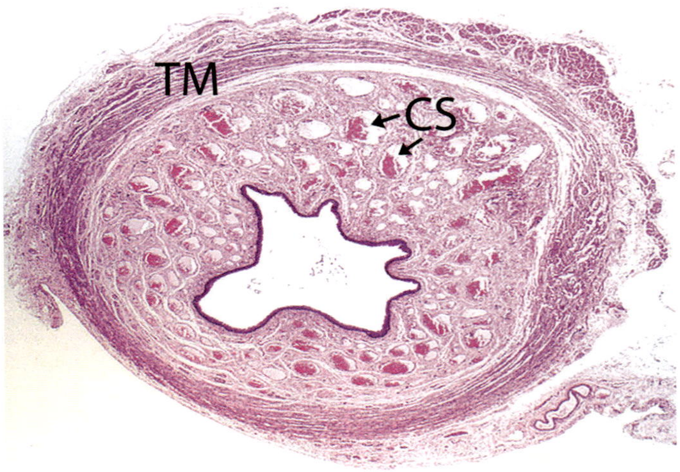

Figure 11-30 Cavernous spaces (CS) of the propria-submucosa of the urethra contain blood and resemble erectile tissue. The tunica muscularis (TM) is primarily smooth muscle. Urethra, female dog. H&E (×250). (Image by W.E. Haensly).

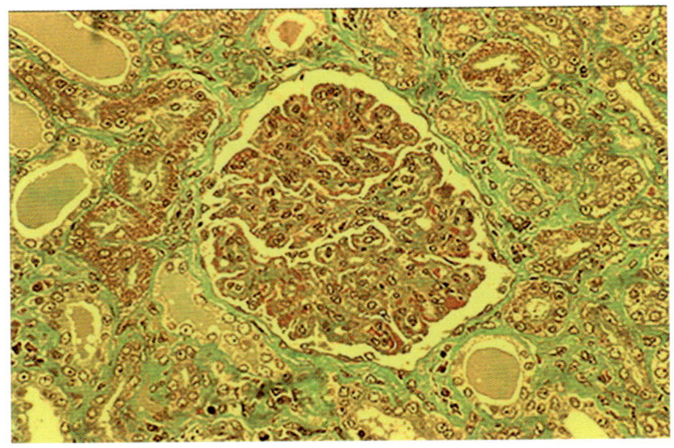

Figure 11-31 Chronic glomerulonephritis (Dog). Shown is a thickening of the glomerular capillary loops, fine interstitial fibrosis, and accumulation of proteinaceous fluid in the tubules. This disease is often immune-mediated and frequently progresses to end-stage kidney failure. Masson's trichrome & Orange G (×250). (Reprinted with permission from Salguero Bodes FJ, Pallares Martinez FJ. Aughey and Frye's Comparative Veterinary Histology with Clinical Correlates. 2nd ed. Boca Raton: CRC Press, 2023.)

transitional cells are connected by numerous desmosomes with long intermediate filaments that extend into the cytoplasm, maintaining epithelial integrity during bladder distention. A lamina muscularis of small, isolated bundles of smooth muscle is present in horses, ruminants, dogs, and pigs but absent in cats. The lamina muscularis divides the loose CT layer into an inner lamina propria and an outer submucosa. The smooth muscle of the tunica muscularis, called the detrusor muscle, is composed of three sometimes ill-defined layers of smooth muscle.

4) **Urethra** (female): The epithelium is primarily transitional near the bladder but changes to stratified squamous near the external urethral orifice. Intermediate areas will have stratified columnar or cuboidal epithelia. Endothelial-lined cavernous spaces are scattered in the CT of the propria-submucosa, resembling erectile tissue. The amount and distribution of cavernous tissue in the urethra vary between species. A few bundles of longitudinally oriented smooth muscle may form a rudimentary lamina muscularis. The smooth muscle in the tunica muscularis includes irregularly arranged circular and longitudinal components. In the distal urethra, bundles of longitudinally and circularly oriented skeletal muscle are mixed with or replace the smooth muscle in the tunica muscularis. A **suburethral diverticulum** lined by transitional epithelium and an underlying loose CT layer is present ventral to the external urethral orifice in pigs and in ruminants. The male urethra is described in Chapter 13.

These passageways serve as conduits and reservoirs for urine, facilitating bladder filling and urine release. Urine is moved from the kidney to the bladder by peristaltic contractions of the smooth muscle in the calyces, renal pelvis, and ureter. The ureters enter the bladder at an acute angle, functioning as a valve to prevent urine reflux back into the ureter. The nervous system regulates the muscular components of the bladder and urethra during both bladder filling and emptying. Bladder filling requires a balance of outflow restriction and bladder wall relaxation. Restriction of outflow is achieved through urethral sphincter constriction via pudendal nerve stimulation of urethral skeletal muscle and sympathetic (hypogastric nerve) stimulation of bladder neck smooth muscle (via α-receptors). Bladder relaxation is facilitated by inhibition of parasympathetic innervation (pelvic nerve) to the detrusor muscle and the inhibition of detrusor muscle contraction by sympathetic nerve stimulation (via β-receptors).

Urine voiding, known as **urination** or **micturition**, is controlled by the caudal brainstem under cortical and cerebellar influence. Normal micturition involves the relaxation of the urethral sphincter and bladder neck, as well as bladder contraction. Urine outflow is permitted through inhibition of pudendal innervation to urethral skeletal muscle and sympathetic innervation to the bladder neck smooth muscle. Bladder contraction is stimulated by parasympathetic stimulation of the detrusor muscle and the inhibition of sympathetic input to the same muscle.

Clinical Correlations

In domestic species, renal disease is often subclinical. A wide variety of developmental, circulatory, metabolic, inflammatory, and neoplastic conditions can affect the kidneys. Glomerulonephritis (Fig. 11-31) is often immune-mediated and is a common cause of chronic renal failure in both dogs and cats. Glomerular damage leads to significant protein loss, which can result in the development of nephrotic syndrome characterized by hypoalbuminemia, generalized edema, and hypercholesterolemia. Renal carcinoma is the most recognized renal neoplasm in dogs, sheep, and cattle, whereas in pigs, blastomas are more frequently seen, especially in younger animals.

Essentials

The major functional unit of the urinary system is the nephron. The nephron has a unique blood flow sequence that starts with an afferent arteriole that flows into the capillaries of the renal glomerulus, exits via an efferent arteriole, passes through a capillary network, and finally enters venules.

The afferent arteriole contains modified smooth muscle juxtaglomerular (JG) cells that produce the hormone renin. The JG complex includes extraglomerular mesangial cells (Lacis cells) and macula densa cells as part of the distal straight tubule (or thick ascending limb, TAL). The JG complex has a role in blood pressure regulation.

Glomerular mesangial cells are found in the interstitial tissue between the capillary loops of the glomerulus, aiding in the turnover of the glomerular basement membrane.

The capillaries of the renal glomerulus are covered by a visceral layer of podocytes that contribute to the filtration barrier essential for urine production.

The glomerulus is contained within the Bowman's (renal) capsule, which is lined by a parietal layer of squamous epithelium and a visceral layer composed of podocytes. The space between the glomerulus and the capsule is the urinary space.

Filtration barrier: It consists of a fenestrated capillary endothelium over a thick basement membrane and podocytes. Podocyte cell processes (pedicels) form filtration slits. This barrier allows water, ions, and small molecules to pass through but restricts large proteins and negatively charged molecules.

Tubule system: The nephron tubules begin at the urinary pole of the renal corpuscle with the PCT. The PCT is lined by simple cuboidal epithelium containing abundant mitochondria, lysosomes and pinocytotic vesicles, and the cell surface has a microvillus brush border. The PCT leads into the loop of Henle.

Loop of Henle – Proximal thick descending tubule: It appears similar to the PCT. *Descending and ascending thin limbs*: Lined with simple squamous epithelium. *Distal straight tubule leading to macula densa*: Lined with simple cuboidal epithelium. *Distal convoluted, connecting tubules, and collecting ducts*: These are lined with simple cuboidal epithelium; the connecting tubules and collecting ducts contain principal and intercalated cells.

Countercurrent multiplier (found in the Loop of Henle) and countercurrent exchanger (involving the vasa recta) functional principle: Different regions of the nephron vary in their permeability to water, sodium chloride, and urea. These three components are exchanged between the capillaries, the renal interstitial tissue, and the nephron tubules to concentrate urine.

- *Proximal convoluted tubule (PCT)*: High percentage of filtrate is reabsorbed along with glucose, amino acids, small proteins, and most NaCl and water. Calcium and water are absorbed in parallel with sodium. Tubular fluid remains essentially isotonic. Na^+/K^+ ATPase at the cell base pumps Na^+ back into the blood.
- *Descending thick limb of Henle's loop (or proximal straight tubule)*: Water is reabsorbed, but NaCl is not.
- *Descending thin limb*: It is permeable to water and the ultrafiltrate equilibrates with the renal interstitium.
- *Ascending thin limb*: It is impermeable to water; NaCl is reabsorbed, and urea is allowed to move into the tubule.
- *Thick ascending limb (TAL)*: Returns to the vascular pole of its own renal corpuscle and at this site forms the macula densa, which is part of the JG apparatus, and acts as an Na^+ sensor.
- *Distal convoluted tubule and part of collecting tubule*: Reabsorb NaCl.

- *Collecting tubule or duct*: Regulates urine composition and maintains acid-base, Na^+, K^+, and water homeostasis. Without ADH, the medullary CD reabsorbs NaCl and is moderately permeable to water and urea, with some urea entering from the interstitium. With ADH, water reabsorption increases, concentrating tubular fluid and raising urea levels due to NaCl reabsorption.

Suggested Readings

Khan ANM, Hard GC, Alden CL. Kidney. In: Haschek WM, Rousseaux CG, Wallig MA, eds. Haschek and Rousseaux's Handbook of Toxicologic Pathology. 3rd Ed. Academic Press, 2013: 1667–1773.

Kriz W, Kaissling B. Structural organization of the mammalian kidney. In: Alpern RJ, Moe OW, Caplan M, eds. Seldin and Giebisch's the Kidney. 5th Ed. Academic Press, 2013: 595–691.

Madsen KM, Verlander JW. Renal structure in relation to function. In: Wilcox CS, Tisher CC, eds. Handbook of Nephrology and Hypertension. 6th Ed. Lippincott Williams and Wilkins, 2008.

Pollak MR, Quaggin SE, Hoenig MP, et al. The glomerulus: the sphere of influence. *Clin J Am Soc Nephrol* 2014;9(8):1461–1469.

Reddi AS, Kuppasani K. Kidney function in health and disease. In: Byham-Gray LD, Chertow GM, Burrowes JD, eds. Nutrition in Kidney Disease. Nutrition and Health. Humana Press, 2008: 3–15.

Salguero Bodes FJ, Pallares Martinez FJ. Urinary System. In: Bodes FJS, Martinez FJP, eds. Aughey and Frye's Comparative Veterinary Histology with Clinical Correlates. CRC Press, 2023: 1–10.

Sands JM, Verlander JW. Functional anatomy of the kidney. In: McQueen CA, ed. Comprehensive Toxicology. 2nd Ed. Elsevier, 2010: 1–22.

Singh B ed. Dyce, Sack, and Wensing's Textbook of Veterinary Anatomy. 5th Ed. Saunders Ltd., 2017.

Verlander JW. Normal ultrastructure of the kidney and lower urinary tract. *Toxicol Pathol* 1998;26(1):1–17.

Verlander JW. Physiology of the kidney. In: Cunningham JG, ed. Textbook of Veterinary Physiology. 3rd Ed. Philadelphia: WB Saunders, 2002.

Verlander JW, Clapp WL. Anatomy of the kidney. In: ASL Y, Chertow GM, Luyckx V, et al., eds. Brenner and Rector's The Kidney. 11th Ed. Vol. 2. Philadelphia: Saunders Elsevier, 2020: 38–79.e12.

12

Endocrine System

John J. Turek and Elikplimi K. Asem

CHAPTER MENU

The endocrine system classically consists of the hormone-secreting, ductless glands, such as the pituitary, thyroid, parathyroid, pineal, and adrenal glands, and the cell clusters (islets of Langerhans) contained within the pancreas. Endocrine function also includes the hormone-secreting cells within the hypothalamus, respiratory, urinary, and digestive tract epithelia; the heart myocardium, and blood vessel baro- and chemoreceptors; liver hepatocytes; renal cells in the kidney; and the male and female gonadal systems. In addition, hormone-secreting adipocytes are considered both connective tissue (CT) cells and integral components of the endocrine system.

Hormones produced by endocrine cells diffuse locally in the interstitial fluid and can act locally in an autocrine or paracrine manner. Hormones also enter the blood or lymph capillaries where they circulate to distant target cells. Circulating hormones are diluted by tissue fluids to relatively low concentrations (10^{-9} to 10^{-11} M) and bind to their receptors with high affinity, typically G-protein-coupled receptors (GPCRs).

Dellmann's Textbook of Veterinary Histology, Seventh Edition. Edited by Marxa L. Figueiredo and John J. Turek.

Companion website: www.wiley.com/go/figueiredo/vethistology7e

Hypothalamus–Hypophyseal System

The controlling structure for many endocrine functions is the hypothalamus–hypophysis (pituitary) system or axis (Fig. 12-1). The hypothalamus lies ventral to the diencephalon within a region of the sphenoid bone called the sella turcica. The hypothalamic neurons in this region regulate vital body functions such as temperature, blood volume and osmolarity, and food intake. These neurons include the paired supraoptic, paraventricular, and arcuate nuclei. They receive afferent neural inputs from many regions of the brain, spinal cord, and special senses. In this circumventricular region, the blood–brain barrier is reduced or absent and this allows the neurons to easily respond to ionic and hormonal signals in the blood.

The pituitary is composed of the *adenohypophysis* (pars distalis, pars intermedia, and pars tuberalis) and a *neurohypophysis* (infundibulum and pars nervosa) (Fig. 12-2). During development, the pars nervosa develops from neural ectoderm growing down from the floor of the future diencephalon. The pars nervosa is connected to the hypothalamus median eminence by a stalk of neural tissue called the infundibulum (Fig. 12-2A). The adenohypophysis is derived from oral ectoderm. The pars tuberalis portion of the adenohypophysis partially envelopes the infundibulum. The pars distalis extends from the pars tuberalis. The pars intermedia is between the pars distalis and the pars nervosa. The stimulating (releasing) or inhibiting factors (hormones) produced by hypothalamic neurons are listed in Table 12-1. These hormones are transported within the axons near the median eminence and released into a primary capillary plexus of the hypothalamo–hypophyseal portal system. The hormones are then distributed through the pars tuberalis via hypophyseal venules to the secondary capillary plexus in the pars distalis where they exit and bind to their target cells. The hormones produced and released by cells of the adenohypophysis are distributed systemically and act on the target cells of other organs, also stimulating the production of effector hormones. The pars nervosa is not a site for hormone synthesis, but rather the hormones in this portion of the

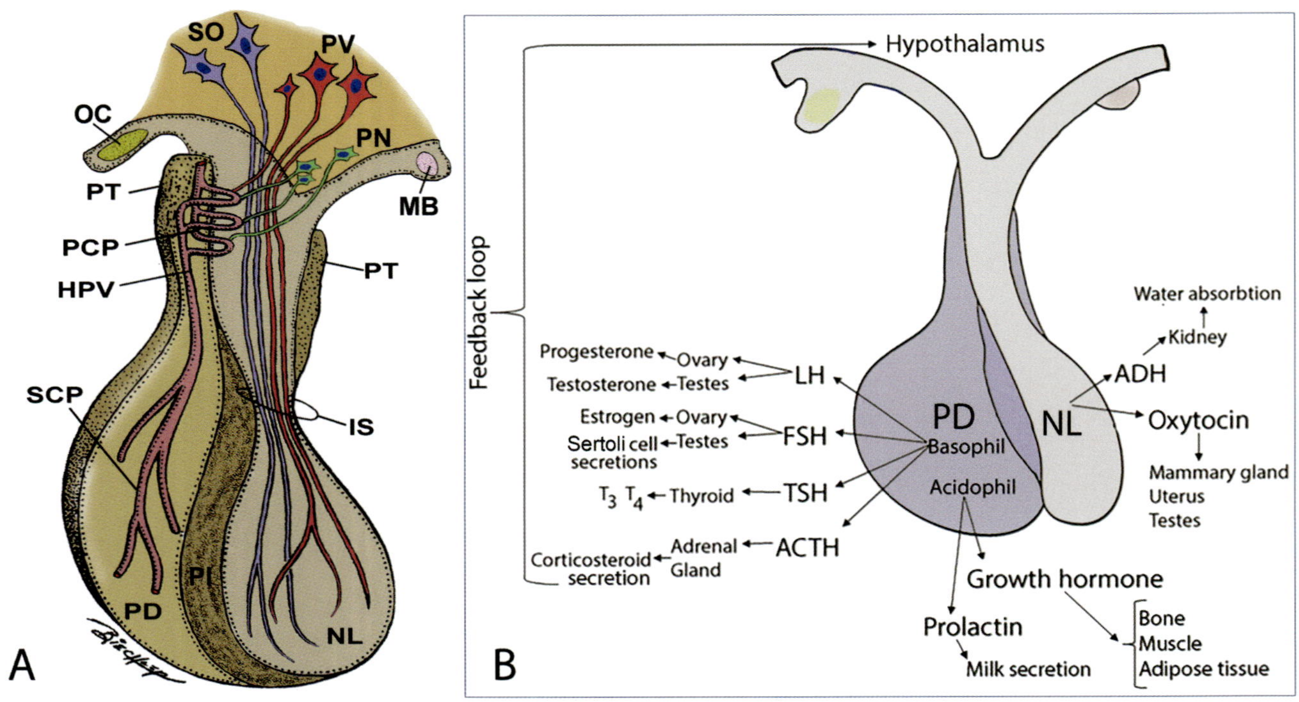

Figure 12-1 **A.** Schematic drawing of the hypothalamo–adenohypophysial and the hypothalamo–neurohypophysial systems. Optic chiasm (OC), mamillary body (MB), and parvocellular neurons (PN) of the hypothalamus terminate near the primary capillary plexus (PCP) of the hypophysial portal system in the median eminence where they secrete releasing or inhibiting factors (hormones). The hormones are carried to the pars distalis (PD) through the hypophysial portal venules (HPV) and gain access to the cells of the pars distalis via a secondary capillary plexus (SCP). Pars intermedia (PI) and pars tuberalis (PT). Axons originating from the magnocellular hypothalamic supraoptic (SO) and paraventricular (PV) nuclei course through the median eminence (ME) and the infundibular stalk (IS) to terminate in the pars nervosa or neural lobe (NL), where oxytocin and vasopressin are stored and released. (Modified and redrawn from original.) **B.** Schematic showing target tissues or functions for hormones produced by the pars distalis (PD) and the neural lobe (NL).

pituitary are produced in the hypothalamic neurons, transported down their axons, and stored in neurosecretory bodies (Herring bodies) prior to release.

Adenohypophysis Regions

The three regions of the adenohypophysis are the **pars distalis, pars intermedia**, and **pars tuberalis**. The relative size and orientation of each part is species dependent (Fig. 12-3).

The pars distalis is the largest part of the adenohypophysis. The pars tuberalis contacts the base of the brain (median eminence) and partially envelops the infundibulum portion of the pars nervosa. In some species, there may be a **hypophyseal cavity** between the pars intermedia and the pars distalis.

Pars Distalis

The cells of the **pars distalis** surround a fenestrated capillary network called the **secondary capillary plexus**. The cell types vary in size, shape, number, and position depending on species, gender, age, and physiologic status (e.g., during pregnancy and lactation or after gonad removal). Secretions are stored in dense secretory granules prior to release via exocytosis (Fig. 12-4). There are six secretory cell types within the adenohypophysis. Postnatally, an organ-specific stem cell population is also present.

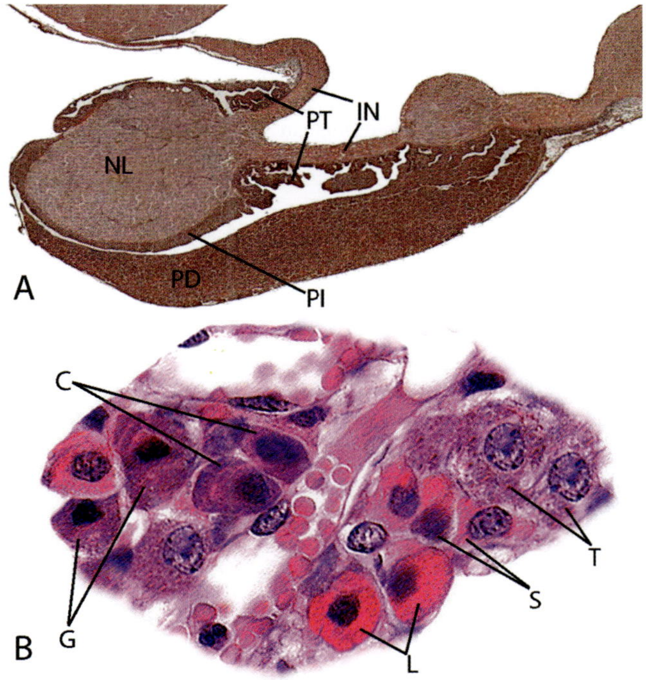

Figure 12-2 **A.** Midsagittal section of the pituitary gland of a puppy. Pars distalis (PD), neural lobe (NL), pars intermedia (PI), pars tuberalis (PT), and infundibulum (IN) (×4.5). Adenohypophysis contacting neural lobe (×40). **B.** Parenchyma of the adenohypophysis. Corticotroph (C), gonadotroph (G), lactotroph (L), somatotroph (S), and thyrotroph (T) (×100). Hematoxylin and eosin (H&E).

Pars Intermedia

The pars intermedia is quite variable among species. It may appear as a simple columnar epithelium or as a pseudostratified columnar epithelium that invades the neural lobe. In some species, such as horses, this region is extensively developed. The pars intermedia has a high concentration of melanotrophs (see below).

Pars Tuberalis

The **pars tuberalis** is a highly vascular region containing veins of the hypophyseal portal system. These vessels receive blood from the primary capillary plexus in the median eminence and transport it to the secondary capillary plexus in the pars distalis. This region contains cell clusters that may form a folded tissue with occasional small cysts. The parenchymal cells have melatonin receptors and likely have a role in the seasonal reproductive cycle of certain domesticated mammals. Other cells include some gonadotrophs and thyrotrophs.

Cells of the Adenohypophysis

Typical hematoxylin and eosin (H&E) staining reveals that the cells display acidophilic, basophilic, or poor staining characteristics. These cells are classified as **acidophils, basophils**, or **chromophobes**.

Acidophils. A common stem cell gives rise to the polypeptide hormone-secreting acidophils (Figs. 12-2B and 12-5). The **somatotrophs** secrete growth hormone (**GH**) and the **lactotrophs** secrete prolactin (**PRL**). Growth hormone–releasing hormone (**GHRH**) from hypothalamic neurons stimulates somatotrophs to release GH. The secretory granules of somatotrophs stain with eosin and orange G dye. Growth hormone has a role in anabolic metabolism by stimulating the production of insulin-like growth factor 1 (IGF-1) in the liver. IGF-1, in turn, stimulates cell differentiation, proliferation, and tissue growth. An important effect of IGF-1 is promoting the growth of chondroblasts during skeletal growth. A negative feedback loop effect of IGF-1 is to inhibit the release of both GH and GHRH to maintain homeostasis. GH secretion is also

Table 12-1 Relationship of Hypothalamic Releasing Hormones, Hormones Released from Adenohypophysis, and Hormones Released by Target Cells

Hypothalamus Secretion	Cell of Origin in Hypothalamus	Hormone from Adenohypophysis, Pars Distalis	Cell of Origin in Adenohypophysis	Chief Target Cell	Hormone Released by Target Cell
Growth hormone-releasing hormone (GHRH)	Hypothalamic neuron	Growth hormone (GH)	Somatotroph	All cells Hepatocyte	— Insulin-like growth factor 1 (IGF-1)
Prolactin-releasing factor (PRF)	Hypothalamic neuron	Prolactin (PRL)	Lactotroph	Mammary ductal/alveolar epithelium	—
Thyrotropin-releasing hormone (TRH)	Hypothalamic neuron	Thyroid-stimulating hormone (TSH)	Thyrotroph	Thyroid follicular epithelium	Triiodothyronine (T_3) and tetraiodothyronine (T_4)
Gonadotropin-releasing hormone (GnRH)	Hypothalamic neuron	Follicle-stimulating hormone[a] (FSH)	Gonadotroph[a]	Ovarian follicular cells	Estrogen, inhibin, and activin
				Testicular Sertoli cell	Estrogen, inhibin, and activin
		Luteinizing hormone (LH)[a]	Gonadotroph[a]	Corpus luteum	Progesterone
				Ovarian internal thecal cell	Testosterone
				Testicular Leydig cell	Testosterone
Corticotropin-releasing hormone (CRH)	Hypothalamic neuron	Adrenocorticotropin (ACTH)	Corticotroph	Zona glomerulosa[b]	Mineralocorticoid
				Zona fasciculata	Glucocorticoid
				Zona reticularis	Androgen

[a] FSH and LH are coexpressed by the same gonadotroph.
[b] Cells of the zona glomerulosa are 10-fold less responsive than those of the zona fasciculata.

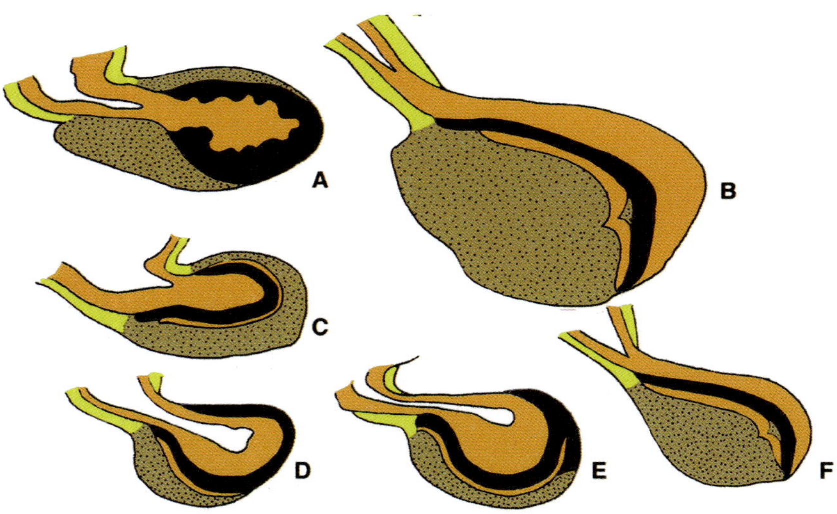

Figure 12-3 Schematic drawings of midsagittal sections of the hypophysis cerebri. **A.** Horse. **B.** Cow. **C.** Dog. **D.** Pig. **E.** Cat. **F.** Sheep. Orange: Neurohypophysis with infundibular recess; yellow: pars tuberalis adenohypophysis; tan with dots: pars distalis adenohypophysis; black: pars intermedia adenohypophysis. (Modified from original by colorization. From Dellmann H-D. *Veterinary Histology: An Outline Text–Atlas*. Philadelphia, PA: Lea & Febiger, 1971.)

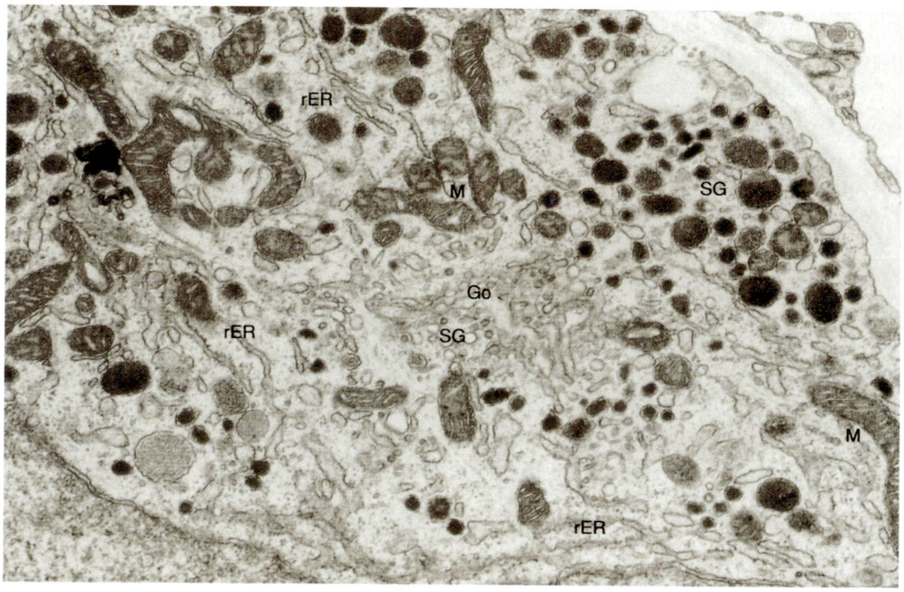

Figure 12-4 Organelles typical of an adenohypophyseal cell: rough endoplasmic reticulum (rER), Golgi complex (Go), mitochondria (M), and secretory granules (SG) of varying maturational stages (×28,000).

regulated by hypothalamic production of somatostatin (SST). SST binds to its receptors (i.e., GPCRs) and decreases intracellular cyclic AMP and calcium, which inhibits GH secretion.

Lactotrophs, which produce **PRL**, stain lightly with eosin. Lactotroph cell size and dye affinity increase during pregnancy and lactation. The cells are round to oval or polyhedral in shape. Location can vary with species, but in rats, they cluster in a band adjacent to the pars intermedia. The pituitary is the primary site of PRL production, but it is also synthesized within the central nervous system, the immune system, the uterus, the placenta, and the mammary gland. In the mammary gland, PRL stimulates mammary epithelial cell proliferation and differentiation into milk-synthesizing cells. In addition to its role in lactation, it is now recognized to have as many as 300 biological functions. A prolactin-releasing peptide (**PRL-RP**) has been identified, but it has multiple functions and is not the primary stimulator of PRL release. PRL-RP appears to have a role in regulation of food intake, energy expenditure, stress regulation, sleep promotion, and may have neuroprotective effects. Thyrotropin-releasing hormone (**TRH**), as well as releasing hormones for follicle-stimulating hormone (**FSH**) and luteinizing hormone (**LH**), stimulates the release of PRL, as well as neurogenic stress or the suckling sensory stimulus. Regulation of PRL involves a combination of stimulatory signals and inhibition by dopamine released from the hypothalamus. When dopamine binds to the membrane receptor on lactotrophs, it uncouples cAMP (cyclic adenosine monophosphate), and lowers intracellular calcium, thus inhibiting the release of PRL.

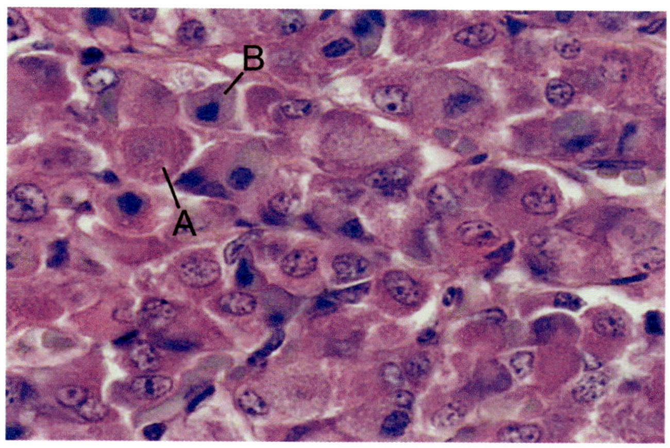

Figure 12-5 Appearance of acidophils (A) and basophils (B) in an H&E-stained section of a mammalian pars distalis (×40).

Basophils. Thyrotroph cells, which secrete the glycoprotein **thyroid-stimulating hormone (TSH)**, are more numerous mid-ventrally and may be detected with aldehyde–fuchsin dye. **TRH** is released from neurons in the paraventricular nucleus. TRH binding to the thyrotrophs promotes the exocytosis of **TSH** (thyrotropin). TSH, in turn, stimulates the synthesis and storage of thyroglobulin and the release of thyroid hormones, **triiodothyronine** (T_3) and **tetraiodothyronine** (T_4). Negative feedback of the T_3 or T_4 to the hypothalamus and the pars distalis regulates the production of TRH and TSH, respectively.

Gonadotrophs are relatively small in size and secrete both **FSH** and **LH**. They stain with aldehyde–thionine dyes. **Gonadotropin-releasing hormone** (GnRH) is released from neurons diffusely scattered in the hypothalamus. GnRH signals the coexpression, synthesis, and release of the glycoprotein hormones FSH and LH. In the female, FSH stimulates ovarian follicle development by targeting **follicular epithelial cells**. In the male, FSH stimulates **Sertoli cells** (sustentacular cells) of the testis to produce androgen-binding protein (ABP). FSH also stimulates **estrogen** production in both sexes. In the ovary, LH targets **internal thecal cells**, signaling the production of **testosterone**, and acts on follicular and thecal cells of the postovulatory follicle, signaling the production of **progesterone**. Cells of the ovarian interstitial stroma in the pig, dog, cat, rabbit, and human also produce testosterone. In the male, LH targets the Leydig interstitial endocrine cells to produce testosterone. The gonadal steroids negatively regulate the production of GnRH and gonadotropins by binding to cells of the hypothalamus and pars distalis. FSH stimulates follicular cells, corpus luteal cells, and Sertoli cells to synthesize **inhibin** and **activin**. Inhibin and activin are members of the TGF-β superfamily of growth factors and either inhibit or activate the production of FSH from the pars distalis.

Corticotrophs, along with closely related cells called **melanotrophs**, constitute the central melanocortin system. While these cells share a common stem cell, melanotrophs follow an alternate differentiation pathway compared to corticotrophs and express different transcription factors. Corticotrophs are dispersed throughout the pars distalis, while melanotrophs cluster in the pars intermedia. Both cell types produce pro-opiomelanocortin (**POMC**). POMC is also produced in peptidergic neurons in the arcuate nucleus of the hypothalamus. POMC is a precursor hormone that is cleaved into a number of peptide hormones that are stored in dense core granules within the cells. In the pars distalis, the POMC is cleaved into pro-ACTH, which is then cleaved into **adrenocorticotropic hormone (ACTH) and ß-lipotropic hormone (ß-LPH)**. In the pars intermedia, ACTH is further cleaved into α-melanocyte stimulating hormone (**α-MSH**), and the ß-LPH is cleaved into **ß-MSH**. **Corticotropin-releasing hormone** (CRH) released from neurons in the paraventricular nucleus stimulates exocytosis of hormones from these cells. These basophils stain with periodic acid-Schiff and Alcian blue dyes. The corticotrophs are part of the hypothalamic–pituitary–adrenal axis. ACTH acts on cells of the zona fasciculata of the adrenal gland to produce cortisol. Inflammatory cytokines such as interleukins (IL-1 and IL-6) and tumor necrosis factor-α (TNF-α) act on the hypothalamus to enhance CRH production. Antidiuretic hormone (ADH) released from the neurohypophysis also stimulates the release of ACTH from corticotrophs. Glucocorticoids negatively regulate hypothalamic CRH production, POMC synthesis, and ACTH release in the pars distalis. Stress can increase neurogenic input to the hypothalamus and overcome glucocorticoid inhibition of ACTH.

Chromophobes. **Chromophobes** stain poorly with dyes typically used to identify acidophils and basophils. These cells are considered to be either degranulated cells or undifferentiated stem cells. These cells may also occasionally form a simple epithelium that lines cysts of unknown significance. Still, other stellate-shaped chromophobes are sometimes interspersed among the other cells of the pars distalis.

Neurohypophysis (Pars Nervosa)

Hypothalamo–neurohypophyseal tract Large (magnocellular) neurons in the hypothalamus make up the majority of the **supraoptic** and **paraventricular nuclei**. Afferent synaptic input to the neurons signals the exocytosis of secretory vesicles from their axons. Bundles of these axons and their glial support cells (pituicytes) make up the median eminence, infundibulum, and neural lobe of the **neurohypophysis**. The pars nervosa contains the axons of hypothalamic neurons and pituicytes but lacks neuron cell bodies. The neuron cell bodies of the supraoptic and paraventricular nuclei in the hypothalamus synthesize **oxytocin** and ADH (Fig. 12-6). ADH is also called arginine vasopressin; however, in pigs, lysine is substituted for arginine, producing lysine vasopressin.

Oxytocin is produced as a prepropeptide (preprooxytocin) in the hypothalamic nuclei and undergoes modification during axonal transport. Along with its carrier protein neurophysin, oxytocin is stored in secretory granules at the axon terminals of the pars nervosa (Fig. 12-7). Accumulations of these secretory granules are located within neurosecretory or Herring bodies. Release of oxytocin is triggered by reproductive and maternal stimuli via brainstem sensory networks (e.g., sensory input from washing the cow's udder during milking or sounds from the sow's litter). When oxytocin binds to mammary alveoli myoepithelial cells, resulting cell contraction induces "milk letdown." Similarly, binding to receptors on myometrial smooth muscle cells leads to uterine contractions during parturition. In addition to its reproductive role, oxytocin, along with ADH, is also regulated by stressors, such as dehydration, hypervolemia, hyperosmolarity, and hemorrhage. In response to hypoxia, stress, hypertensive conditions, or cardiac insufficiency, oxytocin release is decreased while ADH release is increased.

ADH differs from oxytocin by two amino acids, and it is synthesized as a prepropeptide (preprovasopressin). It is modified and packaged into secretory granules during axonal transport along with the carrier protein neurophysin and the

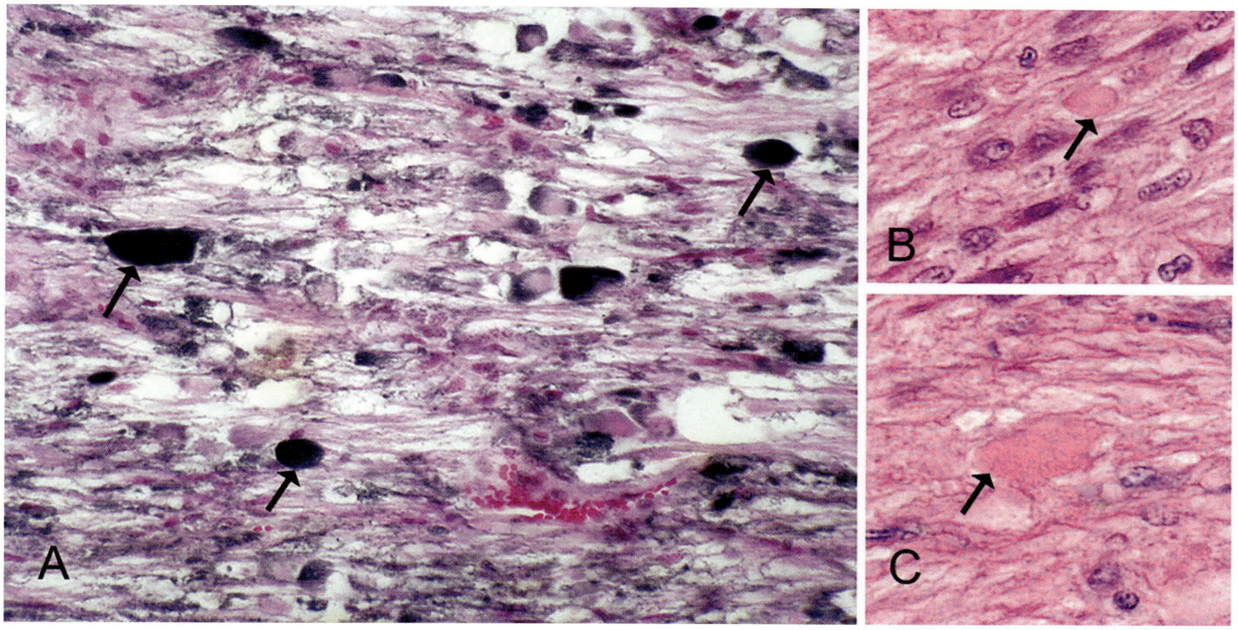

Figure 12-6 **A.** Neurosecretory or Herring bodies in the neural lobe (arrows) containing oxytocin and antidiuretic hormone, visualized using a special stain. Neurohypophysis, ox, and Bargmann's chrome hematoxylin (×250). (Image by W.E. Haensly.) **B and C.** Appearance of neurosecretory bodies (arrows) in H&E-stained sections of a mammalian neural lobe (×400).

glycopeptide copeptin. Like oxytocin, the release of ADH is signaled by sensory synapses from neurons monitoring properties of the internal environment. In cases of dehydration, ADH acts on the kidney by activating water channels (aquaporin 2) in collecting tubule cells, reducing water loss through the urine. ADH also binds to its V1 receptor on vascular smooth muscle, causing increased myocyte tone, vascular constriction, and elevated blood pressure. In addition, binding of ADH to the V3 receptor on hypophyseal corticotrophs stimulates the release of ACTH and a rise in aldosterone secretion.

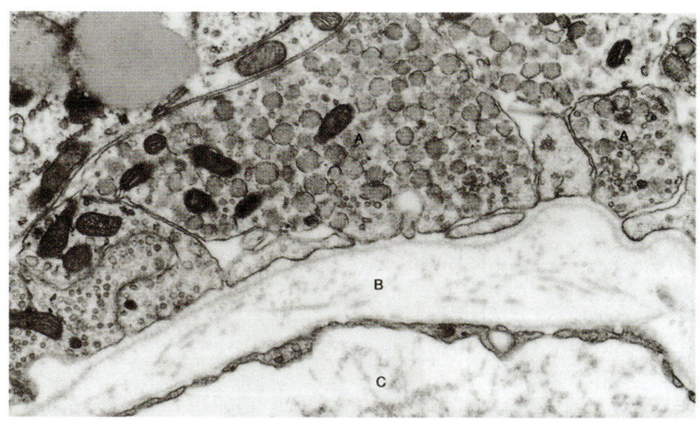

Figure 12-7 Axons of neurosecretory neurons (A) adjacent to a basal lamina, interstitial connective tissue (CT) (B), and a fenestrated capillary (C) in the neurohypophysis. Axon terminals have large electron-dense, hormone-containing secretory vesicles; upon depolarization of the neuron, the contents of the vesicles are released by exocytosis (×31,500).

Epiphysis Cerebri (Pineal Gland)

The pineal gland is a melatonin-producing organ that is responsive to photoperiod environment, and the nocturnally generated melatonin regulates circadian rhythms in animals. An interesting feature in vertebrates and mammals is that the size of the organ is correlated with the harshness of the environment. Generally, the pineal gland increases in size in vertebrates from south to north (equator to poles). Melatonin from the pineal gland is associated with the 24-hour biological clock wake–sleep cycle and regulates breeding cycles for seasonal breeders. For photoperiod-sensitive breeders, melatonin regulates the breeding cycle by inhibiting the release of hypothalamic gonadotropic-releasing hormone, which in turn inhibits LH and FSH secretion from the adenohypophysis. Mitochondria produce melatonin in all cells; interestingly, pineal melatonin is only a small fraction of total melatonin production. As much as 500 times more melatonin is produced by enteroendocrine cells of the gastrointestinal (GI) system, where it acts locally. In the GI system, melatonin functions as an antioxidant and may have a role in the healing of GI lesions and in gut motility. Melatonin is also produced by epithelial hair follicles, salivary glands, platelets,

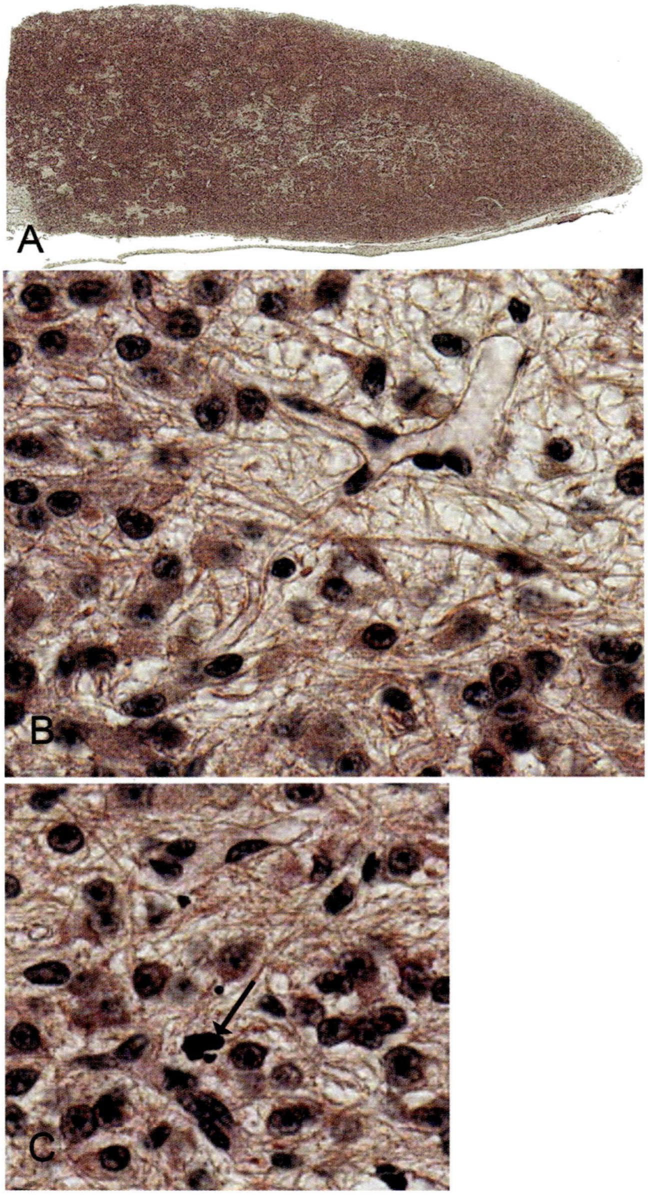

Figure 12-8 **A.** Bovine pineal gland. **B.** Pinealocytes and neuropil. **C.** Corpora arenacea (brain sand) indicated by the arrow. (Courtesy of Purdue College of Veterinary Medicine.)

and lymphocytes. The role of extra-pineal melatonin production is currently an area of extensive research.

The development of the pineal gland is similar across mammalian species, although cell types and morphology can vary. The gland is connected to the epithalamus by a stalk of tissue and is bathed in cerebrospinal fluid from the third ventricle of the brain. This pine cone-shaped organ (*Latin, pinea* or pine cone) (Fig. 12-8A) receives its blood supply from the pia-arachnoid. The clusters and cords of cells within the gland are primarily **pinealocytes** (Fig. 12-8B), and the gland also contains microglia and **glial-like interstitial cells** similar to astrocytes. These glial cells stain positive for glial fibrillary acidic protein. The gland lacks a blood–brain barrier, allowing gland secretions to access fenestrated blood capillaries and the cerebrospinal fluid. In older animals, calcified protein deposits termed **corpora arenacea** ('brain sand') may be present (Fig. 12-8C). The cause of the deposits is unknown, but they do not appear to affect gland function. These calcified deposits are readily observed in histologic slides and serve as a radiographic marker for the brain midline.

The pinealocyte cytoplasm is lightly basophilic, and the nuclei can be irregular and lobulated. The cytoplasm has well-developed Golgi complex and rough endoplasmic reticulum (rER), and many vesicles. Nonmyelinated nerve fibers form synapses with some pinealocytes. **Pinealocytes** are interconnected via gap junctions and extend processes to other pinealocytes, nearby capillaries, and the base of the ependymal lining of the ventricular recess. The suprachiasmatic nuclei (**SCNs**) of the hypothalamus are considered the central circadian clock. When light is received by retinal ganglion cells, they send a signal via the optic nerve to the SCN. In some species, a blue light–sensitive photopigment called melanopsin initiates the light-inhibiting melatonin response, although evidence suggests there are other pigments involved. From the SCN, the signal is transmitted to the spinal cervical ganglia and then, via postganglionic nerve fibers, back to the pineal gland, where it inhibits melatonin production. At the beginning of a dark cycle, the sympathetic pathway nerve supply from the SCN to the pineal gland releases norepinephrine (NE). The NE binding to adrenergic receptors on the pinealocytes activates N-acetyltransferase that converts serotonin to melatonin. Melatonin is released as it is synthesized rather than stored.

Thyroid Gland

The hypothalamus–pituitary–thyroid axis is essential for the regulation of energy metabolism. TRH from the hypothalamus stimulates the release of TSH from the adenohypophysis. The thyroid gland is derived from the endoderm cephalic portion of the alimentary canal. The two lobes are joined by a central isthmus. The gland has an extensive fenestrated blood capillary network and many lymph capillaries. During development, a later migration of cells from pharyngeal pouch IV forms the ultimo-branchial body. As this body fuses with the developing thyroid, it is colonized by neural crest cells. These neural crest cells differentiate within the thyroid as parafollicular (calcitonin-producing, "C") cells (Fig. 12-9B).

The **thyroid follicles** are lined by a simple epithelium (Fig. 12-9A). Typically, these cells have a cuboidal morphology but can become more squamous or columnar depending upon synthetic activity. The size of follicles varies widely, ranging from a few to several hundred micrometers in diameter. Columnar cells indicate highly secretory follicles, whereas squamous cells are associated with follicles in a resting state. Follicular cell cytoplasm has abundant rER, Golgi complex, and secretory vesicles. Gap junctions synchronize the activity of all cells lining a follicle.

Thyroglobulin, a glycoprotein, is exocytosed into the follicle lumen, where it forms a substance referred to as **colloid**. Inorganic iodide is actively transported (iodide symporter) from the blood into the cytosol of the follicular cells. Within the cytoplasm, iodide is oxidized and then enters the colloid, where it iodinates thyroglobulin tyrosine residues. When TSH binds to its receptors on follicle cells, colloid is endocytosed, and the endosomes fuse with lysosomes. Iodinated residues are cleaved from the thyroglobulin, releasing T_3 and T_4 into the cytosol. These hormones then diffuse through the plasma basal membrane. The majority of the hormone released is in the form of T_4, which is converted to the active form, T_3, within cells by deiodinases (Fig. 12-10).

Both TSH and adrenergic input stimulate GPCRs, leading to an elevation of intracellular cAMP, which mediates both the synthesis of thyroglobulin and the release of thyroid hormone. Thyroglobulin is a glycosylated dimer containing tyrosyl sites capable of being iodinated. The enzymes participating in the iodination of thyroglobulin include the iodide symporter and thyroid peroxidase.

Thyroid peroxidase is expressed and incorporated into the apical membrane. In the presence of hydrogen peroxide, iodide is converted to iodine, and one or two ions are incorporated into each tyrosyl residue, forming **mono-** or **diiodotyrosine** (T_1 or T_2). The peroxidase catalyzes the coupling of iodotyrosyl residues within the thyroglobulin dimer, forming **tri-** or **tetraiodothyronine** (T_3 or T_4). T_4 is commonly called **thyroxine**.

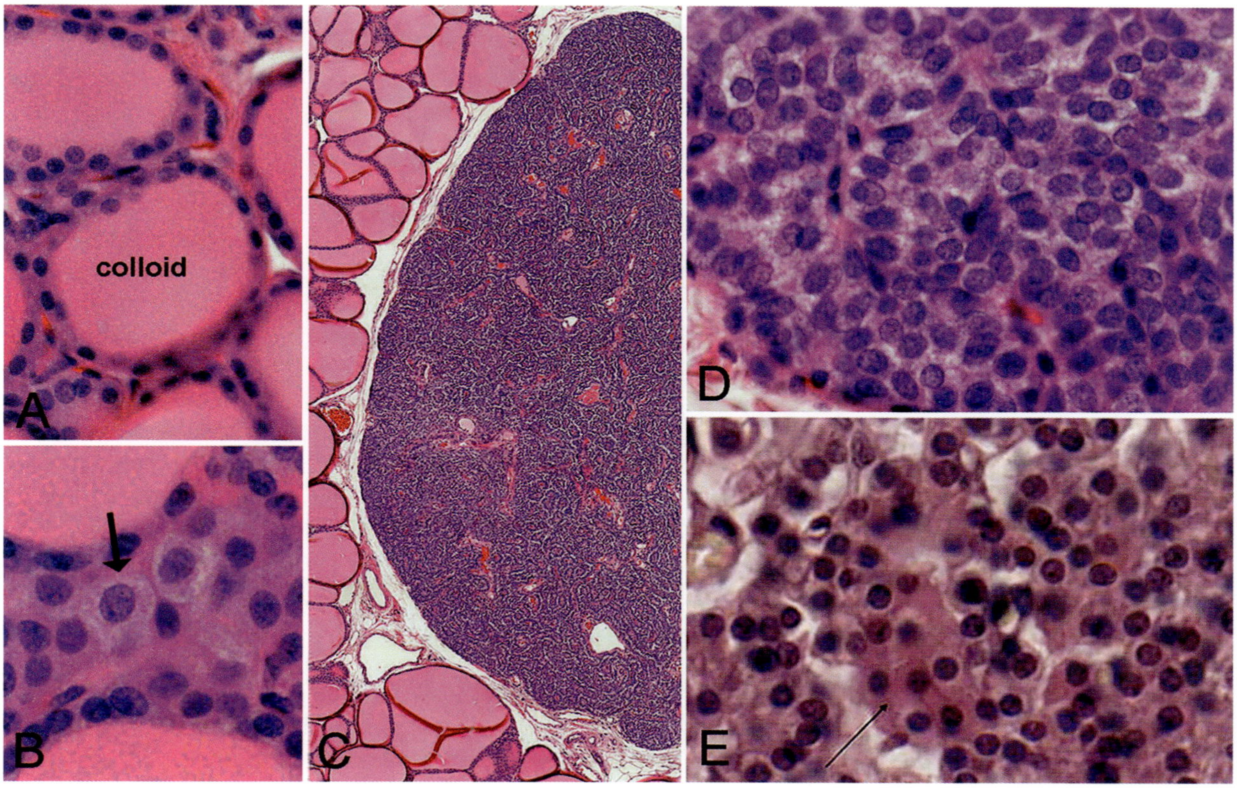

Figure 12-9 **A.** Thyroid follicles filled with colloid, surrounded by a simple epithelium (which can vary from squamous to cuboidal to columnar depending upon synthetic activity). **B.** Calcitonin-secreting parafollicular cells (arrow). **C.** Thyroid gland (left) adjacent to the parathyroid gland (right). **D.** Parathyroid parenchyma primarily composed of chief cells. **E.** Oxyphil cells present in small clusters within the parathyroid gland (arrow).

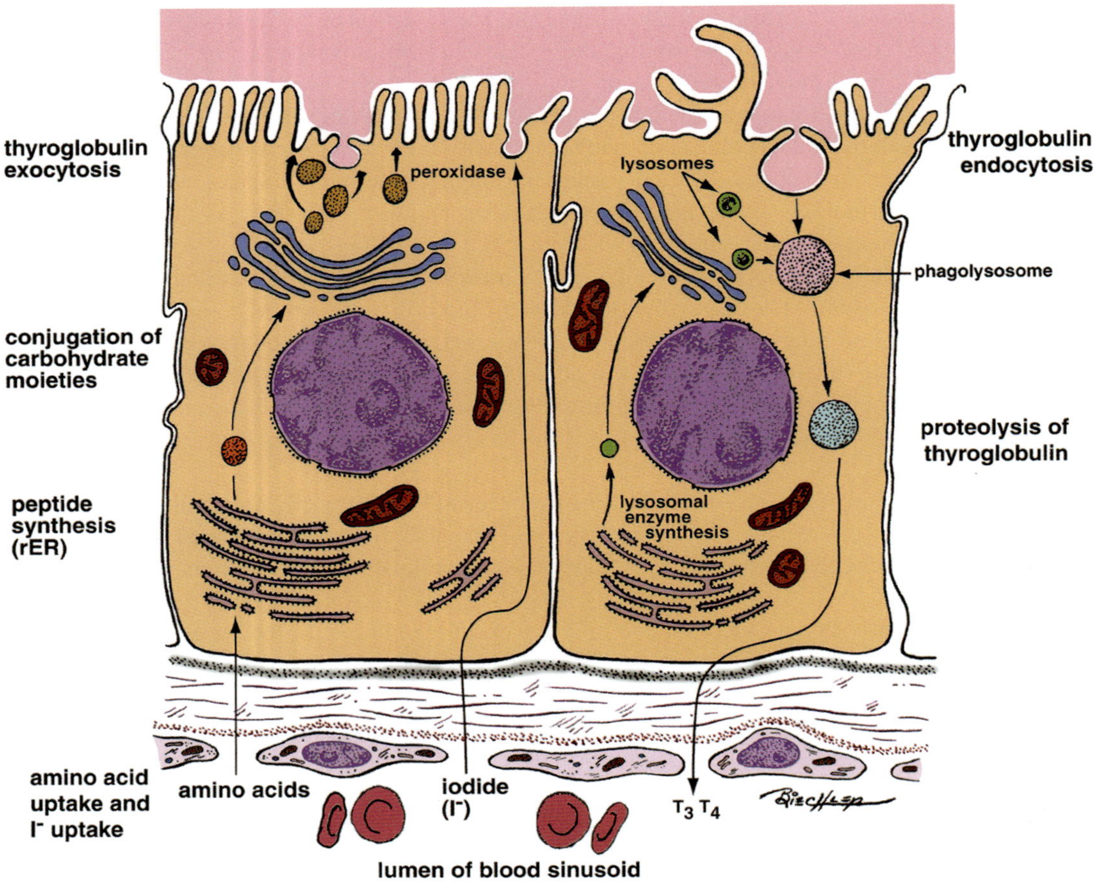

Figure 12-10 Schematic drawing of the biosynthesis of thyroglobulin in one cell (left) and its resorption, proteolysis, and release as T_3 and T_4 in another cell (right).

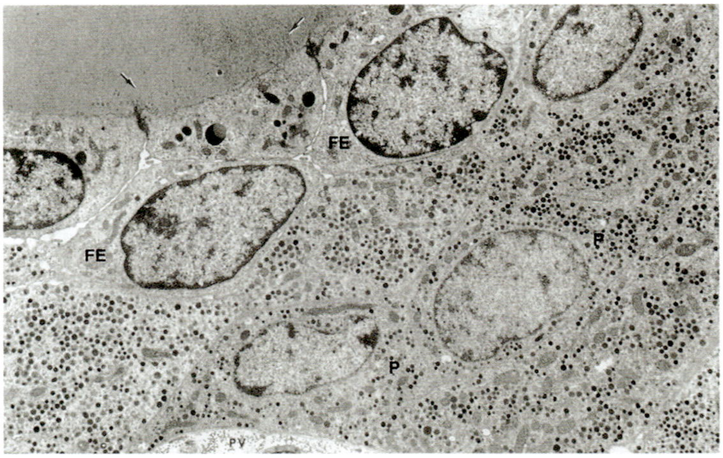

Figure 12-11 Thyroid parenchyma, dog. Follicular epithelial cells (FE) line the follicle. Microvilli (arrows) project into the colloid. Calcitonin-producing parafollicular cells (P) lie near a pericapillary space (PV) (×7900). (Courtesy of K.R. Moore and S.L. Teitelbaum).

The T_3 receptor is a ligand-induced transactivator, and the genes transcribed affect basal metabolic rate, thermogenesis, and gluconeogenesis. In the median eminence and pars distalis, T_3 acts to negatively regulate the release of TRH and TSH, respectively.

The parafollicular cells are often positioned in the basolateral compartment between follicular epithelial cells and within the basal lamina, while others form clusters between the follicles (Figs. 12-9B and 12-11).

These large epithelioid cells (prominent in dogs) synthesize **calcitonin** and are *a*mine *p*recursor *u*ptake and *d*ecarboxylation (APUD) cells (see the "Diffuse Neuroendocrine System Cells" section below). The synthesis and release of calcitonin is regulated by the concentration of calcium in the intercellular fluid. When the intercellular calcium concentration rises, the calcium-sensing receptor on the parafollicular cell detects the increase and triggers calcitonin release. Gastrin also promotes calcitonin release (see the "Enteroendocrine Cells" section). Calcitonin binds to its receptor on osteoclasts and kidney epithelium, lowering the calcium concentration in blood and interstitial fluid by inhibiting osteoclast activity and reducing tubular resorption of calcium, respectively.

Parathyroid Gland

Parathyroid glands are derived from the endoderm of the third and fourth pharyngeal pouches. The cranial external parathyroid forms from pouch III, while the caudal internal parathyroid forms from pouch IV. The glands have a capsule, and the parenchyma has an extensive capillary plexus (Fig. 12-9C). Delicate trabeculae penetrate the gland from the fibrous capsule. The parenchyma is arranged as uniform clusters of small **principal** (chief) **cells** separated by fine collagenous bands (Fig. 12-9D). Variations in the staining affinity of the principal cells likely indicate differences in the secretory cycle, with light-staining cells having a less prominent rER and Golgi complex. The parathyroid glands of horses, cows, and humans contain scattered small clusters of **oxyphil cells** (Fig. 12-9E), which have more acidophilic staining compared to the principal cells. In humans, their numbers increase with age and have been shown to secrete parathyroid hormone (PTH) in some cases of parathyroid hyperplasia; however, their function is otherwise unknown.

The principal cell synthesizes **PTH**, which is stored within cytoplasmic granules 200 to 400 nm in diameter. PTH elevates and maintains normal calcium concentration in both blood and interstitial fluid. Its synthesis and release are regulated by the calcium concentration in the extracellular fluid. A calcium-sensing receptor on principal cells monitors extracellular calcium concentrations. PTH has multiple mechanisms for maintaining calcium homeostasis through endocrine feedback loops. When calcium levels are within normal values, unbound extracellular ionic calcium binds to the calcium-sensing receptor on the parathyroid cells. Signaling from the receptor causes an increase in intracellular calcium that suppresses PTH secretion. However, when low levels of calcium are detected, inhibition of PTH secretion is lifted and this increases both synthesis and secretion of PTH.

Low serum-free calcium initiates PTH release to elevate calcium by acting primarily on three organ systems. PTH is a main factor in initiating osteoclastogenesis to release calcium from the skeleton. PTH stimulates osteoblasts to secrete receptor activator of nuclear factor-kappa B ligand (**RANKL**). RANKL induces differentiation of osteoclast precursors into mature bone-resorbing osteoclasts and also inhibits the release of osteoprotegerin. PTH enhances the reabsorption of calcium from the kidney distal tubules while increasing phosphate excretion. PTH also increases intestinal absorption of Ca^{2+} indirectly by stimulating vitamin D synthesis, which stimulates synthesis of calcium-binding protein in the intestine.

Adrenal Gland

The adrenal glands are part of the hypothalamic–pituitary–adrenal axis. The outer cortex is derived from mesoderm, while the inner medulla is derived from neural crest ectoderm. A thin CT layer separates the cortex and medulla (Fig. 12-12). The gland has a dense irregular collagenous CT capsule that extends thin trabeculae toward the medulla. Branches of the suprarenal arteries distribute to capillaries within the capsule, to sinusoidal fenestrated capillaries of the cortex, and to medullary arterioles and sinusoidal capillaries. The cortical and medullary blood circulations merge in the medulla, forming medullary sinusoids, venous sinuses, and eventually the medullary vein. Preganglionic sympathetic axons course within the parenchyma adjacent to the circulatory elements. Lymphatic vessels are contained within the capsule and some of the sparse stromal tissues.

Adrenal Cortex

The zona glomerulosa/arcuata, zona fasciculata, and zona reticularis are the three regions of the outer cortex. The arrangement of cells in the zona glomerulosa varies between species (Figs. 12-12C and 12-13). In ruminants and humans, the cells of outermost zone are arranged in ovoid cell clusters (**zona glomerulosa**), whereas in horses, pigs, and carnivores, they appear as arches of columnar cells (**zona arcuata**). The mineralocorticoid **aldosterone** is produced in this outer cortex region. The cells in this region have round nuclei and less cytoplasm compared to the adjacent zona fasciculata region. The cells of all three zones within the cortex have extensive smooth endoplasmic reticulum, typical of steroid hormone-producing cells, and the mitochondria have tubular cristae that contain the enzymes necessary for steroid biosynthesis.

The zona glomerulosa cells **release aldosterone** in response to angiotensin II signaling (renin–angiotensin–aldosterone system). **Renin** release (see the "Heart and Kidney" section below and Chapter 11) is triggered by lowered blood perfusion pressure in glomerular arterioles. The plasma protein **angiotensinogen** is the substrate for renin. The peptide **angiotensin I** is cleaved from angiotensinogen, and angiotensin I is converted enzymatically to **angiotensin II** in the pulmonary circulation.

Aldosterone acts on the collecting tubules and distal convoluted tubules to increase Na^+ reabsorption and increase K^+ excretion. When aldosterone diffuses into the kidney tubule cells, it binds to its cytosolic receptor and is transported into the nucleus to its hormone response elements on target genes. This increased expression of target genes in the collecting

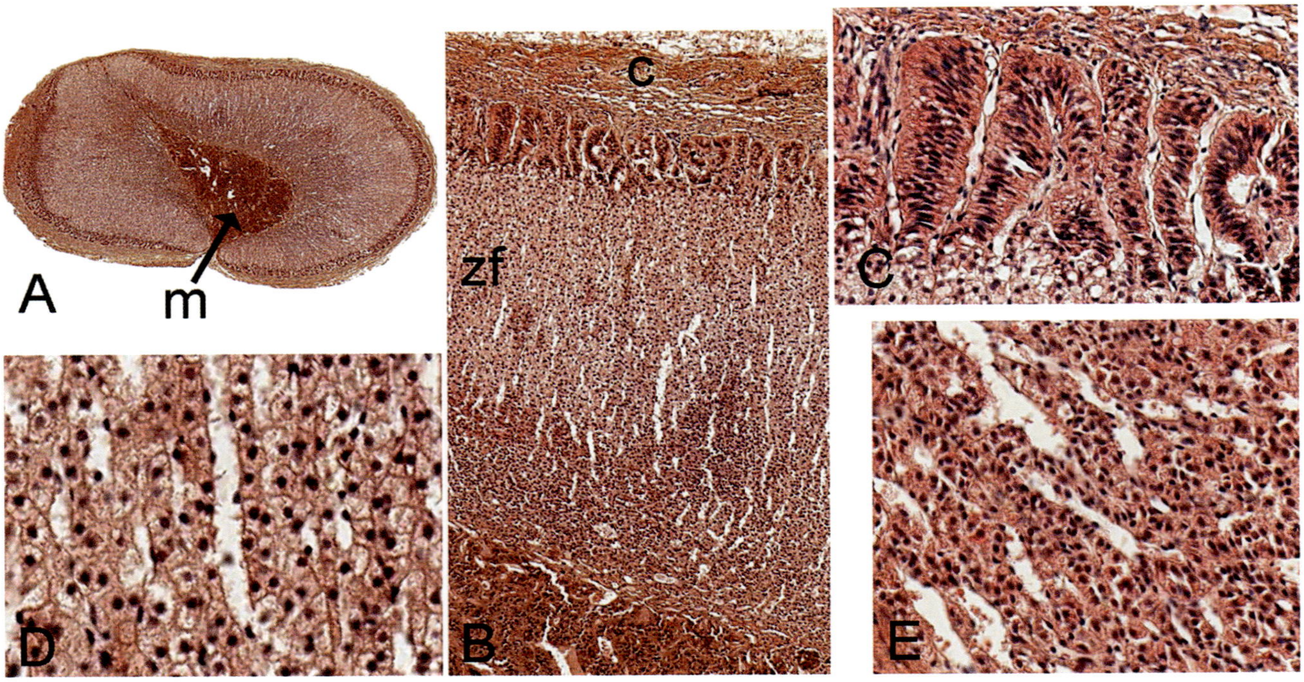

Figure 12-12 Canine adrenal gland. **A.** Cross section of gland showing the medulla (m). **B.** Gland capsule (c) and zona fasciculata (zf). **C.** Zona glomerulosa. **D.** Zona fasciculata. **E.** Zona reticularis. (Courtesy of Purdue College of Veterinary Medicine.)

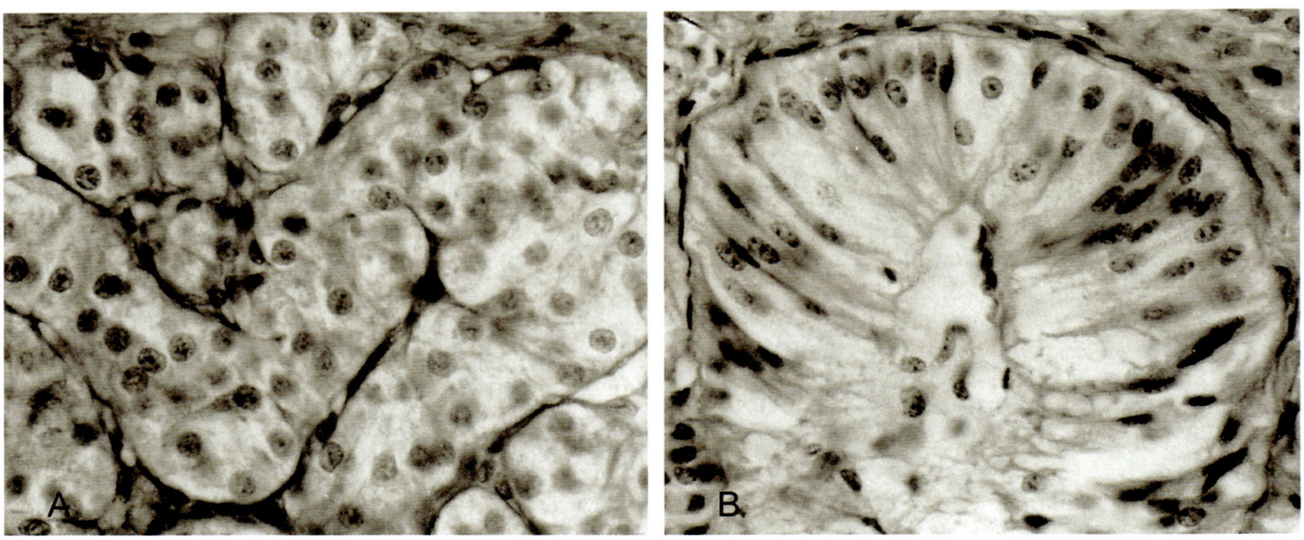

Figure 12-13 In the bovine adrenal cortex (**A**), the outermost zone is formed of cell clusters or tufts (glomeruli), whereas in the donkey (**B**), the cells are arranged in arcs. H&E (×20). (From Dellmann H-D. *Veterinary Histology: An Outline Text–Atlas*. Philadelphia, PA: Lea & Febiger, 1971.)

and distal convoluted tubule cells produces more Na^+–K^+ ATPase transporters in the basolateral cell membrane and more sodium channels in the apical membrane. The resulting increased K^+ release and increased Na^+ sodium retention helps to maintain blood volume. The increased fluid volume and reduction of K^+ concentration then create a negative feedback loop that suppresses the release of renin and aldosterone. While aldosterone is released primarily in response to angiotensin II, it is also released to a lesser extent in response to elevated potassium levels (a chemoreceptor signal) and ACTH. Chronic stimulation of the zona glomerulosa (e.g., kidney disease) leads to cell proliferation within the zona intermedia, growth of the zona glomerulosa, invasion of parenchyma into and through the capsule, and the formation of accessory nodules of the parenchyma.

The **zona fasciculata** (Figs. 12-12D and 12-14B) is the middle zone of the cortex and is made of columns or cords of cells separated by large fenestrated capillaries and a fine collagenous stroma. The cell cytoplasm is more abundant compared to that of the zona glomerulosa, and the cells are pale staining and have a foamy appearance with many lipid droplets. The glucocorticoid **cortisol** is produced by zona fasciculata cells in humans and most mammals via the enzyme 17 α-hydroxylase. Rodents lack this enzyme and instead produce the glucocorticoid **corticosterone**.

Glucocorticoids are released in a circadian manner and also in response to physiological stress signals in the hypothalamus, resulting in ACTH release from corticotrophs in the pars distalis. ACTH binds to its receptor and activates proteins that increase the transcription of enzymes for steroid hormone synthesis. Cortisol is produced via a cascade of enzymatic reactions from cholesterol to progesterone, then to 17-hydroxyprogesterone, and ultimately to cortisol.

Most cortisol circulates in an inactive form bound to carrier proteins such as corticosteroid-binding globulin or albumin. When freed from the carrier, cortisol diffuses into the target cell and binds to its intracellular glucocorticoid receptor. The ligand–receptor complex enters the nucleus via nuclear pores and binds to the hormone response elements on target genes to activate gene transcription. Cortisol has both metabolic and immune anti-inflammatory effects. Cortisol release in response to stress alters energy metabolism. It stimulates lipolysis and fatty acid release and glucose uptake by adipocytes, while also stimulating their differentiation and proliferation. In muscle, protein synthesis is suppressed, preventing the production of new myofibrillar protein. Cortisol also antagonizes the anabolic effects of insulin in muscle, which can lead to further loss of protein and muscle mass. In hepatocytes, glucocorticoids act to favor glycogen storage and gluconeogenesis.

Glucocorticoids also exert anti-inflammatory effects. Cortisol downregulates inflammatory transcription factors such as NK-κB that can inhibit cytokine synthesis. In addition, glucocorticoids exert negative feedback to the pars distalis and inhibit POMC synthesis. In the hypothalamus, they inhibit CRH and ADH synthesis.

The **zona reticularis** (Figs. 12-12E and 12-14B) is a thin band of small polygonal cells arranged as irregular cords or plates. This zone contains many large sinusoids. The cells within it have fewer lipid vesicles than the adjacent zona fasciculata and stain darker. They primarily synthesize **androgen sex hormones** (dehydroepiandrosterone and androstenedione), while also producing a small amount of glucocorticoids. These androgens can be converted to testosterone and estrogen by some other tissues. Cells in the zona reticularis often contain brown lipofuscin granules and pyknotic nuclei, indicative of apoptosis.

Adrenal Medulla

The majority of the cells in the adrenal medulla are the chromaffin cells, which secrete the catecholamines epinephrine and norepinephrine. These cells, derived from the neural crest, are considered to be modified sympathetic ganglion cells. They synthesize **epinephrine** and **norepinephrine** and store these neurotransmitters in dense secretory granules (Fig. 12-14C). Fixatives with potassium dichromate oxidize the catecholamines in the cells to a brown color. These cells, and others, that contain catecholamine-like molecules are referred to as **chromaffin cells**. The chromaffin cell clusters in the parenchyma are separated by sinusoids along with preganglionic sympathetic nerve fibers and occasional sympathetic neurons. At the periphery of the medulla and adjacent to medullary sinusoids, columnar cells (in horses, ruminants, and pigs) produce epinephrine, whereas rounded cells of the medulla produce norepinephrine. Norepinephrine is then converted to epinephrine by the enzyme phenylethanolamine N-methyltransferase.

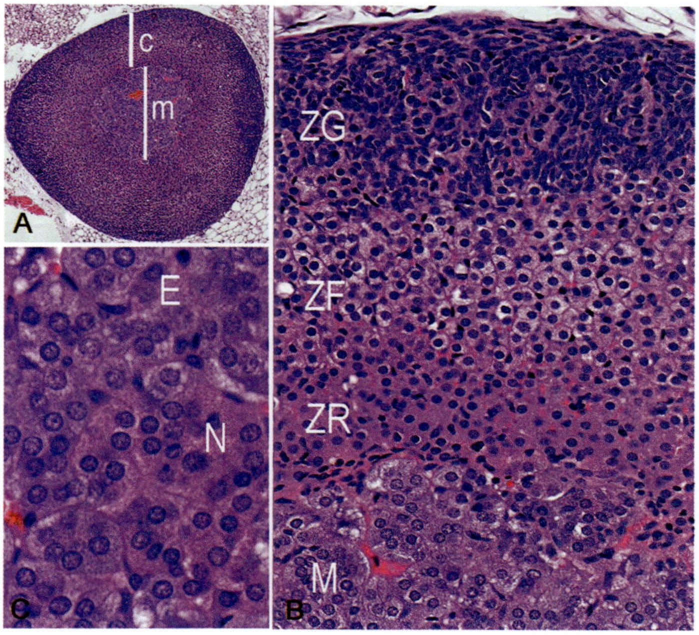

Figure 12-14 Adrenal gland of mouse. **A.** Cross-section through the gland showing the cortex (c) and the medulla (m). **B.** Zona glomerulosa (ZG), zona fasciculata (ZF), zona reticularis (ZR), and medulla (M). **C.** Epinephrine (E) and norepinephrine (N) secreting cells of the adrenal medulla.

The preganglionic sympathetic axons that extend along the trabeculae from the capsule synapse with multiple medullary cells. The neurotransmitter acetylcholine is released at the synapse to trigger exocytosis of epinephrine and norepinephrine from secretory granules. The release of epinephrine and norepinephrine by the sympathetic nervous system constitutes a secondary stress response axis. Epinephrine and norepinephrine both bind to GPCR family α- and β-adrenergic receptors in a variety of tissues and organs. Epinephrine and norepinephrine are mediators of the fight-or-flight mechanism that results in an increased heart rate and the breakdown of glycogen in skeletal muscle and the liver.

Endocrine Tissues and Cells

Pancreatic Islets

The endocrine cells of the pancreas form islets with their own vasculature within the exocrine pancreatic tissue (Fig. 12-15). Venules leaving an islet supply neighboring exocrine pancreas acini. Islets vary in size from a few endocrine cells to clusters of several thousand cells. The primary cells of the islets include glucagon-secreting **alpha (α) cells**, insulin-secreting **beta (β) cells**, and somatostatin (SST)-secreting **delta (δ) cells**. There are also small numbers of γ-pancreatic peptide-secreting pancreatic polypeptide (PP) cells and epsilon (ε) cells that secrete ghrelin. Standard H&E staining cannot distinguish between these cell types, and immunocytochemistry is the most accurate method to identify secretory granule contents.

The alpha and beta cells affect each other in a paracrine manner to maintain glucose homeostasis. Beta cell insulin inhibits alpha cell function, while alpha cells release factors (glucagon and acetylcholine) that stimulate beta cell function and increase glucose-stimulated insulin secretion. SST from delta cells can inhibit the activity of both alpha and beta cells in a paracrine manner.

Alpha cells synthesize and store **glucagon**, representing 5 to 30% of the islet cell population. In pigs, the number of α cells decreases from nearly 50% at birth to 8 to 20% in the adult. In horses, α cells are in the center of the islet, while in cattle, they are more peripheral. Islets in the ventral area of the right lobe of the canine pancreas lack α cells. Glucagon release occurs in response to hypoglycemia (low blood sugar). Upon release, glucagon binds to its receptors on hepatocytes, skeletal myocytes, and adipocytes, activating adenylate cyclase and elevating the concentration of cAMP. This process promotes glycogenolysis and gluconeogenesis, opposing hypoglycemia.

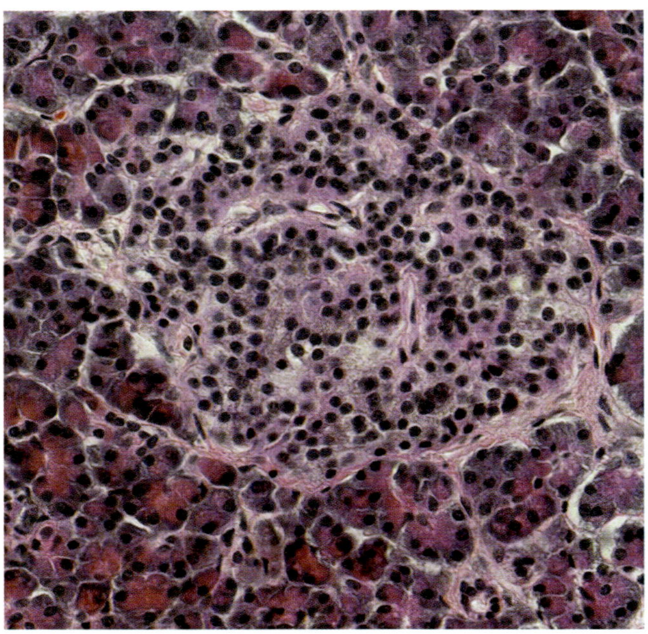

Figure 12-15 Canine pancreatic endocrine islet. An endocrine islet (central and lightly stained) is surrounded by exocrine acini. The acinar cells have eosinophilic dark-staining zymogen granules. The islet primarily contains β-cells (insulin), α-cells (glucagon), and δ-cells (SST), with small numbers of pancreatic polypeptide (PP) cells and ε-cells (ghrelin). The islet is perfused by blood sinusoids (×100). (Courtesy of Purdue College of Veterinary Medicine.)

Beta cells that synthesize and store **insulin** constitute the majority of islet cells (60 to 80%), with a higher proportion observed in sheep (98%). Elevated blood sugar levels signal β cells to release insulin, and this response is potentiated by other nutrients (amino acids and free fatty acids). Glucose is transported by GLUT-2 into the β cell. Glucose metabolism within the β cell generates ATP and closes ATP-sensitive K^+ channels, causing a membrane depolarization that activates voltage-gated Ca^{2+} channels. The increased intracellular calcium concentration triggers exocytosis of insulin. Insulin binds to its ligand-activated tyrosine kinase receptor on hepatocytes, skeletal myocytes, and adipocytes. The activated receptor initiates phosphorylation of insulin receptor substrate proteins (1 and 2) and signals downstream via protein kinases and phosphatases. Insulin promotes the synthesis of enzymes that favor anabolism and oppose hyperglycemia.

The SST synthesized (and stored) by delta cells exerts broad endocrine and neural effects. As mentioned, SST inhibits alpha and beta cells in a paracrine manner, but it can also act in an autocrine mode by inhibiting its own secretion. SST is expressed in hypothalamic neurons and can inhibit the release of GHRH and TRH. SST also functions as a neurotransmitter centrally and regulates the secretion from enteroendocrine cells in a paracrine manner. The lowering of intracellular Ca^{+2} when SST binds to its receptor inhibits hormone release. This mechanism also downregulates mitogen-activated kinases in target cells and suppresses their entry into the mitotic cycle.

Paraganglia

Small clusters of catecholaminergic cells arranged in a nest or glomeruli pattern are called **paraganglia**. The most studied paraganglion is the **carotid body**, located in the adventitia at the bifurcation of the common carotid artery. The size of the highly vascular carotid body is species dependent. The cells of the carotid body include a neuron-like chemoreceptor cell called a **glomus type I** cell and a glia-like **glomus** type II cells (or sustentacular cells). The carotid-sinus nerve sends multiple nerve fibers to the carotid body which terminate on glomus cells. The type I glomus cells are a source of catecholamines like dopamine and the neurotransmitters such as acetylcholine, serotonin, gamma-aminobutyric acid, and substance P. Functioning as chemoreceptors, the type I glomus cells monitor O_2 and CO_2 tension, pH, as well as glucose and lactate levels in blood flowing to the brain. Type I glomus cells are activated by hypoxia or hypercapnia, and afferent nerve fibers then stimulate brainstem neurons to elicit a compensatory response of hyperventilation or sympathetic activation to increase blood pressure and heart stroke volume. Small clusters of chemoreceptor cells are also found in the **aortic body** and other neck paraganglia.

Diffuse Neuroendocrine System Cells

Diffuse neuroendocrine system (DNES) cells are scattered in the epithelium throughout the respiratory, urinary, reproductive, and digestive systems. These cells contain dense secretory granules in their cytoplasm and express the neuroendocrine markers chromogranin A and synaptophysin. Subpopulations of these neuroendocrine cells were originally classified based on staining reactions. Cells that reacted to chromium salts were called chromaffin cells. Likewise, those that reacted to silver stains were called argentaffin cells. Some DNES were classified by their ability to take up and decarboxylate amines and were thus called **APUD cells**.

Enteroendocrine cells make up about 1% of the epithelium in the GI lining. These cells are dispersed among other epithelial cells and adhere to the basal lamina. Most are pyramidal in shape, with cytoplasm extending toward the lumen, while secretory granules are stored nearer to the base. Immunocytochemistry can be used to identify secretions from these cells. The list of hormones produced by enteroendocrine cells is under constant revision with research. Some of the hormones produced include gastrin, secretin, motilin, pancreatic polypeptide, glucagon, glucagon-like peptide 1, insulin, vasoactive intestinal polypeptide, somatostatin, ghrelin, histamine, neuropeptide Y (NPY), neurotensin, peptide YY, and cholecystokinin. Collectively, these hormones inhibit or stimulate processes affecting food intake, digestion, and absorption of nutrients, as well as basal metabolism.

Pulmonary neuroendocrine cells (about 0.5% of the lung epithelium) occur as single cells or may be in clusters called neuroepithelial bodies. They are located at branch points in the airways and are directly innervated. The role of these cells in health and disease is a current topic of research. They appear to function as chemosensors for hypoxia and also as sensors that affect immune responses via secretion of neuropeptides.

Other Endocrine Cells

Adipocytes

Unilocular (white) adipose tissue (see Chapter 3) was once viewed primarily as an energy storage type of CT. However, the discovery of leptin in 1994 began an expansion of our understanding, revealing that adipocytes have major endocrine functions with wide-ranging impacts on glucose and lipid metabolism, appetite regulation, coagulation and fibrinolysis, immune and reproductive functions, and vascular homeostasis. Adipocytes have receptors for insulin, GH, norepinephrine, and glucocorticoids. Some of the factors produced by adipocytes include leptin, interleukin (IL)-6, TNF-α, adiponectin, resistin, PAI-1, angiotensinogen, VEGF, and IGF-1. Leptin, a 16 kDa cytokine peptide of the IL-6 family, plays a central role in regulating hunger and feeding behavior by acting on cells in the hypothalamus. When leptin binds to its hypothalamic receptor, it inhibits the effects of hunger-promoting **NPY** and **agouti-related peptide** and also promotes the synthesis of the hunger suppressant, α-MSH.

Endocrine Cells of the Heart and Kidney

Maintenance of blood pressure and blood volume is critical for circulatory homeostasis. In addition to ADH released from the neurohypophysis, specialized cells of the heart produce peptides, and the kidney produces proteolytic enzymes and glycoprotein cytokines to maintain blood pressure and volume. In the atrial myocardium, some cardiac myocytes synthesize and store in secretory vesicles the peptide hormone **atrial natriuretic peptide** (ANP) (see Chapter 7). When blood volume is increased beyond normal levels, the increased stretch of the atrial myocytes initiates a cascade of effects. Membrane calcium channels open, and this triggers exocytosis of ANP. ANP binds to its receptor on target cells, activating guanylyl cyclase and increasing the concentration of cyclic guanosine 3′,5′-monophosphate (cGMP). cGMP activates a phosphodiesterase that deactivates cAMP, inhibiting cell functions driven by cAMP. In the kidney, ANP acts in the collecting tubule to antagonize the effect of ADH and upon juxtaglomerular cells to inhibit the release of renin. In the brain, ANP inhibits ADH release.

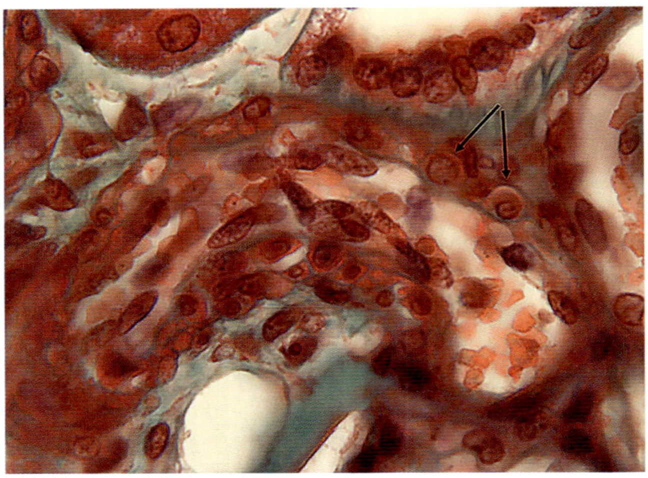

Figure 12-16 Renin-secreting juxtaglomerular cells in the wall of the afferent arteriole of the kidney glomerulus (×400).

In the tunica media of glomerular afferent arterioles, there are modified smooth myocytes (juxtaglomerular cells) that synthesize and store **renin** granules (Fig. 12-16). These cells are part of the renin–angiotensin–aldosterone system (see Chapter 11). Decreased blood perfusion in the glomerulus triggers a baroreceptor signal and subsequent renin release. This signal arises from either a mechanical perturbation of the arteriole myocyte membrane or a chemoreceptor response by the macula densa cells to certain signals (e.g., elevated [K^+], synthesis of prostaglandin E_2, or release of ATP). Renin release triggers an enzymatic cascade that creates angiotensin II. Angiotensin II binds to the AT1 receptor in the zona glomerulosa of the adrenal cortex, releasing aldosterone. Aldosterone increases expression of Na^+–K^+ ATPase transporters and Na^+ channels in the epithelium of the distal tubule and collecting duct, thereby increasing fluid volume and reducing K^+ levels.

Endocrine Cells of the Ovary

The ovarian follicle contains endocrine cells, including granulosa and theca cells, as well as a gamete cell (ovum or oocyte) (see Chapter 14). A basal lamina (basement membrane) separates the avascular granulosa cell layer from the vascularized theca layer, which consists of the endocrine theca interna and the nonendocrine theca externa layers (Fig. 12-17). The endocrine cells in the ovary, granulosa and theca cells, arise from the embryonic mesoderm. During embryonic development, primordial germ cells (oogonia) migrate from the umbilical vesicle (yolk sac) and colonize the gonadal ridge, contributing to the formation of the ovary. In the embryonic ovary, a primordial germ cell (oogonium) is surrounded by mesenchymal cells that later differentiate and transform into epithelial cells designated as follicular cells (granulosa cell precursors). A basal lamina (basement membrane) encloses the entire structure to form a primordial follicle.

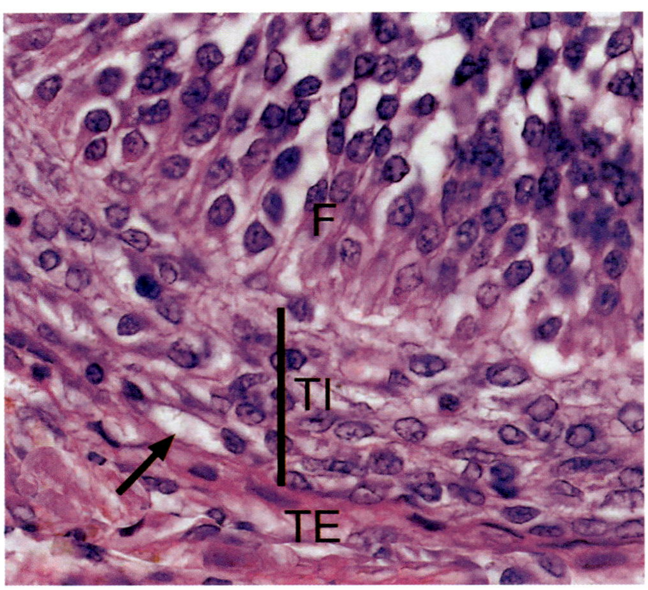

Figure 12-17 Follicular cells (F) of a tertiary follicle, ovary. The theca interna (TI) cells may have a clear cytoplasm (arrow) due to the lipid content in these steroid-producing cells. The theca externa (TE) cells are fibroblast-like CT cells (×400).

The adult ovary contains follicles at different stages of development, including primordial, primary, secondary, and tertiary (Graafian) follicles. The ovary may also contain active or regressing corpora lutea, as well as atretic follicles. Developing ovarian follicles produce estradiol (estrogen), and this process requires the combined actions of theca and granulosa cells.

Theca cells produce androgens, which are converted to estrogens by granulosa cells because granulosa cells lack the enzyme 17 alpha-hydroxylase/C17, 20-lyase (CYP17) needed for androgen production, and theca cells lack aromatase (CYP19) activity.

FSH stimulates granulosa cells in small follicles to proliferate, express aromatase (CYP19), and produce estrogen. In combination with estrogen, FSH induces the expression of LH receptors in granulosa cells of larger follicles. Granulosa cells also secrete the polypeptide hormones inhibin and activin. Luteinizing hormone stimulates theca cells to produce androgens. In large ovarian follicles, LH stimulates granulosa cells to convert androgens to estrogens.

After ovulation, the granulosa and theca cells proliferate, and the entire wall of the ovarian follicle transforms into a corpus luteum, which acts as a temporary endocrine organ producing large amounts of progesterone (corpus luteum cyclicum or corpus luteum of cycle). Initially, the developing corpus luteum contains two main types of endocrine cells: small luteal cells and large luteal cells. Later, the small luteal cells hypertrophy and transform into large luteal cells. The corpus luteum is highly vascularized. If there is pregnancy, trophoblast cells of the conceptus secrete hormones (e.g., chorionic gonadotropin) or factors that act to enhance the functions of the corpus luteum, allowing it to persist as the corpus luteum of pregnancy (corpus luteum graviditas). In the absence of pregnancy, the corpus luteum regresses to form a corpus albicans.

Steroid hormones from the ovary regulate the functions of the uterus and mammary glands and exert negative feedback control on the secretion of GnRH from the hypothalamus and on LH and FSH from the anterior pituitary. Inhibin and activin inhibit or stimulate FSH secretion, respectively.

Endocrine Cells of the Placenta

The placenta, which develops during pregnancy, is a temporary organ like the corpus luteum (see Chapter 15). It has maternal and fetal sections (**fetal placenta** and **maternal placenta**). In species with invasive implantation (e.g., humans, rodents), the maternal placenta, called the **decidua**, is formed from the transformation and differentiation of cells in the stroma of the endometrium. Conversely, in species with noninvasive implantation (e.g., ruminants, horses, and pigs), portions of the endometrium constitute the maternal placenta. The trophoblast layer or its derivative, the villous chorion, forms the fetal placenta. Both the fetal and maternal portions of the placenta synthesize and secrete several protein or peptide hormones that are similar in structure and/or function to hormones secreted by the hypothalamus or anterior pituitary gland (e.g., placental lactogen, PRL, and POMC peptides; oxytocin; leptin; and adiponectin) and steroid hormones produced in the ovary (e.g., progesterone and estrogen). In humans, trophoblast cells of the fetal placenta secrete **human chorionic gonadotropin**, which acts as LH. Further, trophoblast cells of the equine embryo detach and invade the endometrium, where they proliferate, and form clusters called **endometrial cups** that secrete **equine chorionic gonadotropin** (eCG). eCG, which was previously called "**pregnant mare's serum gonadotropin**", acts as FSH when injected into other species. The targets of placental hormones include the fetal gonads, maternal uterus, ovary, mammary glands, and maternal glucose metabolism, among others.

Endocrine Cells of the Testis

The testis contains endocrine cells (Leydig cells), nurturing or sustentacular cells (Sertoli cells), and gamete cells at different stages of development (see Chapter 13). There are different spaces in the testis, namely, interstitial, basal, and adluminal compartments. Both basal and adluminal compartments are located within the seminiferous tubules. A basement membrane (containing myoid cells) surrounds seminiferous tubules and separates the basal and interstitial compartments. Myoid cells are contractile cells that resemble smooth muscle and provide structural support to the seminiferous tubules, and they are often considered to be modified peritubular cells. Zonula junctions between adjacent Sertoli cells separate the basal and adluminal compartments. Sertoli cells lie on the periphery of seminiferous tubules, while Leydig cells (interstitial cells) are located in the interstitial compartment. The primordial germ cells (spermatogonia) are found in the basal compartment. The developing spermatocytes, round spermatids, and elongated spermatids are attached to Sertoli cells in the adluminal compartment, which extends into the lumen of the seminiferous tubule.

The Leydig and Sertoli cells arise from the embryonic mesoderm. During embryonic development, primordial germ cells (spermatogonia) migrate from the umbilical vesicle (yolk sac) and colonize the gonadal ridge during the formation of the testis. Leydig cells mainly produce testosterone (androgen) in response to LH. They also synthesize other hormones such as oxytocin. FSH stimulates Sertoli cells to synthesize and secrete ABP, which acts to sequester large amounts of testosterone in the lumen of seminiferous tubules. Sertoli cells also secrete inhibin and activin.

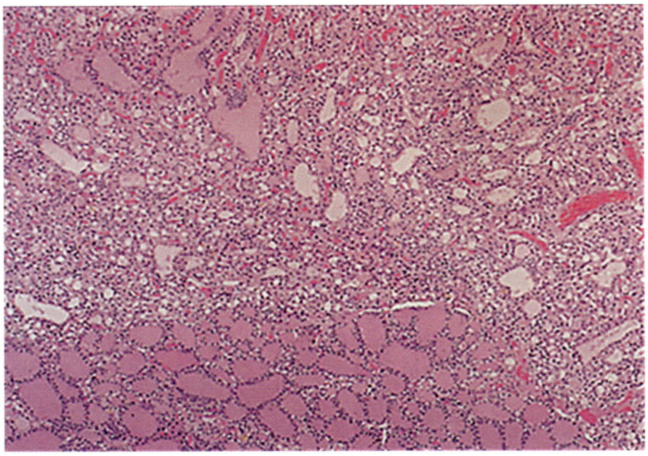

Figure 12-18 **Feline hyperthyroidism**, a prevalent endocrine condition in older cats, manifests as weight loss, increased appetite, vomiting, and diarrhea. It stems from excessive thyroid hormone production due to thyroid gland enlargement, palpable as a goiter. (Reprinted with permission from Salguero Bodes FJ, Pallares Martinez FJ. Aughey and Frye's Comparative Veterinary Histology with Clinical Correlates. 2nd ed. Boca Raton: CRC Press, 2023.)

Testosterone, in combination with FSH, regulates the development of spermatozoa (spermatogenesis). It also regulates the functions male accessory sex organs (e.g., prostate gland) and the expression of male secondary sex characteristics (e.g., development of musculature). Testosterone exerts negative feedback control on the secretion of GnRH from the hypothalamus and on LH and FSH from the anterior pituitary. Inhibin and activin inhibit or stimulate FSH secretion, respectively.

Clinical Correlations

Adult-onset panhypopituitarism: Compression or damage (usually adenoma) leads to inadequate adenohypophysis hormones and downstream effects on other endocrine organs. It is common in dogs/cats. **Juvenile-onset panhypopituitarism**: The adenohypophysis does not fully develop or compromised by a tumor. **Diabetes Insipidus**: The pituitary does not secrete enough ADH (central diabetes insipidus), or there is a poor kidney response to ADH (nephrogenic diabetes insipidus). It is common in dogs/cats. Both **hypo- and hyperthyroidism** occur in domestic species. Canine hypothyroidism is indicated by hair coat thinning/loss, weight gain, and lethargy. Canine hyperthyroidism is rarer, while more prevalent in cats (Fig. 12-18). **Hypercortisol secretion (Cushing's) (polydipsia and polyuria):** It can be caused by a pituitary tumor (most common) or adrenal tumor. **Hypoadrenocorticism (Addison's disease):** It can affect both cortisol and aldosterone levels.

Essentials

Pituitary: It is attached to the hypothalamus by the infundibulum. It contains glandular (adenohypophysis) and neural (neurohypophysis) portions. The **adenohypophysis** contains **basophils**, such as corticotrophs (ACTH), thyrotrophs (TSH), gonadotrophs (FSH and LH), and melanotrophs (α-MSH), and **acidophils**, such as somatotrophs (GH and somatotropin) and mammotrophs (PRL). Hormone production is regulated by releasing and/or inhibiting factors released by the hypothalamus into the primary capillary plexus. The **neurohypophysis** is the site of hormone release from the hypothalamus (ADH and oxytocin). It contains Herring bodies (axon terminals with neurosecretory granules).

Thyroid: Follicular cells secrete thyroglobulin into the follicle lumen where it is iodinated, then endocytosed, digested in lysosomes, and T_3 and T_4 are released at the base of the cell. Parafollicular cells (C cells) secrete calcitonin.

Parathyroid: It contains chief cells that secrete PTH.

Adrenal Glands: The ***cortex*** contains three zones producing mineralocorticoids, glucocorticoids, and gonadocorticoids.

The ***Medulla*** contains ganglion neurons and cells producing adrenaline (epinephrine) and noradrenaline (norepinephrine).

Pineal gland: Pinealocytes produce melatonin. Secretion is regulated by light via the retina, with light-inhibiting melatonin secretion.

Endocrine pancreas: It contains alpha cells (glucagon), beta cells (insulin), delta cells (SST), PP cells, and epsilon cells (ghrelin).

DNES of the GI tract: It includes the regulation of gastric acid and gut motility. **Kidney endocrine cells**: It includes the regulation of blood volume/pressure through the secretion of ***erythropoietin*** and ***renin*** (by modified smooth muscle cells).

Heart: Modified atrial cardiac muscle cells produce **ANP** for blood pressure regulation. **Adipose tissue** regulates appetite through the hormone ***leptin***.

Suggested Readings

Andreoli TE, Reeves WB, Bichet DG. Endocrine control of water balance. In: Goodman HM, ed. Handbook of Physiology. Vol. 3. New York: Oxford University Press, 2000.

Bringhurst FR, Demay MB, Kronenberg HM. Hormones and disorders of mineral metabolism. In: Kronenberg HM, Melmed S, Polonsky KS, et al., eds. Williams Textbook of Endocrinology. 11th Ed. Philadelphia: Saunders, 2008.

Chester-Jones I, Ingleton PM, Phillips JG. Fundamentals of Comparative Vertebrate Endocrinology. New York: Plenum Press, 1987.

Cone RD. Neuroendocrinology. In: Larsen PR, Kronenberg HM, Melmed S, et al., eds. Williams Textbook of Endocrinology. 10th Ed. Philadelphia: Saunders, 2002.

Constanti A, Bartke A, Khardori R. Basic Endocrinology for Students of Pharmacy and Allied Health Sciences. Amsterdam: Harwood Academic Publishers, 1998.

De Bold AJ, Bruneau BG. Natrurietic peptides. In: Goodman HM, ed. Handbook of Physiology. Vol. 3. New York: Oxford University Press, 2000.

Denef C. Autocrine/paracrine intermediates in hormone action and modulation of cellular responses to hormones. In: Goodman HM, ed. Handbook of Physiology. Vol. 1. New York: Oxford University Press, 1998.

Ganguly A. Aldosterone. In: Goodman HM, ed. Handbook of Physiology. Vol. 3. New York: Oxford University Press, 2000.

Halász B. The hypothalamus as an endocrine organ. In: Conn PM, Freeman ME, eds. Neuroendocrinology in Physiology and Medicine. Totowa, NJ: Humana Press, 2000.

Harno E, Ramamoorthy TG, Coll AP, et al. POMC: the physiological power of hormone processing. *Physiol Rev* 2018;98:2381–2430.

Hullinger RL. The endocrine system. In: Evans HE, ed. Miller's Anatomy of the Dog. 3rd Ed. Philadelphia: W. B. Saunders, 1993.

Kaplan NM. The adrenal glands. In: Griffin JE, Ojeda SR, eds. Textbook of Endocrine Physiology. 4th Ed. New York: Oxford University Press, 2000.

Lavine JE. The hypothalamus as a major integrating center. In: Conn PM, Freeman ME, eds. Neuroendocrinology in Physiology and Medicine. Totowa, NJ: Humana Press, 2000.

Lightman SL, Birnie MT, Conway-Campbell BL. Dynamics of ACTH and cortisol secretion and implications for disease. *Endocr Rev* 2020;41(3):bnaa002 https://doi.org/10.1210/endrev/bnaa002.

Low MJ. Neuroendocrinology. In: Kronenberg HM, Melmed S, Polonsky KS, et al., eds. Williams Textbook of Endocrinology. 11th Ed. Philadelphia: Saunders, 2008.

Melmed S, Kleinberg D. Anterior pituitary. In: Kronenberg HM, Melmed S, Polonsky KS, et al., eds. Williams Textbook of Endocrinology. 11th Ed. Philadelphia: Saunders, 2008.

Mendelson CR. Mechanisms of hormone action. In: Griffin JE, Ojeda SR, eds. Textbook of Endocrine Physiology. 4th Ed. New York: Oxford University Press, 2000.

Nilsson M, Fagman H. Development of the thyroid gland. *Development* 2017;144:2123–2140.

Robinson AG, Verbalis JG. Posterior pituitary gland. In: Kronenberg HM, Melmed S, Polonsky KS, et al., eds. Williams Textbook of Endocrinology. 11th Ed. Philadelphia: Saunders, 2008.

Salguero Bodes FJ, Pallares Martinez FJ. Aughey and Frye's Comparative Veterinary Histology with Clinical Correlates. 2nd ed. Boca Raton: CRC Press, 2023.

Sehgal A. Molecular Biology of Circadian Rhythms. Hoboken, NJ: John Wiley & Sons, Inc., 2004.

Szczepanska-Sadowska E, Wsol A, Cudnoch-Jedrzejewska A, et al. Complementary role of oxytocin and vasopressin in cardiovascular regulation. *Int J Mol Sci* 2021;22:11465.

Tucker HA. Neuroendocrine regulation of lactation and milk ejection. In: Conn PM, Freeman ME, eds. Neuroendocrinology in Physiology and Medicine. Totowa, NJ: Humana Press, 2000.

Willis TL, Lodge EJ, Andoniadou CL, et al. Cellular interactions in the pituitary stem cell niche. *Cell Mol Life Sci* 2022;79:612.

Zeidel ML. Physiologic responses to natriuretic hormones. In: Goodman HM, ed. Handbook of Physiology. Vol. 3. New York: Oxford University Press, 2000.

13

Male Reproductive System

Carlos E. Fonseca Alves and John J. Turek

CHAPTER MENU

Dellmann's Textbook of Veterinary Histology, Seventh Edition. Edited by Marxa L. Figueiredo and John J. Turek.

Companion website: www.wiley.com/go/figueiredo/vethistology7e

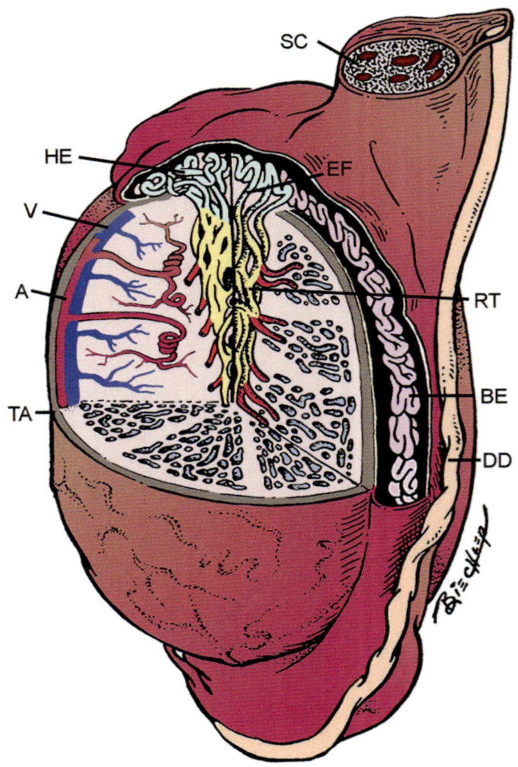

Figure 13-1 Schematic drawing of bovine testis. Tunica albuginea (TA), spermatic cord (SC), head of epididymis (HE), efferent ducts (EF), rete testis (RT), body of epididymis (BE), ductus deferens (DD), arteries (A), and veins (V).

The male reproductive system consists of (a) the testes surrounded by the connective tissue (CT) tunics (tunica albuginea and tunica vaginalis), (b) the epididymis, (c) the ductus deferens, (d) the accessory glands (ampulla of the ductus deferens, vesicular and bulbourethral glands, and prostate), (e) the urethra, and (f) the penis surrounded by the prepuce.

Testis

Connective Tissue

The testes are enclosed by a dense irregular CT capsule called the **tunica albuginea (TA)** (Fig. 13-1). A posterior thickening of the TA forms the **mediastinum testis (MT)**, which contains the **rete testis (RT)**. The TA is primarily composed of collagen fibers with a few elastic fibers. Some interstitial (Leydig) cells occur in the cat. The inner surface of the TA contains the vascular layer (tunica vasculosa) with branches of the testicular artery and a plexus of anastomosing veins. Partially covering the anterior and lateral surfaces is a mesothelial-lined serous sac derived from the peritoneum called the **tunica vaginalis**.

A visceral layer of the tunica vaginalis (TV) covers the testis, while a parietal layer lines the scrotum. The two layers are separated by a space called the vaginal cavity. CT trabeculae extend from the TA as septae (septula testis) to subdivide the testis into **lobules**. The trabeculae form complete septa in dogs and boars, but in other domestic animals, they are fine CT strands that surround intratesticular vessels.

Each lobule contains one to four convoluted seminiferous tubules (Fig. 13-2). The MT contains blood and lymph vessels and the channels of the rete testis. The MT of stallions and many rodents is relatively small and located in a marginal position. In ruminants, pigs, cats, and dogs, the RT occupies a central position along the testis's longitudinal axis.

Interstitial Leydig Cells

The tissue surrounding the seminiferous tubules contains loose CT, blood and lymph vessels, free mononuclear cells, and **Leydig** (interstitial endocrine) cells. Leydig cells make up approximately 1% of the entire testicular volume in adult rams, 5% in bulls, and 20 to 30% in boars. In seasonally breeding males (e.g., camels), Leydig cell volume and number change throughout the year. The cells occur in cords or clusters and are large and polymorphous with a spherical nucleus. Smooth endoplasmic reticulum (sER) (in bulls, a granular endoplasmic reticulum) is abundant as the sER membranes contain the enzymes necessary for steroid biosynthesis.

The mitochondria of Leydig cells have tubular cristae, similar to mitochondria in cells of the adrenal cortex. These cells produce testosterone when stimulated by luteinizing hormone (LH). They also transport cholesterol to the mitochondria, where it is transformed into pregnenolone. The small Golgi complex does not participate in androgen secretion. Lipid inclusions are found in all species but are especially abundant in cats (Fig. 13-3). There are intercellular canaliculi and gap junctions between adjacent cells.

Leydig cells develop from mesenchyme-like precursors. Leydig cells produce testicular androgens (testosterone) and, in boars, they also produce estrogen. More than 90% of all androgens are produced by the testis. Testosterone and its 5-α reductase byproduct of dihydrotestosterone function to (a) promote secondary sex characteristics and sexual behavior, (b) trigger growth and maintenance of penis function and male accessory glands, (c) control spermatogenesis along with follicle-stimulating hormone (FSH), (d) affect feedback inhibition on the hypophysis and hypothalamus, (e) promote general anabolic effects, and (f) maintain the mesonephric duct during development and its differentiation into the epididymis and ductus deferens.

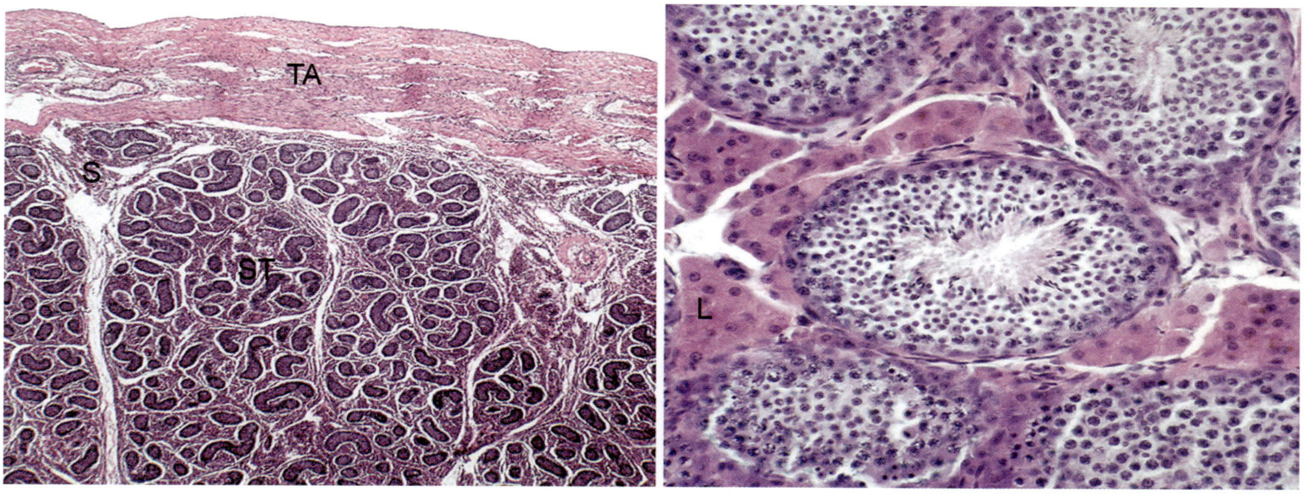

Figure 13-2 Left: The testis is covered by a dense irregular connective tissue (CT) capsule called the tunica albuginea (TA); seminiferous tubules (ST) are contained within lobules separated by CT septae (S). Right: Eosinophilic Leydig endocrine cells (L) are contained in the CT surrounding the seminiferous tubules. A lamina propria of collagen and elastic fibers with flat peritubular cells surrounds the epithelium. Testis, horse. Hematoxylin and eosin (H&E) (×250). (Image by W.E. Haensly.)

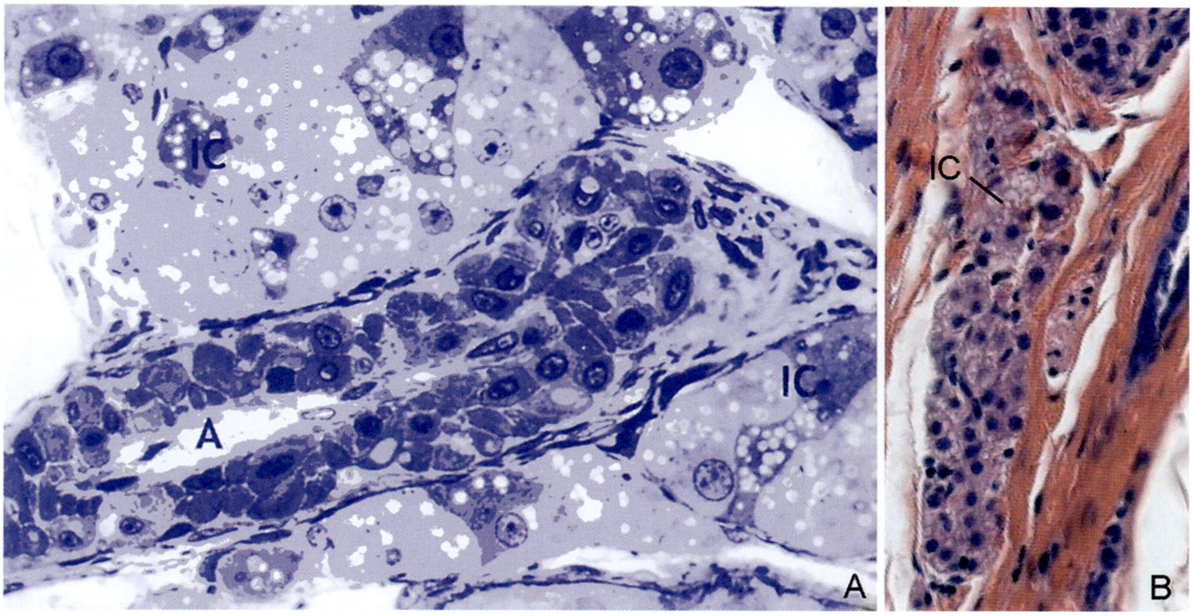

Figure 13-3 **A.** Intertubular region of the cat testis. The Leydig or interstitial endocrine cells (IC) have round nuclei and lipid inclusions. Small artery (A). Semithin section (×450). **B.** Leydig cells in the feline tunica albuginea. H&E.

Seminiferous Tubules

The **seminiferous tubules** in most mammals are convoluted two-ended loops with a diameter between 150 and 300 μm. They are lined by a **spermatogenic cell layer** consisting of spermatogenic cells and **Sertoli** (sustentacular) cells, surrounded by a lamina propria. The tubule epithelium is unique in that the Sertoli cells do not attach basally via hemidesmosomes or laterally via desmosomes and also do not contain intermediate filaments. However, desmosomes have been reported in nonmammalian vertebrates. The adherens junctions are also biochemically unique. The tubules are connected at both ends to straight testicular tubules by a specialized terminal segment. In adult bovines, the combined length of all seminiferous tubules amounts to approximately 5000 m.

Lamina Propria

The lamina or tunica propria surrounds the seminiferous tubule. Its innermost layer is a basement membrane. In some species (i.e., bovine), the basal lamina indents into the Sertoli cell layer and it does so slightly in human and porcine tubules. The peritubular wall, situated beneath the basement membrane, contains layers (1 to 5, depending on the species) of flattened peritubular smooth muscle cells alternating with an extracellular matrix containing collagen and elastic fibers.

At birth, the peritubular cells resemble mesenchymal cells, which later differentiate into contractile smooth muscle cells postnatally. The peritubular cells contain all markers of smooth muscle, including smooth muscle α-actin, smooth muscle myosin, desmin, vimentin, and smoothelin. These cells are responsible for tubular contractions and are connected by cadherin-based adherens junctions. A thin monolayer of cells separates the seminiferous tubules from the interstitial space. Previously, this layer was considered to be a lymphatic endothelium, but recent studies show that these cells lack endothelial markers and may represent a unique cell type. The peritubular smooth muscle cells participate in the transport of tubule contents and in the release of spermatozoa into the lumen.

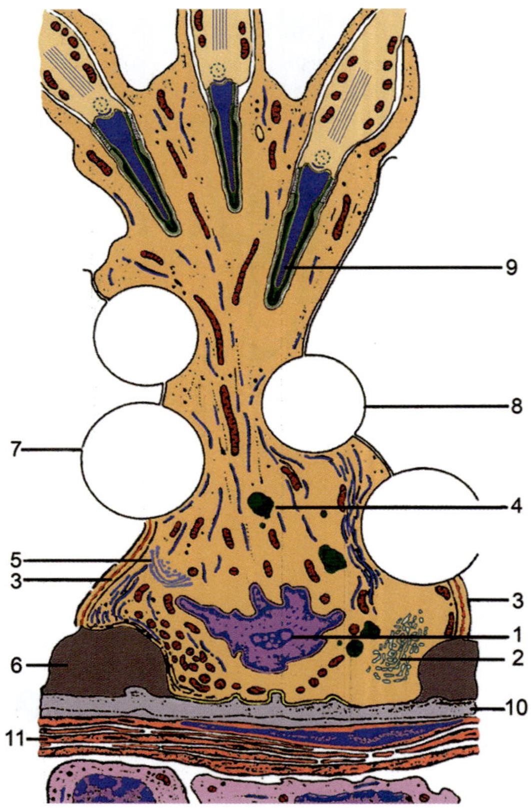

Figure 13-4 Diagram showing the Sertoli cell interrelationships in the bull. 1. Sertoli cell nucleus. 2. Smooth endoplasmic reticulum. 3. Tight junctions between adjacent Sertoli (sustentacular) cells, constituting the morphologic equivalent of the blood–testis barrier. 4. Phagolysosomes. 5. Golgi complex. 6. Space occupied by a spermatogonium. 7. Space occupied by a primary spermatocyte. 8. Space occupied by a spherical spermatid. 9. Elongated spermatid within the apical recess of Sertoli cell. 10. Basement membrane. 11. Peritubular cell. (With permission from Mosimann M, Kohler T. *Zytologie, Histologie und mikroskopische Anatomie der Haussäugetiere*. Hamburg: Paul Parey, 1990. Modified from the original.)

Sertoli Cells

The Sertoli cells are the **sustentacular** (support) cells of the testis (Figs. 13-4 and 13-5). Molecular analysis of developing **Sertoli** cells indicates that they are likely derived from coelomic epithelial somatic cells that undergo differentiation through an epithelial–mesenchymal transition. In the indifferent gonad, undifferentiated Sertoli cells are mitotically active and produce a glycoprotein hormone of the transforming growth factor beta (TGF-ß) superfamily called **antiparamesonephric hormone**. This hormone suppresses the development of uterine tubes, uterus, and vagina in males. Sertoli cells are mitotically active until puberty. At puberty, they undergo a terminal differentiation step and no longer undergo mitosis.

The base of the Sertoli cell lies on the basement membrane without hemidesmosome attachments, and its branched cytoplasm extends toward the tubular lumen. These cells are rather evenly spaced across the tubule, and their cytoplasmic processes fill the

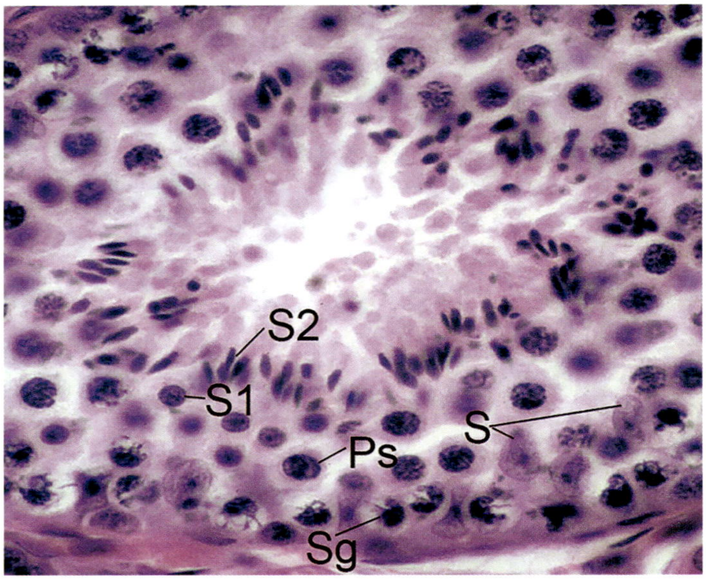

Figure 13-5 Horse seminiferous tubule epithelium. Sertoli cells (S), spermatogonia (Sg), primary spermatocyte (Ps), early spermatid (S1), and late spermatid (S2). H&E (×400). (Image by W.E. Haensly.)

spaces between adjacent spermatogenic cells. The oval, indented nucleus is located in the basal portion of the cell and contains a large nucleolus. Membranous organelles (smooth and rough ER, mitochondria, and Golgi complex) cluster in the basal and central regions of the cell, with only a few organelles present in the lateral and apical Sertoli cell processes.

The Sertoli cell shape and volume change during a spermatogenic cycle. Temporary junctions with adjacent germ cells are important for active vertical displacement and release of the spermatozoa into the tubule lumen. Adjacent Sertoli cells are joined by a unique adherens junction based on N-cadherin, anchored in cytoplasmic plaques. These junctions are biochemically distinct from the E-cadherin-containing adherens junctions of epithelial tissues. These junctions separate a **basal compartment** from an **adluminal compartment**, creating a **blood–testis barrier**. The blood–testis barrier selectively prevents substances from entering the adluminal compartment and also prevents autoimmune reactions against developing germ cells. Early spermatocytes pass through these specialized Sertoli cell junctions without interrupting the physiological blood–testis barrier.

Sertoli cells are nutritive, protective, and supportive for the spermatogenic cells. They phagocytize degenerating spermatogenic cells and detached spermatid residual bodies. The cells also receive hormonal signals from testosterone, FSH, and thyroid triiodothyronine (T_3). FSH regulates the secretion of androgen-binding protein (ABP), which has a high affinity for androgens. ABP aids in the concentration of testosterone in the tubule lumen, essential for germ cell development. Sertoli cells also secrete inhibin, activin, and transferrin. Inhibin is resorbed in the efferent ductules and the epididymis initial segment and provides negative feedback for gonadotropin-releasing hormone (GnRH) by the hypothalamus and subsequent FSH release by the adenohypophysis. Activin, on the other hand, provides positive feedback on FSH release. While Sertoli cells have little steroidogenic function, Sertoli cell tumors may aberrantly produce large amounts of estrogen, leading to feminization of the affected animal.

Spermatogenic Cells

Spermatogenic cells at different stages of development and differentiation are located between the Sertoli cells. The development of spermatozoa from spermatogonia is referred to as **spermatogenesis** and is subdivided into three phases: (a) spermatocytogenesis (the spermatogonial proliferative phase), (b) the spermatocyte meiotic phase, and (c) spermatid development (spermiogenesis after meiosis). The duration of spermatogenesis varies among species: approximately 39 days in boars, 61 days in bulls, 50 days in rams and stallions, and 55 days in dogs.

Spermatocytogenesis

Spermatocytogenesis begins with retinoic acid signaling acting on Sertoli cells and spermatogenic stem cells (As). The As cells give rise to prospermatogonia (Apr), which in turn give rise to the differentiating type-A spermatogonia. The differentiating type-A spermatogonia form syncytia of 4, 8, or 16 cells, which progress to type-B spermatogonia connected by cytoplasmic bridges. The type-B spermatogonia detach from the basal lamina and become preleptotene primary spermatocytes. The primary spermatocytes will then undergo two meiotic divisions, which result in a fourfold increase in the number of germ cells.

Type-A spermatogonia are in contact with the basement membrane. Some of these cells are mitotically inactive (G_0 phase of cell cycle) and have dark basophilic nuclei. When entering the cell cycle, these spermatogonia have prominent nucleoli and a pale-staining nucleus. The small **B-spermatogonia** have spherical nuclei containing numerous chromatin particles and less prominent nucleoli. Preleptotene primary spermatocytes are passively translocated into the adluminal compartment through intercellular junctions between the Sertoli cells. In preleptotene primary spermatocytes, the nuclear DNA is replicated, resulting in all chromosomes consisting of two sister chromatids.

Meiosis

During **meiosis**, a primary spermatocyte undergoes two nuclear divisions without DNA replication, and this results in the formation of four haploid spermatids. **Primary spermatocytes** are the largest spermatogenic cells. The prophase of the first meiotic division is subdivided into five stages: leptotene, zygotene, pachytene, diplotene, and diakinesis. Each stage has characteristic changes in nuclear chromatin (Fig. 13-6). During the prophase of the first meiotic division, the cells grow considerably.

For example, ovine primary spermatocytes increase in volume 4.8 times, and the nuclei increase in volume 3.3 times between the preleptotene and diplotene stages. Toward the end of prophase, the nuclear membrane disappears. During the **leptotene stage**, the maternal and paternal homologous chromosomes appear as thin, threadlike strands. In the **zygotene stage**, the synaptonemal complex (observed with the electron microscope) develops between homologous chromosomes

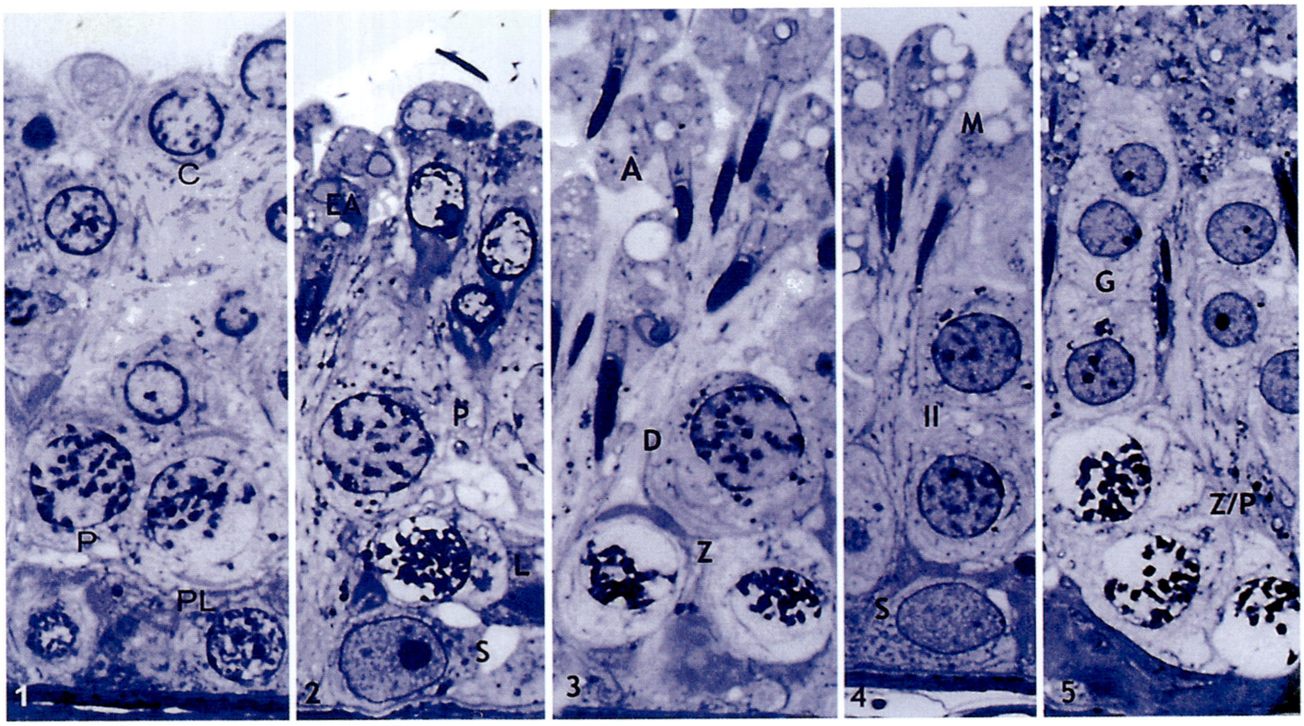

Figure 13-6 Typical morphology of the various cells in the spermatogenic epithelium (water buffalo). The numbers on the images correspond to the stages of the epithelial cycle (compare to Fig. 13-9). Spermatogonia (S), preleptotene primary spermatocytes (PL), leptotene primary spermatocytes (L), zygotene primary spermatocytes (Z), zygotenes entering pachytene (Z/P), pachytene primary spermatocytes (P), diplotene primary spermatocytes (D), secondary spermatocytes (II), Golgi-phase spermatids (G), cap-phase spermatids (C), early acrosome-phase spermatids (EA), acrosome-phase spermatids (A), and maturation-phase spermatids (M). Semithin sections (×1560).

and tetrads of four chromatids emerge. By the completion of pairing in the **pachytene phase**, genetic crossing over occurs between the nonsister chromatids of the chromosomes.

Primary spermatocytes are easily identified during this phase of meiosis. During the **diplotene phase**, the paired chromosomes separate, although sister chromatids remain attached by one or more chiasmata, where crossing over occurs. The centrioles duplicate prior to metaphase, and during **diakinesis**, chromosomes shorten and broaden, with the four separate chromatids becoming evident. Simultaneously, a microtubule spindle begins to develop.

The metaphase, anaphase, and telophase of the first reductional division occur rapidly. During these phases, the paired chromosomes align at the equatorial plate. Homologous chromosomes then move to opposite poles of the cell to be distributed to the secondary spermatocytes, each containing half the number of chromosomes, with two chromatids each. **Secondary spermatocytes** are short-lived (a few hours) and are intermediate in size between diplotene primary spermatocytes and spherical spermatids.

After a short period of interphase, secondary spermatocytes undergo the **second maturation division**, with a short prophase followed by metaphase, anaphase, and telophase stages, which are similar to those of mitotic divisions. During this division, the centromeres divide, and the sister chromatids of the secondary spermatocytes separate, being distributed to each of the spermatids resulting from that division. These cells then possess a haploid set of chromosomes, with 1N DNA each.

Spermiogenesis

The newly formed spermatids resulting from the second meiosis are joined by intercellular bridges and will undergo a transformation from round haploid spermatids into spermatozoa (Fig. 13-7). Testosterone is required for successful completion of this process. During spermiogenesis, morphological changes include formation of the acrosome, condensation of nuclear chromatin, outgrowth of a motile tail, and loss of excess spermatid material.

Spermiogenesis is divided into the Golgi phase, cap phase, acrosomal phase, and maturation phase. In histologic sections, the Golgi and cap phases are characterized by spherical nuclei, whereas the acrosomal and maturation phases have elongated nuclei.

During the **Golgi phase**, pro-acrosomal vesicles bud from the trans-Golgi network. These vesicles accumulate in a concave region of the nucleus and fuse together to form a large acrosomic granule, with its central part bound to the nuclear membrane. Simultaneously, a pair of centrioles begins to migrate toward the pole opposite the acrosome.

During the **cap phase**, the acrosome grows and spreads over one to two-thirds of the nucleus to form a head cap. This cap attaches to the nuclear envelope via an F-actin cytoskeletal plate called the acroplaxome. Meanwhile, the Golgi complex moves to the future neck region, and the axoneme begins to assemble from the proximal centriole. The axoneme is the internal microtubule cytoskeletal structure of the flagellum. In addition, the development of the second distal centriole and surrounding matrix begins, marking the initiation of the head-tail connecting piece formation. The spherical spermatid becomes polarized, and the developing spermatids rotate so that the acrosome is oriented toward the base of the seminiferous tubule.

In the **acrosomal phase**, the nucleus and cell body start to elongate, a process facilitated by a temporary cylinder of microtubules called the manchette. As the nucleus elongates, the chromatin undergoes a higher order of packaging where DNA nuclear histones are replaced by arginine and lysine-rich protamines, which allow dense packing of the chromatin. After repackaging, the DNA becomes transcriptionally inactive. The spermatids are now embedded within apical recesses of Sertoli cells.

During the **maturation phase**, nuclear condensation is completed, and the acrosomal granule spreads to cover the entire acrosomal membrane. The manchette disassembles when elongation is complete. Excess cytoplasm and organelles (mitochondria, ribosomes, and vesicles) are discarded as a residual body. The residual bodies are engulfed and digested by Sertoli cells. In the region of the future spermatozoon middle piece, the mitochondria gather around the axoneme in a helical manner. The outer fibers and the fibrous sheath of the future principal piece develop. Finally, a small remaining portion of spermatid cytoplasm, the cytoplasmic droplet of young spermatozoa, is lost during passage through the epididymis. Although testicular spermatozoa are morphologically differentiated, they remain functionally immature.

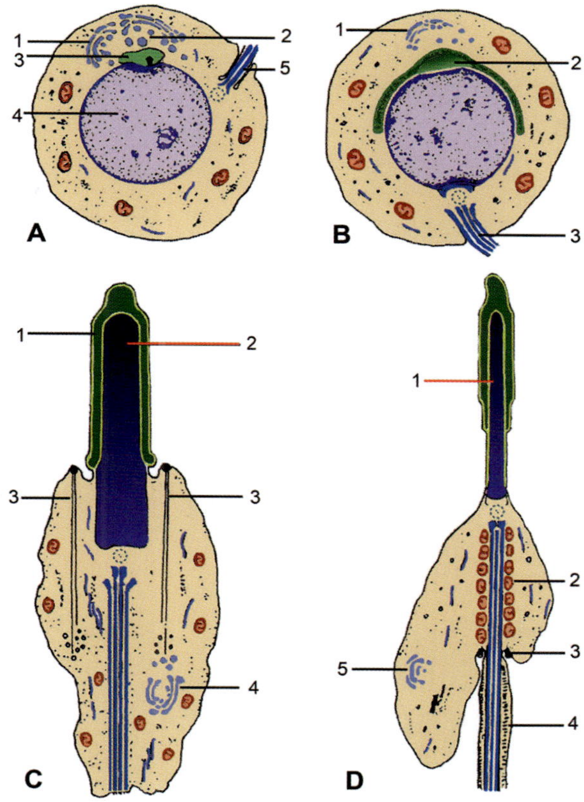

Figure 13-7 Spermiogenesis (bull). **A.** Spherical spermatid, Golgi phase. 1. Golgi complex. 2. Golgi vesicle. 3. Acrosomal vesicle containing acrosomal granule. 4. Nucleus. 5. Developing tail. **B.** Spherical spermatid, cap phase. 1. Golgi complex. 2. Head cap containing acrosome. 3. Developing tail. **C.** Elongated spermatid, acrosomal phase. 1. Acrosomal cap containing acrosome. 2. Nucleus. 3. Manchette. 4. Golgi complex. **D.** Elongated spermatid, maturation phase. 1. Nucleus. 2. Middle piece with mitochondrial sheath. 3. Annulus. 4. Principal piece. 5. Golgi complex. (With permission from Mosimann W, Kohler T. *Zytologie, Histologie und mikroskopische Anatomie der Haussäugetiere*. Hamburg: Paul Parey, 1990. Modified from the original.)

Spermatozoon

Spermatozoa vary in length from approximately 60 µm (boars and stallions) to 75 µm (ruminants). The spermatozoon consists of two major portions: the head and the tail. The tail is further subdivided into the neck, middle piece, principal piece, and end piece (Fig. 13-8).

Head The shape of the head is determined by the shape of the nucleus and the acrosome, varying significantly across species. The anterior pole of the nucleus is covered by the **acrosomal cap**, with outer and inner acrosomal membranes that fuse at the caudal end. The acrosomal cap contains hydrolytic and proteolytic enzymes, which are set free during the **acrosome reaction** of capacitated spermatozoa in the uterine tube. Acrosomal enzymes facilitate the penetration of the zona pellucida

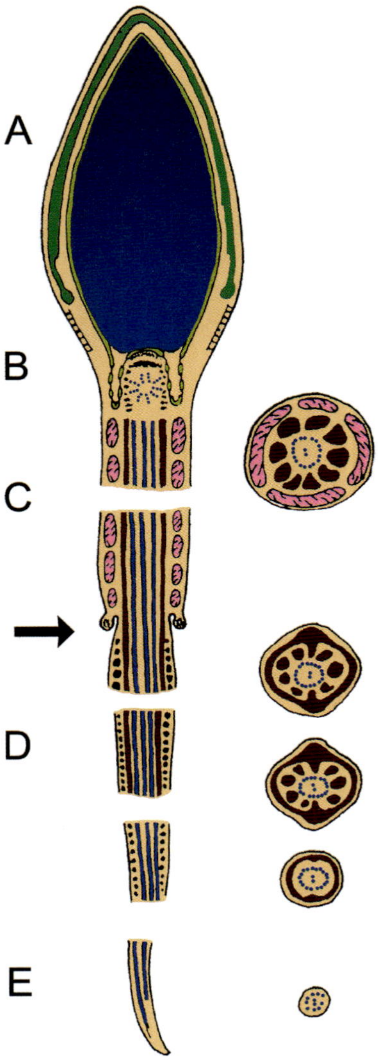

Figure 13-8 Schematic drawing of a spermatozoon. Left: Longitudinal section. Right: Cross sections located at the levels from which they are taken. **A.** Head containing the nucleus covered by the acrosome. Note the equatorial segment of the acrosome and the postacrosomal sheath. **B.** Neck. **C.** Middle piece with central axial filament complex, nine outer dense fibers, and the surrounding mitochondria. The middle piece terminates at the annulus (arrow). **D.** Principal piece in which the outer dense fibers are surrounded by the fibrous sheath; they terminate before the end of the principal piece. **E.** In the end piece, the microtubules of the axial filament complex terminate at various levels.

during fertilization. The base of the nucleus is encased by the postacrosomal sheath, which consists of sulfur-rich fibrous proteins. In dead spermatozoa, this sheath stains intensely with eosin or bromophenol blue. This reaction can be used to evaluate the spermatozoa quality.

Neck The **neck** is a short structure between the head and middle piece. It has a centrally located centriole and nine longitudinally oriented coarse fibers (connecting piece). These fibers extend peripherally and connect with the outer dense fibers of the middle piece.

Middle Piece The core of the **middle piece** has the characteristic structure of a flagellum with two central microtubules and nine peripheral microtubule doublets. These are surrounded by nine longitudinally oriented, tapered outer fibers that are connected to the fibers of the connecting piece in the neck. These, in turn, are surrounded by the mitochondria in a helical arrangement. In ruminants, the mitochondrial helix consists of approximately 40 turns. A ring-shaped thickening of the plasma membrane (annulus) of the middle piece marks the limit between the middle piece and the principal piece.

Principal Piece The **principal piece** is the longest part of the spermatozoon. The axial filament complex has a structure identical to that of the middle piece and is surrounded by the continuing outer fibers of the middle piece. The fibers vary in size and shape and gradually taper toward the end of the principal piece. Semicircular ribs of structural proteins, arranged helically, fuse with two of the outer fibers to form the peripheral fibrous sheath of the principal piece.

End Piece The end of the fibrous sheath marks the beginning of the **end piece**, which contains the axial filament complex. Proximally, in this complex has nine peripheral doublets; distally, these doublets become reduced progressively to singlets and terminate at various levels.

Cyclic Events in the Seminiferous Tubules

New generations of developing spermatozoa begin before one spermatogenic series is completed. This results in successive cell generations following each other at regular intervals of constant duration.

Within a region of the seminiferous tubule, changes in the shape and staining of the nuclei during cell division, and the release of spermatozoa into the lumen can be classified histologically. Eight stages have been identified for the spermatogenic cycle of bulls, rams, and boars. There are variations in the literature regarding how this process is described. However, the overlay of several developing generations will result in the following differentiating cells being observed during the eight stages below, as follows in this sequence: (a) Type-A spermatogonia, (b) Intermediate (In) spermatogonia, (c) Type-B spermatogonia, (d) Primary Spermatocytes (Leptotene, Zygotene, Pachytene, Diplotene), (e) Secondary spermatocytes, and (f) Spermatids (Sa-round spermatids and elongating to fully elongated spermatids Sb_1, Sb_2, Sc, Sd_1, and Sd_2).

Stage 1. Type-A and type-B spermatogonia, preleptotene/leptotene spermatocytes, pachytene primary spermatocytes, and Sb_1 spermatids.
Stage 2. Type-A spermatogonia, zygotene primary spermatocytes, pachytene primary spermatocytes, and Sb_2 spermatids.

Stage 3. Two generations of Type-A spermatogonia, zygotene primary spermatocytes, diplotene primary spermatocytes, and Sc spermatids.

Stage 4. Elongated spermatids are arranged in bundles and lie in deep apical recesses of the Sertoli cells. Also present are zygotene primary spermatocytes, diplotene, and spherical secondary spermatocytes.

Stage 5. Type-A spermatogonia, intermediate spermatogonia produced by asynchronous division, pachytene primary spermatocytes, and two generations of spermatids. New spherical spermatids (Sa) and older elongated spermatids (Sd_1)

Stage 6. The bundles of older spermatids have moved away from the vicinity of the Sertoli cell nuclei. Type-A spermatogonia, intermediate spermatogonia, pachytene primary spermatocytes, and Sa and Sd_1 spermatids.

Stage 7. The maturation-phase spermatids achieve a position close to the tubular lumen. Also present are type-A and type-B spermatogonia, pachytene primary spermatocytes, and Sa and Sd_2 spermatids.

Stage 8. Type-A spermatogonia, type-B_1 and -B_2 spermatogonia, pachytene primary spermatocytes, and Sa and Sb_2 spermatids. Spermatozoa that separate from their residual bodies leave the tubular epithelium (spermiation).

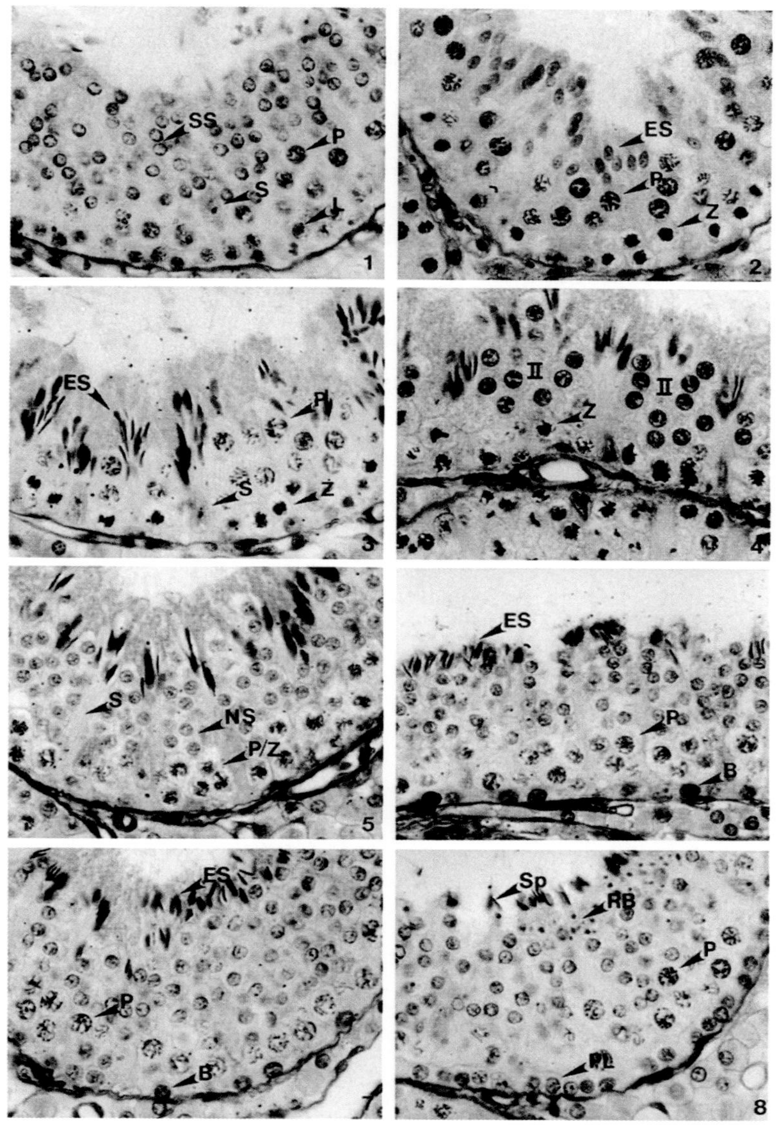

Figure 13-9 The eight stages of the spermatogenic cycle (boar). B spermatogonia (B), elongated spermatids (ES), leptotene primary spermatocytes (L), newly formed spermatids (NS), pachytene primary spermatocytes (P), preleptotene primary spermatocytes (PL), primary spermatocytes leaving zygotene and entering pachytene (P/Z), zygotene (Z), residual bodies (RB), sustentacular cell (S), spermatozoa in spermiation (Sp), spherical spermatids (SS), and secondary spermatocytes (II). Periodic acid-Schiff (×500).

The production of mature spermatozoa, as described above, occurs in cycles within regions of the seminiferous tubule (Fig. 13-9). Spermatogonia initiate the cell divisions of spermatogenesis at time intervals of constant duration. New generations of cells start the process of spermatogenesis before the succeeding generation finishes the process. The cell–cell associations within regions of the tubule allow for synchronized development of mature spermatozoa. Sertoli cells and spermatogonia respond to pulses of retinoic acid that move along the seminiferous tubule epithelium. The retinoic acid signal initiates the development of spermatozoa from undifferentiated spermatogonia. These regularly timed cycles of cell division occur within regions or segments of the seminiferous tubule and are referred to as spermatogenic waves. In the bull, segments of tubule approximately 10 mm in length cycle to produce the spermatogenic wave.

Straight Testicular Tubules

In all domestic mammals and rodents, the convoluted seminiferous tubules feed into a straight tubule segment (**transitional region**) that connects to the rete testis (Fig. 13-10). In stallions and boars, some seminiferous tubules terminate at the periphery of the testis and join the rete testis by long, straight testicular

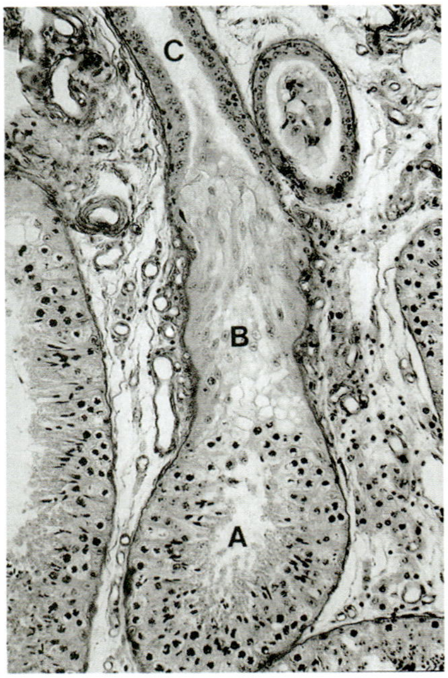

Figure 13-10 Convoluted seminiferous tubule (A), terminal segment (B) surrounded by a vascular plexus, and straight testicular tubule (C) in the bovine testis. Iron hematoxylin (×140).

tubules within the CT septa. The terminal segment or transition region of the convoluted seminiferous tubules contains modified Sertoli cells that form a valve or plug-like structure that partially occludes the tubular lumen. The region also contains high numbers of macrophages. All spermatozoa pass through the narrow intercellular slits between adjacent modified Sertoli cells on their way to the straight tubule. The terminal segment may further function as a valve that prevents reflux of rete testis fluid into the seminiferous tubules.

The straight testicular tubules are lined with a simple squamous to columnar epithelium. In bulls, a simple cuboidal epithelium lines the proximal portion of the straight tubules, while a simple columnar epithelium lines the distal portion. This epithelium contains numerous macrophages and lymphocytes and is capable of phagocytizing spermatozoa.

Rete Testis

The rete testis is formed by a plexus of anastomosing channels surrounded by loose CT (Fig. 13-11). Most of the rete is within the MT, but smaller intratunical and extratesticular portions are also present. The rete testis is lined by a simple squamous or cuboidal to columnar epithelium. Elastic fibers and contractile cells are present under the epithelium. The rete testis produces testicular fluid (in the ram, approximately 40 mL/day) that is largely reabsorbed in the head of the epididymis. Rete testis fluid differs in composition from seminiferous tubular fluid, testicular lymph, and blood plasma.

Testicular Blood Supply and Testicular Innervation

The testicular artery is a branch off the abdominal aorta that becomes highly coiled after reaching the spermatic cord. The coiled portion gives rise to small branches and larger epididymal arteries. In the testis, the artery is embedded in the tunica albuginea and courses parallel to the epididymis. The testicular artery divides at the caudal testicular pole to form the arterial contributions to the vascular layer of the tunica albuginea. Within the septula testis, centripetal septal arteries course to the MT, where they form convoluted coils in ruminants. From these convoluted coils or from the septal arteries, smaller arterial vessels deviate to supply the testicular parenchyma (Fig. 13-12).

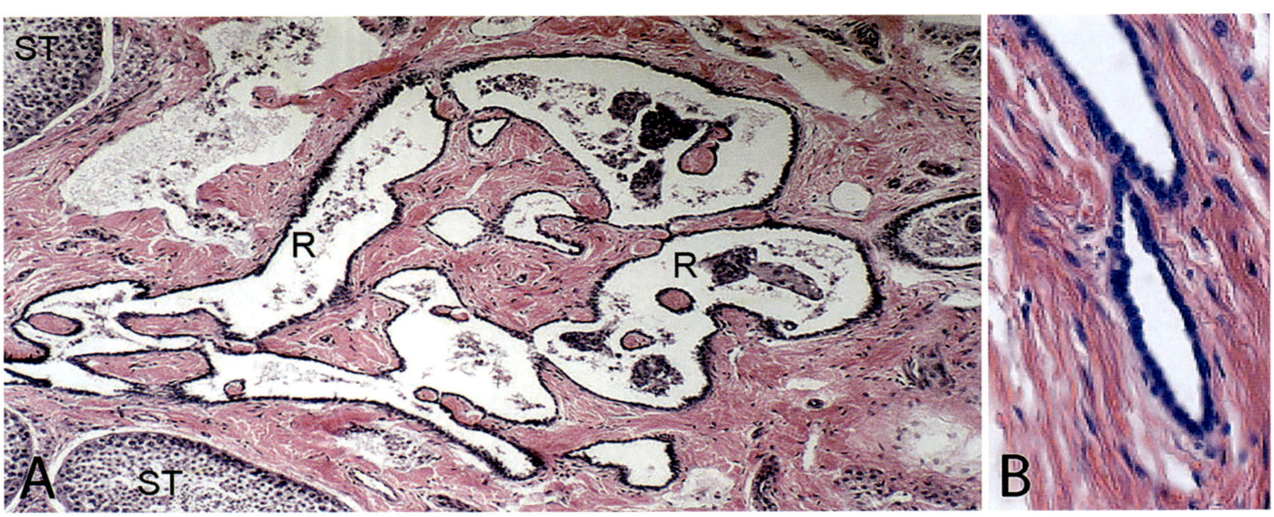

Figure 13-11 **A.** The seminiferous tubules (ST) terminate as straight testicular tubules that empty into the anastomosing channels of the rete testis (R). Simple squamous to columnar epithelium lines the rete tubules, which are surrounded by CT. Testis, cat. H&E (×100). (Image by W.E. Haensly.) **B.** Rete testis in the mediastinum testis of the cat. H&E (×400).

Most of the testicular veins empty into superficial veins in the vascular layer of the tunica albuginea. The albugineal veins converge at the base of the spermatic cord to form the **pampiniform plexus**, which surrounds the windings of the testicular artery. This vascular arrangement functions as a heat exchanger to cool arterial blood and may allow for venous-arterial steroid hormone transfer. Valves are present in the veins of the spermatic cord in all domestic species and in the septal veins of the porcine testis.

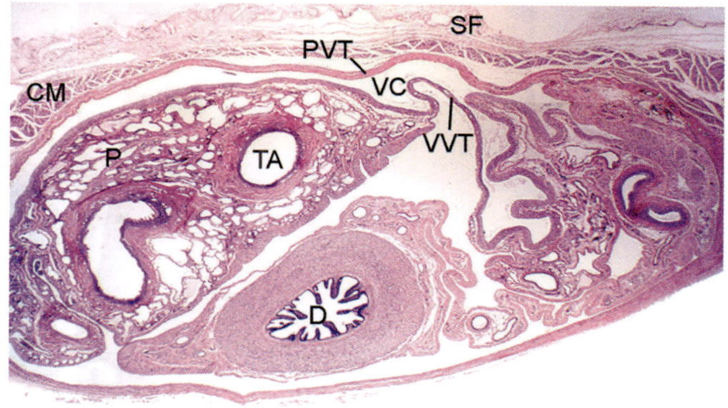

Figure 13-12 The spermatic cord contains the testicular vein, which coils to form the pampiniform plexus (P), the ductus deferens (D), and the testicular artery (TA). A peritoneal process, the vaginal tunic, encloses the testis and the spermatic cord. The visceral vaginal tunic (VVT) surrounds the ductus deferens and blood vessels and reflects as the parietal vaginal tunic (PVT), with the vaginal cavity (VC) located between the layers. The skeletal muscle of the cremaster muscle (CM) lies outside the parietal vaginal tunic. Spermatic fascia (SF) CT surrounds the entire spermatic cord. Spermatic cord, dog. H&E (×16). (Image by W.E. Haensly.)

The scrotal area is innervated by myelinated and nonmyelinated branches of the lumbosacral plexus. Considerable species-specific differences exist in the testicular innervation pattern. In the cat, many nerves are present in the tunica albuginea, septula, mediastinum, and lobuli testis, but the large testis of the adult boar is not innervated at all. In the testis of the bull and donkey, large areas of the testicular interior are devoid of nerve fibers. The majority of the intrinsic testicular nerve fibers are postganglionic sympathetic fibers. In the cat, medium-sized arterioles within the mediastinum, septula, and testicular lobules receive dual innervation by both noradrenergic and cholinergic axons. The testis of most species contains sensory nerves that are calcitonin gene-related peptide (CGRP)-positive axons. The autonomous innervation of testicular interstitial endocrine cells and the functional correlations between neural and endocrine regulation in the testis are still a matter of debate. In the camel testis, volume changes occur over the year, and an inverse relationship between neural and endocrine activities has been reported. The greatest volume and highest 3-β-hydroxysteroid-dehydrogenase (3-β-HStDH) content of the interstitial Leydig cell compartment in the winter is paralleled by a regression of testicular innervation. Conversely, weak or absent 3-β-HStDH activity and a decreasing volume of the interstitial endocrine cells in summer is accompanied by an increase in intertubular nerve fibers.

Epididymis

The mammalian **epididymis** is dependent on testicular androgens for the maintenance of its differentiated epithelium. It comprises a number of efferent ductules and a long, coiled ductus epididymis. The epididymis is divided into a head, body, and tail (Fig. 13-13). It is surrounded by a thick TA of dense irregular CT covered by the visceral layer of the TV. In stallions, the TA has a few smooth muscle cells scattered throughout the dense CT.

Efferent Ductules

Between 8 and 25 efferent ductules with regionally varying diameters connect the rete testis to the ductus epididymis. The ductules are gathered in small lobules with distinct boundaries of CT. The simple squamous to columnar epithelium of the rete testis transitions to simple columnar epithelium with ciliated and nonciliated principal cells in the efferent ductules (Fig. 13-14). Scattered free mononuclear immune cells may be present in the ductules. The ciliated cells with apical nuclei help move the spermatozoa toward the ductus epididymis.

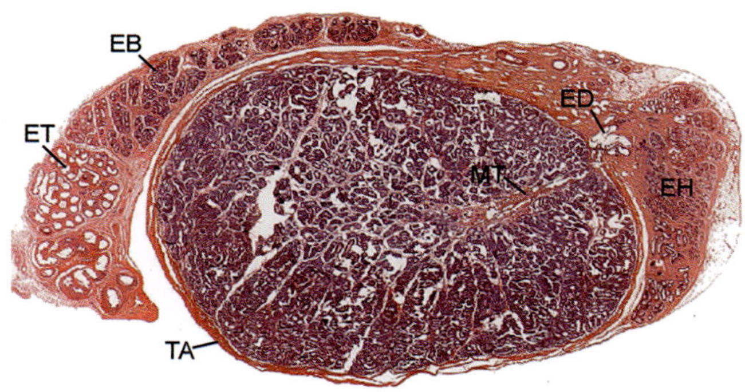

Figure 13-13 Cat testis. Tunica albuginea (TA), mediastinum testis (MT) containing rete testis, efferent ductules (ED), epididymis head (EH), epididymis body (EB), and epididymis tail (ET). H&E. (Courtesy of Purdue College of Veterinary Medicine.)

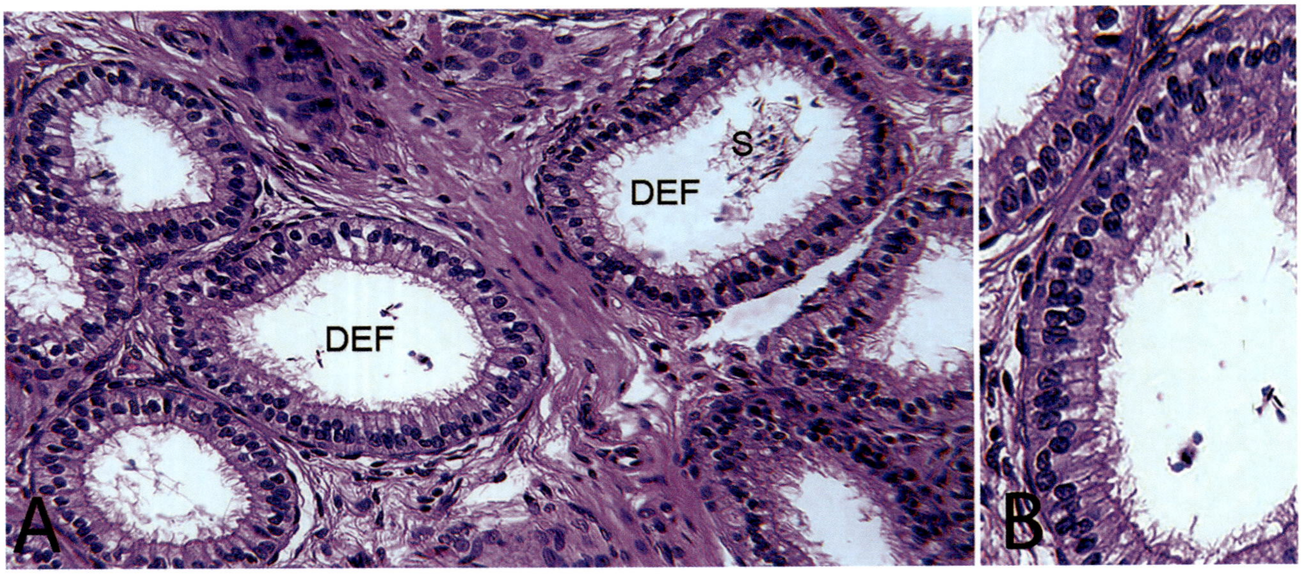

Figure 13-14 **A.** Between 8 and 25 ductules (DEF) form the ductuli efferentes. Simple columnar epithelium with ciliated and nonciliated cells helps propel spermatozoa (S) through the lumen of the ductules. In addition, the epithelium resorbs fluid from the ductular contents. Myofibroblasts and CT surround the epithelium. Ductuli efferentes, rat. H&E (×250). (Image by J. Eurell.) **B.** Higher magnification view of rat efferent ductule epithelium.

The nonciliated principal cells (basal row of nuclei) have a microvillus brush border and are active in the endocytosis of testicular fluid. Besides generating an osmotically driven water flow by transcellular transport of ions, most nonciliated principal cells are involved in resorptive processes. After the resorption and digestion of ductular fluid and macromolecules, they may contain globular Periodic Acid-Schiff (PAS)-positive residual bodies; others may have secretory activity. Intermediate forms between ciliated and nonciliated epithelial cells are occasionally observed. The ratio between ciliated and nonciliated principal cells varies along the ductule, with ciliated cells increasing in number toward the epididymal duct. The ductular epithelium is surrounded by three to six loosely arranged layers of myofibroblasts and CT. The efferent ductules and the initial portions of the ductus epididymis constitute the head of the epididymis.

Ductus Epididymis

The **epididymis** (Figs. 13-15 to 13-17) is extremely tortuous and coiled and the length of the duct varies among species. The length can be as much as 40 m, such as in bulls and boars, and can extend to 80 m in stallions. Spermatozoa acquire motility and fertilizing ability during the 9 to 15 days that they transit through the epididymis.

The epididymis is lined by a pseudostratified columnar epithelium surrounded by loose CT and a smooth muscle layer. This muscle layer is thinnest at the head and gets progressively thicker toward the tail. The epithelial height and innervation density of the muscle layer change in seasonal breeders (i.e., camel). Two cell types are present in the epididymal epithelium of all domestic mammals: columnar principal cells and small, polygonal basal cells. In many species, additional cell types, such as apical, narrow, clear, and halo cells are present.

The **principal cells** are the most abundant cell type found throughout the epididymis, and they are generally taller in the head region. These cells have high secretory and endocytic absorptive capacity. Their apical surface has branching microvilli (stereocilia) that becomes gradually shorter toward the epididymal tail. The principal cells are a source of vesicular epididymosomes secreted via an apocrine mechanism.

The epididymosomes are important for sperm maturation, and their content (e.g., lipids, proteins, enzymes) varies among species (Fig. 13-17). There are hundreds of proteins in epididymosomes, and their composition changes within different regions of the epididymis. The apical and narrow cells in the initial epididymal segment of the head are endocytic, with narrow cells secreting H^+ ions into the lumen to control pH. The clear cells also have high endocytic activity and are primarily responsible for endocytosis of cytoplasmic droplets released by spermatozoa during maturation. While these cells are not present in the initial segment, they are found throughout other epididymal regions. The halo cells are not part of the epithelium and represent immune cells (monocytes and various lymphocyte subtypes) that migrate into the epithelium. These immune cells are involved in regulating local immune tolerance and are found throughout the epididymis. In disease states, these cells can change phenotype to defend against pathogens and self-antigens.

The endocytic nature of the various cells lining the efferent ductules and the epididymis results in most of the testicular fluid (>90%) being reabsorbed. ABP and inhibin produced by the Sertoli cells are also reabsorbed in the initial segment of the ductus epididymis. In addition to the epididymosomes, substances such as glycerophosphoryl choline, phosphatase, and glycosidase are also secreted.

Based on histology (Fig. 13-18), histochemistry, ultrastructure, and patterns of gene expression, the ductus epididymis may be subdivided into several segments. The distribution and number of segments are characteristic for each species (six in bulls).

The proximal parts of the duct (initial segment, head, and body) are involved in the maturation process of spermatozoa. The tail of the epididymis serves as their main storage place (e.g., 45% of bovine epididymal spermatozoa are stored here). Spermatozoa are immotile and infertile when they leave the testis and acquire motility and fertility in the epididymis. During their passage through the ductus epididymis, spermatozoa undergo a series of morphologic and functional changes that lead to the acquisition of full fertilizing ability by the time they reach the tail. The change in the functional status of the spermatozoa is reflected in (a) the development of progressive motility, (b) modification of their metabolism, (c) alteration of the plasma membrane surface characteristics (activation of membrane-bound molecules necessary for recognition processes during fertilization), (d) stabilization of the plasma membrane by oxidation of incorporated sulfhydryl groups, and (e) caudad movement (i.e., toward the tail end of the sperm cell) and eventual loss of the cytoplasmic droplet, a remnant of the spermatid cytoplasm. Spermatozoa with persisting droplets are probably infertile. Fully mature spermatozoa can be stored in the tail of the epididymis for a long period. Epididymal spermatozoa have a wide range of potent antigens that can trigger an autoimmune response by antisperm antibodies, but this is prevented or attenuated by a blood–epididymal barrier similar to the apical epithelial junctional complex.

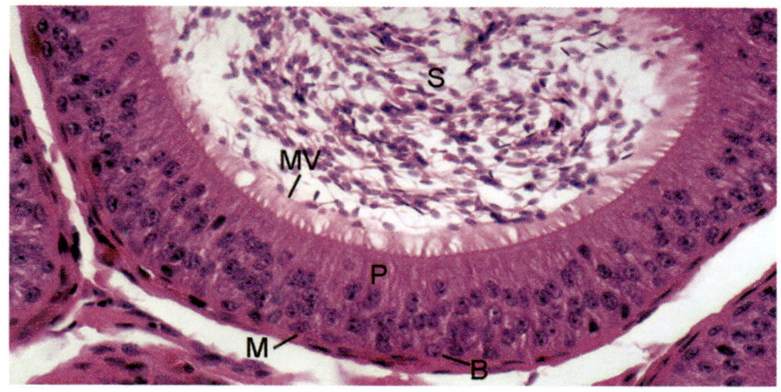

Figure 13-15 The ductus epididymis is lined by pseudostratified columnar epithelium comprised of columnar principal cells (P) and small, polygonal basal cells (B). The principal cells have long, branching microvilli (MV), also called stereocilia. The epithelium is surrounded by circular smooth muscle (M) that increases in thickness toward the tail of the epididymis. While passing through the ductus epididymis, spermatozoa (S) develop progressive motility, modify their metabolism, and alter their cell membrane in preparation for fertilization. Epididymis, dog, H&E (×400). (Image by W.E. Haensly.)

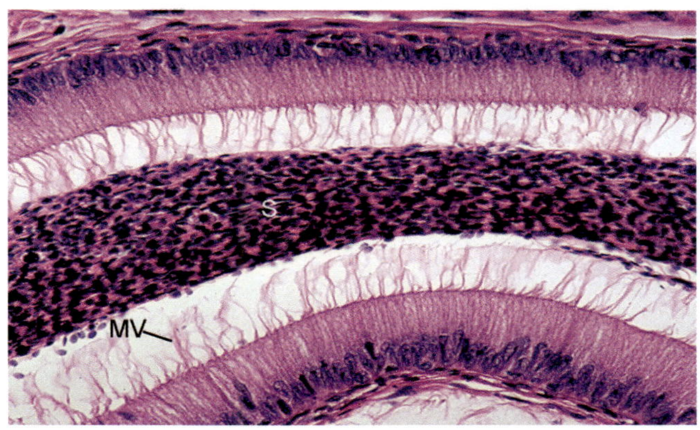

Figure 13-16 The branching microvilli (MV), or stereocilia, on the epithelial cells of the ductus epididymis are longest near the head of the epididymis and shortest at the tail. As spermatozoa move through the ductus, considerable testicular fluid is removed, and the spermatozoa (S) are concentrated. Epididymis, dog. H&E (×250). (Image by W.E. Haensly.)

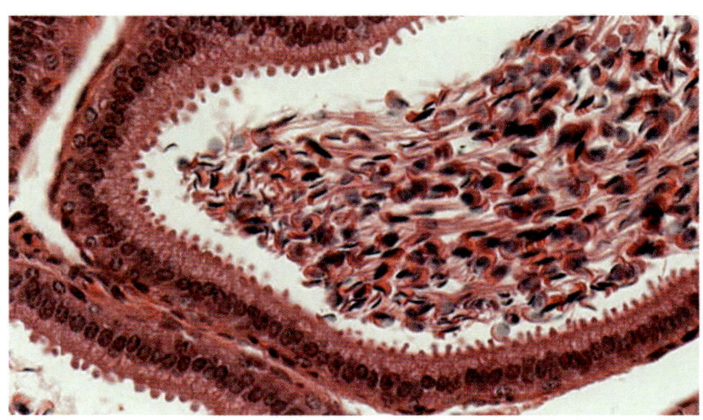

Figure 13-17 Ductus epididymis epithelium in the guinea pig H&E (×400). (Courtesy of Purdue College of Veterinary Medicine.)

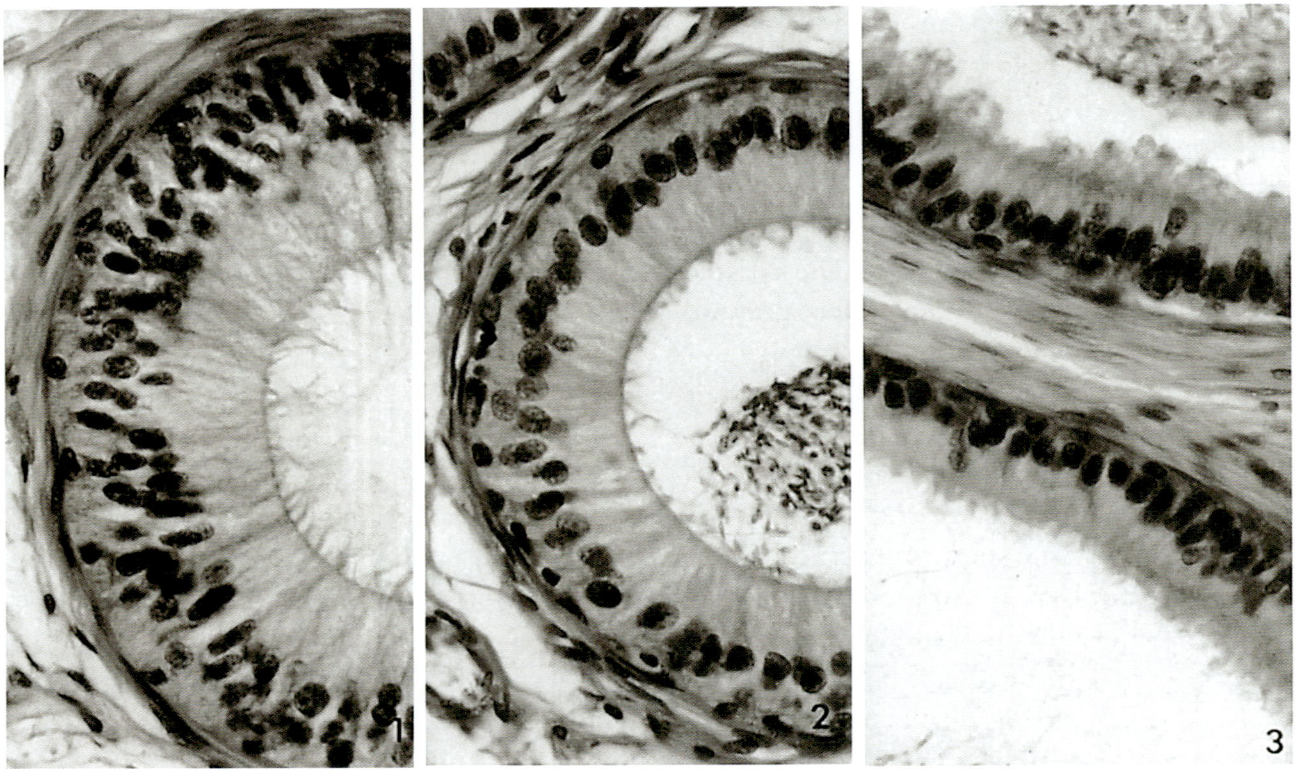

Figure 13-18 Sections through the wall of the feline ductus epididymis taken at the level of the head (1), body (2), and tail (3) of the epididymis. Note the variations in the position of the nuclei, height of the pseudostratified columnar epithelium, length of the microvilli, and thickness of the muscular coat. H&E (×435).

Ductus Deferens

There is a sharp bend at the tail of the epididymis that straightens and leads into the ductus deferens. In stallions and ruminants, the ductus deferens joins the excretory duct of the vesicular gland to form a short ejaculatory duct, which opens at the colliculus seminalis into the urethra. The pseudostratified lining epithelium of the bovine ejaculatory duct contains engulfed spermatozoa. In boars, the ductus deferens and the excretory duct open separately into the urethra. Carnivores lack vesicular glands and the ductus deferens joins the urethra alone.

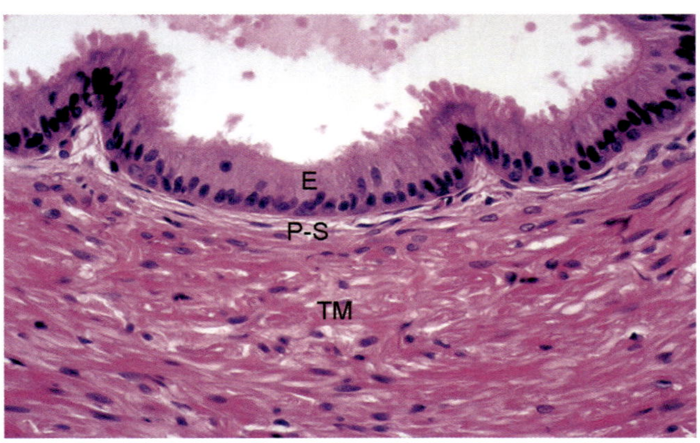

Figure 13-19 Pseudostratified columnar epithelium (E) lines the ductus deferens. Beneath the epithelium lies a propria-submucosa (P-S) of loose CT. Variable layers of smooth muscle form the tunica muscularis (TM). Ductus deferens, cat. H&E (×400). (Image by W.E. Haensly.)

The ductus deferens is lined by a pseudostratified columnar epithelium similar to that of the ductus epididymis but with more basal cells (Fig. 13-19). Toward the end of the duct, it may transition to a simple columnar epithelium. At the beginning of the duct the columnar cells possess short, branched microvilli. In bulls, small lipid droplets are present in the basal cells. The loose CT of the lamina propria-submucosa is highly vascularized (Fig. 13-20, low magnification), rich in fibroblasts and elastic fibers, and contains a network of cholinergic nerves, whereas the tunica muscularis is densely innervated by postganglionic sympathetic fibers.

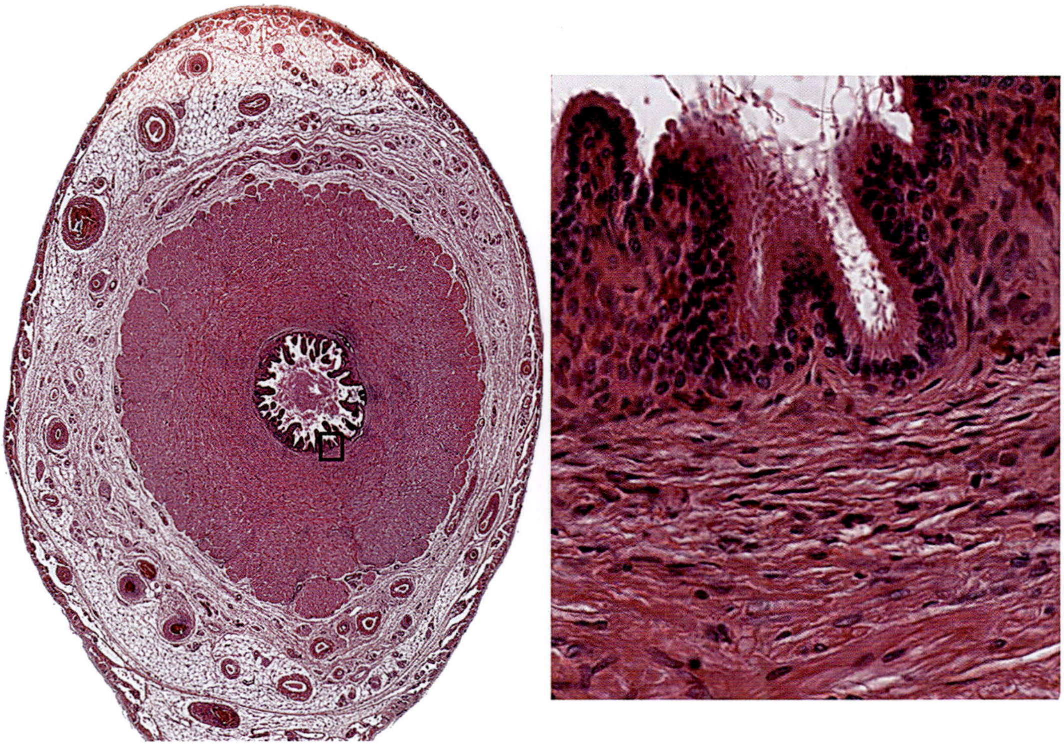

Figure 13-20 Equine ductus deferens. High-magnification view in the right panel is from the boxed area on the overview image. H&E (×250). (Courtesy of Purdue College of Veterinary Medicine.)

In stallions, bulls, and boars, the tunica muscularis consists of intermingled circular, longitudinal, and oblique layers; in small ruminants and carnivores, an inner circular layer and an outer longitudinal layer are present. A tunica serosa covers the organ.

The terminal portion of the ductus deferens functions as a male accessory gland. In stallions, ruminants, and dogs, it forms an **ampulla**, but not in boars and cats (Fig. 13-21). The ampulla contains simple branched tubuloalveolar glands in the lamina propria-submucosa. In stallions, bulls, and rams, these glands occupy a large portion of the lamina propria-submucosa, which is rich in smooth muscle cells.

In dogs and bucks, the glands are surrounded by CT lacking smooth muscle cells. The glands are lined by cells that vary from tall columnar cells with ovoid nuclei to cuboidal cells with spherical nuclei. Spherical to polyhedral basal cells are distributed irregularly between the columnar cells. In ruminants, the glandular epithelium is rich in glycogen, and the basal cells contain lipid droplets of variable size. Lipid droplets are also present in the columnar cells of bulls. The lipids in bovine basal cells may coalesce, thereby giving these cells the appearance of fat cells. The tunica muscularis of the terminal portion of the ductus deferens consists of variably arranged smooth muscle bundles surrounded by the highly vascularized loose CT of the tunica adventitia.

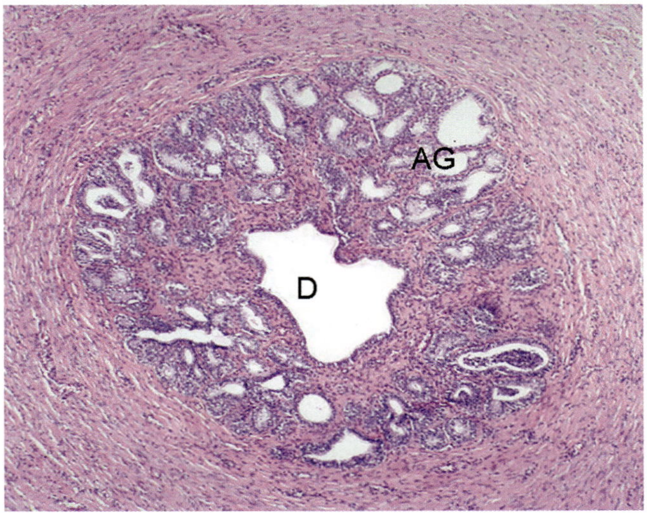

Figure 13-21 In the dog, ampullary glands (AG) are located beneath the epithelium of the terminal ductus deferens (D). Tall simple columnar epithelium lines the secretory units, and periglandular CT, which is devoid of smooth muscle, surrounds them. Ampulla, dog. H&E (×40). (Image by W.E. Haensly.)

Accessory Glands

The accessory glands of the male reproductive system function to secrete fluids containing structural proteins, forming the seminal plasma. These glands include the glandular portion of the ductus deferens, the vesicular glands (seminal vesicles), prostate gland, and the bulbourethral gland. They secrete fluids that enter the urethra and compose the ejaculate, which consists of spermatozoa and seminal plasma containing secretions from the epididymis and male accessory glands. All accessory glands are present in stallions, ruminants, and boars; the vesicular glands are absent in carnivores, and the bulbourethral gland is absent in dogs. In cats, the prostate and bulbourethral glands are the only accessory glands.

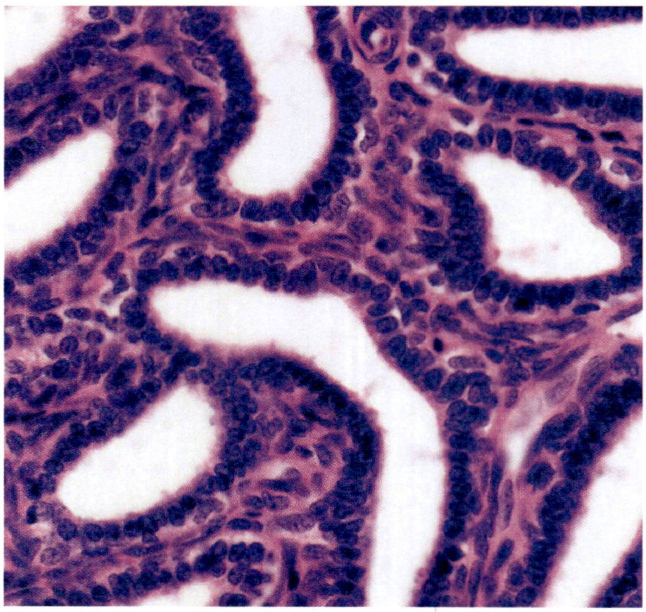

Figure 13-22 The epithelium of the vesicular gland is classified as pseudostratified columnar with mostly tall columnar cells and few basal cells. The epithelium is often folded and projects into the wide lumens of the tubuloalveolar secretory units. Vesicular gland, pig. H&E (×400).

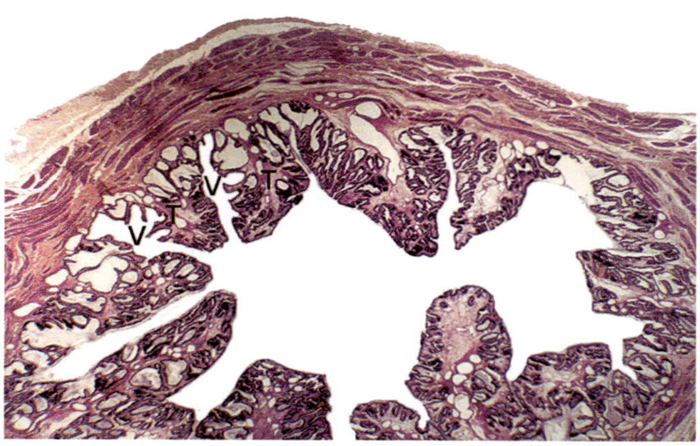

Figure 13-23 Vesicular gland of a stallion with true vesicles (V) containing short, branched tubuloalveolar glands that open into central ducts. The vesicles are separated by thin CT trabeculae (T). The structure of the gland in other species is variable. H&E (×16). (Image by W.E. Haensly.)

Vesicular Glands

The **vesicular glands** are typically paired tubular or tubuloalveolar structures with papillary projections into the lumen (Fig. 13-22). They are located laterally to the ampullae and adjacent to the neck of the bladder. The glandular epithelium is pseudostratified, with tall columnar cells and basal cells that are sparse and spherical. The abundant CT has fibroblasts, collagen fibers, and small vessels scattered in the stroma.

The intralobular and main excretory ducts are lined by a simple cuboidal epithelium, or by a stratified columnar epithelium in horses. The gland can be subdivided into lobes and lobules, composed of highly vascular CT (Fig. 13-23). The propria-submucosa is continuous with the denser CT of the trabeculae, which may subdivide the organ into lobes and lobules. A tunica muscularis of varying thickness and arrangement surrounds the organ, covered by a tunica serosa or adventitia. In the peripheral region, it is possible to see larger-caliber blood vessels and peripheral innervation.

Species Differences

The vesicular glands are prominent in stallions and boars and have a sac-like morphology in both species. They are considered true vesicles in stallions, with short, branched tubuloalveolar glands that open into wide central ducts. These ducts are separated by thin CT trabeculae with irregularly arranged smooth muscle cells.

Boars have two large and lobulated vesicular glands with a common CT capsule and a thin tunica muscularis. The interlobular CT septa have a few smooth muscle cells. The tubular lumina are wide and the secretory epithelium is folded.

In bulls and rams, the vesicular glands are compact and lobulated. In bulls, the ducts drain the slightly coiled tubular portions of the gland and, in turn, are drained by the main excretory duct. Large amounts of citrate are found in the secretions in all species, although in bulls and small ruminants, fructose is also present. In the secretory columnar tissue, small lipid droplets are present, and these cells have a positive reaction for alkaline phosphatase due to the presence of glycogen. Some of the columnar cells possess light, bleb-like apical projections. The vesicular glands of bulls have a high amount of lipids, with approximately 50% being cholesterol. The remaining lipid component consists of triglycerides and phospholipids. The interlobular septa are muscular, derived from the thick tunica muscularis, which is surrounded by a capsule of dense irregular CT with a few smooth muscle cells.

In rams and bucks, the vesicular glands are morphologically similar to that of bulls, and lipid droplets are present in the basal cells of the buck's vesicular gland but absent in rams. During the breeding season of bucks, the gland epithelium increases in height. The vesicular glands produce part of the ejaculate, and the proportion of its fluid in the total ejaculate varies among species. The gland fluid is usually a gelatinous, white, or yellowish-white secretion and is approximately 25 to 30% of the total ejaculate in bulls, 10 to 30% in boars, and 7 to 8% in rams and bucks. The gland secretions contain a high amount of fructose, which is an energy source for ejaculated spermatozoa.

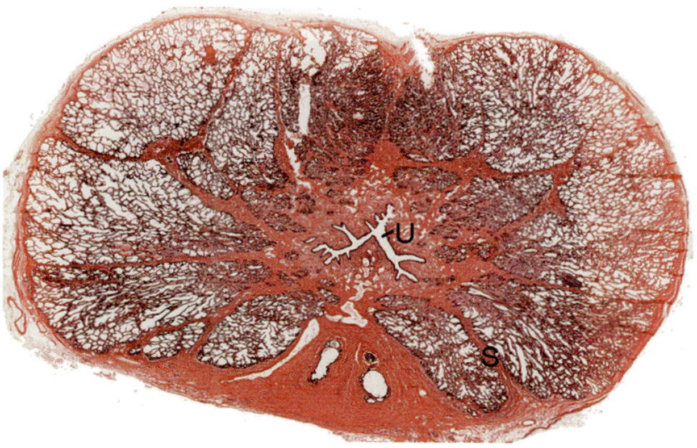

Figure 13-24 Canine prostate gland. Prostatic urethra (U) and septa (S). H&E. (Courtesy of Purdue College of Veterinary Medicine.)

Prostate

The **prostate** is a tubuloalveolar encapsulated gland surrounded by a fibromuscular capsule, which encloses the pelvic urethra (Fig. 13-24). It can be divided into two portions: the **body** (corpus prostatae) and the **disseminate** part (pars disseminata prostatae). The body either entirely surrounds the pelvic urethra at the level of the colliculus seminalis or covers part of its dorsal aspect. The prostate gland is composed of luminal, basal, and neuroendocrine cell populations. The disseminate part is located in the propria-submucosa of the pelvic urethra.

The stroma is fibromuscular and supports a moderate amount of tubulo-acinar glands with simple cuboidal or columnar epithelium (Fig. 13-25). The simple epithelium changes to stratified columnar or transitional epithelium toward the terminal portions of the ducts. The prostate glands exhibit a basal layer composed of cells with oval nuclei and scant cytoplasm. The basal cells are usually scattered, forming a discontinuous basal cell layer in dogs.

The epithelial columnar prostate cells (luminal) produce and secrete proteins, resulting in a positive mucous reaction in the cytoplasm (proteinaceous secretory granules). Luminal cells are the most abundant cell subtype, forming a columnar-shaped cell layer responsible for producing serine proteases called kallikreins. This cell layer is usually arranged in a tubular form, with columnar cells showing microvilli and sometimes bleb-like apical protrusions. A common feature in the tubules and alveoli are concretions of lamellar secretory material (**corpora amylacea**). The duct system of the prostate possesses saccular dilations in which secretory material may be stored.

The urethra histologically consists of urothelial (transitional) tissue arranged in multiple layers of cells with scant cytoplasm. The prostatic capsule contains large-caliber arteries and peripheral nerves.

The prostate gland capsule is dense irregular CT enriched with smooth muscles cells and elastic fibers. Large trabeculae

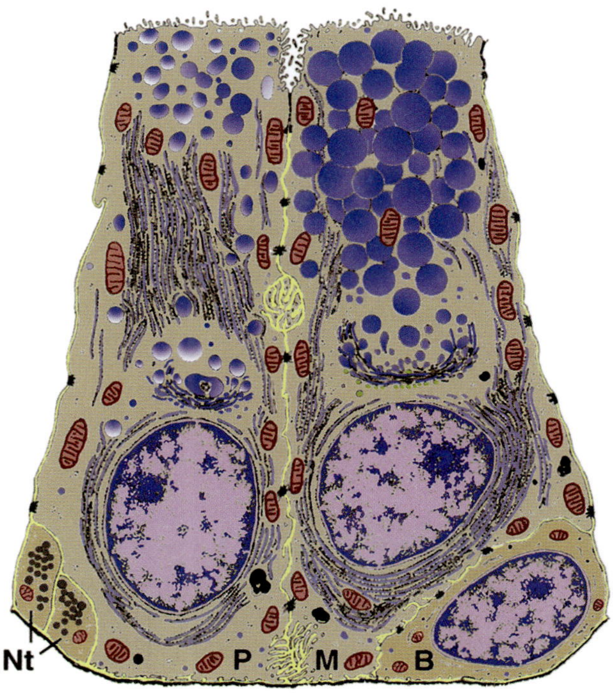

Figure 13-25 Ruminant prostatic epithelium. The cell (P) on the left side is a specific secretory cell containing proteinaceous granules. The cell on the right secretes mucus (M). Basal cell (B); intraepithelial autonomic nerve terminals (Nt). Modified from the original.

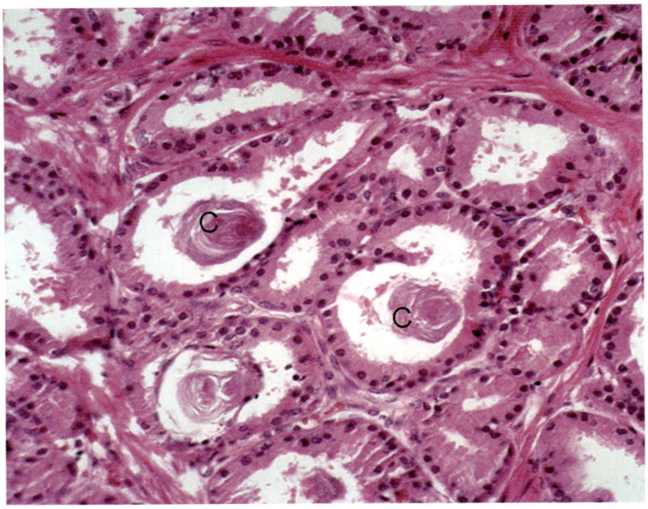

Figure 13-26 The prostate is a tubuloalveolar gland lined by simple cuboidal or columnar epithelium. Tall columnar cells have microvilli, and bleb-like apical protrusions are often present. Concentrically laminated concretions of secretory material, called corpora amylacea (C), are sometimes found in the lumen of the tubules. Prostate, pig. H&E (×250). (Image by W.E. Haensly.)

extend from the capsule, separating the body and the disseminate part into individual lobules. They are predominantly muscular in the body of the gland.

Secretory portions and ducts of the prostate are surrounded by loose CT containing smooth muscle cells that are abundant in the body of the gland. Corpora amylacea may be found in the lumen of the tubules (Fig. 13-26).

Species Differences

The prostate gland is present in all domestic and wild mammals and is usually subdivided in two distinct lobes. In dogs, the prostate is surrounded by a fibrovascular capsule, located immediately caudal to the bladder, completely surrounding the pelvic urethra. In cats, the prostate is positioned caudally compared to dogs, located behind the cranial border of the pelvic symphysis under the ventral wall of the rectum. The disseminate part in dogs consists of a few glandular lobules, while in cats, individual lobules of the disseminate part are scattered between the colliculus seminalis and the bulbourethral glands. Lamellar corpuscles may be observed in the interstitium.

In stallions, the gland is located in the retroperitoneal region composed of right and left lobes dorsal to the pelvic urethra. The capsule, trabeculae, and interstitial CT have a large amount of smooth muscle. In ruminants, the prostate is an unpaired gland, with some differences reported between bulls and small ruminants. In bulls, the gland is relatively inconspicuous and small compared to other domestic species. The disseminate portion encircles the urethra in bulls; however, in small ruminants, the prostate is not grossly visible and consist of internal glandular tissue.

The main role of the prostate gland is the production of prostatic fluid, and its contribution to the total ejaculate varies among species. In dogs, prostatic fluid is responsible for 90% of the ejaculate volume; in ruminants, it is 4 to 6%; in stallions, 25 to 30%. One of the functions of the prostate is to neutralize the seminal plasma, made acidic by accumulation of metabolic carbon dioxide and lactate, and to initiate active movements of the ejaculated spermatozoa. The prostate gland is hormonally dependent, and castration induces its atrophy. In castrated subjects, the glandular tissue will appear atrophic with more abundant intertubular CT.

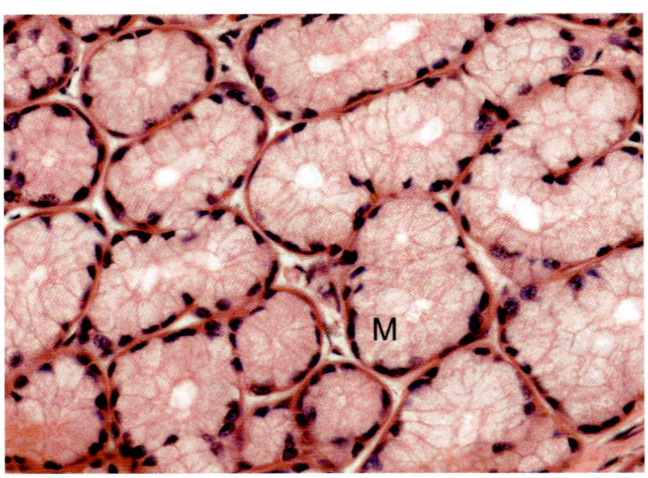

Figure 13-27 The secretory units of the bulbourethral gland contain mucous-producing (M) simple columnar epithelial cells. The combined mucous and proteinaceous secretions help lubricate and neutralize the urethra and vagina environment. Bulbourethral gland, bull. H&E (×400).

Bulbourethral Gland

The **paired bulbourethral** glands (Fig. 13-27) attach to the dorsolateral surface of the bulb of the penis and caudal to the prostate gland. The gland is compound tubular (boars, cats, bucks) or tubuloalveolar (stallions, bulls, and rams); it is absent in dogs. The bulbourethral gland is multilobular, with each lobule formed by acini opening to a central duct. The bulbourethral ductal epithelium presents one layer of cuboidal cells with dark cytoplasm. The secretory portions of the gland are lined with a tall simple columnar epithelium. The glands are divided into lobes by CT septa consisting of elastic fibers and both smooth and striated muscle. A thin basal (myoepithelial) cell layer surrounds each acinus.

The acini open into ducts, and different ducts join each other to form the central excretory duct, which is a larger intraglandular duct. The ducts connected with each acinus are lined by simple cuboidal or columnar epithelium. In contrast, the larger intraglandular ducts are lined by pseudostratified columnar epithelium, and they open into a single (or multiple) duct(s) lined by urothelial epithelium.

The gland is enveloped by a fibroelastic capsule containing an adaptable mixture of striated muscle. Extending outward from this capsule are dense irregular CT trabeculae, accompanied by a combination of smooth and striated muscle fibers. The interstitial space is composed of loose CT, with a few smooth muscle fibers.

Species Differences

In cats, the bulbourethral glands are paired circular glands, approximately 4 to 5 mm in diameter. The gland consists of spacious, sinus-like intraglandular ducts and short, narrow, mostly unbranched tubular end pieces. The secretory cell surface is increased by a well-developed system of intercellular canaliculi. In stallions, they are not rectally palpable since the urethralis and bulboglandularis muscles completely surround the gland. Three to four individual bulbourethral ducts can exist.

In boars, the glands are prominent and large and surrounded by the bulboglandularis muscle. Histologically, few smooth muscle cells are found on the gland interstitium, and the collecting ducts are characterized by a simple columnar epithelium. In ruminants, the gland is surrounded by the bulbospongiosus muscle. In bulls and rams, short connecting pieces link the secretory portions to the collecting ducts, which are lined with simple cuboidal epithelium and sometimes also have a secretory function. In bucks, the secretory fraction flows directly into these channels. Smooth muscle cells are particularly common in the stroma.

The bulbourethral gland produces a secretion that is a combination of mucous and protein. In ruminants, this secretion is released prior to ejaculation, where it appears to have a dual role: neutralizing the urethral environment and providing lubrication for both the urethra and the vagina. In boars, the secretion is predominantly mucous and rich in sialic acid, constituting a significant portion of the ejaculate (15 to 30%). This secretion may play a role in sealing the cervix after insemination to prevent sperm loss. In cats, the secretory product is primarily composed of mucus and also contains glycogen. In the absence of a vesicular gland, this bulbourethral glycogen may serve as an alternative energy source for sperm metabolism.

Urethra

The male urethra is a tubular organ divided into three parts: prostatic, pelvic, and penile portions. The prostatic portion extends from the urinary bladder to the caudal edge of the body of the prostate gland, crossing through the prostate parenchyma. The pelvic urethra begins at the end of the prostatic portion and extends until the bulb of the penis. The penile portion of the urethra begins in the penile bulb and continues to the external urethral opening.

The mucosal lining of the urethra forms longitudinal folds that become flattened or disappear during erections and urination. A distinct and permanent dorsomedial fold called the urethral crest is present in the prostatic urethra. This crest extends to an enlargement called the **colliculus seminalis**. At this point, various ducts open into the urethra depending on the species: in ruminants and stallions, these are the ejaculatory ducts; in boars, these are the ductus deferens and excretory ducts of the vesicular glands; and in carnivores, these are the deferent ducts. Among these ducts, remnants of the fused paramesonephric ducts, referred to as the uterus masculinus, may be observed as either a solid epithelial cord or a short canal.

The urethral lining presents a transitional epithelium (urothelium), characterized by variably sized patches of simple columnar epithelium that can change into pseudostratified columnar epithelium in the pelvic and prostatic urethra. In the penile urethra, in the region of the external penile urethral orifice, the cells will modify to stratified squamous cells at the external meatus (Fig. 13-28).

The propria-submucosa layer is composed of loose CT containing numerous elastic fibers, smooth muscle cells, and, in the case of dogs, occasional scattered lymphatic tissue or lymphatic nodules. In stallions and cats, the tissue contains simple tubular mucous glands. Additionally, the epithelia of the urethra and urogenital sinus-derived glands, such as the prostate and bulbourethral gland, consistently contain cells containing regulatory peptides, which are part of the diffuse neuroendocrine system.

Along the entire extent of the urethra, the propria-submucosa is characterized by its erectile properties due to the presence of variable-sized caverns lined with endothelium. These caverns form what is commonly referred to as the vascular stratum in the prostatic region and pelvic urethra. Surrounding the penile urethra, there is a significant augmentation in the number and size of the cavernous spaces. In this region, the vascular layer is known as the **corpus spongiosum**, commencing at the ischiatic arch and exhibiting a bilobed expansion referred to as the bulb of the penis. In the pelvic section of the urethra, the tunica muscularis is composed of smooth muscle near the bladder and striated muscle in the remaining portion of the urethra. It is encased by a tunica adventitia made up of loose or dense irregular CT.

In the case of ruminants and stallions, the terminal section of the urethra extends partially (bulls) or entirely (stallions, rams, and bucks) beyond the glans penis, forming the urethral process. This structure is lined with transitional or stratified squamous epithelium and is surrounded by a corpus spongiosum, which contains numerous cavernous spaces in stallions and fewer, smaller spaces in ruminants. In bucks and rams, two fibrocartilaginous cords run longitudinally alongside the urethra. The urethral process is covered by a cutaneous mucous membrane.

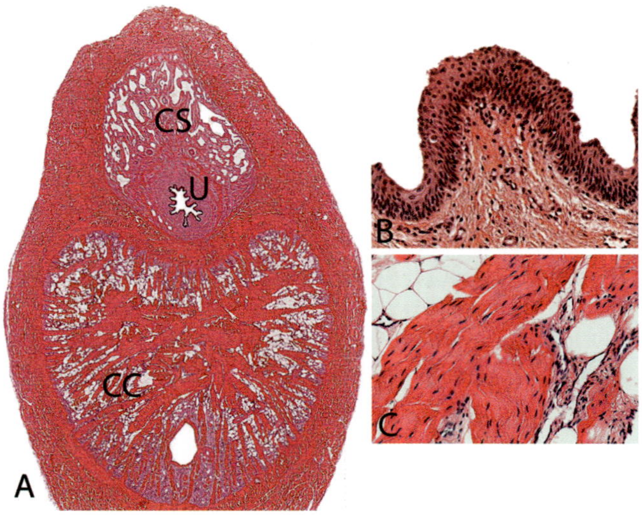

Figure 13-28 **A.** Bull penis. The urethra (U) is surrounded by the cavernous spaces of the corpus spongiosum (CS). The corpus cavernosum (CC) contains fibroelastic CT. **B.** Penile urethra urothelium. **C.** Fibroelastic CT of the corpus cavernosum. H&E. (Courtesy of Purdue College of Veterinary Medicine.)

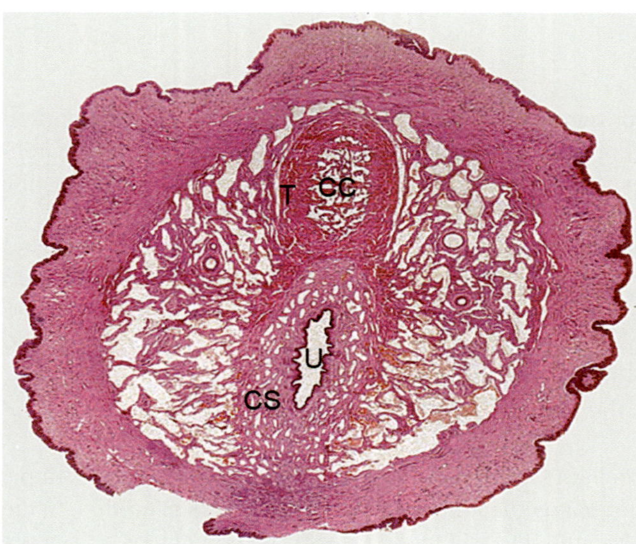

Figure 13-29 The corpus cavernosum (CC) in the musculocavernous penis of the horse forms two ventrolateral and one central median projection for support. The cavernous spaces are lined by endothelium and surrounded by CT. The corpus spongiosum (CS) encases the urethra (U), and a thick tunica albuginea (T) surrounds the cavernous tissue. The equine penis lacks an os penis. H&E. (Image by W.E. Haensly.)

Penis

The penis is a male reproductive organ that ensures the internal fertilization in all mammalian species. Morphologically, it consists of (a) corpus cavernosum, (b) the corpus spongiosum surrounding the penile urethra, and (c) the glans penis (Figs. 13-28 to 13-30).

Corpus Cavernosum

The corpus cavernosum is surrounded by a thick layer of dense, irregular CT containing a variable number of elastic fibers and smooth muscle cells (tunica albuginea). A CT septum completely or partially divides the corpora cavernosa of the penis.

The gaps between the tunica albuginea and the network of trabeculae stemming from the tunica albuginea are occupied by erectile tissue. In stallions and carnivores, this erectile tissue comprises cavities lined with endothelium and encircled by CT, the composition of which ranges from loose to dense irregular, along with the inclusion of smooth muscle cells. In stallions, these muscle bundles align along the lengthwise axis of the penis, frequently leading to nearly complete closure of the lumens within the cavernous spaces. When these muscle cells relax, the penis extends and emerges from the prepuce, typically occurring during the process of urination. In boars and ruminants, the CT surrounding the caverns contains few, if any, smooth muscle cells.

The primary blood supply to the cavernous spaces is provided by the **helicine arteries**. These arteries are distinctive for their epithelioid smooth muscle cells within the tunica intima, which extend into the vessel lumens as ridges or pads, resulting in partial constriction. When these smooth muscle cells relax, blood flow into the cavernous spaces increases and leads to an erection. Drainage of the cavernous spaces is facilitated by venules, some of which give rise to veins with thick walls.

Glans Penis

Among animals, a fully developed glans penis is found exclusively in stallions and dogs. Feline species develop keratinized spines on the glans surface (Fig. 13-31). The glans is encircled by a tunica albuginea that is notably abundant in elastic fibers. This tunica albuginea extends into trabeculae, outlining spaces filled with erectile tissue that resembles either the corpus spongiosum penis (in stallions) or a network of sizeable caverns (in dogs) (Fig. 13-32). The glans penis is covered by the prepuce (as discussed in a later section of this chapter).

Species Differences

The corpora cavernosa penis in dogs (Fig. 13-32) are entirely separated by a CT septum and extend cranially to the **os penis**, which terminates in a fibrocartilaginous tip. The glans penis comprises the bulbus glandis and the pars longa glandis, both of which almost entirely encircle the os penis and the distal part of the penile urethra, along with its accompanying corpus spongiosum. The **bulbus glandis** is made up of sizable venous cavities separated by CT trabeculae rich in elastic fibers. **The pars longa glandis** constitutes the upper part of the glans penis and shares an identical structure with the bulbus.

Among felines, numerous adipose cells are present within the cavities of the corpus cavernosum penis. Their quantity increases toward the tip of the corpus cavernosum, where there is relatively less erectile tissue. Additionally, a diminutive os penis is encircled by the corpus spongiosum of the glans.

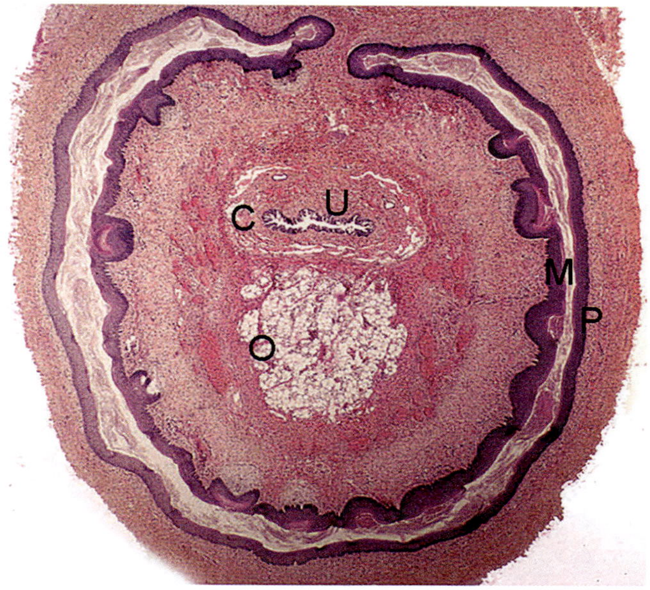

Figure 13-30 The cat penis is covered by a mucosa (M) consisting of keratinized stratified squamous epithelium. Erectile tissue of the corpus spongiosum (C) surrounds the penile urethra (U). A remnant of the os penis (O) lies ventral to the urethra. The prepuce (P) forms a thick circular fold around the penis. H&E (×25). (Image by W.E. Haensly.)

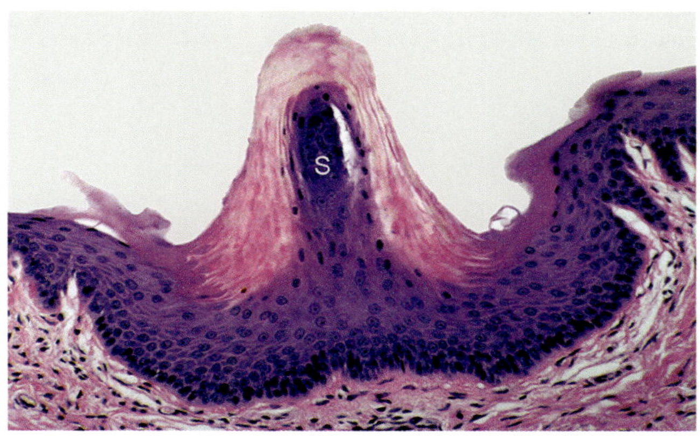

Figure 13-31 Penile spines (s) in the cat arise from the keratinized squamous epithelium of the free portion of the penis. They develop at sexual maturity and regress after castration. Penis, cat. H&E (×250). (Image by W.E. Haensly.)

The CT within the corpus cavernosum of stallions is rich in elastic fibers and smooth muscle cells. The glans envelops the cranial portion of the corpus cavernosum penis and features a long **dorsal process** extending caudally. It also exhibits an enlargement known as the corona glandis, which is covered with epithelium containing cylindrical papillae. Within the glans, there is a concavity referred to as the fossa glandis, housing the slightly protruding end of the urethra, known as the urethral process. At the level of the glans, the bundles of the bulbospongiosus muscle are interrupted by the retractor penis muscle.

The cranial third of the boar's penis is characterized by a distinctive leftward corkscrew-like spiral. The structure of the remainder of the porcine penis closely resembles that of a bull's penis. In bulls, the corpus cavernosum penis features a central strand of CT formed by the converging trabeculae. The tip of the penis, known as the glans, is composed of

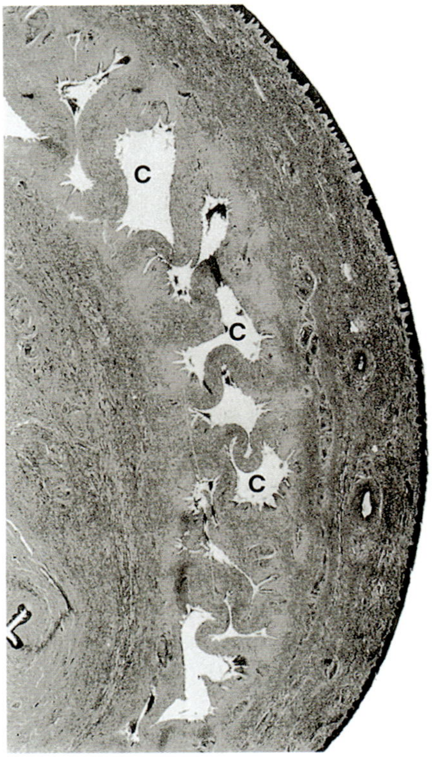

Figure 13-32 Glans penis, pars longa (dog). Note the large cavernous spaces (C) in the erectile tissue. H&E (×11).

gelatinous CT, adipose cells, and spacious intercellular areas. It includes an expansive venous plexus for erectile function. The structure of the penis in bucks and rams is similar to that of bulls, with a similarly large, cap-like glans. The urethra extends from the glans as a spiral-shaped urethral process.

Mechanism of Erection

In animals with a vascular or intermediate-type penis, erection leads to an increase in size and firmness of the organ. When the smooth muscle cells within the helicine arteries relax, this facilitates an influx of blood into the sinuses of the corpora cavernosa. This heightened blood volume exerts pressure on the veins, reducing the outflow of blood and ultimately filling the erectile tissue spaces in the corpora cavernosa, corpus spongiosum, and glans penis.

The process of detumescence begins with the contraction of the musculature within the helicine arteries, reducing arterial blood flow. The smooth muscle cells within the tunica albuginea, trabeculae, and erectile tissue contract, causing the penis to revert to its flaccid state. In species with a fibroelastic penis, erection primarily leads to an elongation of the penis extending from the prepuce. In the case of ruminants and boars, the retractor penis muscle plays a crucial role in the detumescence process by retracting the penis back into the prepuce.

During copulation, the constrictor vestibuli muscle in female dogs constricts the veins that drain the entire glans and especially the bulbous glandis. This constriction causes the bulbous to enlarge to such a degree that immediate withdrawal of the penis from the vagina is impossible; consequently, coitus is prolonged.

Prepuce

The **prepuce** represents the upper part of the penile body, and the glans penis is enclosed within a tubular extension of the skin (Fig. 13-33). The prepuce consists of an external and an internal layer. The external layer curves inward at the preputial opening, forming the internal layer, which wraps around the front part of the penis and is firmly connected to the glans penis.

The external layer is typical skin, and at the preputial opening, it has numerous sebaceous glands that may be associated with hair follicles. In ruminants and boars, there are long, bristle-like hairs present. In stallions, ruminants, boars, and dogs, fine hairs, along with sebaceous and sweat glands, are distributed over varying distances within the internal layer. Stallions also have occasional hairs in the penile skin, which is rich in sebaceous and sweat glands. Dogs and ruminants, on the other hand, have solitary lymphatic nodules in both the internal layer of the prepuce and the penile skin. In boars, these lymphatic nodules are found exclusively in the internal layer. In cats, the mucosa covering the glans penis features numerous keratinized papillae.

In boars, there is an upward protrusion of the inner layer of the prepuce known as the preputial diverticulum. This structure is partially divided into two lateral sections by a central septum. It is common for the keratinized cutaneous mucous membrane to exhibit folds. A mixture of desquamated epithelial cells and urine forms smegma, which collects in the diverticulum and is odoriferous.

Clinical Correlations

The clinical significance of the different pathologies that affect domestic animals is variable, with different organs of the male reproductive system being more affected by certain diseases depending on the species. In boars and ruminants, infertility is common and is usually associated with infectious pathogens (i.e., brucellosis, leptospirosis, and toxoplasmosis).

The stallion can present with several diseases that cause infertility (associated with nutrition, trauma, toxic, and genetic causes). The stallion also can present other pathologies, such as vesiculitis (bacterial infection of seminal vesicle), balanitis, and preputial tumors. In dogs, different pathologies will be important only in noncastrated intact animals. Prostate gland disorders are the most common cause of reproductive disease, including prostatic hyperplasia, paraprostatic cysts, and prostatitis. Testicular tumors are also common, and usually, dogs can present different histological subtypes in the same testicle (i.e., seminoma and Leydig cell tumor). In tropical countries, transmissible venereal tumors are common, particularly as penile tumors. In cats, disorders of the reproductive system are very rare.

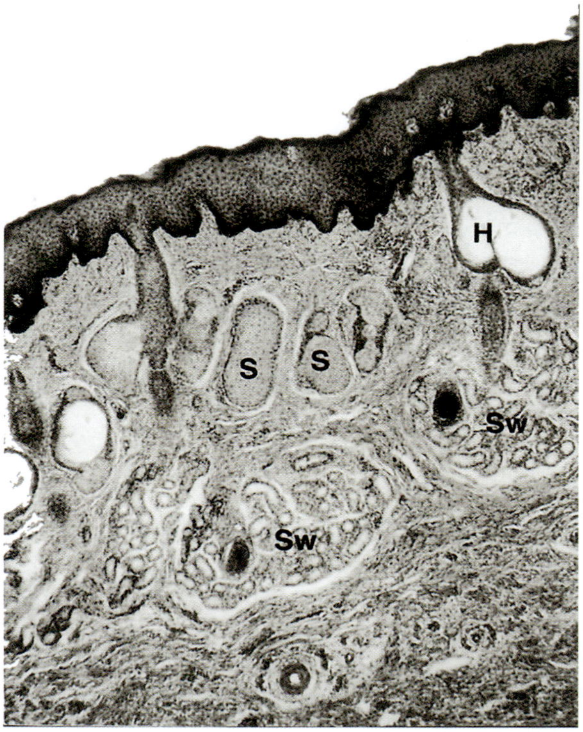

Figure 13-33 Skin with hair follicles (H) and sebaceous (S) and sweat (Sw) glands covering the corpus penis (stallion). H&E (×40).

Essentials

Fertility is closely related to endocrine regulation. In mammals, GnRH from the hypothalamus stimulates the release of LH and FSH from the adenohypophysis. LH stimulates Leydig cells to produce testosterone, while FSH induces Sertoli cells to produce ABP and inhibin B. ABP concentrates testosterone, necessary for sperm maturation, within the seminiferous tubule lumen. Testosterone produced by Leydig cells provides negative feedback regulation to both the hypothalamus and cells of the adenohypophysis. Inhibin B provides negative feedback to the adenohypophysis to regulate levels of FSH.

Sertoli (sustentacular) cells are important for spermatozoa development and maturation. The cells form unique tight junctions with each other to maintain a basal and adluminal compartment that provides a blood–testis barrier to protect developing spermatozoa from autoimmune reactions. The **epididymis** is important for spermatozoa maturation and regulating capacitation prior to ejaculation. Additionally, the **prostate gland** and **vesicular glands** contribute to the production of semen and to sperm viability by secreting fluids that nourish and support spermatozoa during ejaculation. Finally, the penis exhibits species-specific variations in morphology and function across domestic species.

Suggested Readings

Aumüller G. Prostate gland and seminal vesicles. In: Handbuch der mikroskopischen Anatomie des Menschen. Vol. 7. Berlin: Springer-Verlag, 1979 (6).

Barrachina F, Battistone MA, Castillo J, et al. Sperm acquire epididymis-derived proteins through epididymosomes. *Hum Reprod* 2022;37(4):651–668.

Cole HH, Cupps PT. Reproduction in Domestic Animals. 3rd Ed. New York: Academic Press, 1977.

Domke LM. The cell-cell junctions of the mammalian testes – a summary. *Cell Tissue Res* 2020;379:73–74.

Fawcett DW, Bedford JM eds. The Spermatozoon. Maturation, Motility, Surface Properties and Comparative Aspects. Baltimore: Urban and Schwarzenberg, 1979.

Guraya SS. Biology of Spermatogenesis and Spermatozoa in Mammals. New York: Springer-Verlag, 1987.

Knobil E, Neill JD eds. The Physiology of Reproduction. 4th ed. New York: Raven Press, 2014.

Russell LD, Griswold MD eds. The Sertoli Cell. Clearwater, FL: Cache River Press, 1993.

Setchell BP. The Mammalian Testis. London: Paul Elek, 1978.

Steinberger A, Steinberger E. Testicular Development, Structure and Function. New York: Raven Press, 1980.

Van Blerkom J, Motta P eds. Ultrastructure of Reproduction. Boston: M. Nijhoff, 1984.

14

Female Reproductive System

Christopher Premanandan

CHAPTER MENU

Dellmann's Textbook of Veterinary Histology, Seventh Edition. Edited by Marxa L. Figueiredo and John J. Turek.

Companion website: www.wiley.com/go/figueiredo/vethistology7e

The female reproductive system consists of bilateral ovaries, uterine tubes (oviducts), uterus, cervix, vagina, vestibule, vulva, and associated glands. Its functions include the production and transport of ova, the transport of spermatozoa, fertilization, and the accommodation of the conceptus until birth.

Ovary

The ovary produces ova and ovarian hormones, chiefly estrogens and progesterone (endocrine secretion). The structure of the normal ovary varies with the species, age, and phase of the estrous cycle. It is an ovoid structure divided into an outer cortex and an inner medulla (Fig. 14-1). In the mature mare, these areas are reversed, and the cortical tissue remains on the surface only in the ovulation fossa, the site of ovulation.

Cortex

The cortex is a broad peripheral zone containing **follicles** in various stages of development, **corpora lutea**, **and corpora albicans** embedded in a loose connective tissue (CT) stroma (Fig. 14-1). It is covered by **a surface epithelium** (also referred to as **germinal epithelium**). This epithelial cell layer is cuboidal in young animals and flattens to squamous epithelium with age. A CT layer, the **tunica albuginea**, lies beneath the surface epithelium. It is disrupted by the growth of ovarian follicles and corpora lutea and may be difficult to visualize during increased ovarian activity. In the ovary of rodents, bitches, and queens, the cortical stroma contains cords of polyhedral **interstitial endocrine cells**, also referred to as interstitial or granulosa rests (Fig. 14-2). In the ovary of bitches, **subepithelial surface structures** are also prominent; these are narrow channels lined by a cuboidal epithelium that can be continuous with the surface epithelium (Fig. 14-3).

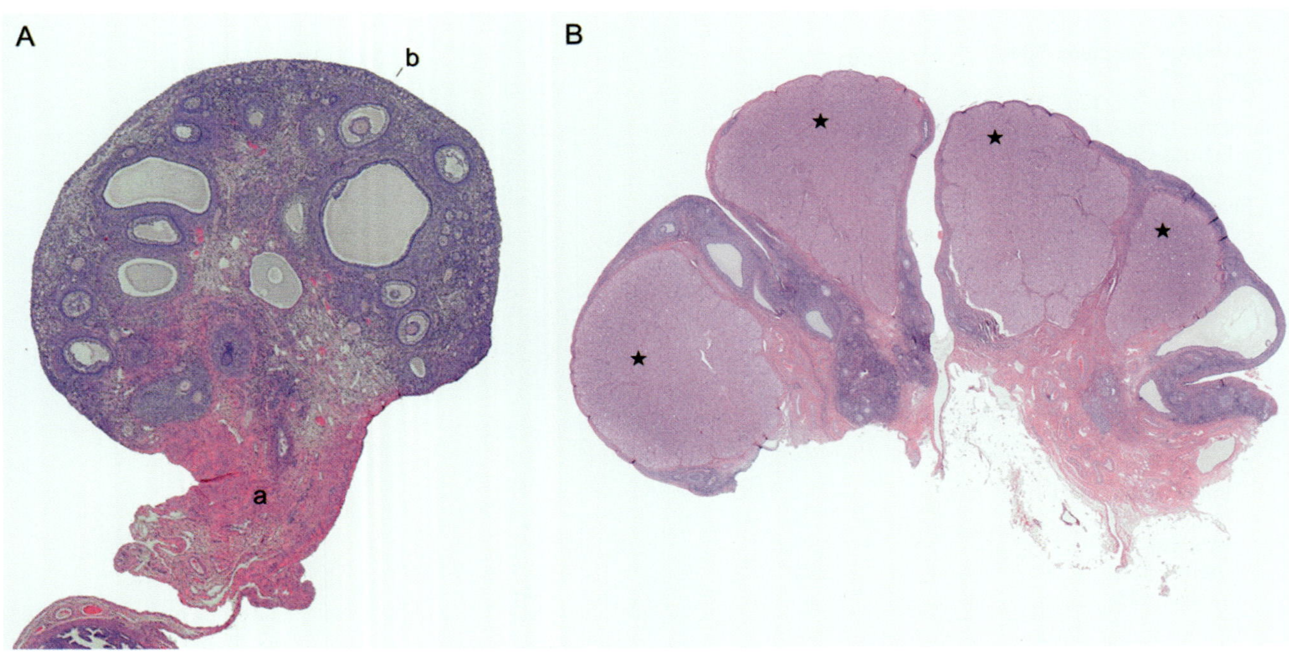

Figure 14-1 **A.** Ovary of a queen showing the development and regression of follicles in the ovarian cortex. The ovarian medulla contains blood vessels (a) that enter the ovary at the hilus from the mesovarium and (b) surface (germinal) epithelium. **B.** Ovary of a bitch depicting multiple well-developed corpora lutea (stars). H&E.

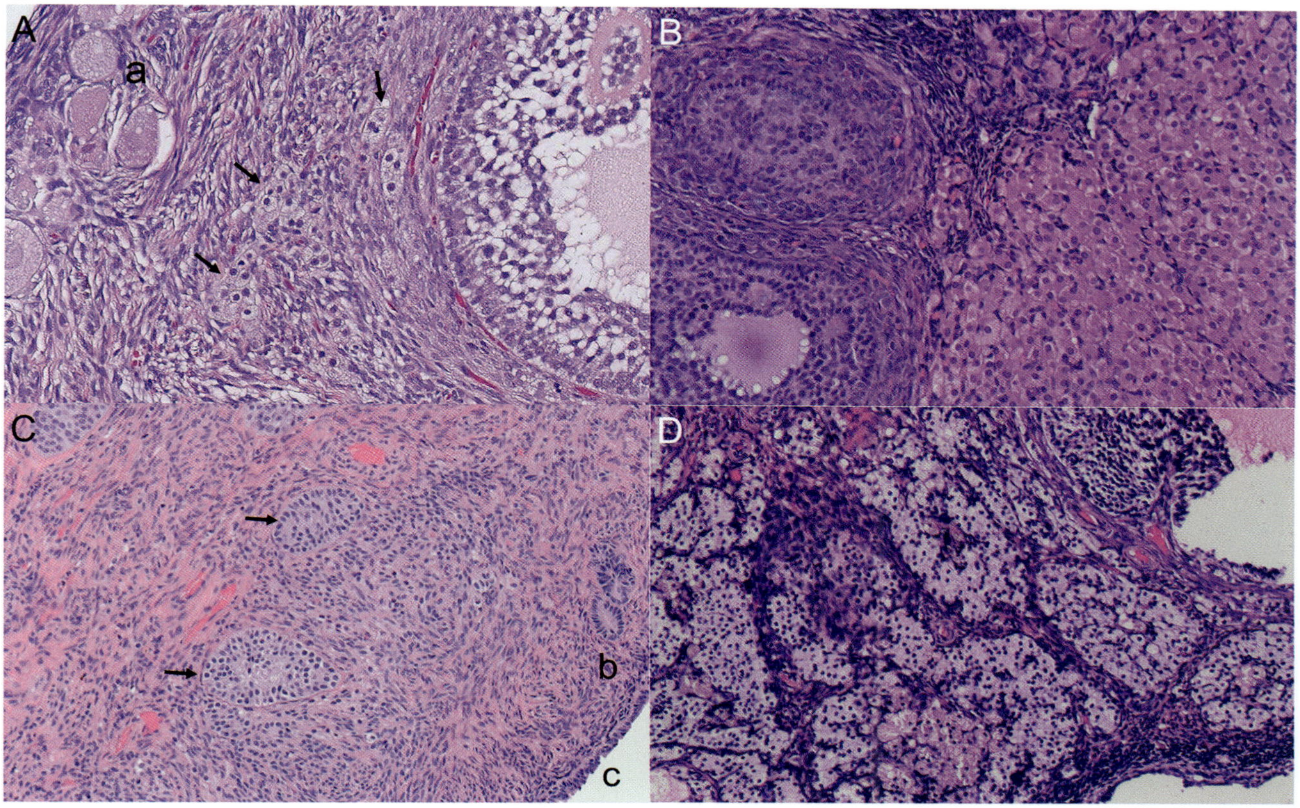

Figure 14-2 Ovarian cortex from multiple species depicting interstitial endocrine cells or granulosa rests (arrows). Primordial follicles (a), canine subepithelial surface structures (b), and germinal epithelium (c) can be observed also. **A.** Feline. **B.** Rabbit. **C.** Canine. **D.** Rat. H&E.

Follicular Development

An **ovarian follicle** is a structure composed of an oocyte surrounded by specialized epithelial cells. During follicular development, the epithelial cells become surrounded by specialized stroma cells, and a fluid-filled cavity develops among the epithelial cells.

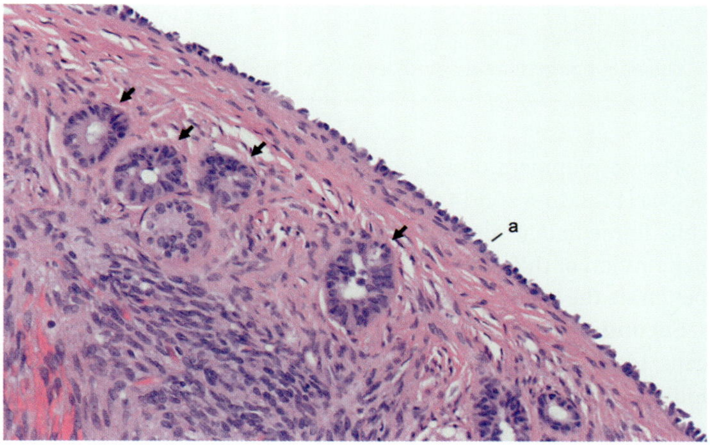

Figure 14-3 Ovarian cortex from a canine depicting multiple subepithelial surface structures (arrows) and the germinal epithelium (a). H&E.

Primordial follicles are composed of a primary oocyte surrounded by a flattened epithelium of follicular cells (Fig. 14-4). The oocytes within primordial follicles arise prenatally by mitotic proliferation of migrated germ cells in the ovarian cortex. In some species (e.g., bitches), primordial follicles also may arise postnatally. During ovarian development, protuberances of tissue referred to as the gonadal ridge arise from the dorsal body wall within the embryonic coelomic cavity. **Primordial germ cells** migrate to the gonadal ridge from the wall of the yolk sac. A proportion of the epithelium overlying the gonadal ridge surface interacts with the primordial germ cells and penetrates into the stroma of the gonadal ridge, aggregating into clusters referred to as ovigerous cords. The central cell of a cluster becomes the **oogonium**. The oogonia enlarge, enter the prophase of the first meiotic division, and are then termed **primary oocytes**, measuring approximately 20 μm in diameter in most species. The primary oocytes go through the leptotene, zygotene, pachytene, and diplotene stages and then remain in a prolonged diplotene stage referred to as the dictyotene stage. As the primary oocyte develops, the surrounding cells form a single layer of flat follicular cells resting on a basal lamina. Together, these components constitute the primordial follicle, approximately 40 μm in diameter. Primordial follicles are located mainly in the outer cortex. They are evenly distributed in ruminants and the sow and occur in clusters in carnivores. In mares, a majority are found in the ovulation fossa but can also be found individually in the ovarian stroma.

Key Concept:

Primary follicles are composed of a primary oocyte surrounded by a simple cuboidal epithelium of follicular cells (Figs. 14-4 and 14-5). The primary oocytes begin the first meiotic division before birth, but the completion of prophase does not occur until the time of ovulation. Therefore, the primary oocytes remain arrested in prophase (dictyotene stage) until after puberty. Several hundred thousand to one million potential oocytes may be present at birth in a single ovary. However, most of these undergo atresia before or after birth, and only several hundred ovulate during a normal lifetime. The processes involved in the selection of follicles for growth from a pool of nonproliferating primordial follicles are poorly understood.

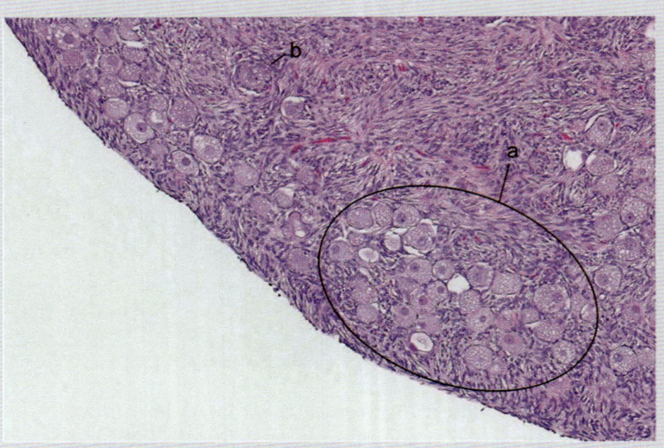

Figure 14-4 Ovary of a queen showing numerous primordial follicles (a), which consist of primary oocytes surrounded by a simple squamous epithelium. The simple squamous epithelium undergoes hypertrophy to become cuboidal epithelium in a primary follicle (b). H&E.

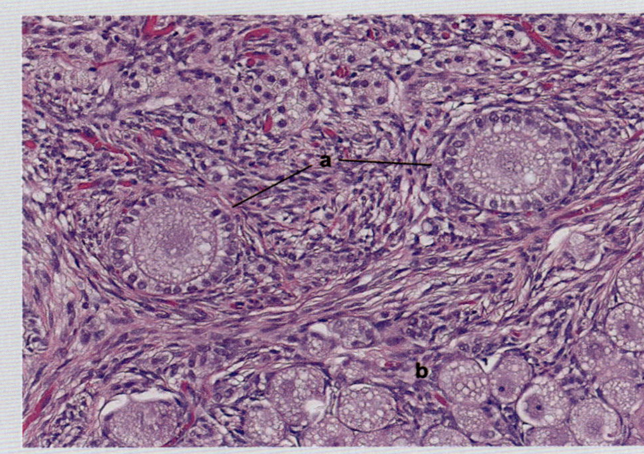

Figure 14-5 Two primary follicles (a) in the ovarian cortex of a queen. Below the primary follicles, there is a group of primordial follicles (b), located close to the surface of the ovary (not shown). H&E.

The development of a 3- to 5-μm-thick glycoprotein layer, the **zona pellucida**, around the plasma membrane of the oocyte (Figs. 14-6 and 14-7) can be seen in the primary or secondary follicle. The zona pellucida is secreted by the granulosa cells immediately surrounding the oocyte and, in part, by the oocyte itself, depending on the species. There is partial penetration of this zone by the oocyte microvilli. Cytoplasmic extensions of the granulosa cells situated around the oocyte penetrate the zona pellucida and closely associate with these microvilli.

Secondary follicles are composed of a primary oocyte surrounded by a stratified epithelium of polyhedral follicular cells, termed **granulosa cells** (Figs. 14-6 and 14-7). The multilaminar stratum of granulosa cells arises from proliferating follicular cells of the primary follicle. In carnivores, sows, and ewes, polyovular follicles may develop, each containing several oocytes. In cows, the late secondary follicle is approximately 120 μm in diameter and contains an oocyte of approximately 80 μm in diameter. As follicular development continues, small fluid-filled clefts are formed among the granulosa cells. A vascularized multilaminar layer of spindle-shaped stroma cells, termed **theca cells**, begins to form around the granulosa cell layer in late secondary follicles.

Primary follicles can be classified as structures associated with a single layer of cuboidal granulosa cells, and secondary follicles as those with multiple layers of granulosa cells prior to any follicular antrum development. However, some variation exists regarding the classification of primary and secondary follicles in the literature. The most prominent variation concerns the differentiation of **primary follicles** into two types: those characterized by a single layer of cuboidal granulosa cells (unilaminar or early primary follicles) and those with multiple layers of cuboidal granulosa cells (multilaminar or late primary follicles). **Secondary follicles** are defined as follicular structures composed of multiple layers of cuboidal granulosa cells. Within these layers, spaces form due to the secretion and accumulation of liquor folliculi (follicular fluid). They can be further classified as preantral (with small fluid-filled spaces among granulosa cells) and antral follicles (with a well-defined central cavity).

Tertiary follicles, also termed **Graafian follicles**, are composed of a **primary oocyte** surrounded by a stratified epithelium of granulosa cells. These granulosa cells are further enveloped by a multilaminar layer of specialized stromal cells called the **theca**, while a fluid-filled cavity, the **antrum**, develops among the granulosa cells (Figs. 14-8 and 14-9). The antrum, a defining feature of tertiary follicles, forms when small, fluid-filled clefts among the granulosa cells of secondary follicles coalesce to form a *single large cavity* filled with **liquor folliculi** (follicular fluid). Late tertiary follicles, just before ovulation, are termed **mature or preovulatory follicles** (Fig. 14-10). In mature follicles, the primary oocyte completes the first meiotic division, just before or after ovulation, depending on the species. This process gives rise to a secondary oocyte and the **first polar body**.

The primary oocyte in tertiary follicles measures 150 to 300 μm in diameter, depending on the species. It has a spherical, centrally located nucleus with a sparse chromatin network and a prominent nucleolus. The Golgi complex, initially dispersed in the cytoplasm, becomes concentrated near the plasma membrane. Lipid granules and lipochrome pigment occur in the cytoplasm. As the antrum enlarges through the accumulation of liquor folliculi, the oocyte is displaced eccentrically (Figs. 14-8 to 14-10). The oocyte then lies in an accumulation of granulosa cells, the **cumulus oophorus** (Figs. 14-9 and 14-10). In large tertiary follicles, the granulosa cells immediately surrounding the oocyte are arranged in a radial fashion termed the **corona radiata** (Fig. 14-9). The corona radiata cells are believed to provide nutrient support for the oocyte and generally persist after ovulation until just before fertilization in most species.

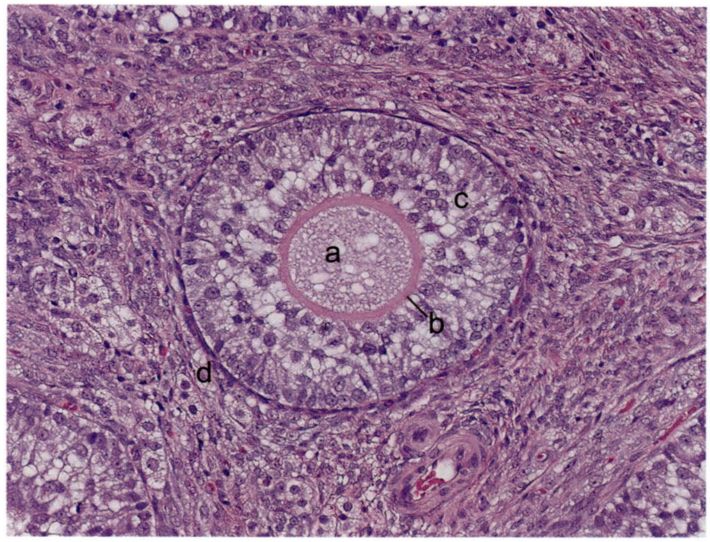

Figure 14-6 Ovary of a queen showing a secondary follicle (also referred to as multilaminar primary follicle), in which the primary oocyte (a) is surrounded by a thin zona pellucida (b) and a stratified epithelium of polyhedral cells (c). The CT cells that surround the follicle will form the theca interna (d). H&E.

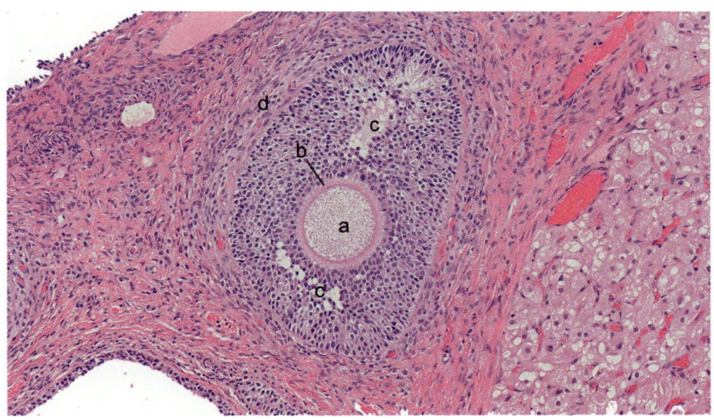

Figure 14-7 Ovary of a queen showing a secondary follicle. The follicle contains a primary oocyte (a) associated with a zona pellucida (b). Spaces (c) are forming between granulosa cells, which will eventually form the follicular antrum. The cells surrounding the granulosa cells are beginning to organize into thecal structures (d). H&E.

In tertiary follicles, the granulosa cells form a parietal follicular lining, the **stratum granulosum** (Figs. 14-8 and 14-11). Most of the parietal granulosa cells are polyhedral, but the basal layer may be columnar. In the large tertiary follicle, the granulosa cells have the fine structural characteristics of protein-secreting cells, notably an extensive granular endoplasmic reticulum (ER). Before ovulation, the granulosa cells of the mature follicle assume the characteristics of steroid-secreting cells, especially an agranular ER and mitochondria with tubular cristae.

The stratum granulosum is surrounded by the theca, which in tertiary follicles differentiates into two layers: an inner vascular **theca interna** and an outer supportive **theca externa** (Figs. 14-9 and 14-11). The **theca interna** cells are spindle shaped in early tertiary follicles and located in a delicate reticular fiber network. An extensive blood and lymph capillary network is present in the theca interna, but it does not penetrate the stratum granulosum (Fig. 14-12). Sympathetic nerve

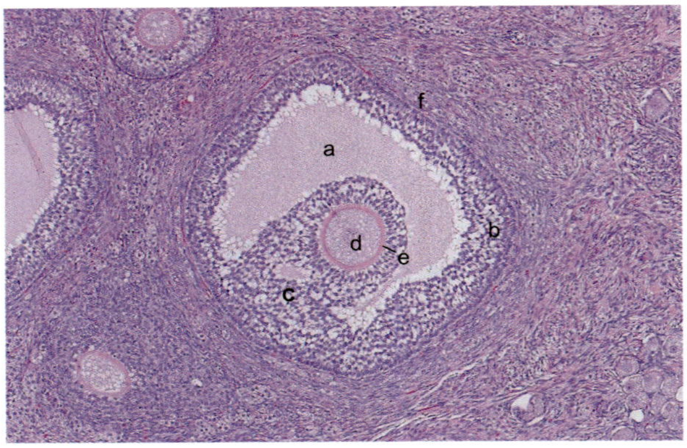

Figure 14-8 Early tertiary follicle from a feline ovary, which contains an antrum (a) and a multilayered epithelium, the stratum granulosum (b). A cumulus oophorus (c) enclosing the primary oocyte (d) with associated zona pellucida (e) forms in the stratum granulosum. The antrum contains a flocculent liquor folliculi (follicular fluid). A CT layer, the theca (f), surrounds the stratum granulosum. H&E.

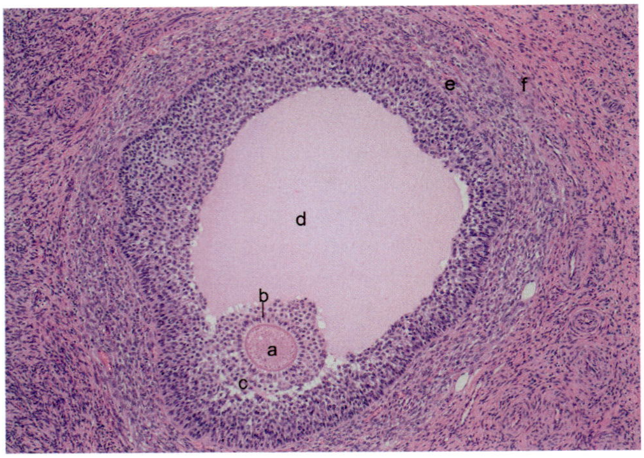

Figure 14-9 Growing tertiary follicle from a bovine ovary. The follicle contains a primary oocyte (a) surrounded by a circumferential row of granulosa cells called the corona radiata (b). The cumulus oophorus consists of all the granulosa cells surrounding the oocyte (c). The antrum (d) is larger. The theca layer can be divided into an inner theca interna (e) and an outer theca externa (f). H&E.

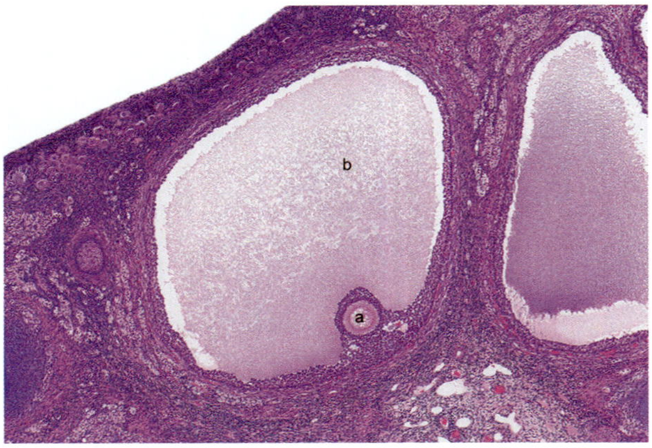

Figure 14-10 Preovulatory follicle from a feline ovary, showing the oocyte (a) and a very large antrum (b). H&E.

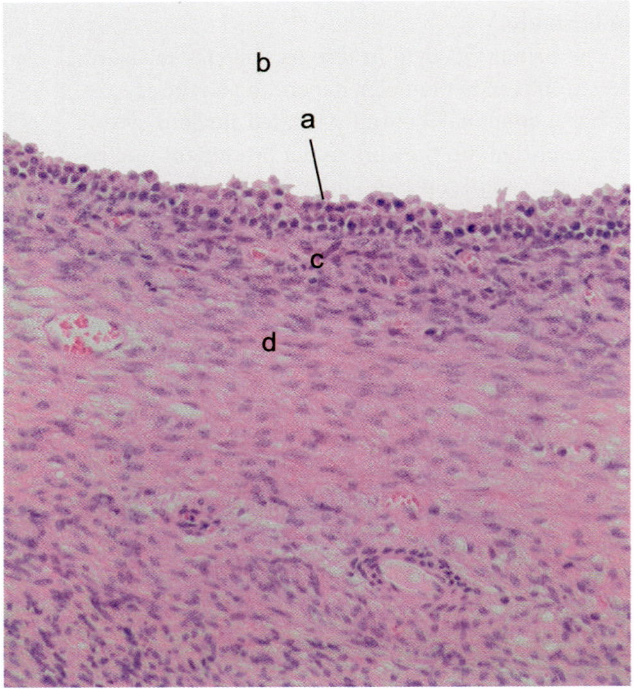

Figure 14-11 Equine preovulatory follicle. In large preovulatory follicles, the stratum granulosum (a) is only a few layers thick when the follicular antrum (b) develops. The theca interna (c) lies closest to the stratum granulosum, and the theca externa lies outside the theca interna. H&E.

endings are present around the larger follicles. In mature follicles, many of the spindle-shaped theca interna cells adjacent to the stratum granulosum increase in size and become polyhedral and epithelioid. The nuclei of the epithelioid cells have a lighter chromatin pattern and more distinct nucleoli than those of the spindle-shaped cells. Cytoplasmic organelles in the epithelioid cells become typical of steroid-secreting cells: the mitochondria with tubular cristae, agranular tubular ER, and lipid inclusions are present. The epithelioid cells are abundant in mature follicles during proestrus and estrus and during their early regression.

The **theca externa** consists of a thin layer of loose CT, with fibrocytes arranged concentrically around the theca interna. Blood vessels of the theca externa supply capillaries to the theca interna. The cells and CT associated with the theca externa blend into the ovarian interstitium.

One or more mature follicles reach maximal development near the time of ovulation. The primary oocyte within these follicles completes the first meiotic division to become a secondary oocyte (containing a haploid number of chromosomes). During this division, chromosome pairs are established, and a mixture of parental genetic material occurs. The separation of the chromosome pairs and the production of the secondary oocyte, along with the first polar body (which also contains a haploid number of chromosomes but little cytoplasm), occur as the division is completed. In domestic animals, the first meiotic division is completed shortly before ovulation, except in the bitch, in which it is completed shortly after ovulation, resulting in the ovulation of a primary oocyte. The second meiotic division begins immediately after the first but is arrested in metaphase and remains incomplete unless fertilization occurs. Upon fertilization, the second meiotic division resumes, transforming the secondary oocyte into an ovum and generating a second polar body (also with little cytoplasm). The ovum becomes a **zygote** when the male and female chromosomes come together, establishing a diploid number of chromosomes.

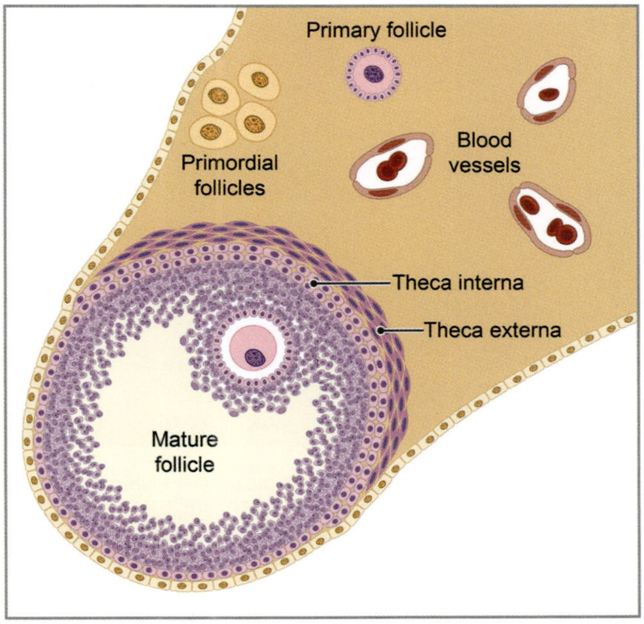

Figure 14-12 A schematic drawing of the follicle shows the oocyte ready to disengage itself from the stratum granulosum at a site opposite the thinned, protruding follicular wall at the ovulation site, the stigma. Note the theca interna, theca externa, primordial follicles, primary follicle, and blood vessels. (Illustration by Tim Vojt, courtesy of The Ohio State University®.)

Ovulation

When the follicle is fully developed, it protrudes from the surface of the ovary in most species. Abundant blood and lymph vessel networks surround the follicle, leading to an increased secretion rate of a thin follicular fluid. This increased secretion rate is facilitated by increases in the follicular blood capillary pressure and permeability during proestrus and estrus. As a result, the follicles swell due to the increased accumulation of follicular fluid, though intrafollicular pressure does not significantly increase. Small hemorrhages may occur in the follicular wall, which becomes thin and transparent at the future site of follicular rupture, the **stigma** (Fig. 14-12). The mature ovulatory follicles attain a size of 15 to 20 mm in cows; 50 to 70 mm in mares; approximately 10 mm in ewes, goats, and sows; approximately 5 to 8 mm in bitches; and approximately 3 mm in queens.

Changes in the wall of the follicle preceding rupture are caused by the release of collagenases. Luteinizing hormone (LH) stimulates the production of prostaglandins (PG) F_2 and E_2. PGF_2 is believed to release collagenases from follicular cells, causing digestion of the follicular wall and its distension at the stigma. The process of digestion also releases proteins that provoke an inflammatory response with leukocytic infiltration and the release of histamine. All of these processes degrade the CT of the follicular wall and the ground substance of the cumulus oophorus so that the follicle ultimately ruptures at the stigma and the oocyte is released. The oocyte, usually surrounded by the corona radiata, escapes into the peritoneal cavity, from which it is swept directly into the infundibulum of the uterine tube. In most species, the corona radiata cells disperse in the uterine tube upon contact with spermatozoa. The oocyte generally remains fertilizable for less than 1 day; when not fertilized, it degenerates and is resorbed. Most domestic animals ovulate spontaneously, but in some species, ovulation is induced by a copulatory stimulus (queens and rabbits).

Follicular Atresia and Interstitial Endocrine Cells

Most follicles regress at some time during their development, and only a small percentage of all potential oocytes are ovulated from the ovary. This regression is called **atresia**; many more follicles become atretic than ever attain maturity. Prominent signs of atresia in follicular wall cells are nuclear pyknosis and chromatolysis (Fig. 14-13). During atresia, the basal lamina of the granulosa layer may fold, thicken, and hyalinize; it is then called the **glassy membrane** (Fig. 14-14). Eventually, atretic follicles are resorbed, except that small fibrous tissue scars may remain after atresia of large follicles. The remnants of the zona pellucida may also be observed in the cortical stroma.

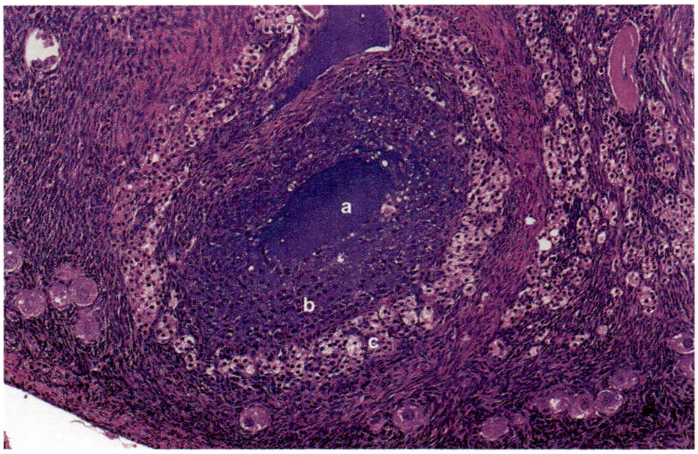

Figure 14-13 Atretic tertiary follicle (queen). The antrum (a) begins to collapse and the cells of stratum granulosum (b) detach and fall into the former antrum. The theca (c) has been replaced by epithelioid interstitial endocrine cells. H&E.

In cows, during atresia of primary and secondary follicles, the oocyte commonly degenerates before the follicular wall, whereas in tertiary follicles, the reverse is true. Atretic changes in bovine tertiary follicles may result in the formation of two different morphologic types of atretic follicles: obliterative and cystic. In **obliterative atresia**, both the granulosa and theca layers infold, hypertrophy, and extend inward to occupy the antrum. In **cystic atresia**, both the granulosa and theca layers may atrophy, or only the granulosa layer may atrophy, and the theca layer may luteinize, become fibrotic, or hyalinize around the antrum (Fig. 14-14). In cystic atretic follicles, the theca interna cells containing LH receptors may continue to synthesize androgens after the regression of the granulosa cells, which convert the androgens to estrogens.

In the ovaries of the bitch, the queen, and rodents, **interstitial cells** (also referred to as granulosa rests) are prominent; they chiefly arise from the epithelioid theca interna cells of atretic antral follicles or from hypertrophied granulosa cells of atretic preantral follicles (Fig. 14-2). They are usually absent from the ovaries of other adult domestic animals. The interstitial endocrine cells are polyhedral and epithelioid and contain lipid droplets. In species such as rabbits and hares, they show an abundance of steroid-synthesizing organelles and can comprise a large portion of the ovarian interstitium.

Corpus Luteum

At ovulation, the follicle ruptures, collapses, and shrinks as the liquor pressure is reduced. The follicular wall forms extensive folds as it collapses. The ruptured follicle is referred to as a **corpus hemorrhagicum** because of the blood that may fill the antrum. Bleeding after rupture of the follicle in mares, cows, and sows is greater than in carnivores and small ruminants. Immediately before ovulation, some cells of the stratum granulosum exhibit signs of pyknosis. After ovulation, the stratum becomes vascularized by an extensive capillary network originating from blood vessels in the theca interna. The granulosa cells enlarge, luteinize, and contribute to the **large luteal cell** population of the corpus luteum. Simultaneously, folding of the follicular wall results in the incorporation of the theca interna into the corpus luteum, and, in most species,

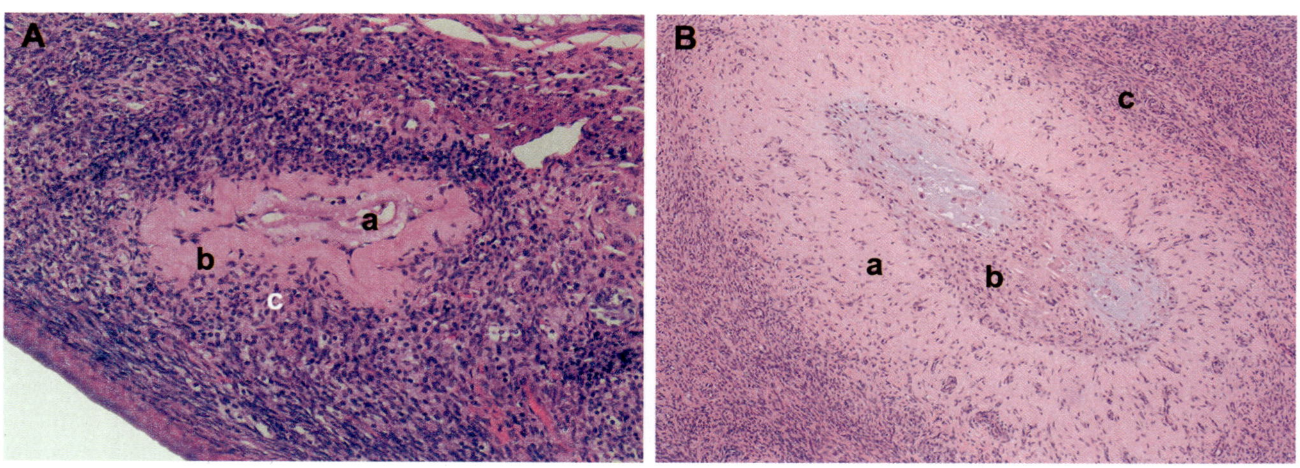

Figure 14-14 **A.** Atretic tertiary follicle (mature bitch). The oocyte (a) and granulosa layer have degenerated, the basement membrane has condensed to form a "glassy membrane" (b), and the theca layer (c) has fibrosed. **B.** Atresia of a large tertiary ovarian follicle (cow). Extensive hyalinization of theca interna (a) and loss or pyknosis of granulosa cells (b). Theca externa (c). H&E.

the theca interna cells contribute initially to the **small luteal cell** population of the corpus luteum. The distinction between small and large luteal cells is more pronounced in small ruminants, cattle, and some camelids than in other domestic animal species.

Luteinization is the process by which the granulosa and theca cells transform into luteal cells (Fig. 14-15). It involves hypertrophy and hyperplasia of both cell types. A yellow pigment, lutein, appears in the luteal cells in cows, mares, and carnivores; it is absent in ewes, goats, and sows. The increase in size of the corpus luteum, after the period of mitotic activity, mainly results from hypertrophy of the large luteal cells. The small luteal cells make up a minor part of the corpus luteum and mainly occupy trabecular and peripheral areas.

The large luteal cells are polygonal and have a large spherical vesicular nucleus. They contain numerous metabolic lipid inclusions (Figs. 14-15 and 14-16). During metestrus and diestrus, the cells contain organelles characteristic of steroid-synthesizing cells, such as mitochondria with tubular cristae and abundant tubular agranular ER. The small luteal cells have more lipids but fewer steroid-synthesizing types of organelles than the large luteal cells (Fig. 14-16). The two luteal cell types eventually become mixed in the corpus luteum and are then difficult to distinguish. Both types produce progesterone.

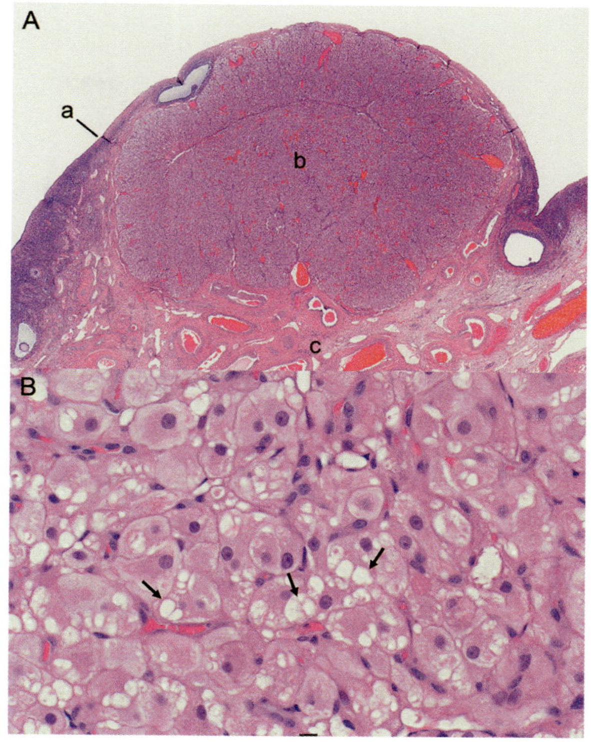

Figure 14-15 **A.** Canine ovary showing ovarian surface epithelium and adjacent tunica albuginea (a), mature corpus luteum (b), and medulla (c). **B.** Higher magnification of the corpus luteum, showing luteal cells containing lipid droplets (arrows). H&E.

The first sign of luteal regression is seen in late diestrus and involves the condensation of lutein pigment, which then appears reddish, followed by fibrosis and resorption of most of the corpus luteum. In cows, these signs are first observed 15 days after ovulation. Further shrinkage of the corpus luteum rapidly occurs after day 18, and regression is completed 1 to 2 days after estrus. Large lipid droplets and crystalloid inclusions are typical of regressing luteal cells (Fig. 14-17). The vascular CTs of the corpus luteum become conspicuous in regression, with muscle cells in the walls of luteal arteries transformed by cellular hypertrophy and sclerosis. The CT scar remaining after luteal regression is called the **corpus albicans** (Fig. 14-18). In older ovaries, there is an abundance of such scars.

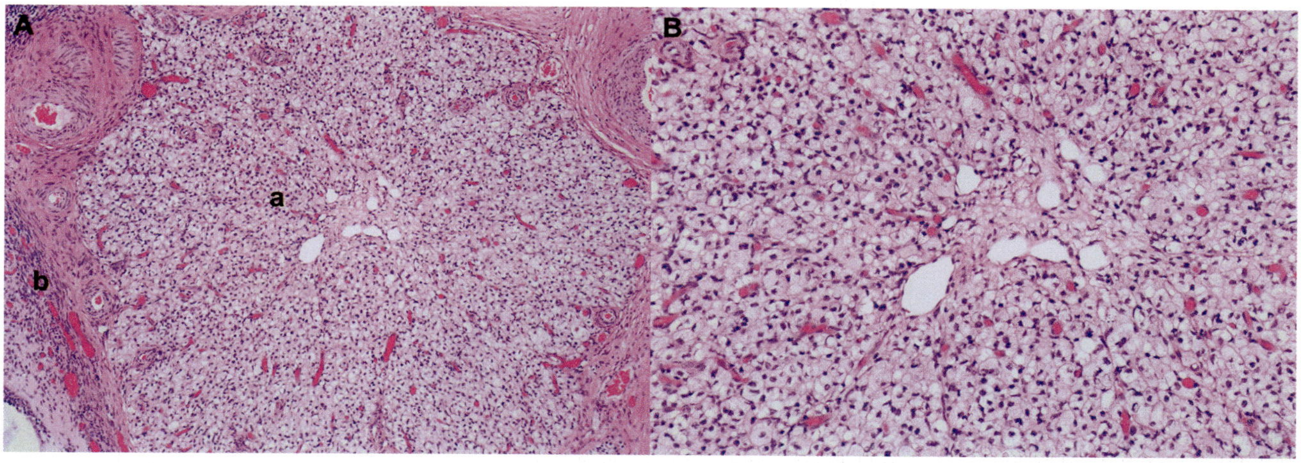

Figure 14-16 **A.** Corpus luteum (bitch) in regression (corpus regressivum) (a) with adjacent CT of theca origin (b). **B.** Lipid droplets of varying sizes are typical of regressing luteal cells. H&E.

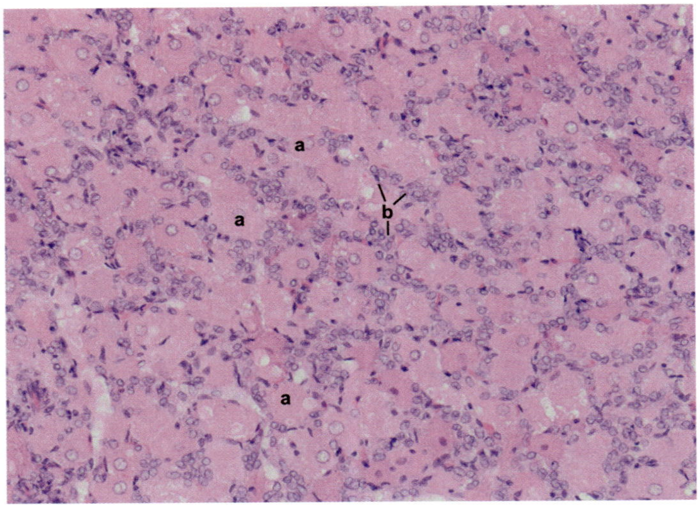

Figure 14-17 Mature corpus luteum (alpaca) with distinct large (a) and small (b) luteal cells. H&E.

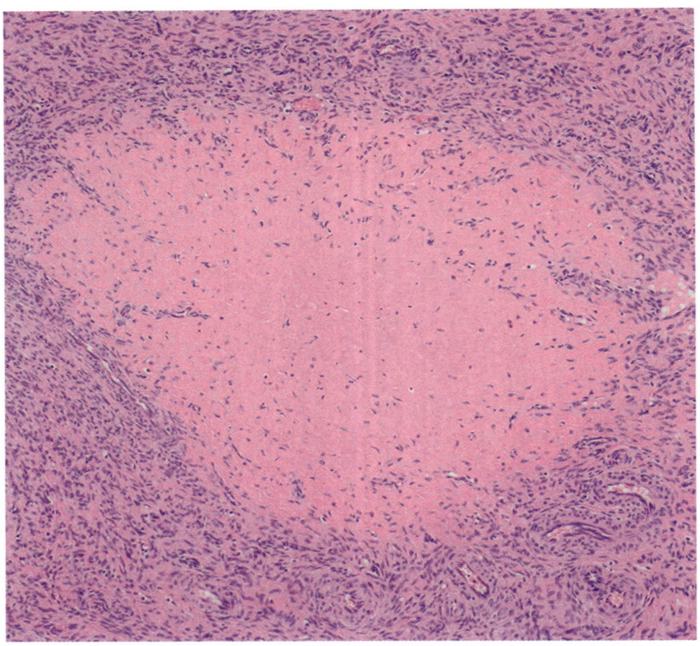

Figure 14-18 Corpus albicans from a bovine ovary, showing a regressed structure with fibrous tissue and degenerating luteal cells. The corpus albicans forms after the involution of the corpus luteum, marking the final stage of the ovarian cycle. H&E.

Medulla

The medulla is the inner area of the ovary containing nerves, many large and coiled blood vessels, and lymph vessels (Fig. 14-1). It consists of loose CT and strands of smooth muscle continuous with those in the mesovarium. Rete ovarii are located in the medulla; they are solid cellular cords or networks of irregular channels lined by cuboidal epithelium. They are prominent in carnivores and ruminants.

Blood Vessels, Lymphatics, and Nerves

Arteries enter the ovary at the hilus. In the medulla, they form plexuses and give off branches to the theca cells, corpora lutea, and stroma. Around the larger follicles, arterial branches form a capillary wreath. During cyclic regression of the corpora lutea and the follicles, muscle hypertrophy and sclerosis occur in the walls of the arteries supplying these structures. The venous return is parallel to the arterial supply. Lymph capillaries accompany blood vessels in the follicular thecae and corpus luteum.

The nerves that supply the ovary are generally nonmyelinated. They are vasomotor in nature but include some sensory fibers. The nerves follow blood vessels and terminate in the walls of the vessels and around the follicles, in the corpora lutea, and in the tunica albuginea. They are mainly derived from the sympathetic system through renal and aortic plexuses, but vagal supply of the ovary has also been claimed.

Uterine Tube

The uterine tubes are bilateral, tortuous structures that extend from the region of the ovary to the uterine horns and convey ova, spermatozoa, and zygotes. Three segments of the uterine tube can be distinguished: (a) the **infundibulum**, a large funnel-shaped portion (Fig. 14-19); (b) the **ampulla**, a thin-walled section extending caudally from the infundibulum (Fig. 14-20); and (c) the **isthmus**, a narrow muscular segment joining the uterus (Fig. 14-21). In domestic mammals, the uterine tube is relatively short, whereas in species with a simplex uterus (e.g., primates), the uterine tubes are longer.

Histologic Structure

The epithelium of the uterine tube is simple or pseudostratified columnar with motile cilia on most cells (Fig. 14-19). Both ciliated and nonciliated cell types possess microvilli. Morphologic signs of secretory activity are evident only in the nonciliated cells. During the luteal phase, the secretory cells become taller than the ciliated cells. Their secretion provides the ovum and zygote with the necessary nutrients.

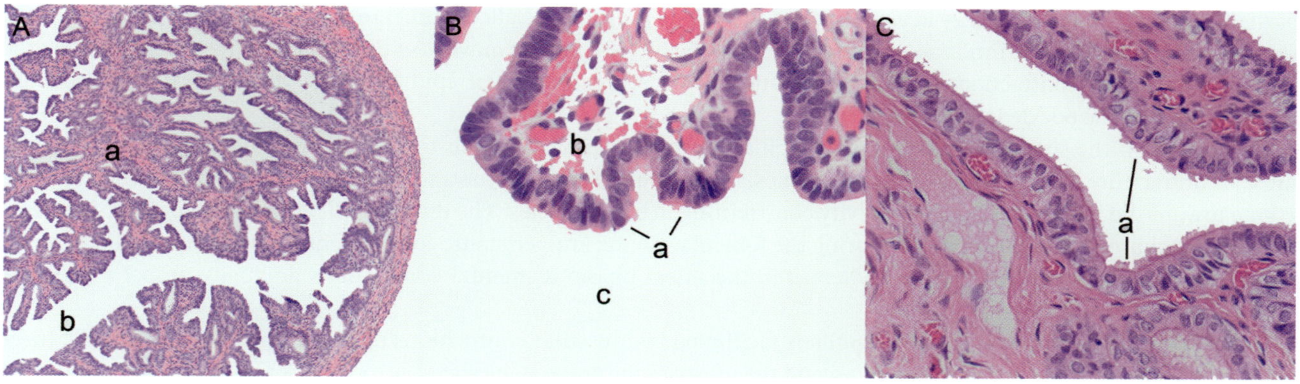

Figure 14-19 **A.** Cross section of infundibulum (queen). This structure contains numerous folds (a) extending into the lumen (b) with secondary and tertiary folds. **B.** Columnar epithelium of the infundibulum of the uterine tube (queen) (a). The epithelium overlies a stroma with numerous capillaries and venules (b). Lumen (c). **C.** Columnar epithelium of the infundibulum (bitch) with cilia (a) extending from the apical surface. A tunica serosa is present and contains many blood vessels and nerves.

The mucosa is continuous with the submucosa in the female reproductive tract because the thin lamina muscularis (that separates these tunics in other tubular structures) is absent. The tunica mucosa-submucosa of the ampulla is highly folded (Fig. 14-20), especially in sows and mares. In cows, approximately 40 primary longitudinal folds are present in the ampulla, each with secondary and tertiary folds. In the isthmus, with increasing distance from the ampulla, secondary and tertiary folds gradually disappear, and at the isthmus–uterus junction, where the isthmus is embedded in the uterine wall, only four to eight primary folds and no secondary or tertiary folds are present.

The tunica muscularis chiefly consists of circular smooth muscle bundles, although isolated longitudinal and oblique bundles also are present. The muscle layer gives off radial strands into the mucosa-submucosa. In the infundibulum and ampulla, the tunica muscularis is thin (Figs. 14-19 and 14-20). In the isthmus, the inner muscle layer is prominent and blends with the uterine circular muscle (Fig. 14-21).

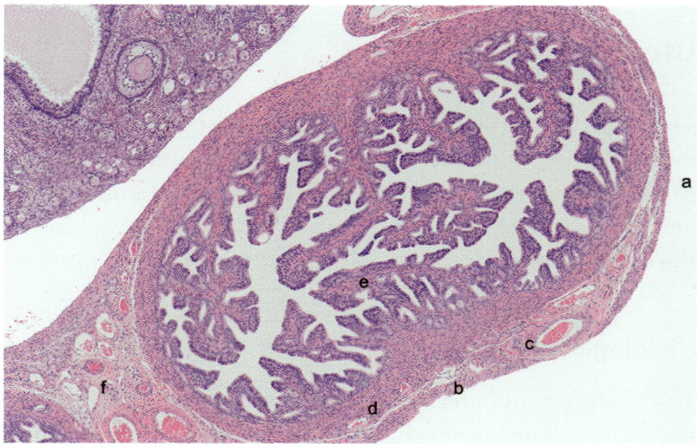

Figure 14-20 Cross section of the ampulla (queen). Tunica serosa (a), longitudinal muscle layer (b), stratum vasculare (c), circular muscle layer (d), mucosal-submucosal folds (e), and mesosalpinx with blood vessels (f). H&E.

Blood Vessels, Lymphatics, and Nerves

The blood vessels form subepithelial vascular plexuses and proliferate during pregnancy. The lymph vessels have capillary networks in the mucosal and serosal layers and drain into the lumbar lymph nodes.

Both myelinated and nonmyelinated nerve fibers with many subepithelial branches are present. They are derived mainly from the sympathetic system.

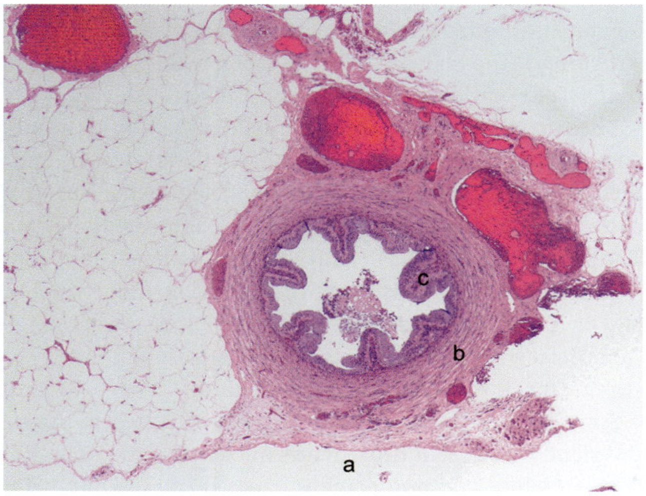

Figure 14-21 Cross section of the isthmus (rabbit). Tunica serosa (a), muscle layer (b), and mucosal-submucosal folds (c). H&E.

Function

The infundibulum secures oocytes extruded from the ovary. It is enclosed in the ovarian bursa or, in species without a definite ovarian bursa (e.g., the mare and queen), it is partially applied around the ovary at estrus. It has finger-like projections called **fimbriae**. At the time of ovulation in most species, blood vessels in the fimbriae become engorged. The turgid fimbriae move over the surface of the ovary due to rhythmic smooth muscle contractions. At the same time, cilia of the infundibular epithelial cells, mostly beating toward the uterus, transport the oocyte into the ampulla.

The ampulla is the site of fertilization, where ciliary activity primarily propels the oocyte or zygote toward the isthmus; muscle contractility is also involved in some species. In the isthmus, muscle contractility is the primary force propelling the zygote toward the uterus, with ciliary activity contributing in some species. The directionality of isthmus contractions varies with the phase of the estrous cycle. During the follicular phase, antiperistaltic contractions of the isthmus tend to move luminal contents toward the ampulla, whereas in the luteal phase, segmental contractions gradually propel the zygote toward the uterus.

The passage of spermatozoa to the ampulla is facilitated by muscular contractions of the uterine and tubal walls. Inert particles and nonmotile spermatozoa can ascend the uterine tube at the same speed as motile spermatozoa, suggesting that sperm transport is not solely due to their innate motility. In cows, spermatozoa can reach the ampulla within 5 minutes after mating, a rate too rapid to be solely accounted for by sperm motility or ciliary movement of tubal cells.

Although spermatozoa develop in the male reproductive tract, their ability to fertilize is attained in domestic animals only after capacitation in the uterine tube.

Uterus

The uterus is the site of attachment of the conceptus. It undergoes a distinct sequence of changes during both the estrous cycle and pregnancy. In most species, it consists of bilateral horns (cornua) connected to the uterine tubes, along with an unpaired body (corpus) and a neck (cervix) that joins the vagina, collectively referred to as a bicornuate uterus. The length and development of the uterine horns vary among species. The cervix is considered separately in this chapter. In primates, the entire uterus forms a single tube, called the simplex uterus.

Histologic Structure

The uterine wall consists of three layers (Figs. 14-22A and 14-23): (a) the mucosa-submucosa or **endometrium**, (b) the muscularis or **myometrium**, and (c) the serosa or **perimetrium**. The perimetrium, the longitudinal layer of the myometrium, and the vascular layer of the myometrium continuously extend into corresponding structures in the broad ligament of the uterus.

Endometrium

The endometrium is composed of two zones that differ in structure and function. The superficial layer partially or fully degenerates after pregnancy or estrus. A thin deep layer persists following these events, from which the superficial tissue regenerates. In mares, the superficial region is referred to as the **stratum compactum**, where the density of glandular structures is the highest. The region below the stratum compactum is referred to as the **stratum spongiosum**, characterized by a lower density of glandular profiles.

The surface epithelium (or luminal epithelium) is simple columnar in the mare, the bitch, and the queen. It is pseudostratified columnar and/or simple columnar in sows and ruminants, with isolated areas exhibiting simple cuboidal epithelium. The height and structure of the epithelial cells correlate with the secretion of ovarian hormones throughout the cycle. The superficial epithelium of the canine endometrium develops marked cytoplasmic vacuolization during diestrus. The subepithelial, superficial part of the endometrium consists of a richly vascular, loose CT with many fibrocytes, macrophages, and mast cells. Neutrophils, eosinophils, lymphocytes, and plasma cells also are present, while sheep additionally have melanophores. The deeper region of the endometrium consists of loose CT that is less cellular than that of the superficial part. In ruminants, during estrus, large irregular fluid-filled interstitial spaces are present in the endometrial stroma; this is termed **endometrial edema**.

Simple coiled, branched tubular glands are present throughout the endometrium in most species (Fig. 14-22). However, the glands are absent from the caruncles of ruminants (Fig. 14-23). The simple columnar glandular epithelium includes both secretory and nonsecretory ciliated cells. While rising estrogen levels stimulate the growth and branching of the glands, coiling and a copious secretion typically do not occur until progesterone stimulation ensues. The branching and

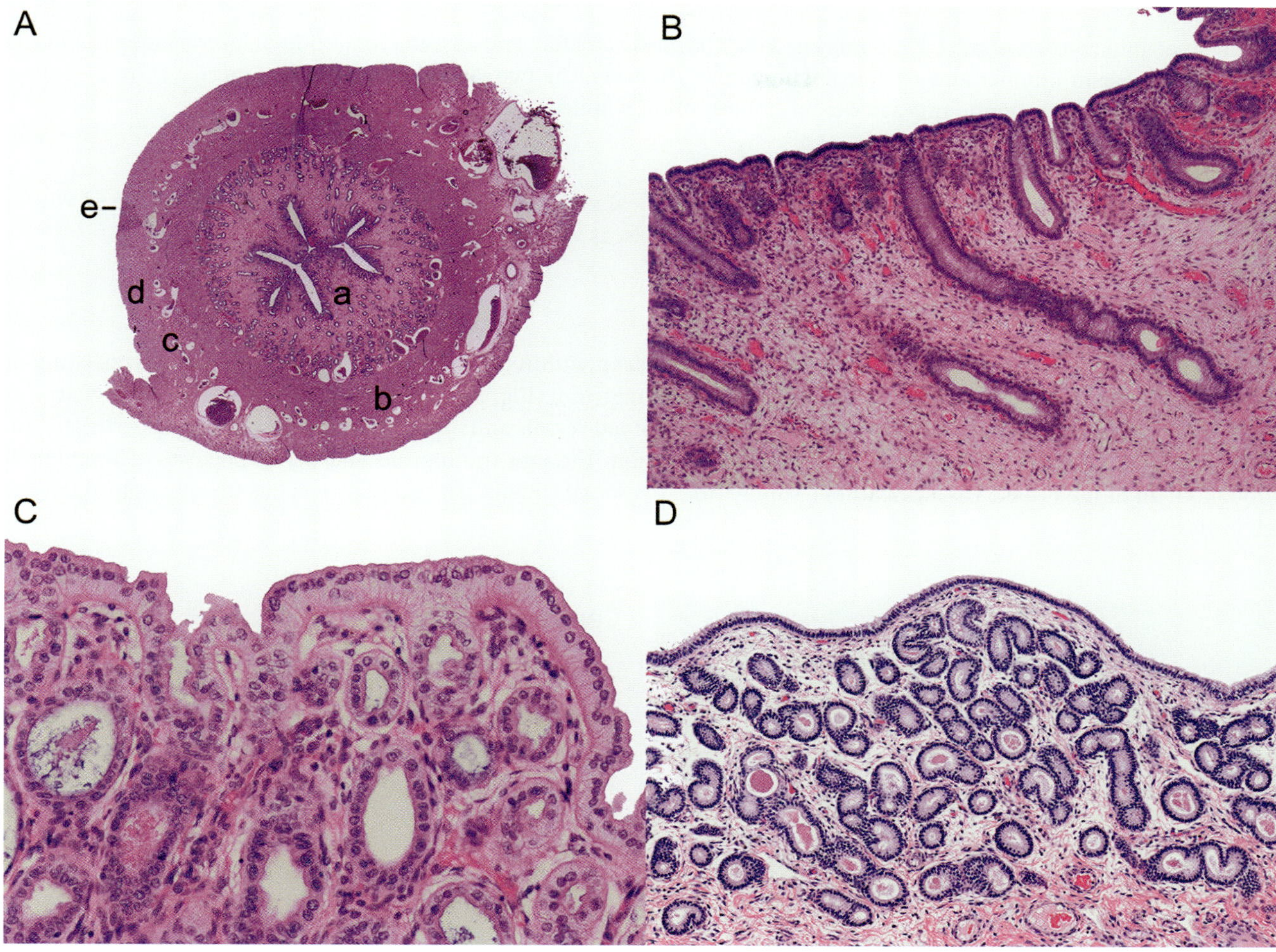

Figure 14-22 **A.** Cross section of uterine body (bitch). Endometrium (a) with numerous glands (coiled and straight). Myometrium consists of an inner muscle layer (b), a stratum vasculare (c), and an outer muscle layer (d). Perimetrial surface (e). **B.** Endometrium (bitch) exhibiting straight glands typical of proestrus and estrus. **C.** Endometrium (bitch) exhibiting coiled dilated glands and highly vacuolated epithelium typical of diestrus. **D.** Endometrium (mare) with columnar epithelium and coiled endometrial glands. H&E.

coiling of the glands are extensive in mares, whereas less branching is seen in carnivores. **Endometrial cups** develop in mares during early pregnancy after endometrial invasion by fetal trophoblasts (see Chapter 15).

In ruminants, circumscribed thickenings of the endometrium, known as **caruncles**, are present (Fig. 14-23). They are rich in fibrocytes and have an extensive blood supply. Each uterine horn in cows, does, and ewes contains approximately 15 caruncles in each of four rows. In cows, they are dome shaped, while in does and ewes, they are cup shaped, resembling a dome with a central depression. Caruncles are the endometrial structures providing attachment of the maternal placenta to the corresponding structures of the fetal placenta, the cotyledons (see Chapter 15).

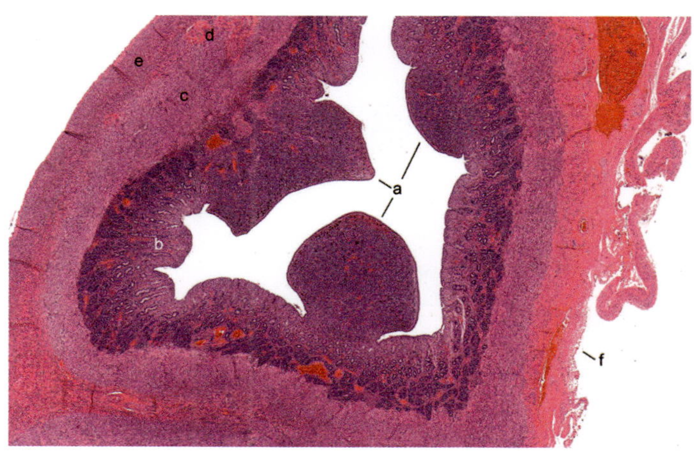

Figure 14-23 Cross section of the uterine horn (cow). Endometrium forms three caruncles (a). Glands (b) are present between the caruncles. Myometrium consists of an inner muscle layer (c), a stratum vasculare (d), and an outer muscle layer (e). Perimetrium or serosa (f). H&E.

Myometrium

The myometrium consists of a thick inner layer, which is mostly circular, and an outer longitudinal layer of smooth muscle cells that increase in number and size during pregnancy. Between the two layers, or within the inner layer, is a vascular layer (stratum vasculare) containing arteries, arterioles, veins, venules, and capillaries.

Perimetrium

The perimetrium consists of loose CT covered by the peritoneal mesothelium. Smooth muscle cells are dispersed within the perimetrium, alongside numerous lymph and blood vessels, as well as nerve fibers.

Blood Vessels, Lymphatics, and Nerves

Between the inner and outer layers of the myometrium, or deep within the inner layer, is a vascular layer consisting of large arteries, veins, and lymph vessels that supply the endometrium (Fig. 14-22 and 14-23). They are especially large in the caruncular regions of ruminants. Numerous lymph and blood vessels and nerve fibers are present in the perimetrium.

The nerves are derived mainly from the sympathetic system through the uterine and pelvic plexuses. They branch throughout all of the tunics. Parasympathetic supply from the sacral spinal cord segments reaches the uterus through the pelvic plexus.

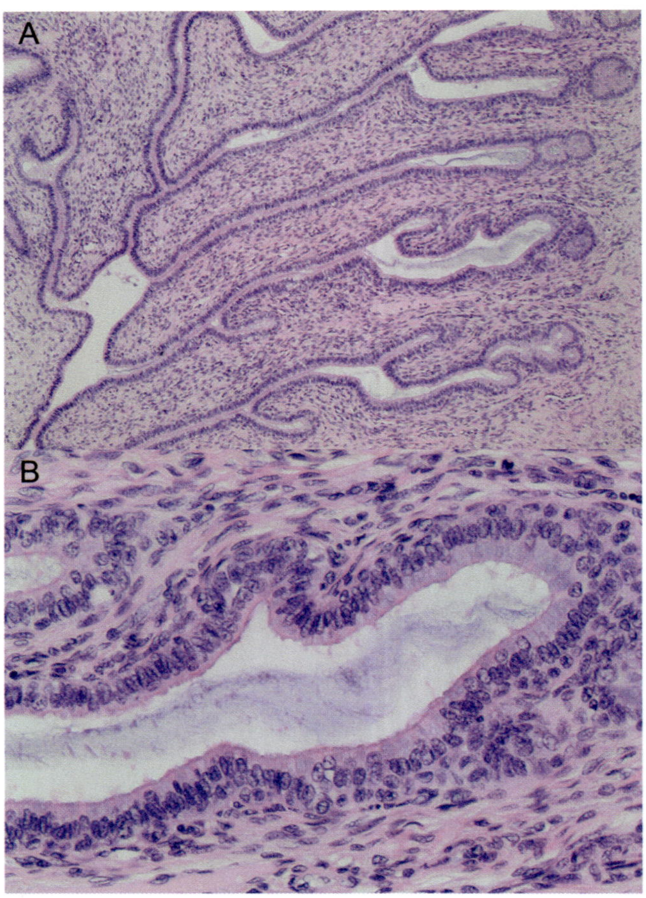

Figure 14-24 Cervix uteri (goat). **A**. Section of a large primary mucosal-submucosal fold with small secondary and tertiary folds projecting into the cervical lumen. **B**. Note the mucous secretory activity of the epithelial cells as evidenced by the coagulated mucus in the cervical lumen. H&E.

Cervix

The cervix, or neck of the uterus, is thick-walled, muscular, and rich in elastic fibers. The mucosa-submucosa forms high primary folds with secondary and tertiary folds. In cows, large circular and longitudinal primary folds, each with many secondary and tertiary folds, are present (Fig. 14-24A). These folds may give a false impression of glandular structure. While glandular elements present in the cervix are mostly mucigenous (Fig. 14-24B), uterine glands do not extend into this region.

Histologic Structure

In most species, the epithelium consists of simple columnar cells, with many mucigenous cells, including goblet cells. Increasing quantities of mucus are secreted during estrus, and much of the mucus passes to the vagina. In pregnancy, the mucus thickens to form the cervical seal. A small proportion of epithelial cells is ciliated in some species. Intraepithelial and simple tubular glands may be present in ruminants. In sows, more than 90% of the cervix may have a vaginal type of mucosa with stratified squamous epithelium that undergoes cyclic alterations as in the vagina. These features and alterations have relevance for the porcine copulatory mechanism.

The propria-submucosa consists of dense irregular CT, which becomes edematous and assumes a loose areolar structure during estrus. In mares and bitches, venous plexuses are present in the deep part of the propria-submucosa.

The tunica muscularis consists of an inner circular and an outer longitudinal layer of smooth muscle. Elastic fibers are prominent in the circular layer. Both muscle and elastic fibers are important in re-establishing cervical structure after parturition. The muscle layers of the cervix are continuous with those of the body of the uterus and the vagina. The cervical circular muscle layer is variously modified in different species. Thickening and infolding of the circular layer occurs in the region of the circular folds or prominences in the small ruminants and sows. In mares and cows, the thickened circular layer forms the body of the vaginal portion of the cervix. The orifice of the vaginal portion of the cervix in bitches is surrounded by a loop of vaginal muscle.

The tunica serosa of the cervix consists of loose CT covered by mesothelium.

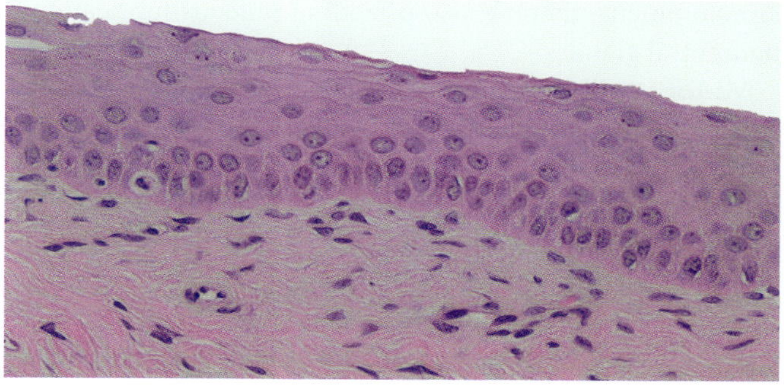

Figure 14-25 Canine vaginal mucosal epithelium. This photomicrograph depicts the epithelial lining in a nonkeratinized state. H&E.

Vagina

The vagina is a muscular tube extending from the cervix to the vestibule. Flat longitudinal mucosal-submucosal folds extend throughout its length, with prominent circular folds present in the cranial portion of the vagina in cows. Cyclic variations occur in epithelial height and structure, and intraepithelial glands are present in some species. The increased amounts of vaginal mucus during estrus mainly originate in the cervix.

Histologic Structure

The vaginal mucosa is lined mostly by a stratified squamous epithelium that increases in thickness during proestrus and estrus (Fig. 14-25). In the cranial part of the bovine vagina, the stratified squamous epithelium is overlaid by a surface layer of columnar and goblet cells that contain Periodic Acid-Schiff stain (PAS)-positive mucosubstances. In mares, the epithelial cells are generally polyhedral, with a few layers of flattened cells on the surface. The propria-submucosa consists of loose or dense irregular CT, containing lymphatic nodules in the caudal part of the vagina.

The tunica muscularis consists of two or three layers, with a thick inner circular smooth muscle layer separated into bundles by CT and surrounded by a thin outer longitudinal smooth muscle layer. In sows, bitches, and to a small extent in queens, an additional thin layer of longitudinal smooth muscle is present inside the circular layer.

Cranially, the vagina is covered by a typical tunica serosa (loose CT covered by mesothelium). Caudally, it is covered by a tunica adventitia, also composed of loose CT. Both the serosa and adventitia contain large blood vessels and extensive venous and lymphatic plexuses. Numerous nerve bundles and ganglia occur in the tunica serosa and adventitia, with innervation primarily sympathetic, derived from the pelvic plexus.

Vestibule, Clitoris, and Vulva

The wall of the **vestibule** is similar to that of the caudal portion of the vagina, except for the presence of more subepithelial lymphatic nodules, especially in the region of the clitoris. Blood vessels, erectile cavernous tissue, venous plexuses, and small lymph vessels are abundant in the vestibular wall and become congested during estrus. A discrete mass of erectile tissue, called the **bulbus vestibuli**, is present on each side beneath the vestibular mucosa in mares and bitches, resembling the corpus spongiosum penis.

The **major vestibular glands** are bilateral compound tubuloacinar mucous glands located in the deep part of the propria submucosa. They occur in cows, sheep, and queens. The terminal secretory acini contain large mucigenous cells, while the small ducts draining the acini are lined by columnar mucous cells, with isolated areas of goblet cells. The large ducts leading to the vestibule are lined by a thick stratified squamous epithelium, and individual or aggregated lymphatic nodules may surround them. These glands provide mucous lubrication for the vestibule and may be compressed during coitus and secrete mucus, thereby also providing mucous lubrication of the caudal vagina. They are homologous to the male bulbourethral glands.

Minor vestibular glands are bilateral small, branched, tubular mucous glands scattered in the vestibular mucosa in most domestic animals. They are homologous to the male urethral glands.

The **clitoris** consists of paired, joined erectile corpora cavernosa clitoridis, a rudimentary glans clitoridis, and a preputium clitoridis. The corpus cavernosum clitoridis, homologous to the corpus cavernosum penis, is well developed in mares. The glans clitoridis, homologous to the glans penis, is functionally erectile only in mares. A nonerectile fibroelastic tissue cover replaces the glans clitoridis in queens, sows, and ewes. In ewes, this cover contains a venous plexus. The clitoris contains many lymphatic nodules and is richly supplied with sensory and autonomic nerve endings.

The **vulva** is formed by the labia vulvae, which are covered by skin that is richly supplied with apocrine and sebaceous glands. Striated muscle fibers of the constrictor vulvae are found in the hypodermis. The labia are well supplied with small blood and lymph vessels, which become congested during estrus, especially in sows and bitches.

The Estrous Cycle

Hormones of the Ovary

The ovary has important endocrine functions, secreting essential sex hormones. **Estrogens** are produced primarily during estrus by the granulosa cells, which convert androgens secreted by the theca interna cells into estrogens. **Progesterone**, on the other hand, is produced primarily by the luteal cells during metestrus, diestrus, and pregnancy, and by the placenta in some species. Estrogen induces the growth and development of the female reproductive tract and estrous behavior. Progesterone stimulates the development of uterine glands, induces them to produce secretory products, and renders the endometrium receptive to the attachment or implantation of the developing conceptus. In addition, progesterone inhibits follicular maturation and estrus, and promotes behaviors appropriate to pregnancy. Both estrogens and progesterone contribute to the development of the mammary gland.

The growth and maturation of ovarian follicles, as well as their estrogen secretion, are controlled by pituitary **gonadotropins**. Both the granulosa and theca cells of late secondary or early tertiary follicles become responsive to gonadotropic hormones. The granulosa cells develop follicle-stimulating hormone (FSH) receptors, while the theca cells develop LH receptors. In mature tertiary follicles, the granulosa cells also are induced by FSH to develop LH receptors.

In tertiary follicles, LH interacts with receptors on the theca interna cells to stimulate the production of androgens and small amounts of estradiol. These androgens are secreted either into capillaries or traverse the basal lamina to reach the granulosa cell layer. Receptors on the granulosa cells interact with FSH to activate the aromatase enzyme system, which converts the thecal androgens (testosterone and androstenedione) into estrogens (estradiol-17 and estrone). Granulosa cells themselves are unable to produce androgens. The estrogens are then secreted into the follicular fluid and enter capillaries. The antral concentration of estradiol-17 is approximately 1000 times greater than that in the bloodstream. This high local concentration of estrogens maintains a favorable environment for follicular maturation. The action of FSH and LH on follicular cells is mediated by increased production of cyclic adenosine-3′,5′-monophosphate, which acts as an intracellular "second messenger." The process of estrogen production in this scenario is referred to as the two-cell, two-gonadotropin theory.

Immediately before ovulation, the ovulatory surge of LH interacts with its receptors on the granulosa cells to induce events leading to ovulation. In addition, the LH surge seems to inhibit the aromatase activity of granulosa cells and thus diminishes estrogen secretion. In the mature preovulatory follicle, LH is involved also in the induction of oocyte maturation (i.e., the completion of the first meiotic division). Several other physiologically active substances accumulate in the fluid of the mature preovulatory follicle, including inhibin, a large protein that selectively suppresses pituitary FSH secretion.

Ovarian secretion of estrogens reaches a threshold and stimulates the release of an ovulatory surge of LH, thereby inducing the processes leading to ovulation. Pituitary LH also initiates the formation of the corpus luteum. LH interacts with receptors on the cells of the ruptured follicular wall to initiate luteinization and progesterone secretion. In some species, such as rats and mice, prolactin is needed to maintain the corpus luteum and its progesterone secretion. The expression of progesterone receptors in and on luteal cells during metestrus, diestrus, and pregnancy suggests that local luteal autoregulatory mechanisms may also control progesterone production.

Luteal cells produce progesterone during late metestrus and most of diestrus, with secretion peaking in late diestrus shortly before luteal regression sets in. In cells of the developing and the mature corpus luteum, lipids are mostly phospholipids with traces of triglycerides and cholesterol and its esters. During regression, cholesterol accumulates in the luteal cells, suggesting decreased utilization for steroid hormone synthesis. In active luteal cells, the lipid droplets are small and even in size and distribution, whereas during regression, they are large and unevenly distributed. With the light microscope, they appear as large vacuoles (Fig. 14-16). The mechanism of luteolysis varies between species, with the main luteolytic factor being prostaglandin $F_2\alpha$ ($PGF_2\alpha$). If pregnancy occurs, the corpus luteum persists as the corpus luteum of pregnancy for varying periods of time across species. In cows and does, progesterone production by the corpus luteum continues throughout gestation, supported by luteotropic hormones from the pituitary, placenta, and local luteal autoregulatory mechanisms. In later stages of pregnancy in some species, the corpus luteum becomes less important as the placenta secretes sufficient progesterone for maintaining pregnancy. Ovarian and placental steroid hormones, in turn, influence pituitary gonadotropin secretion through feedback effects on the hypothalamus, mainly regulating the release of gonadotropin-releasing hormones. Other structures of the central nervous system, such as the pineal gland, also influence gonadotropic functions.

Phases of the Estrous Cycle

The estrous cycle is regulated by an intrinsic hypothalamo–hypophyseal–ovarian rhythm, which is influenced by environmental and internal neuroendocrine factors. In domestic animals, the estrous cycle is generally divided into the following sequential phases.

1) **Proestrus** is the phase of follicular maturation and endometrial proliferation following regression of the corpus luteum of the previous cycle. During this phase, the progesterone level falls, thus allowing release of FSH. Rising estrogen levels lead to estrus.
2) **Estrus** is the phase of sexual receptiveness, often coinciding with ovulation in most species. Ovulation is preceded by a surge of LH. At the end of estrus, estrogen levels decline.
3) **Metestrus** is the phase of corpus luteum development and initial progesterone secretion.
4) **Diestrus** is the phase of the active corpus luteum, with luteal progesterone predominating. Endometrial glandular hyperplasia and secretion peak during diestrus. Toward the end of diestrus, however, the corpus luteum regresses, leading to endometrial involution, including glandular regression. Diestrus extends into pseudopregnancy or gestational and lactational diestrus.
5) **Anestrus** is the prolonged period of sexual inactivity.

Cyclic Changes of the Endometrium

The cyclic changes in the endometrium, largely governed by ovarian hormones such as estrogens and progesterone, play a significant role in reproductive processes. During pregnancy, these hormones are produced primarily by the placenta.

Some animals (e.g., bitches) are **monestrous** and have one or two estrous cycles per year, followed by a long anestrous period. Continuously cycling animals, without an anestrous period (e.g., cows and sows), or seasonally cycling animals (e.g., queens, mares, ewes, and goats) are **polyestrous**. Uterine regenerative changes are induced by estradiol and continued by progesterone, which induces glandular secretory activity and causes the endometrium to produce a maternal placenta when stimulated by the presence of the blastocyst. A detailed description of the cyclic changes in the cow and the bitch follows.

Cow

In the cow, the estrous cycle lasts 21 days (Fig. 14-26). Ovulation occurs on the day after estrus or approximately 30 hours after its onset. Estrus may be designated as "day 0" or "day 21" of the cycle, while the last day of proestrus may be referred to as "day 20." During the last 3 to 4 days of **diestrus**, the endometrial stroma shrinks, and the epithelium becomes lower. The glands become shorter, their epithelium becomes lower, and their secretions cease. During **proestrus**, under the influence of estrogens, the endometrium is restored; the mucosa becomes thickened, congested, and edematous with a predominance of mucin-filled epithelial cells. However, glandular proliferation is limited to straight lumen growth without significant branching or coiling. During **estrus**, endometrial edema and hyperemia are maximal. During **metestrus**, the edema lessens, and a breakdown occurs in some of the congested endometrial blood vessels. Upon the onset of **diestrus**, under the influence of progesterone, the endometrium transforms from a proliferative to a secretory type, with glandular epithelial growth and glandular branching, coiling, and secretion. During the first 11 days of diestrus, endometrial glandular secretion is greatest. If pregnancy does not occur, the glands again regress along with the corpus luteum during the last 3 days of diestrus.

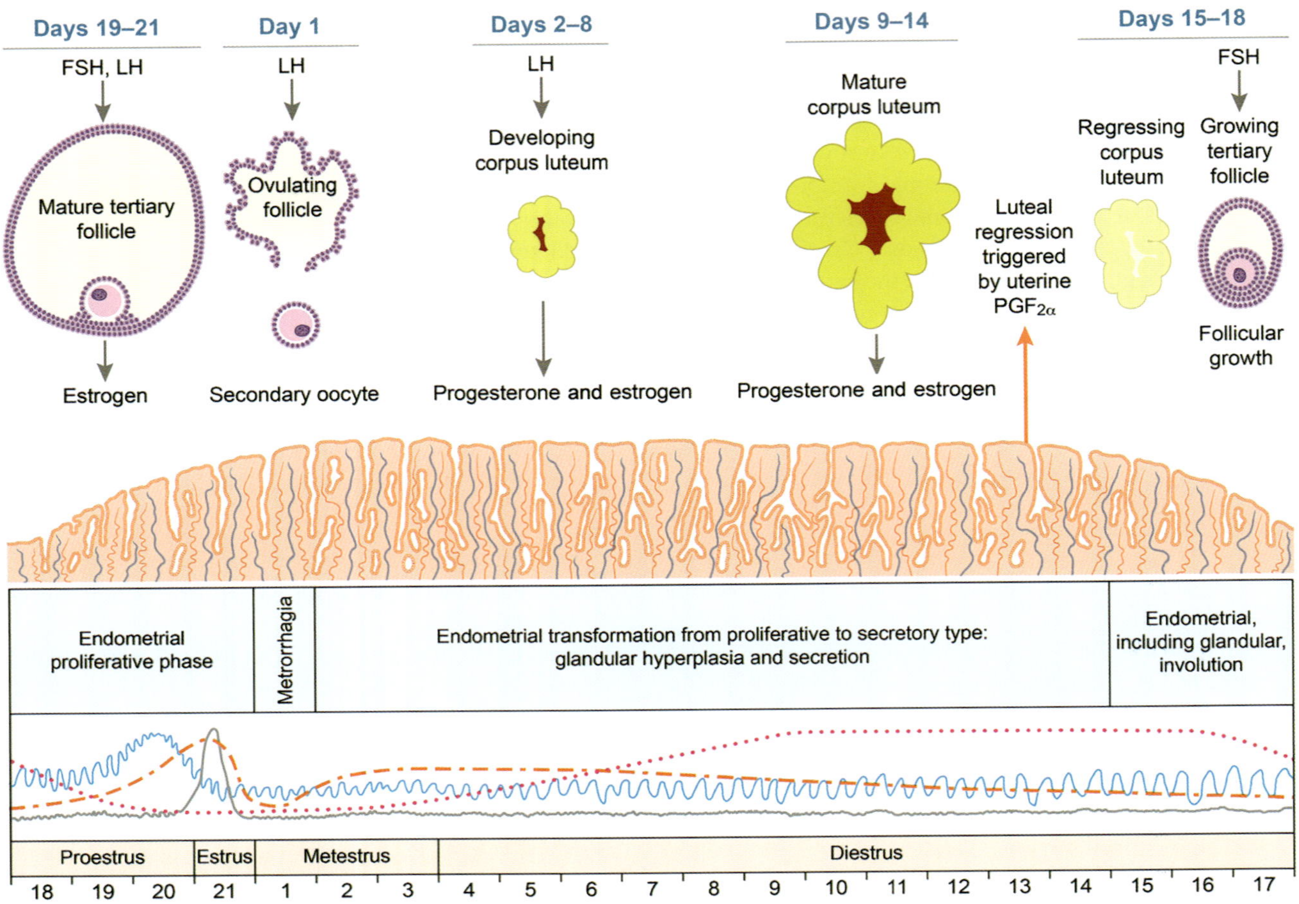

Figure 14-26 The ovarian and uterine changes during the estrous cycle in the cow are shown schematically. The ovarian follicular (days 15 to 21) and luteal (days 1 to 14) phases, along with the endometrial proliferative and secretory stages, characterized by maximal glandular branching and activity on days 8 to 12, are shown. Additionally, endometrial involution triggered by local prostaglandin $F_2\alpha$ is indicated. The relative blood levels of key hormones are diagrammed (blue line: estrogens, dotted red line: progesterone, grey: LH, dashed orange line: FSH). The scale indicates days 1 to 21 of the estrous cycle. (Illustration by Tim Vojt, courtesy of The Ohio State University®.)

Mitotic activity begins in the surface and glandular epithelia, along with the interstitial elements, during estrus and continues for approximately 6 days after estrus. Neutrophils invade the lamina propria, epithelia, and uterine lumen from late proestrus to approximately day 3 or 4 after estrus. Agranulocytes, mainly lymphocytes, invade from day 3 to 5 postestrus and are especially abundant in the basal zone of the endometrium. An eosinophilic invasion may occur from estrus to midcycle. Mast cells increase in number at the time of maximal edema, especially in the caruncular areas. **Metrorrhagia** refers to the microscopic hemorrhages in the functional zone of the endometrium, which begin shortly before ovulation in cows. At ovulation, metrorrhagia becomes widespread and is prominent in the pitted central areas of the caruncles. It peaks immediately after maximal endometrial edema. Capillaries rupture within the mucosa, leading to blood accumulating in "blisters" beneath the surface epithelium. The blisters rupture, releasing blood and shreds of mucosa into the uterine lumen. Although blood in the caruncular areas is mainly phagocytized and resorbed, it generally does not reach the uterine lumen. However, tissue fluid, along with blood, may be lost at rupture points in the intercaruncular areas. Metrorrhagia ends abruptly near the end of day 2 after estrus. A bloody vulvar discharge occurs at this time.

Bitch

Proestrus and estrus each lasts approximately 9 days in bitches. If pregnancy does not follow estrus, pseudopregnancy and anestrus ensue. Endometrial edema, congestion, and hemorrhages occur during proestrus. Ovulation occurs shortly after the onset of estrus. Progesterone begins to rise before ovulation, serving as a rough marker to estimate a time of ovulation in bitches. Around day 6 of estrus, corpora lutea become functional, and uterine glands and interstitial elements begin to proliferate. The glandular epithelium becomes tall, columnar, and vacuolated, while the glands become coiled. In the non-pregnant state, involution of the endometrial glands and stroma begins approximately 20 to 30 days after the onset of estrus. During anestrus, the endometrium is thin and regressed, with mainly cuboidal epithelium.

Primates

Menstruation in primates is an entirely different phenomenon from the uterine bleeding seen in bovines. The uterine hemorrhages in cows occur during a **regenerative phase** of the endometrium near estrus.

Menstruation, on the other hand, occurs during a **degenerative phase** of the endometrium, precipitated by the withdrawal of estrogens and, more importantly, of progesterone after the involution of the corpus luteum. The occurrence of hemorrhage in primates has been attributed to special coiled arteries in the endometrial functional zone, which periodically constrict and dilate as progesterone and estrogen support wanes. The arterial constriction causes ischemia and necrosis of tissue, while the dilation that follows leads to blood vessel rupture, hemorrhage, and loss of functional zone tissues.

In bitches, pseudopregnancy invariably follows estrus and spontaneous ovulation if the animal has not become pregnant. In other animals, pseudopregnancy follows estrus and ovulation only if a mating stimulus resulting in a corpus luteum of pseudopregnancy has occurred (i.e., a corpus luteum of prolonged and sometimes greater activity than that of the corpus luteum of diestrus). Regression of the corpus luteum results in decreased progesterone and estrogen supply, leading to the regression of the endometrium and termination of pseudopregnancy. Although no external bleeding occurs in bitches at this time, microscopic hemorrhages of the endometrium have been observed.

Cyclic Changes of the Vaginal Epithelium

Cow

The epithelium varies with the site and hormonal status of the animal. Under the influence of **progesterone**, the epithelium in the cranial part of the vagina consists of approximately 3 layers of cells and increases to approximately 10 layers in the caudal part.

Under the influence of **estrogens**, the rate of epithelial cell proliferation increases throughout the vagina, and the epithelium thickens. In early estrus, the superficial layer of columnar and goblet cells in the cranial part of the vagina attains maximal height as a result of stored mucus. The epithelium of the caudal part is at maximal height from 2 days after estrus until midcycle, during which period the surface cells are more squamous than at other times, and desquamation occurs. True keratinization (cornification) of the superficial epithelial cells is not observed, however.

Neutrophils invade the vaginal epithelium from estrus until 2 days after estrus. Lymphocytes and plasma cells are more common under the influence of progesterone.

Bitch

Cyclic cellular changes that occur in the vaginal epithelium of the bitch are clinically useful and important for estimating the times of estrus and breeding (Fig. 14-27). The assessment of these changes through the vaginal smear method is widely used. After staining, vaginal smears appear as follows:

1) **Proestrus** (~9 days in duration): Numerous erythrocytes (of uterine origin) and many large, flat, keratinized cells are present.
2) **Estrus** (~9 days in duration): Some erythrocytes and numerous keratinized cells are present. As estrus progresses, the keratinized cells become wrinkled and distorted and are frequently invaded by bacteria.
3) **Diestrus** (~2 months in duration): Epithelial cells are less keratinized and appear more like unstained living cells. Neutrophils are numerous on day 3 of diestrus and gradually disappear until day 10 to 20 of diestrus.
4) **Anestrus** (~2 months in duration): Numerous unstained nonkeratinized epithelial cells, a few large, stained cells with pyknotic nuclei, and a few neutrophils and lymphocytes are present.

Although the epithelial lining of the vagina is thin during anestrus, with only approximately two to three layers of cells, it proliferates during proestrus and may reach a thickness of 12 to 20 cells at the beginning of estrus, accompanied by keratinization of the surface layers (Fig. 14-28). By late estrus, desquamation of the keratinized layers begins (Fig. 14-28). Intraepithelial glands are common during estrus.

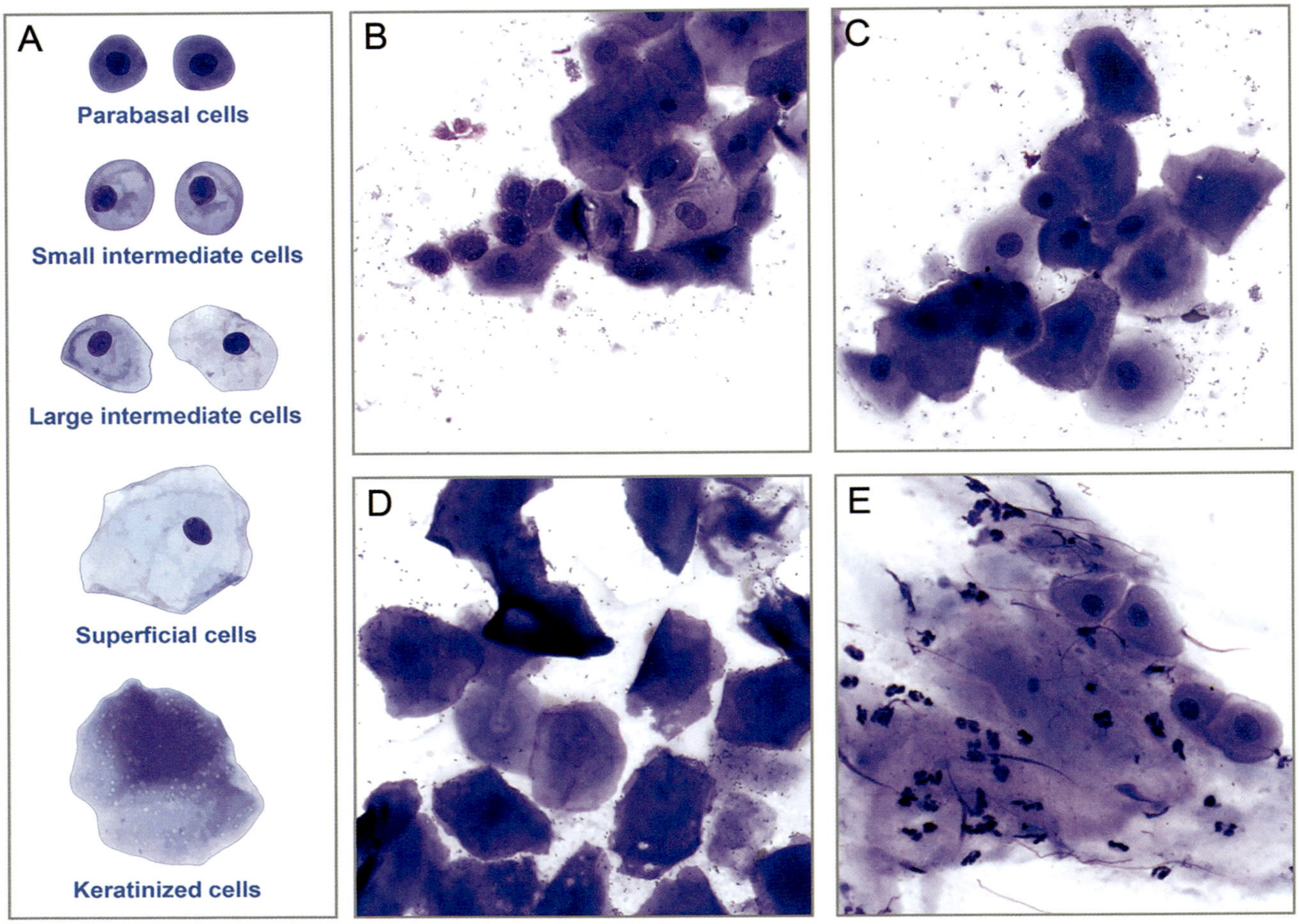

Figure 14-27 **A.** Cyclic cellular changes of the vaginal epithelium in the bitch illustrated by a scheme of epithelial cells. Vaginal smears (epithelial and blood cells). **B.** Anestrus: note parabasal cells. **C.** Proestrus: note small intermediate cells, large intermediate cells, and superficial cells (keratinized). **D.** Estrus: note superficial cells (keratinized). **E.** Diestrus: note small intermediate cells, large intermediate cells, and granulocytes. (Illustration by Tim Vojt / Courtesy of The Ohio State University. Wright-Giemsa stain.)

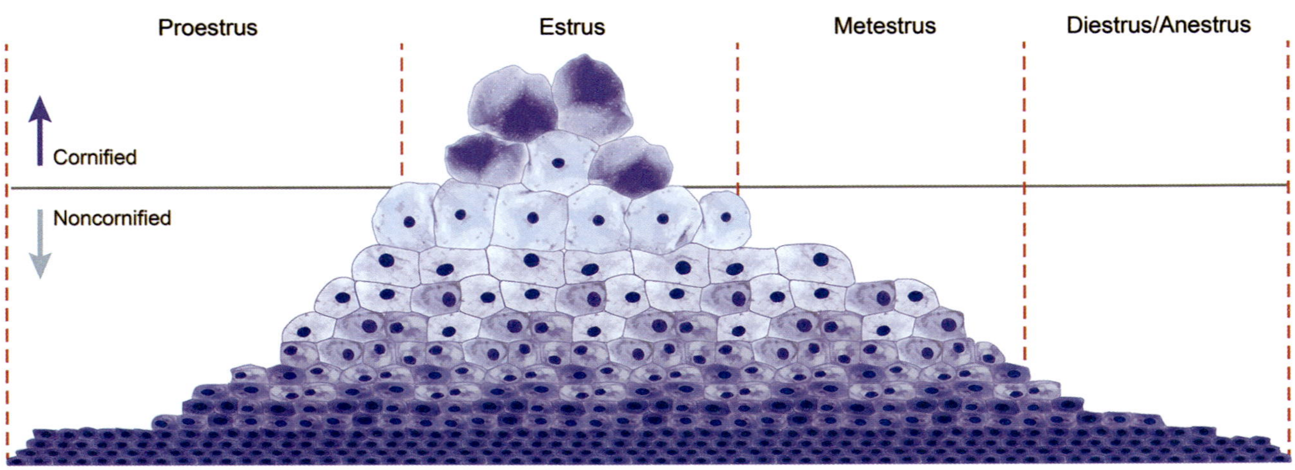

Figure 14-28 Schematic drawing of the cyclic changes of the vaginal epithelium in the bitch. (Illustration by Tim Vojt, courtesy of The Ohio State University®.)

Avian Female Reproductive System

Ovary

In adult birds, only the left ovary is present. The ovarian cortex and medulla are distorted by the presence of large "follicles" in various stages of development or atresia, each attached to the ovary by a peduncle. True follicles are not present in the avian ovary because a fluid-filled follicular antrum does not develop. Within the follicle, the oocyte is surrounded by one or several layers of granulosa cells, which in turn are surrounded by cells of the theca interna and theca externa. The granulosa cells are shed with the oocyte at ovulation, whereas the theca cells remain to form a transient corpus luteum. Interstitial endocrine cells are found at the periphery of the ovary.

Formation of follicles usually begins in the post hatching period, when the oogonia enlarge and become primary oocytes surrounded by follicular cells. These primary oocytes then undergo the first meiotic division. At the time of sexual maturity (5 to 6 months in hens), secondary oocytes are ovulated. The second meiotic division is completed at fertilization, resulting in the formation of an ovum, and then a zygote. While the primary oocyte is primarily protoplasmic, the secondary oocyte contains mainly yolk, with abundant accumulation at one end of the cell and the nucleus situated at the other end. These secondary oocytes and ova are thus termed **macrolecithal, telolecithal cells**. The yolk contains lipids, such as lecithin, cholesterol, and carotene, arranged in concentric layers. The oocyte is surrounded by a plasma membrane, termed the **vitelline membrane**. After ovulation, other layers are added to the outside of the oocyte during its passage through the female reproductive tract.

Oviduct

The term **oviduct** in the bird is used to describe the entire reproductive duct, present only on the left side in adults. The left oviduct consists of the **infundibulum**, **magnum**, **isthmus**, **uterus**, and **vagina** (Fig. 14-29). Although each of these divisions has special structural and functional features, they all have two morphologic elements essential for egg formation: (a) a muscle layer, which supports the oviduct and propels the egg, and (b) a glandular epithelial lining, which secretes all parts of the egg outside the yolk-filled oocyte/zygote. Moreover, the mucous membrane produces a secretion that forms a soft, resilient cushion for the egg as it passes through the oviduct.

The following secretions of the oviduct are added onto the oocyte/zygote:

1) Four layers of albumen are added in the magnum (the cranial part of the oviduct).
2) A shell membrane, consisting of a thin inner and a thick outer layer of protein (mainly keratin) filaments, is added in the isthmus. These layers become separated in the air chamber at the blunt end of the egg.
3) A porous shell is formed in the uterus. This shell consists of an inner layer of conical calcareous masses, surrounded by a spongy organic layer, and an outer shell cuticle. An organic pigment layer may be added externally in some breeds.

Infundibulum

The cranial extremity of the infundibulum is dilated and has long fimbriae that grasp the secondary oocyte as it is released from the ovary. The infundibulum is the usual site of **fertilization**. The mucosa-submucosa is thrown into low longitudinal ridges or primary folds; in addition, secondary mucosal-submucosal folds are present in the caudal infundibulum. The egg remains in the infundibulum for approximately 25 minutes.

The epithelium is ciliated pseudostratified columnar. It contains occasional goblet cells, except at the bottom of the folds, where the epithelium transitions to nonciliated simple columnar. Toward the caudal portion of the infundibulum, glandular cells increase in number and aggregate in **glandular grooves** that resemble the tubular glands of the magnum.

The propria-submucosa consists of loose CT containing many lymphocytes and plasma cells. The tunica muscularis is composed of scattered bundles of longitudinal smooth muscle. The tunica serosa consists of loose CT and mesothelium.

Magnum

The magnum has a thick wall and tall thick longitudinal primary and secondary mucosal-submucosal folds. Here, **albumen**, or egg white, is added to the developing egg, a process taking approximately 3 hours.

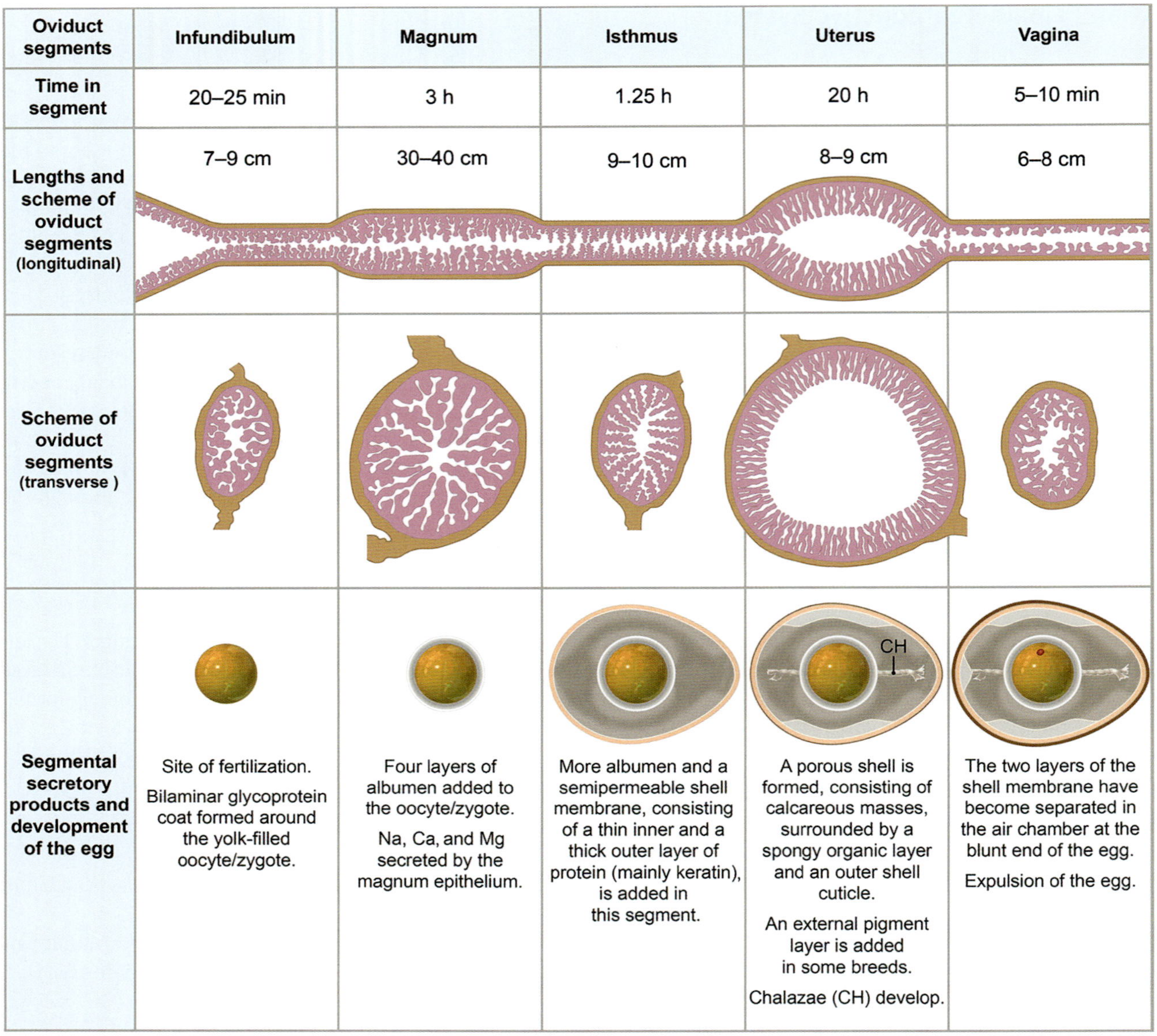

Figure 14-29 Egg development in the laying domestic hen: structural changes of the egg in the various segments of the oviduct. (Image courtesy of Tim Vojt.)

The epithelial lining of the magnum is simple columnar, with close to equal numbers of ciliated cells and goblet cells. The loose CT of the propria-submucosa is packed with many long, branched, coiled tubular glands. The cells are pyramidal and contain coarse basophilic granules. An inner circular and an outer longitudinal smooth muscle layer are present. A thin tunica serosa consists of loose CT and mesothelium. The magnum is sharply divided from the next portion of the oviduct, the isthmus, by a 1- to 3-mm segment devoid of glands.

Isthmus

The isthmus has pronounced longitudinal ridges, where the egg typically remains for approximately 1.23 hours. The bilaminar **shell membrane** is formed in this region.

The epithelium is simple columnar with close to equal numbers of ciliated and goblet cells.

The propria-submucosa is filled with distended branched tubular glands. These glands are lined by pyramidal cells whose cytoplasm contains many acidophilic secretory granules. The tunica muscularis consists of circular and longitudinal smooth muscle layers. The tunica serosa consists of loose CT and mesothelium.

Uterus

The uterus, or **shell gland**, is thick-walled, saclike, and distensible. Primary and secondary longitudinal folds are obscured by a series of primary and secondary circular folds. Rotation of the egg, associated with twisting of the chalazae, occurs here. The egg remains in the uterus for approximately 20 hours, during which time shell components, including the organic matrix, shell cuticle, and inorganic material, are formed.

The epithelium is ciliated pseudostratified columnar. The propria-submucosa contains branched, coiled tubular glands. The cells of these glands are pyramidal and have a diffusely granular and vacuolated cytoplasm. Sparse loose CT separates the glands. The tunica muscularis consists of two layers of smooth muscle, with the inner circular layer being notably thick and forming a sphincter at the boundary with the vagina. The tunica serosa consists of loose CT and mesothelium.

Vagina

The vaginal wall is thick and has low primary and secondary longitudinal folds. The egg remains in the vagina for a short time, and the vagina does not participate in the formation of the egg. It lacks glands except for the so-called **sperm-host glands** at the uterovaginal junction that are used for the storage of spermatozoa.

The epithelium lining the vagina is ciliated pseudostratified columnar with few goblet cells. The propria-submucosa is loose CT, frequently containing lymphocytes, plasma cells, and granulocytes. The tunica muscularis is functional in expelling the egg and consists of a thick inner circular layer and an outer longitudinal layer. The tunica serosa consists of loose CT and mesothelium.

Cloaca

The vagina, colon, and ureters open into the cloaca. The epithelium of the cloaca is simple columnar and contains many goblet cells.

Clinical Correlations

Cystic Endometrial Hyperplasia

Cystic endometrial hyperplasia (Fig. 14-30) is a condition most commonly observed in female dogs. It occurs during diestrus when the endometrium is exposed to and primed by high levels of estrogen followed by progesterone. The lesion is comprised of numerous cystically dilated endometrial glands that, in severe cases, can be seen throughout the uterine body and both uterine horns. Severe cystic endometrial hyperplasia can be observed grossly and detected by ultrasonography of uterine tissue.

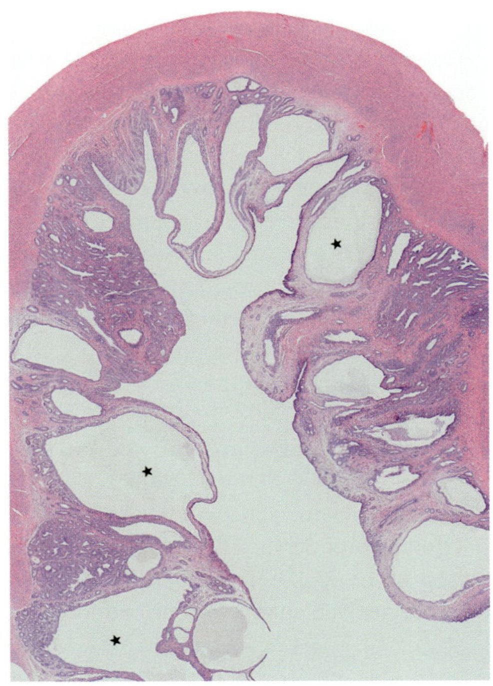

Figure 14-30 Cystic endometrial hyperplasia (bitch). This cross section of uterus exhibits multiple large cystically dilated glands (stars) that distort the endometrium. H&E.

Granulosa Theca Cell Tumor

Granulosa theca cell tumors or granulosa cell tumors are neoplasms arising from the ovary that are classified as sex cord stromal tumors. They can be observed in a variety of domestic animal species. These neoplasms can be associated with a variety of clinical signs associated with autonomous production of hormones. In mares, this can include abnormalities in the estrus cycle such as continuous or intermittent estrus and atypical anestrus periods (Fig. 14-31). Affected mares may also show stallion-like behavior. Treatment typically involves surgical removal of the affected ovary.

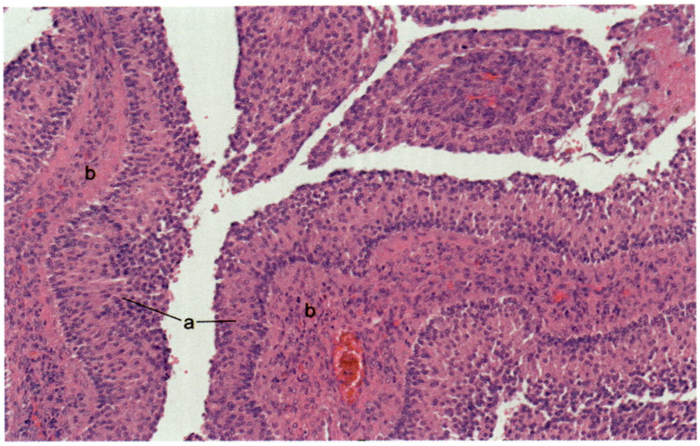

Figure 14-31 Granulosa theca cell tumor (mare). Equine granulosa theca cell tumors typically appear as a large cystic mass that expands the ovary. Microscopically, the neoplasm is composed of granulosa cells arranged haphazardly and forming trabeculae (a) within fibrous CT (b), attempting to mimic follicular structures. H&E.

Essentials

Ovary structure: The cortex is covered by a cuboidal to squamous surface epithelium (germinal epithelium). *The dense irregular* CT tunica albuginea lies beneath the surface epithelium. Follicles progress from primordial to tertiary stages, with granulosa cells forming theca layers and an antrum. Most follicles undergo atresia, with remnants observed in the stroma. *Medulla*: It contains blood vessels, lymphatics, and nerves supporting ovarian function.

Ovary function: The corpus luteum formed after ovulation secretes progesterone until regression, seen as luteinization followed by fibrosis. The ovary secretes predominantly estrogens during estrus and progesterone during metestrus, diestrus, and pregnancy. Estrogens promote reproductive tract growth and estrous behavior, while progesterone prepares the uterus for conceptus attachment. LH induces ovulation and corpus luteum formation, leading to progesterone production. Luteal cells produce progesterone during diestrus, peaking before luteal regression, mainly mediated by $PGF_2\alpha$ if pregnancy does not occur.

Uterine tube (mammals)/oviduct (avian): It facilitates ovum and zygote transport toward the uterus. The segments are the fimbriated infundibulum, ampulla, and isthmus. The epithelium is simple or pseudostratified columnar and has motile cilia and secretory cells. The mucosa folds extensively in the ampulla, diminishing toward the isthmus. The muscularis layer has mainly circular smooth muscle bundles, thicker in the isthmus and merging with the uterine circular muscle. Innervation helps coordinate smooth muscle contractions necessary for gamete and embryo transport.

Uterus: It is vital for conceptus attachment and varies across species but generally contains horns, a body, and a neck. It consists of *three main layers*: *the endometrium, myometrium, and perimetrium*. The endometrium has coiled, branched glands, while the myometrium has inner circular and outer longitudinal smooth muscle layers. The perimetrium consists of loose CT. Blood vessels, lymphatics, and nerves are abundant, especially in caruncular regions of ruminants. Each layer plays distinct roles in the estrous cycle and pregnancy. The endometrium undergoes cyclic changes in response to hormonal fluctuations, preparing for embryo implantation during the receptive phase.

Cervix: It is a muscular neck of the uterus with thick walls and folds in its mucosa-submucosa. It features a simple columnar epithelium, rich in mucigenous cells, and has inner circular and outer longitudinal smooth muscle layers. The tunica serosa is composed of loose CT. It facilitates mucus secretion and sperm transport.

Vagina: It consists of a muscular tube that extends from cervix to vestibule with cyclic epithelial variations, lined by stratified squamous epithelium. It has a tunica muscularis and extensive blood vessels and nerve bundles in serosa and adventitia.

Vestibule, clitoris, and vulva: Vestibule resembles caudal vagina, with abundant blood vessels, erectile tissue, and lymphatic nodules. Major vestibular glands provide mucous lubrication. Clitoris has paired erectile corpora cavernosa and rudimentary glans, rich in nerve endings. Vulva consists of labia vulvae with rich vascularization and striated muscle fibers.

The estrous cycle: The cycle includes proestrus (follicular maturation), estrus (sexual receptiveness and ovulation), metestrus (corpus luteum development), diestrus (luteal progesterone influence), and anestrus (sexual inactivity). Hormone-driven changes in the endometrial epithelium play a crucial role in reproductive processes.

Suggested Readings

Baird DT. The ovary. In: Austin CR, Short RV, editors. *Reproduction in Mammals*. 2nd edition. Vol. 3. Cambridge: Cambridge University Press; 1984. p. 91.

Berisha B, Thaqi G, Sinowatz F, et al. Prostaglandins as local regulators of ovarian physiology in ruminants. *Anatomia, Histologia, Embryologia* 2024;53(1):e12980.

Goodman RL, Karsch FJ. The hypothalamic pulse generator: a key determinant of reproductive cycles in sheep. In: Follett BK, Follett DE, editors. *Biological Clocks and Seasonal Reproductive Cycles*. Colston Papers No. 32. Bristol: John Wright; 1981. p. 223.

Hyttel P. Electron microscopy of mammalian oocyte development, maturation and fertilization. In: Tosti E, Boni R, editors. *Oocyte Maturation and Fertilization: A Long History for a Short Event*. Sharjah, United Arab Emirates (UAE): Bentham Science Publisher; 2011. p. 1–37.

Knobil E, Neill JD. *The Physiology of Reproduction*. 4th edition. New York: Raven Press; 2015.

Liggins GC. The fetus and birth. In: Austin CR, Short RV, editors. *Reproduction in Mammals*. 2nd edition. Vol. 2. Cambridge: Cambridge University Press; 1983. p. 114.

McDonald LE. *Veterinary Endocrinology and Reproduction*. 5th edition. Wiley-Blackwell; 2002.

Mehlmann LM. Stops and starts in mammalian oocytes: recent advances in understanding the regulation of meiotic arrest and oocyte maturation. *Reproduction* 2005;130(6):791–799.

Miyamoto A, Shirasuna K. Luteolysis in the cow: a novel concept of vasoactive molecules. *Animal Reproduction (AR)* 2018;6(1):47–59.

Moore RM, Seamark RF. Cell signaling, permeability and microvascularity changes during antral follicle development in mammals. *J Dairy Sci* 1986;69:927.

Rekawiecki R, Kowalik MK, Slonina D, et al. Regulation of progesterone synthesis and action in bovine corpus luteum. *J Physiol Pharmacol* 2008;59(suppl 9):75–89.

Rodgers RJ, Irving-Rodgers HF. Morphological classification of bovine ovarian follicles. *Reproduction* 2010;139(2):309.

Windsor P. Abnormalities of development and pregnancy. In: Noakes DE, Parkinson TJ, GCW E, editors. *Veterinary Reproduction and Obstetrics*. 10th edition. Amsterdam: Elsevier Health Sciences; 2018. p. 168–194.

15

Placentation

Karl Klisch and Estela Bevilacqua

CHAPTER MENU

Dellmann's Textbook of Veterinary Histology, Seventh Edition. Edited by Marxa L. Figueiredo and John J. Turek.

Companion website: www.wiley.com/go/figueiredo/vethistology7e

Introduction

The placenta is a temporary organ that, during the prenatal period, establishes the exchange of nutrients, gases, and waste products between the mother and the developing embryo/fetus. The placenta is also involved, in a species-specific manner, in the production and release of hormones and the transfer of immunoglobulins. The placental structure is complex and changes over time during gestation. Despite the seemingly similar main functions (molecular exchange), the placenta shows considerable variation between species, which includes macroscopic shape, histological structure, and biochemical composition. The placental characteristics and its species-specific abilities make it the most variable organ in higher mammals.

Embryology

The initial source of nutrition for the mammal embryo while in the uterine cavity is uterine milk, the secretions of the endometrial glands (**histotrophic nutrition**). However, to meet the increasing demand for nutrients, the embryo needs efficient strategies, which include the differentiation of an external membrane capable of carrying out the gaseous and nutritional exchange—**the chorion**—and its lodgment in the endometrium, which occurs during a process called **implantation**. This process establishes a close relationship between fetal and maternal circulatory systems for physiological exchange. As a result, a combined organ, **the placenta**, is formed, which consists of a fetal part (pars fetalis) and a maternal part (pars uterina). The fetus and fetal membranes, including the fetal part of the placenta, are known as the **conceptus**. The manner of attachment and subsequent formation of the placenta is termed **placentation**.

The first events in placentation occur during the development of the blastocyst, a fluid-filled vesicle with an epithelial wall—**the trophoblast**—and an agglomerate of a few cells, **the inner cell mass** (or embryoblast). The outer layer of the blastocyst, the trophoblast, is essential for the transfer of nourishment to the offspring during intrauterine life but has no function after the birth of the young and is expelled with the afterbirth (secundinae). The inner cell mass differentiates into three germ layers in two stages, initially forming **ectoderm** and **endoderm**, and then **mesoderm** between the original layers. These three germ layers not only form the embryo but also participate in developing the fetal membranes.

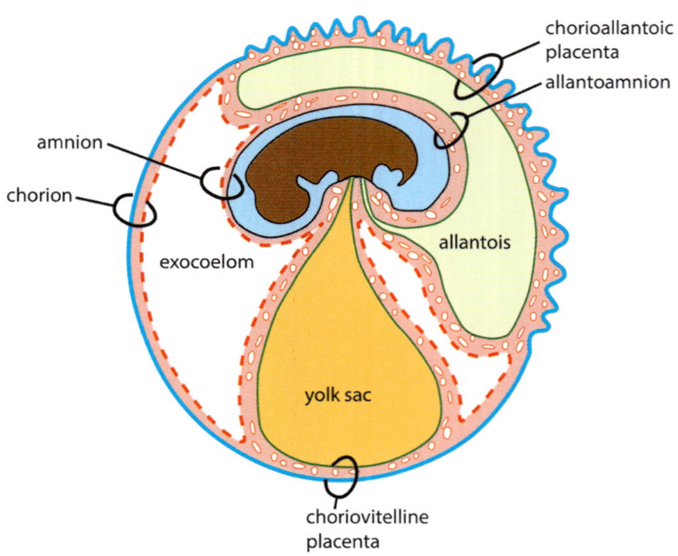

Figure 15-1 Schematic diagram of the fetal membranes. The amnion encloses the amniotic cavity (light blue) and the embryo. The trophoblast (blue line) and the somatic mesoderm (somatopleure) form the primary chorion. The yolk sac and the allantois are formed by the endoderm (green) and the splanchnic mesoderm (splanchnopleure). (From Dellmann H-D, Carithers JR. Cytology and Microscopic Anatomy. Philadelphia: Williams & Wilkins, 1996).

Part of the ectoderm contributes to developing a membrane (**amnion**), which forms a vesicle enclosing the embryo, **the amniotic cavity**. The amniotic cavity provides buoyancy and protected space for embryo development.

The endoderm contributes to the **yolk sac**, which communicates with the midgut, and the **allantois**, a diverticulum from the hindgut (see Fig. 15-1). The allantois forms a sizeable fluid-filled sac in domestic animals, which can be regarded as an extra-fetal urinary bladder. This contrasts with humans, where the allantois only initially develops and does not form a fluid-filled chamber. Consequently, the human fetus is surrounded only by one fluid-filled chamber, the amniotic sac, while in domestic animals, two sacs, the amniotic sac and the allantoic sac, are present.

The further development of the extraembryonic membranes (amnion, yolk sac, and allantois) is achieved after their association with the mesoderm. In the embryonic tissues, after gastrulation, the lateral mesoderm splits into a **somatic** and a **splanchnic** layer. The resulting intramesodermal cleft gives rise to the body cavity (intraembryonic coelom). At this stage, the embryonic mesoderm extends and fuses with the extraembryonic mesoderm that lines the extraembryonic cavity called the **exocoelom**, as well as the amnion, yolk sac, allantois, and trophoblast.

The somatic/extraembryonic mesoderm associated with the trophoblast layer forms the **chorion**, while its association with the ectoderm forms the **amnion**. These membranes constitute the **extraembryonic somatopleure**. The splanchnic/extraembryonic mesoderm lines the endoderm of the yolk sac and the allantois, and together, these layers form the **extraembryonic splanchnopleure**.

The extraembryonic somatopleure, and hence the chorion, is initially avascular. Blood islands and vessels first arise in the extraembryonic splanchnopleure of the yolk sac and later in the allantois. In due course, the chorion's avascular mesoderm fuses with the allantois's mesoderm, forming the **allantochorion**, which then becomes vascularized and filled with allantoic fluid. The placental vessels and the vitelline and allantoic ducts are contained in the body stalk, which later develops into the **umbilical cord**. At birth, the **allantoamnion**, a fusion of the allantois and amnion, protrudes through the ruptured allantochorion and assists in the dilation of the cervix during parturition.

Secretions from the fetal membranes play an essential role in the maternal recognition of pregnancy and its continuation. The secretions alter the endometrial signal to the ovary, leading to the preservation of the corpus luteum. In the pig, estrogen secreted by the blastocyst is antiluteolytic, while in ruminants, interferon τ exerts a similar effect.

Classification

The wide variation of placental structures has led to several types of classifications based on specific aspects. Five commonly used types include (a) contributions of fetal extraembryonic membranes, (b) macroscopic structure of the placenta, (c) three-dimensional structure of the fetal–maternal interface, (d) tissue layers of the fetal–maternal interhemal barrier, and (e) the degree of fetal–maternal anchoring and the fate of maternal tissues at birth.

Contributions of Fetal Extraembryonic Membranes

Based on the contributions of fetal extraembryonic membranes in domestic mammals, two types of placentae can be distinguished: the **choriovitelline placenta** (yolk sac placenta) and the **chorioallantoic placenta** (Fig. 15-1). This differentiation is based on which of the two endodermal structures, the yolk sac or the allantois, comes into contact with the overlying trophoblast layer. Since the yolk sac develops earlier than the allantois, the choriovitelline placenta precedes the chorioallantoic placenta. In early gestation, both placental types coexist temporarily, but the choriovitelline placenta regresses as the exocoelom and allantois expand, separating the yolk sac from the chorion. The chorioallantoic placenta remains and assumes pivotal functions for most of the pregnancy duration.

Choriovitelline Placenta

The **choriovitelline**, or **yolk sac placenta**, is formed when the yolk sac wall (composed of endoderm plus extraembryonic splanchnopleure) associates with the chorion, establishing contacts with the endometrium (see Fig. 15-1). This placenta may be fully or partially vascularized by the vitelline plexus, which connects with the omphalomesenteric vein and supplies blood to the developing heart. Blood returns from the embryo to the vitelline circulation in the yolk sac via the omphalomesenteric artery, which branches from the dorsal aorta.

In sows and ruminants, the chorion, along with the underlying yolk sac wall, simply apposes to the uterine luminal epithelium. In these animals, the yolk sac begins to involute 3 to 4 weeks after conception. However, in carnivores and mares, the yolk sac undergoes more significant development in the early stages and persists throughout gestation. A temporary lamellar choriovitelline placenta, characterized by multiple folds in the chorion, also develops in carnivores. Despite these variations, the choriovitelline placenta remains of minor importance in physiological fetal–maternal exchange in all domestic animals.

Chorioallantoic Placenta

The expanding allantois, upon contact with the chorion, forms the **allantochorion**. The **chorioallantoic placenta** (see Fig. 15-1) results from the attachment of the allantochorion to the endometrium. This placenta is very well vascularized by umbilical arteries, which run along the urinary bladder and the urachus in the fetus. The pathway of these arteries indicates that the vasculature is originally allantoic, even in species like humans, where an allantoic cavity is not well developed. Structural variations in this type of placenta occur among the different species, dictated by the organization of its layers and cell types.

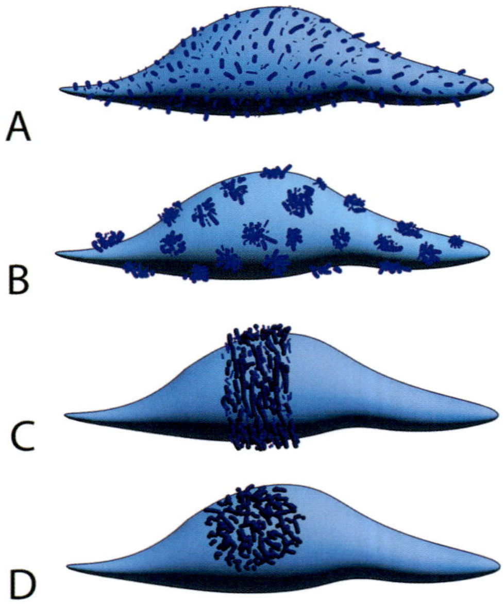

Figure 15-2 Schematic drawings of the chorionic sac to illustrate the macroscopic placental shapes. **A. Diffuse placenta:** The frondose chorion forms small villi or folds, which cover most of the surface of the chorionic sac. This type is found in pigs, equids, and camelids. **B. Cotyledonary placenta (placenta multiplex):** In ruminants, the frondose chorion is concentrated in tufts of chorionic villi (cotyledons), which attach to preformed areas of the endometrium (caruncles). A cotyledon, together with a caruncle, forms a placentome. The intercaruncular surface of the endometrium is covered by the smooth chorion (chorion leave). **C. Zonary placenta:** The frondose chorion forms a band or girdle around the equator of the chorionic sac. Outside this band, the smooth chorion is attached to the endometrium. This placental shape is present in dogs and cats. **D. Discoid placenta:** The frondose chorion forms a disc-shaped area, surrounded by the chorion leave. This type is found in humans and in many rodents and lagomorphs (rabbits and hares).

Macroscopic Structure of the Placenta

Regions where the chorion forms extensive surface area enlargements by developing folds, villi, or lamellae (exchange areas) are called **frondose chorion** (*chorion frondosum*). The remaining chorion, if present, without such projections is referred to as the **smooth chorion** (*chorion laeve*). The macroscopical classification is based on the shape and distribution of the frondose chorion and its uterine counterpart. Types such as **diffuse**, **cotyledonary**, **zonary**, and **discoid** can be differentiated (Fig. 15-2).

Three-Dimensional Arrangement of the Chorion and Endometrium

One adaptation to meet the increasing fetal demands during pregnancy is the expansion of the contact area between the frondose chorion and the endometrium, which is reflected in different shapes of the fetal–maternal contact area.

Folded Placenta

The frondose chorion develops vascularized macroscopic folds (**plicae**) of varying magnitudes and microscopic ridges (**rugae**) of different heights. These folds are attached to the corresponding shapes on the endometrium. This type of placenta is found in **sows**.

Villous Placenta

The villi of the frondose chorion can be simple (fingerlike) or may form larger branched (treelike) structures. The distribution of the villi can be concentrated in specific regions (cotyledons in **ruminants**), or more diffuse, as seen in **camelids** and **equids**. These villi fit into corresponding crypts of the endometrium. **Humans** have a chorionic villous tree extending into the maternal intervillous blood space.

Lamellar Placentation

The trophoblast of the allantochorion forms leaflike lamellar sheets, which envelop the endothelium of maternal endometrial blood vessels (seen in **carnivores**). In **rodents** and **lagomorphs**, these lamellae form trophoblast-lined vascular channels filled with maternal blood.

Microscopic Structure of the Interhemal Barrier

In the placenta, fetal and maternal blood circulate in distinct blood vessels, separated by fetal and maternal tissue layers forming the interhemal barrier. This structure can be reduced to enable the hemotrophic maternal–fetal transfer of substances, with a consequent reduction in the distance between fetal and maternal vessels. In general, the number of maternal tissue layers may be reduced, while the fetal layers (vascular endothelium, connective tissue (CT), and trophoblast) remain present in all placental types. The extent of maternal tissue reduction depends on the grade of trophoblast invasiveness, which varies among different species.

Epitheliochorial Placenta (Placenta Epitheliochorialis)

In this type of placenta (Fig. 15-3A), the trophoblast is noninvasive. All three fetal layers (endothelium, CT, and trophoblast) and three maternal layers (endothelium, CT, and uterine epithelium) are present. Microvilli increase the contact surface area between the trophoblast and the uterine epithelium from both sides, which interdigitate. The CT might be vastly reduced on both sides, with only the vascular and epithelial basement membranes remaining. This type of placenta occurs in **sows**, **mares**, and **camelids**.

Synepitheliochorial Placenta (Placenta Synepitheliochorialis)

This type (Fig. 15-3B) shares many similarities with the simple epitheliochorial type. However, in this variant, specialized trophoblast cells—known as binucleated trophoblast cells—show limited invasiveness. These cells migrate toward the endometrial surface epithelium and fuse with maternal epithelial cells. As a result, the uterine epithelium partially consists of cells of mixed fetal and maternal origin. This placenta type is present in **ruminants**.

Endotheliochorial Placenta (Placenta Endotheliochorialis)

In this type (Fig. 15-3C), the trophoblast is invasive. The endometrial surface epithelium is absent and the underlying maternal CT is vastly reduced, essentially leaving only the endothelium to separate the maternal blood from the trophoblast. This type of placenta is present in **dogs** and **cats**.

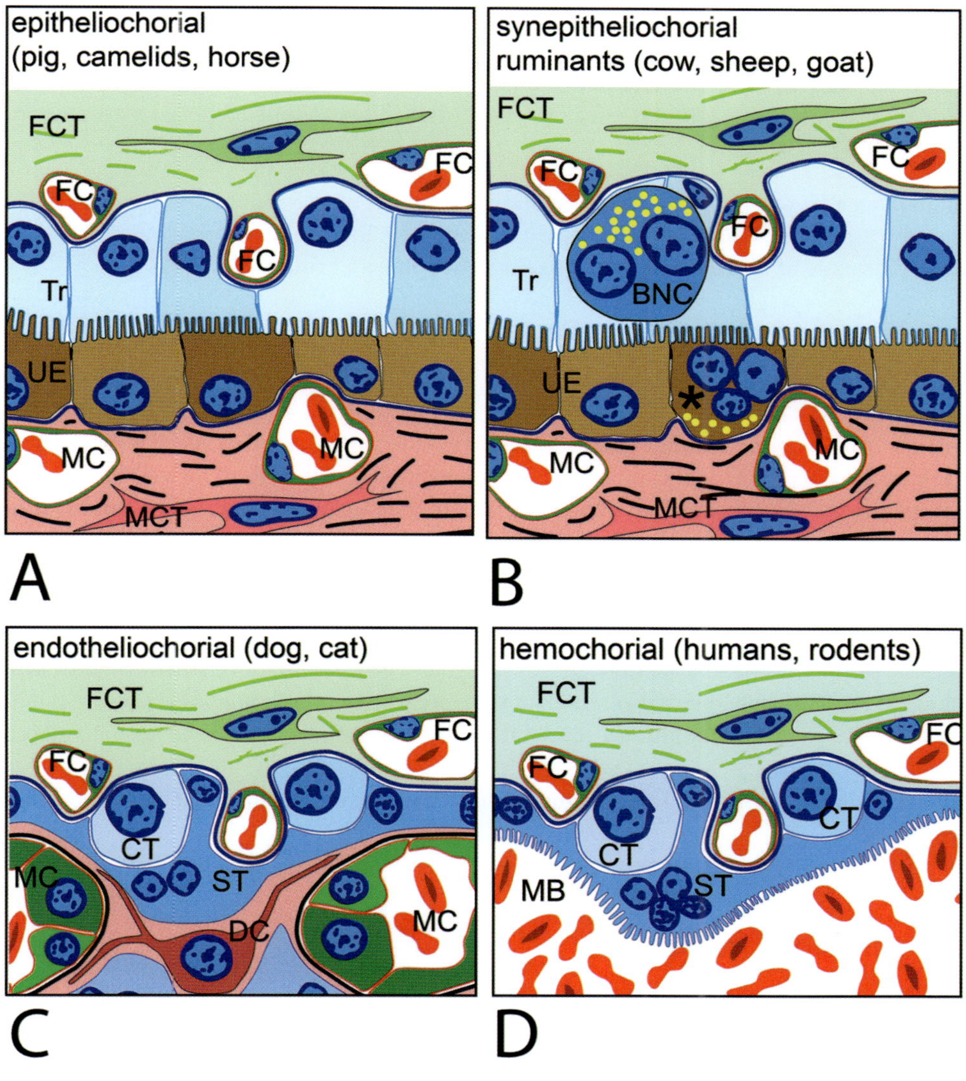

Figure 15-3 Schematic drawings of the tissue layers at the feto-maternal interface. **A.** In the epitheliochorial placenta, the trophoblast (Tr, blue) is connected to the uterine epithelium (UE, brown) by interdigitating microvilli. **B.** The term "synepitheliochorial" primarily indicates an epitheliochorial placenta, where the term "syn" points toward the fusion of specific binucleate trophoblast cells (BNCs) with uterine epithelial cells. In cows, this fusion leads to the formation of trinucleate cells (asterisk), which contain two fetal nuclei and one maternal nucleus. **C.** In the endotheliochorial placenta, cytotrophoblast cells (CTs) proliferate and fuse to generate the multinucleated syncytiotrophoblast (ST), which contacts maternal capillaries (MCs) with a high endothelium (dark green) and a thickened basement membrane (interstitial layer, pink). Modified maternal fibroblast cells (decidual cells [DCs]) are embedded in this interstitial layer. **D.** In the hemochorial placenta, the syncytiotrophoblast (ST) directly contacts maternal blood (MB). FCT, fetal connective tissue (CT); FC, fetal capillary; Tr, trophoblast; BNC, binucleate (trophoblast) cell; CT, cytotrophoblast; ST, syncytiotrophoblast; UE, uterine epithelium; MC, maternal capillary; MCT, maternal CT; DC, decidual cell; MB, maternal blood.

Hemochorial Placenta (Placenta Hemochorialis)

The trophoblast invades the endometrium, causing the opening of maternal endometrial blood vessels. As a result, all three maternal layers are absent, and the chorion is exposed to maternal blood (Fig. 15-3D). This type of placenta is present in **humans**, **rodents**, and **lagomorphs**.

Shedding of Maternal Tissues at Birth

At birth, the complete placenta, or part of it, will be released as the afterbirth. The depth at which the afterbirth separates from the maternal tissues remaining in the womb depends on the trophoblast invasiveness and the anchoring type of fetal tissues on the endometrium. Based on this, two types of placentation are recognized: nondeciduate and deciduate.

Nondeciduate Placentae

Here, the separation happens in the fetal–maternal contact area, and no or very little maternal tissue is shed during the delivery. Nondeciduate placentation is found in the epitheliochorial and synepitheliochorial placentation of **ungulates**.

Deciduate Placentae

This type is found in placentae with an invasive trophoblast, where part of the endometrial stroma undergoes transdifferentiation to form a new tissue—**the decidua**. The decidua is shed with the fetal membranes after parturition. Examples of this type include the placentae of **carnivores**, **humans**, **lagomorphs**, and **rodents**.

Nourishment of the Embryo

The primary function of the chorioallantoic placenta is to provide an efficient molecular exchange surface between maternal and fetal blood to obtain nutrients and oxygen for the embryo and to discard toxic metabolites and CO_2.

Depending on the source of the substances that nourish the embryo, they receive different names. Substances made up of fluids and secretions from maternal tissues or cellular debris that nourish the mammalian embryo are collectively called **embryotrophs**. When the embryotroph is obtained from maternal blood, it is called **hemotroph**; when it comes from uterine glandular secretions or cellular fragments, it is called **histotroph**. Regardless of the origin of the embryotroph, it is always captured and absorbed by the trophoblast.

The histotroph is the primary nutritional source of the embryo before implantation. This substance is present in areolae (specialized exchange areas of the fetal placenta), which appear as chorion indentations aligned with openings of the endometrial glands. Areolae are found in the diffuse placenta of sows, camelids, and mares or the smooth chorion of the cotyledonary placentae of ruminants.

After implantation, the embryo is nourished by hemotrophs, which are metabolites that cross the placental barrier from the maternal circulation.

Placental Vascularity and Circulation

Fetal and maternal blood circulatory systems in epitheliochorial and endotheliochorial placentae are completely separated by maternal and fetal tissues. The tissues that separate the fetal and maternal capillaries are collectively referred to as the *interhemal barrier*. However, the number of layers in this barrier depends on the species (see Fig. 15-3). In these placentae, maternal blood is contained within the uterine capillaries, so that the placental barrier includes not only the fetal vessels and trophoblast but also the endothelium of the maternal vessels.

On the contrary, in hemochorial placentae, the uterine vessels are absent from the placental barrier, so maternal blood flows through trophoblast-lined channels or in intervillous spaces (lacunae) and makes direct contact with the chorion. In this case, the placental barrier reaches its lowest number of layers. However, regardless of the type of chorioallantoic placentation, trophoblast and fetal endothelium are always present in the placental interhemal barrier (see Fig. 15-3).

In carnivores and ruminants, deposits of extravasated maternal blood are also found between the endometrial epithelium and the trophoblast (see section on Dog and Cat placenta). These deposits are called **hematomas** and result from ruptured uterine vessels due to local degeneration of the endometrial tissue. Phagocytosis by adjacent trophoblast cells, mainly of red blood cells, is observed in these areas, raising the possibility of these regions being involved in iron transfer from mother to fetus.

The chorion's capillaries have smaller lumens than the maternal capillaries, are partially fenestrated, and are surrounded by basal laminae.

The endometrial arterial vessels that reach the maternal–fetal interface are branches of the uterine artery, making anastomoses with branches of ovarian and vaginal vessels. The blood is drained back to the maternal systemic circulation via uterine veins. The arteries become dilated during pregnancy, and their placental capillary network develops into a species-specific architecture that reflects the internal three-dimensional structure of the placenta.

Fetal placental vessels absorb oxygen and nutrients from the maternal circulation and release toxic products for metabolism, such as urea and uric acid. In the choriovitelline placenta (when present), deoxygenated blood arrives through the omphalomesenteric arteries, while oxygenated blood returns to the heart through the omphalomesenteric veins. In the chorioallantoic placenta, deoxygenated and nutrient-depleted fetal blood reaches the placenta through the umbilical artery and returns, after molecular exchanges, to the fetal systemic circulation via the umbilical vein.

Specialized Cells of the Placenta

In the endotheliochorial placenta of carnivores and always in hemochorial placentae, changes can occur in the endometrial stroma in contact with the invasive trophoblast. In these placentae, endometrial fibroblasts undergo a transdifferentiation process and generate specialized **decidual cells** (see Fig. 15-3C, 15-16C and E). These cells exhibit new morphology (becoming large and rounded or polyhedral) and content (lipid and glycogen), and assume immune and endocrine functions (hormones, cytokines, and growth factors). In pigs and ruminants, subepithelial endometrial fibroblasts differentiate into contractile **myofibroblasts**.

Migration or redistribution of immune cells in the endometrium is also part of the maternal tissue adaptation to gestation. Although these cells are most studied in human and rodent placentae, where migration of macrophages, uterine natural killer cells, and specific subpopulations of lymphocytes is observed, changes in the distribution and activity of these immune cell populations are also observed in epitheliochorial and endotheliochorial placentae. These cells perform functions closely related to gestational immunoregulation and defense against pathogens in the placental area.

At the fetal side of the placenta, the trophoblast primarily performs chorionic functions, such as gas exchange, absorption of nutrients, excretion of metabolites, secretion of hormones (equine chorionic gonadotropin, progestogens, estrogens, etc.) and signaling molecules, induction of angiogenesis (vessel formation), defense and immunoregulation. Specialized trophoblastic cell types differentiate from the simple layer lining the blastocyst, varying in morphology, density, and functions across different species. These characteristics may also vary throughout gestation, reflecting changes in placental activity over time.

Trophoblast cells can exist as layers of individualized cells called **cytotrophoblast cells** (see Fig. 15-3). Binucleate trophoblast cells (BNCs) (Fig 15-3B) are generated from cytotrophoblast by acytokinetic mitoses (mitoses without subsequent cell division) in ruminants and mares. Cytotrophoblast cells can also fuse to form a syncytial layer—the **syncytiotrophoblast** (Figs. 15-3C and D, 15-16B, C, and E). These cell fusions are facilitated by syncytins, which were originally viral envelope proteins that have been integrated into the mammalian genome (see the Box about syncytins). In addition, cytotrophoblast cells can differentiate into either diploid cells with proliferative activity or polyploid cells. For example, in the placenta of rodents, these cells can reach a ploidy level of 512C, indicating the presence of 512 sets of chromosomes, accomplished without the need for replication.

Cytotrophoblasts and the syncytiotrophoblast may coexist as two-layered membranes in carnivores and humans (Figs. 15-3C and D). In these arrangements, the development of the syncytial form depends on the source of cytotrophoblast cells for fusion and is more differentiated in terms of organelle development.

The presence of binuclear or multinuclear trophoblastic cells correlates with the increasing invasion of the endometrium. In the placentae of ruminants and mares, only the binucleate cells, and not the uninuclear cytotrophoblast, show some invasiveness. This invasion is relatively low compared to the significant endometrial invasion seen with the syncytiotrophoblast in carnivores, rodents, and primates.

Syncytins: The Endogenous Retrovirus-Encoded Envelope Proteins That Altered the Course of Reproduction in Mammals

Viruses that insert their genetic material into the host's genome are called retroviruses, and when they infect germline cells, they can be transmitted to subsequent generations. The incorporated viral DNA fragments are called endogenous retroviruses (ERVs). A significant fraction of our genomic DNA (8% in humans and 12% in cattle) consists of these ERVs, some incorporated more than 100 million years ago. During the infectious process, virus envelope proteins fuse the virus to the host cell membrane. The placenta of many mammals expresses the genes of such envelope proteins, now called "syncytins." Their fusion capacity was co-opted by the placenta for processes such as the fusion of cytotrophoblast into syncytiotrophoblast. Different retroviruses have infected mammals repeatedly throughout evolutionary history, which explains why different groups of mammals often have different placental syncytins. These findings have raised the hypothesis that morphological variations in placentae in different species may have resulted from incorporating different ERVs and expressing different syncytins. The expression of placental syncytins is an example of convergent evolution via the co-option of a retroviral gene for critical biological functions in reproductive biology.

Changes During Placentation

The placenta is a dynamic organ that continually changes size, shape, and internal structure throughout gestation. It grows rapidly during its initial development after implantation, gradually decreasing growth rates in later phases. Depending on the placental type, it may undergo minor involution before term. Rearrangements at the cellular level are reflected in the balance between apoptosis (regulated cell death) and mitotic activity. In addition, the physical barrier between the maternal and fetal circulatory systems may also change with time, undergoing progressive attenuation (for details, see the "Function–Structure Relationships" section below).

Function–Structure Relationships

Transport through the placenta occurs either by diffusion or some type of active or facilitated transport. Structural differences in the various placental types do not necessarily indicate differences in this function. The transfer mechanism of respiratory gases (i.e., oxygen and carbon dioxide) is primarily simple diffusion in all placental types. However, the rates at which gas molecules cross the placental barrier can vary depending on the number of cell layers separating maternal and fetal blood. Therefore, the interhemal distance is of major importance for both diffusion and active transport. In placentae containing several layers (such as epitheliochorial placentae), strategically positioned capillaries from both fetal and uterine sides approach and indent the respective epithelia (see Fig. 15-3). Consequently, despite variations in the number of layers in the interhemal barrier, the diffusion barrier thins to 2 μm, which is similar across species.

To traverse a cell (or syncytium), a substance must pass both the apical and basal plasma membranes and rely on mechanisms within these membranes that facilitate this transfer, such as receptors and other transport mechanisms. In the placenta, the membranes regulate the cellular uptake and transfer of nutrients and export unusable metabolic components. Therefore, the selective barrier and transport function of the placenta critically depend on the number and activity of the plasma membranes that need to be traversed.

A directional preference from mother to fetus generally exists for essential inorganic elements (e.g., calcium, phosphorus, iodine, and iron). This characteristic is especially true for iron, as no retrograde iron transfer occurs from fetus to mother. In different species, however, iron transfer takes place through different mechanisms. In carnivores, and to a lesser extent in ruminants, iron is absorbed from blood hemoglobin in maternal hemorrhages adjacent to the trophoblast (phagocytosis). In sows and mares, and to some extent in ruminants, the source of iron is a glycoprotein complex secreted by the endometrial glands. In hemochorial placentation, the trophoblast takes up iron from circulating maternal transferrin. Calcium is also transferred in different regions of the fetal membranes, depending on the species. In sows, transfer occurs across the folded interhemal barrier of the interareolar area. In contrast, in cows, it occurs at the intercotyledonary region, and in mares, across the areolar-gland complexes.

The transfer of nutritional factors, such as fatty acids and keto acids, depends on the expression and density of transporters to facilitate their uptake, which can vary across placental types. These molecules rapidly cross the hemochorial placenta (found in rodents, rabbits, and primates), whereas uptake in epitheliochorial placentae (typical of ruminants, pigs, and horses) is efficient but slow.

Fetal erythrocyte differentiation is temporally and anatomically regulated, as are the types of hemoglobin. The earliest (nucleated) erythrocytes originate from the yolk sac mesoderm and contain embryonic hemoglobin. Later in intrauterine life, erythrocytes differentiate in hepatic and splenic tissues and carry fetal hemoglobin. Near the time of birth, this differentiation occurs in the bone marrow with a gradual transition to adult hemoglobin expression. Embryonic and fetal hemoglobins have a higher affinity for oxygen than adult hemoglobin, allowing them to extract oxygen more efficiently across the placental barrier. This difference is an adaptation for intrauterine life with low oxygen pressure.

Placental tissues show a very high degree of expression of various genes. The trophoblast secretes hormones, such as chorionic gonadotropin (in mares), placental lactogen (in ruminants), estrogens, and progesterone. Throughout pregnancy, the placenta also produces a broad spectrum of other factors for regulating metabolic activity, growth, and structural changes (paracrine factors). These factors are expressed differently among species to regulate gestation and ensure successful placentation (more in Clinical Correlations below).

Species Differences

The beginning of placentation and the length of pregnancy differs considerably between species. A brief summary is given in Table 15-1.

Pig

The chorioallantoic placenta is diffuse, folded, epitheliochorial, and nondeciduate (Fig. 15-4). The elongated chorionic sacs of the multiple fetuses adhere to the endometrium over their entire area, except at the avascular extremities and over the uterine gland openings, where areolae form at the opening of the endometrial glands (Fig. 15-5).

The blastocysts undergo a very rapid elongation, changing from spheres of 5 mm diameter on day 10 to threads of 1 m in length by day 13. They migrate and distribute evenly across both uterine horns. The trophoblast secretes estrogen, which serves as the signal for maternal recognition of pregnancy. A minimum of four blastocysts is required for successful signaling and the establishment of pregnancy. The blastocyst attaches to the uterine epithelium on days 13 to 14, and interdigitation of fetal and maternal microvilli starts on day 15.

With the progression of pregnancy, the feto-maternal contact area enlarges and becomes more complex. The endometrium, along with the chorion, forms macroscopic circular folds (plicae), which are orientated perpendicular to the long axis of the long tubular uterine horns. At a microscopic level, the endometrium and chorion form small folds (rugae) which intertwine (Fig. 15-6A). In late pregnancy, short bullous villi form on the chorionic rugae.

The chorionic surface of the rugae can be divided into two types. The ridges and flanks of the chorionic rugae are the locations for hemotrophic transfer. The trophoblast cells are cuboidal, and the fetal capillaries deeply indent between the cells (Fig. 15-6B). With increasing gestational age, this indentation becomes deeper, reducing the distance between fetal and maternal blood vessels to about 2 μm. At the ultrastructural level, the contact surface is further enlarged by interdigitating microvilli (Fig. 15-6C).

Table 15-1 Implantation and Gestation in Domestic Animals

	Beginning of Implantation (days)	Gestation Time (days)
Dog	17–18	58–63
Cat	12.5–14	63–65
Horse	35–40	329–345
Pig	13–14	112–115
Alpaca/llama	22–30	340–350
Dromedary/Bactrian camel	12–13	350–410
Cow	16–18	279–285
Sheep/goat	15–20	144–152

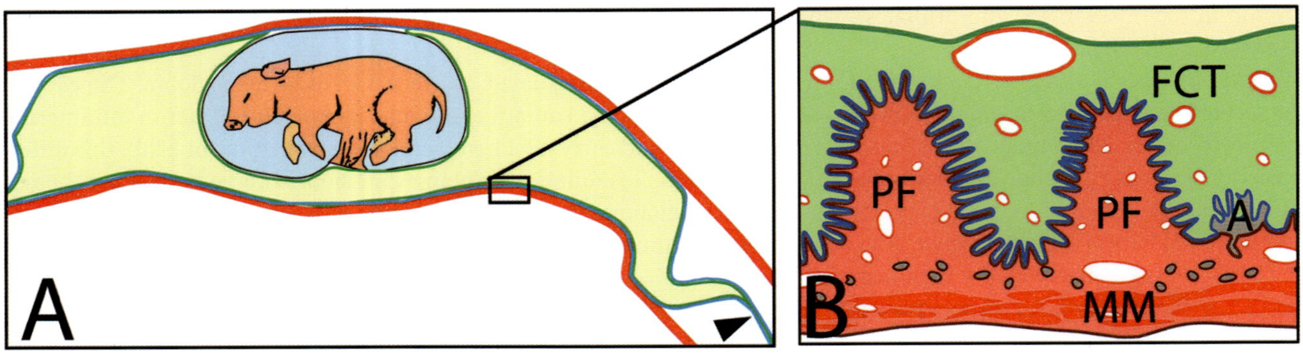

Figure 15-4 Schematic drawing of the porcine placenta. **A.** The fetus is embedded in the amniotic cavity (blue), surrounded by the allantoic cavity (yellow). The tips of the chorionic sac (arrowhead) are not vascularized. The region within the small rectangle is magnified in panel B. **B.** Two primary folds (PFs) of the endometrium are shown, covered by secondary folds/rugae. An areola (A) is shown on the right side of the drawing. FCT, fetal connective tissue; MM, myometrium. The blue line represents trophoblast, and underneath it, the brown line depicts maternal epithelia.

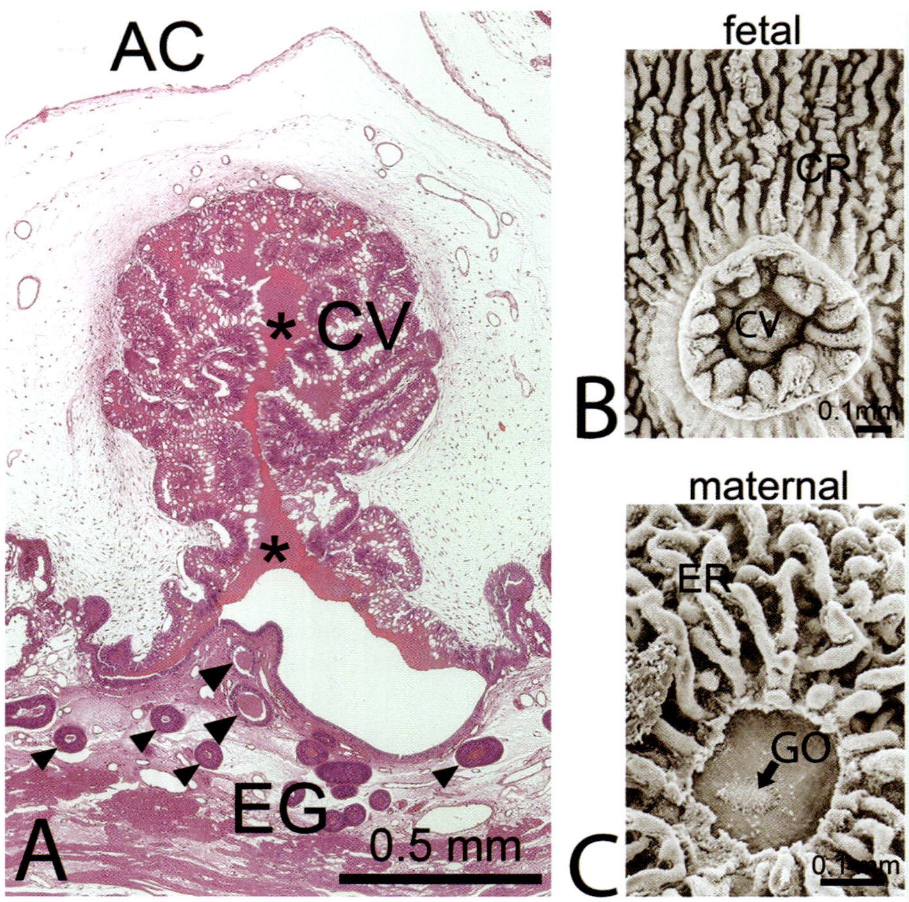

Figure 15-5 Structure of areola in the porcine placenta. **A.** Hematoxylin and eosin (H&E)-stained section showing folded chorionic villi (CV) protruding toward the lumen of the areola, which is partially filled with uterine milk (asterisks). On the fetal side (top) the areola is adjacent to the allantoic cavity (AC). In the endometrium, several uterine glands and excretory ducts (small and large arrowheads, respectively) are visible. **B.** Scanning electron micrograph of the fetal areola, with chorionic villi (CV) visible inside the cavity. The chorionic rugae (CR) radiate from the areola, with long furrows (fossae) between them. **C.** Scanning electron micrograph of the maternal part of the areola, showing endometrial gland opening (GO) covered with glandular secretion. The maternal endometrial rugae (ER) fit into the furrows between fetal chorionic rugae. (B and C: From Dantzer V. Scanning electron microscopy of exposed surfaces of the porcine placenta. Acta Anat 1984;118:96.)

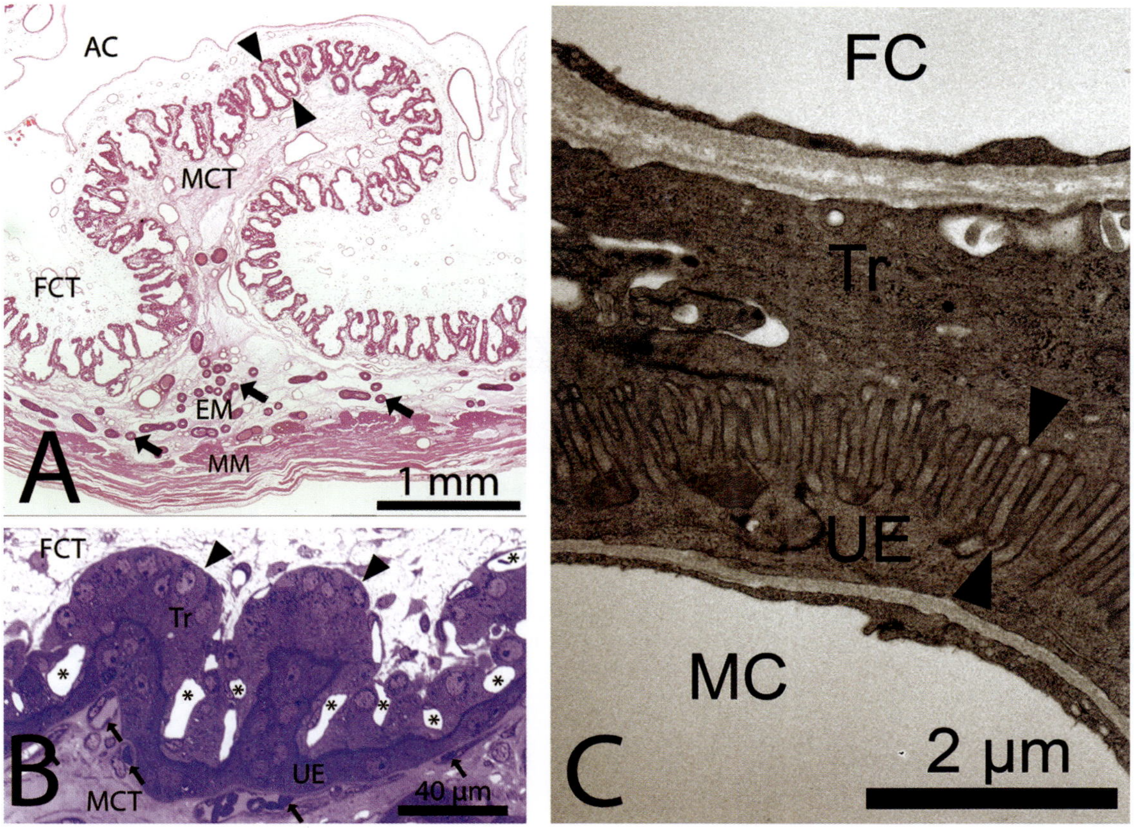

Figure 15-6 Structure of the feto-maternal interface in the pig. **A.** Longitudinal section (H&E-stained) of the uterine horn of a sow in mid-pregnancy. A primary fold (plica) of the endometrium has a core of maternal connective tissue (MCT) containing only a few uterine glands. Uterine glands (arrows) can be seen mainly in the deeper part of the endometrium (EM). The fetal connective tissue (FCT) has a very low content of fibers (compared to the MCT), which is indicated by the weak staining intensity. Trophoblast and uterine epithelium intertwine as secondary folds (rugae) (between arrowheads). MM, myometrium; AC, allantoic cavity. **B.** Early porcine placenta (methylene blue staining) shows fetal capillaries (asterisks) deeply indenting the trophoblast epithelium, while maternal capillaries (MCT, arrows) are less frequent. Two trophoblast (Tr) types can be differentiated. Fetal rugae tips and flanks are covered by trophoblast cells, separated by fetal capillaries. Troughs (fossae) between fetal rugae consist of columnar trophoblast cells (arrowheads) without capillary indentation. **C.** Transmission electron micrograph of the interhemal barrier in a late porcine placenta shows trophoblast (Tr) and uterine epithelium (UE) contact via interdigitating microvilli (between arrowheads). FC, fetal capillary; MC, maternal capillary.

At the troughs (fossae) at the bottom of the chorionic rugae, trophoblast cells are columnar. No indentation of capillaries occurs here, and the distance between fetal and maternal vessels ranges between 20 and 100 µm. These trophoblast cells are involved in hormone (steroid) production.

The areolae are macroscopically visible as small opalescent structures (Fig. 15-5). The lumen between the fetal and maternal surfaces is filled with histotroph (Fig. 15-5A), composed of secretory products and degenerating cell material. The chorion forms a sac with inwardly directed folds (Fig. 15-5B). At the endometrial surface, a small cup surrounds the openings of a uterine gland (Fig. 15-5C). The areolae are the main location for the transfer of iron from the mother to the fetus. The uterine glands secrete an iron-containing glycoprotein, uteroferrin, which is taken up by the areolar trophoblast. The areola–gland complexes also participate in the transfer of vitamin A (retinoids).

Camelids

The placenta of camelids is epitheliochorial, diffuse, villous, and nondeciduate (Fig. 15-7). In camels, the apposition phase starts 14 days after coitus (pc). More complex interactions are not observed until day 75 pc. From this stage onward, typical adhesion areas are observed, represented by the interdigitation between the microvilli of trophoblast and uterine epithelium.

In llamas and alpacas (camelids from the New World), embryo implantation begins around day 30 and 22 of gestation, respectively, with close microvilli interdigitation observed from day 45 onward.

Initially slightly undulating, this interface evolves with progressive trophoblast outgrowth that fits endometrial crypts. The chorion forms simple bullous villi, modified into more prominent tufts of ramified structures as pregnancy progresses (Fig. 15-8A). Areolae at the openings of the endometrial glands are very similar to those in pigs.

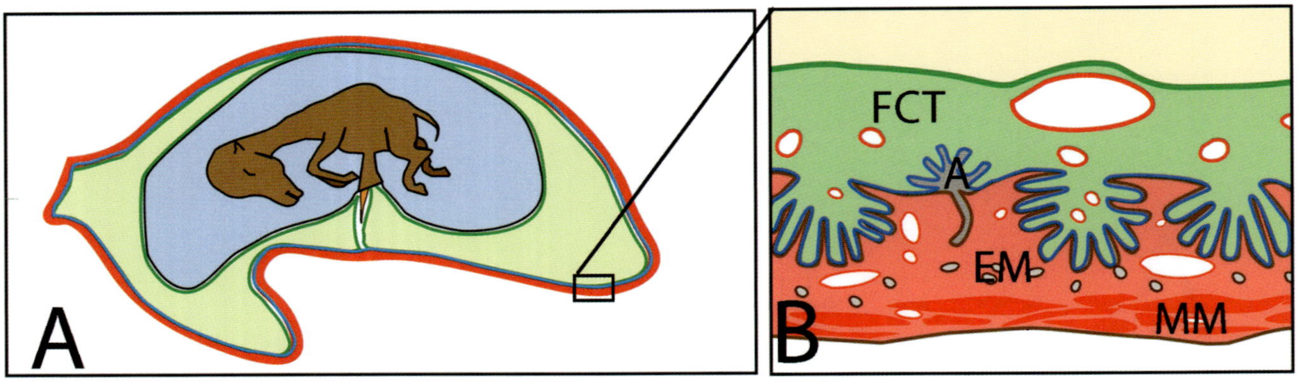

Figure 15-7 Schematic drawing of the camelid placenta. **A.** Overview of the camelid fetus with the fetal membranes (blue for amniotic cavity and yellow for allantoic cavity). **B.** Chorion forms tufts of simple villi, which intertwine with endometrium (EM). Areolae (A) resemble those of the pig. FCT, fetal connective tissue; MM, myometrium. The blue line represents trophoblast, and underneath, the brown line depicts maternal epithelia.

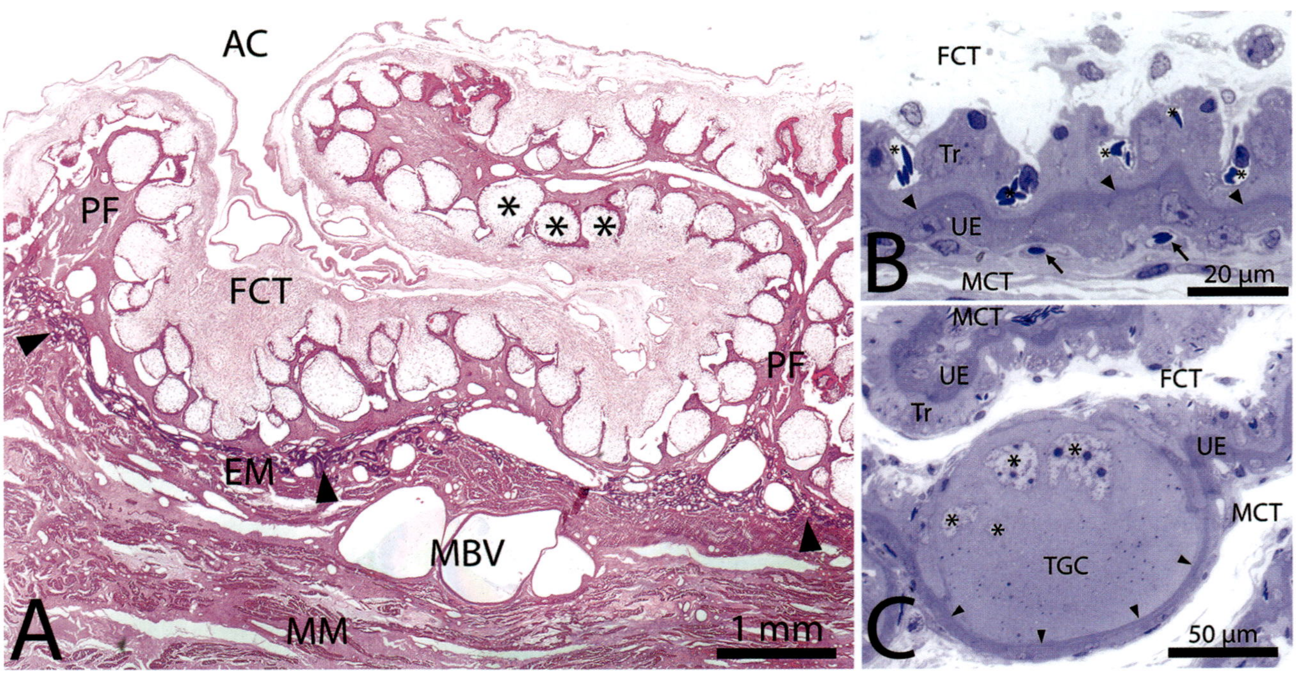

Figure 15-8 Structure of the camelid placenta. **A.** Low magnification image of a Dromedary (*Camelus dromedarius*) placenta in late pregnancy, stained with H&E. Uterine glands (arrowheads) and maternal blood vessels (MBVs) are visible in the endometrium (EM). Primary folds (PFs) of the endometrium enlarge the feto-maternal contact surface, which is further expanded by thin septae of maternal tissue, which separate bullous chorionic protrusions/villi (asterisks). AC, allantoic cavity; MM, myometrium; FCT, fetal connective tissue. **B.** Methylene blue staining of the feto-maternal interface of the alpaca (*Vicugna pacos*). Maternal connective tissue (MCT) shows capillaries (arrow) adjacent to uterine epithelium (UE). Fetal capillaries (asterisks) deeply indent between trophoblast cells (Tr). A vacuolated fetal macrophage (Hofbauer cell) can be seen in fetal connective tissue (FCT) at the upper right corner of the figure. **C.** Throughout pregnancy, large trophoblast giant cells (TGCs) containing highly lobulated nuclei (asterisks) are present. Nuclei are located in the basal part of the cell, adjacent to fetal connective tissue (FCT). The apical part (arrowheads) is covered by microvilli, which interdigitate with microvilli of the uterine epithelium (UE).

Two types of trophoblast cells are found, both participating in the formation of interdigitating microvilli with the uterine epithelium. Cuboidal trophoblast cells cover most of the chorionic surface (Fig. 15-8B). Fetal capillaries indent between these cells, facilitating the transfer of hemotroph. The second type is large trophoblast giant cells (Fig. 15-8C). The giant cells reach a diameter of up to 150 µm and have multiple highly lobulated nuclei. In their development, the cells undergo several rounds of mitoses without subsequent cell division (acytokinetic mitoses), resulting in a highly polyploid cell. The giant cells are predominantly located at the tip of the chorionic villi, and their frequency increases toward parturition. One of the functions of these cells is the production of steroid hormones.

The Epidermal Membrane in Pigs and Camelids

In camelids and pigs an additional fetal membrane, the nonvascularized epidermal membrane (epithelion) envelops the hairy parts of the body of near full-term fetuses, attaching to the fetus at mucocutaneous junctions, the coronary band, footpad, and umbilicus. This membrane is formed by sloughing of superficial skin layers and is composed of squamous epithelium. It likely helps to lubricate the fetus during parturition.

Horse/Donkey

The chorioallantoic placenta of the mare/jenny is diffuse, villous, epitheliochorial, and nondeciduate (Fig. 15-9). In early development, a large yolk sac is present with an essential area for fetal–maternal interchange, characterizing a yolk sac placenta. This placenta has an avascular part (bilaminar omphalopleure) and a part which forms the vascularized choriovitelline placenta (Fig. 15-10A). By the end of week 6, the vitelline circulation transitions to allantoic circulation in the placenta, while the yolk sac, though persisting until term, undergoes gradual involution.

The embryo emerges from the zona pellucida at days 8 to 9 and then becomes completely encapsulated in an acellular glycoprotein capsule, which persists until at least day 21. After a phase of intense migration within the uterine lumen, the equine blastocyst becomes fixed in position at approximately day 16. The conceptus thus remains spherical and unattached in the uterine lumen, held in place merely by a pronounced increase in uterine tone until day 50. The allantochorionic villi aggregate into tufts to form the **microcotyledons** only around day 60 (Fig. 15-11A).

At the junction of the developing allantochorion and the regressing yolk sac, the chorion forms an annulate **chorionic girdle** (Figs. 15-10A to C), consisting of projections of rapidly proliferating trophoblast. Between days 36 and 38, the trophoblast cells of the girdle become binucleate and begin to invade the endometrium through ameboid movements. They destroy the apposed uterine epithelium and implant themselves in the endometrial stroma, where they form **endometrial cups** (Fig. 15-10D). These cups range from a few millimeters to approximately 5 cm in diameter. The endometrial

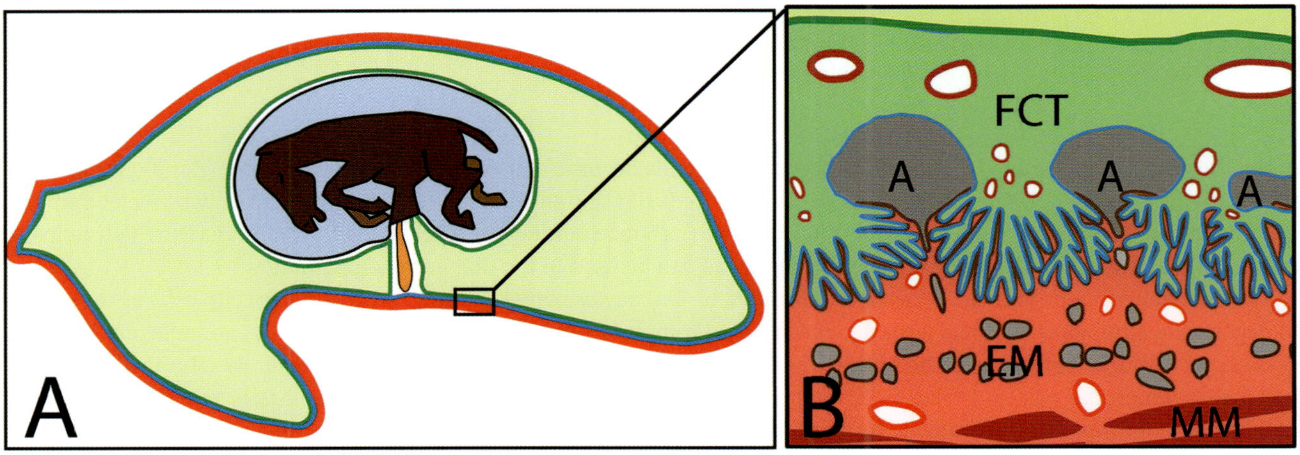

Figure 15-9 Schematic drawing of the equine placenta. **A.** Overview of the equine fetus with fetal membranes (blue for amniotic cavity and yellow for allantoic cavity). **B.** Chorion forms tufts of villi (microcotyledons), which intertwine with the endometrium (EM). Areolae (A) are located above gland openings between microcotyledons. FCT, fetal connective tissue; MM, myometrium. The blue line indicates fetal epithelia, and underneath areolae, the brown line depicts maternal epithelia.

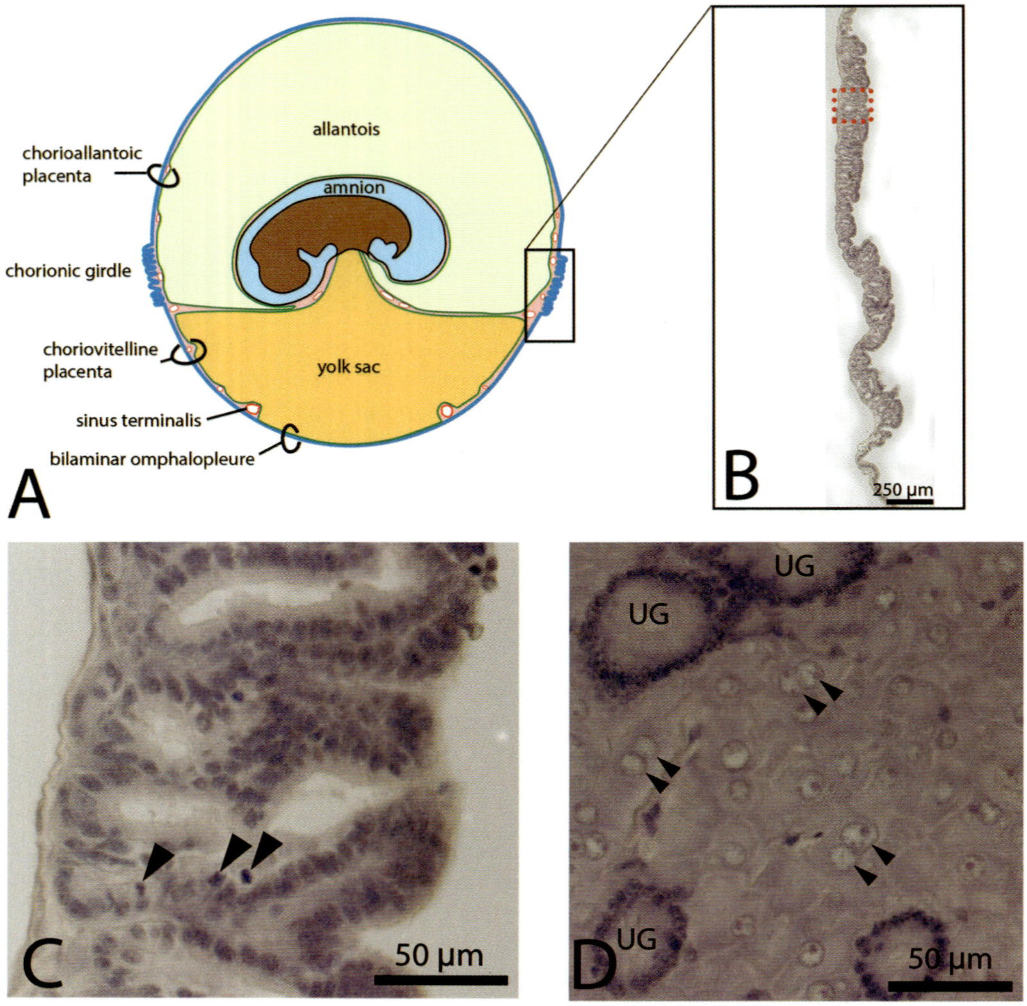

Figure 15-10 **A.** Schematic drawing of an equine conceptus. At the junction between the chorioallantoic and the choriovitelline placenta the chorion differentiates into the chorionic girdle. **B.** The chorionic girdle (gestation day 34) is thickened due to extensive chorion folding. The region marked by the red square is shown in panel C at a higher magnification. **C.** The chorionic girdle is characterized by a high proliferation rate, indicated by frequent mitotic figures (arrowheads). **D.** Endometrial cup (gestation day 45). The space between the uterine glands (UG) is filled with large invasive fetal trophoblast cells producing equine chorionic gonadotrophin. Many of these cells are binucleate (double arrowheads).

epithelium regenerates quickly, and the underlying cup cells become densely packed among uterine glands, supplied by the relatively sparse endometrial vasculature. The cup cells develop into large polyhedral cells with two nuclei and predominant rER. Cup cells act as an endocrine gland and produce equine chorionic gonadotropin (eCG), which helps to stabilize the hormonal function of the corpora lutea and can be used in the diagnosis of pregnancy.

The endometrial cups eventually become infiltrated by leukocytes, which invade and destroy the cup cells as they begin to degenerate after approximately 80 days of gestation. From days 120 to 150, the cellular remnants are rejected. This process aligns with the regression of the primary and secondary corpora lutea (which form concurrently with the cup formation), after which the placenta takes over the production of progestogens at a reduced level. After detachment from the uterine wall, the cups are encapsulated by chorionic folds and form allantochorionic pouches. Also, there are flattened oval bodies of disputed origin known as **hippomanes** that float freely in the allantoic fluid.

Fetal allantochorionic tufts (microcotyledons) and complementary maternal endometrial crypts begin to develop after the initiation of endometrial cups (between days 38 and 40). By approximately day 150, the typical microcotyledonary placenta has formed over the entire surface of the endometrium. The fetal tufts, with a dense capillary system and

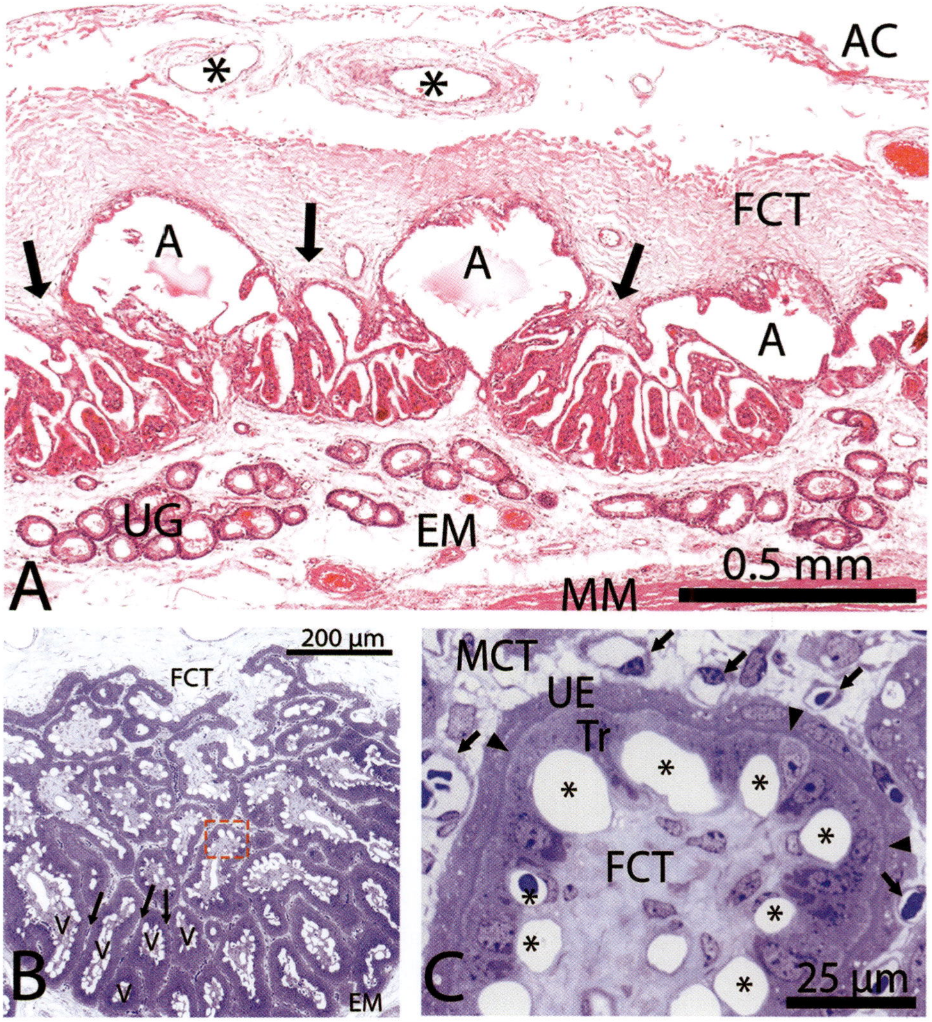

Figure 15-11 Structure of the horse placenta. **A.** H&E-stained section showing three microcotyledons (below arrows) extending into the endometrium (EM) with areolae (A) between them. In the fetal connective tissue (FCT), fetal blood vessels (asterisks) can be seen. AC, allantoic cavity; UG, uterine glands; MM, myometrium. **B.** A microcotyledon (methylene blue staining) shows chorionic villi (V), separated by septae (arrows) of the endometrium (EM). The highlighted central region (red rectangle) is shown at higher magnification in panel C. **C.** Fetal capillaries (asterisks) indent between trophoblast cells (Tr), while uterine epithelium (UE) contacts trophoblast via interdigitating microvilli (arrowheads). In the maternal connective tissue (MCT), maternal capillaries are labeled by arrows.

corresponding crypts, form placental units known as **microplacentomes** (Fig.15-11A). Positioned between these microplacentomes are the areola–gland complexes (Fig.15-11A), with the areolae surrounding the base of the fetal portion of the microplacentomes. Uterine glandular secretory products are released into the areolar cavity between endometrial epithelium and trophoblast cells covering the areolar villi; consequently, these epithelia are not in close contact. The transfer of iron and calcium from mother to fetus occurs in the areolar–gland complexes.

In the microcotyledons, the fetal villi consist of vascular mesenchyme covered with trophoblast (Figs. 15-11B and C). These villi fit into crypts lined with simple columnar uterine epithelium of varying heights. The crypts are separated by septa consisting of vascular uterine CT Indentations of capillaries into the trophoblast (Fig. 15-11C) and, to a lesser degree, into the maternal epithelium are seen in later pregnancy.

The apical surface of the trophoblast and uterine epithelial cells bear microvilli that interdigitate and form a dark border, as evident in both light and electron microscopy (Fig. 15-11C). In the later stages of gestation, preceding placental detachment after delivery, local apoptosis of the trophoblast and cryptal epithelium is indicated by dark-staining epithelial cytoplasm and the presence of cellular debris.

Ruminants

Ruminants (except the most basal phylogenetic branch, the chevrotains [Tragulidae]) have a cotyledonary placenta. This placental type can be further classified as polycotyledonary (with 80 to 120 placentomes in cows, sheep, and goats) and oligocotyledonary (with 4 to 12 placentomes in deer species). In the regions between the placentomes, the smooth chorion is loosely attached to the endometrial epithelium.

Cow

The chorioallantoic placenta is cotyledonary, villous, synepitheliochorial, and nondeciduate (Fig. 15-12). Initially, the yolk sac has a relatively large vascular area and forms a functional choriovitelline placenta. However, the yolk sac is rapidly outgrown by the allantois, and after 3 weeks, it begins to degenerate.

Implantation of the elongated blastocyst begins at day 18. Around day 21, the trophoblast layer develops papillae, which extend into the openings of uterine glands, possibly functioning as an anchor. The blastocyst extends equally into both uterine horns, and by day 27, an overall intimate contact between trophoblast cells and maternal epithelium is established through interdigitating microvilli. A firm fetal–maternal connection is initiated at days 32 to 34. Simple villi develop on areas of the chorionic sac in contact with elevated, convex structures of the maternal endometrium (**caruncles**), which lack uterine glands. The simple chorionic villi ramify and form **cotyledons**, projecting into crypts of the caruncle. Maternal blood vessels enter the caruncle through the caruncular stalk. Together, the fetal cotyledon and maternal caruncle form the mushroom-shaped **placentome** (Fig. 15-13A). During gestation, the placentomes grow to a diameter of about 10 cm and a height of about 4 cm. The number of formed placentomes is limited by the number of endometrial caruncles.

Amniotic plaques (Figs. 15-13A and C) are white/yellow irregular elevations of stratified ectodermal epithelium on the inner surface of the amnion. They typically have a diameter of a few millimeters and contain large quantities of glycogen.

The chorionic villi of the cotyledon consist of vascular mesenchyme covered with a simple layer of trophoblast cells (Fig. 15-13D). These trophoblast cells include columnar or irregularly shaped mononuclear cells and large binucleate cells (Fig. 15-13B). The **mononuclear cells** (Fig. 15-13E) have spherical or irregularly shaped nuclei with large nucleoli. In addition, these cells have sparse rER and relatively numerous apical mitochondria. **Binucleate trophoblast cells** (Figs. 15-13E and F) have spherical nuclei with conspicuous nucleoli, and their cytoplasm is voluminous. At the ultrastructural level (see Fig. 15-14C), the cell surface lacks microvilli. The cytoplasm contains a great diversity of organelles and inclusions. The Golgi complex is well developed, and the cells produce granules containing placental lactogen, prolactin-related proteins, and pregnancy-associated glycoproteins. In contrast to the mononuclear cells, giant cells show no morphologic evidence of absorption. Furthermore, these giant cells lack desmosomes and are mobile within the chorionic epithelium. They migrate toward the uterine epithelium, where they fuse with uterine epithelial cells to form trinucleate hybrid cells, thereby transferring hormone-containing granules from the fetal to the maternal

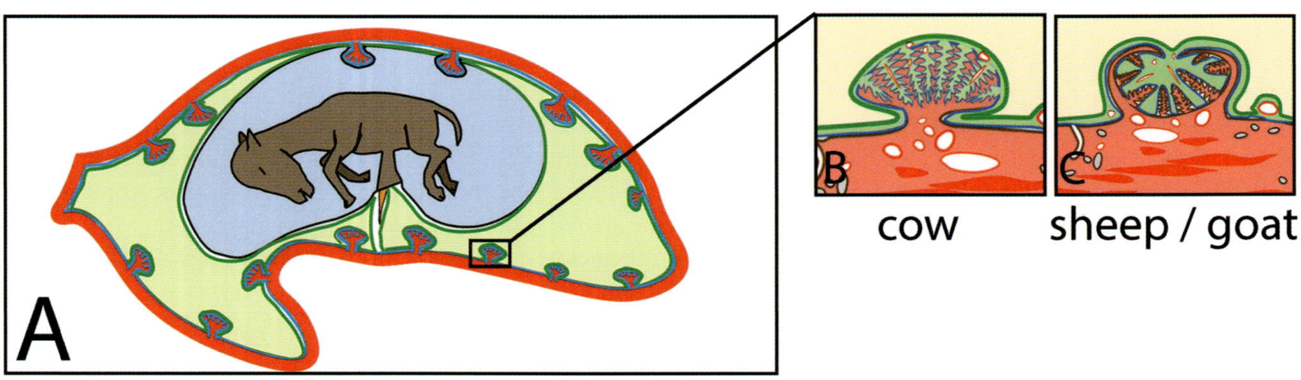

Figure 15-12 Schematic drawing of the ruminant placenta. **A.** Overview of ruminant fetus with the fetal membranes. Amniotic cavity (blue) and allantoic cavity (yellow). **B.** In cows, placentomes have a convex shape, each comprising fetal part (cotyledon) and maternal (caruncle) parts. Within the placentome, complex branched chorionic villi converge toward the base of the placentome. **C.** In small ruminants (sheep and goats), the shape of the placentomes is concave.

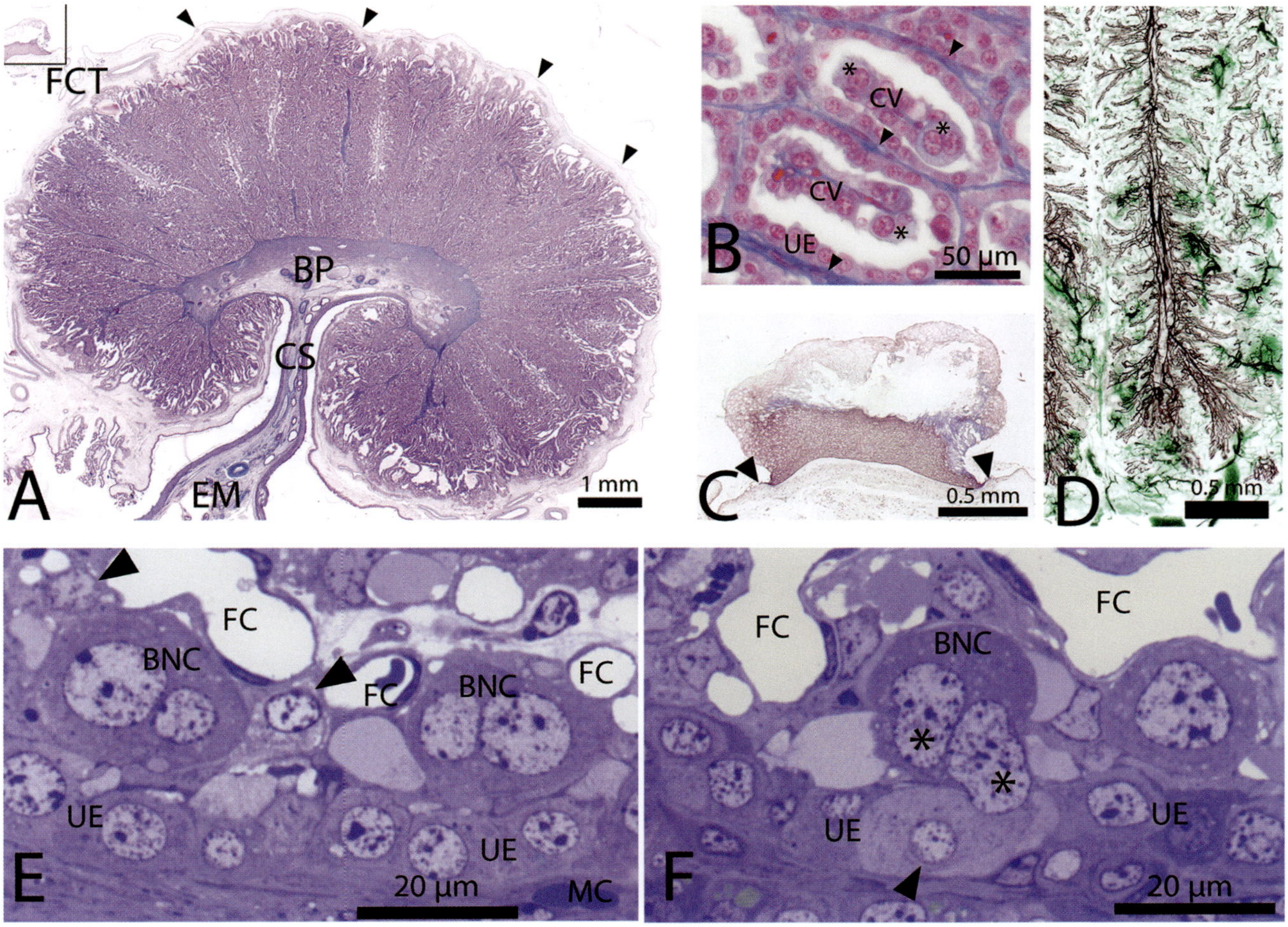

Figure 15-13 Structure of the bovine placenta. **A.** Bovine placentome (Azan staining). Convex surface is covered by amniochorion (arrowheads), with complex branched chorionic villi converging toward the center. The fetal part (cotyledon) and the maternal part (caruncle) are attached to the basal plate (BP), which is attached to the endometrium (EM) by the caruncular stalk (CS). The maternal tissue also forms crypts, which surround the fetal villi. One amniotic plaque (rectangle in the left upper corner) is shown in C at higher magnification. **B.** Section (Azan staining) from the inner placentome. Two shrunken chorionic villi (CV) are detached from the uterine epithelium (UE) at the feto-maternal contact zone, a typical artifact in formaldehyde-fixed paraffin-embedded tissues. Binucleate trophoblast cells (asterisks) are present within the chorionic villi. Maternal connective tissue (arrowheads) forms a net around the fetal villi. **C.** Amniotic plaque (magnified from panel A). Amniotic plaques are whitish regions on amniotic epithelium found in many species, where the epithelium abruptly changes (arrowheads) into a multilayered structure. **D.** Ink injection into the fetal (burgundy) and maternal (green) vasculature of a bovine placentome. One vertical stem villus is shown, from which the secondary villi branch. **E.** Semithin section (methylene blue staining). The trophoblast consists of two distinct cell types, uninucleate trophoblast (arrowheads) and binucleate trophoblast cells (BNCs). The uterine epithelium (UE) consists of individual cells. FC, fetal capillary; MC, maternal capillary. **F.** Semithin section (methylene blue staining). Fusion of a binucleate trophoblast cell (BNC) with a cell (arrowhead) of the uterine epithelium (UE). The two nuclei of the BNC (asterisks) are pushed into the uterine epithelial cell below, forming a trinucleate cell, with two fetal nuclei and one maternal nucleus. FC, fetal capillary.

compartment. Pregnancy-associated glycoproteins from these granules are detected in the blood or milk of cows for pregnancy diagnosis.

The maternal uterine epithelium of the caruncle is cuboidal or flattened (Figs. 15-13E and F). These cells have spherical nuclei with distinct nucleoli. Among them are cryptal giant cells with three or more nuclei, generated by hybridization with trophoblast binucleate cells. Most uterine epithelial cells also contain lipid inclusions in the infranuclear region.

The apical borders of the trophoblast and the cryptal epithelial cells have interdigitating microvilli, which are more irregular in cows than in mares or sows.

Hematomas develop at the convex side of the placentome between the fetal side of the caruncular crypt walls and the base of the chorionic villi. They form in the later part of gestation. Blood collects in the fetal tissues surrounding leaky vessels.

Erythrocytes are phagocytized by the trophoblast and broken down by lysosomes. Hemoglobin from the erythrocytes is digested, and iron is released. These areas may be subject to bacterial infections during pregnancy.

In the intercotyledonary area, a smooth chorion adheres to the endometrium, except over the glandular openings, where areolae are formed. The simple columnar cells of the trophoblast and the uterine epithelium have interlocking brush borders (microvilli). Interdigitations are tight during early pregnancy and become less pronounced as pregnancy advances. In the intercotyledonary area, BNCs are also frequent. After parturition, the chorionic villi are released from the crypts. This separation occurs between the interdigitating microvilli, leaving both the trophoblast and the uterine epithelium intact. Failure of this separation is a common problem in bovine reproduction (see the Box about retention of fetal membranes).

Sheep and Goat

The placentae of ewes and goats show many similarities to the bovine placenta but differ in some respects. Implantation begins at days 14 to 15, and the development of interdigitating microvilli between trophoblast cells and maternal epithelium occurs at days 16 to 18. Chorionic villi are seen from days 13 to 20. Grossly, the placentome has a concave surface (Figs. 15-12C and 15-14A). The placentome of goats is flatter than that of ewes but has a similar internal structure.

Microscopically, the chorionic villi are more irregular than those of the bovine placenta (Figs. 15-14A and B). The trophoblast layer also has uninucleate cells, giving rise to the typical ovoid binucleate cells. The cryptal lining mainly consists of multinucleated cell masses arranged as syncytial plaques (Fig. 15-14B), formed by subsequent fusions of BNCs (Fig. 15-14C) with the caruncular epithelium.

Hematomas are more pronounced and located in the central concave area of the placentome; they occur earlier than in cows. Amniotic plaques are also present in ewes.

Dog and Cat

The yolk sac forms a choriovitelline placenta, with trophoblastic villi invading eroded uterine mucosa. This transient lamellar placenta is initially extensive but eventually disappears. The yolk sac, however, persists until term.

The chorioallantoic placenta is zonary, lamellar, endotheliochorial, and deciduate (Fig. 15-16). Implantation occurs at day 17 in bitches and at day 13 in cats with the formation of gap junctions between the trophoblast and maternal epithelium. The frondose chorion and uterine capillaries form the **placental labyrinth** (lamellar zone), with tightly arranged **lamellae** (Figs. 15-15, and 16A-C), localized in a girdle around the equator of the chorionic sac. In the girdle, a **junctional zone** containing terminal parts of placental lamellae, maternal vessels, cell debris, and glandular secretions is located beneath the placental labyrinth (lamellar zone). The junctional zone is specifically enlarged in bitches and located adjacent to the dense CT of the **supraglandular layer** (Fig. 15-16A). The **glandular zone**, formed by the dilated lower parts of the uterine glands, lies just above the myometrium (Fig. 15-16A). In the late stages of gestation, the invasion into the glandular zone progresses almost to the deep part of the glands, where histotroph and cell debris accumulate. Remnants of the glandular zone are left at parturition. Outside the girdle, a chorion laeve is apposed to the uterine surface epithelium, and here the glandular development is restricted.

Hemorrhage of uterine blood within and at the fringe of the placental girdle gives rise to hematomas. In bitches, distinct **marginal hematomas** with large blood compartments are formed (Fig. 15-16A). In queens, smaller hemorrhages occur in irregular positions in the placental girdle and between the smooth chorion and endometrium along the girdle. The columnar trophoblast cells lining the compartments of the hematoma have phagocytic characteristics believed to be involved in the absorption of large molecules and iron from destroyed maternal erythrocytes. After the breakdown of the blood, the hematomas become brown (in queens) or green (uteroverdin in bitches) because of degradation of hemoglobin.

The fetal part of the placenta is composed of trophoblast-covered mesenchymal lamellae, which contain small thin-walled capillaries (Figs. 15-16B to E). In bitches, the lamellae are branched (Fig. 15-16B), whereas in queens, the lamellae are more regularly stacked (Fig. 15-16C). Relatively wide and thick-walled maternal capillaries are enclosed by trophoblast and surrounded by a mesh of fetal capillaries (Figs. 15-16B to D), giving a labyrinthine appearance in histologic sections. The maternal capillaries are surrounded by a thick layer of amorphous material, the **interstitial layer**, which is especially irregular in queens (Fig. 15-16C). Modified maternal endometrial fibroblasts, the giant decidual cells, form an incomplete layer around the maternal capillaries. These cells are very large and often binucleated in cats (Fig. 15-16C). In dogs, the decidual cells are less noticeable and have several cellular processes embedded in the interstitial layer (Fig. 15-16E).

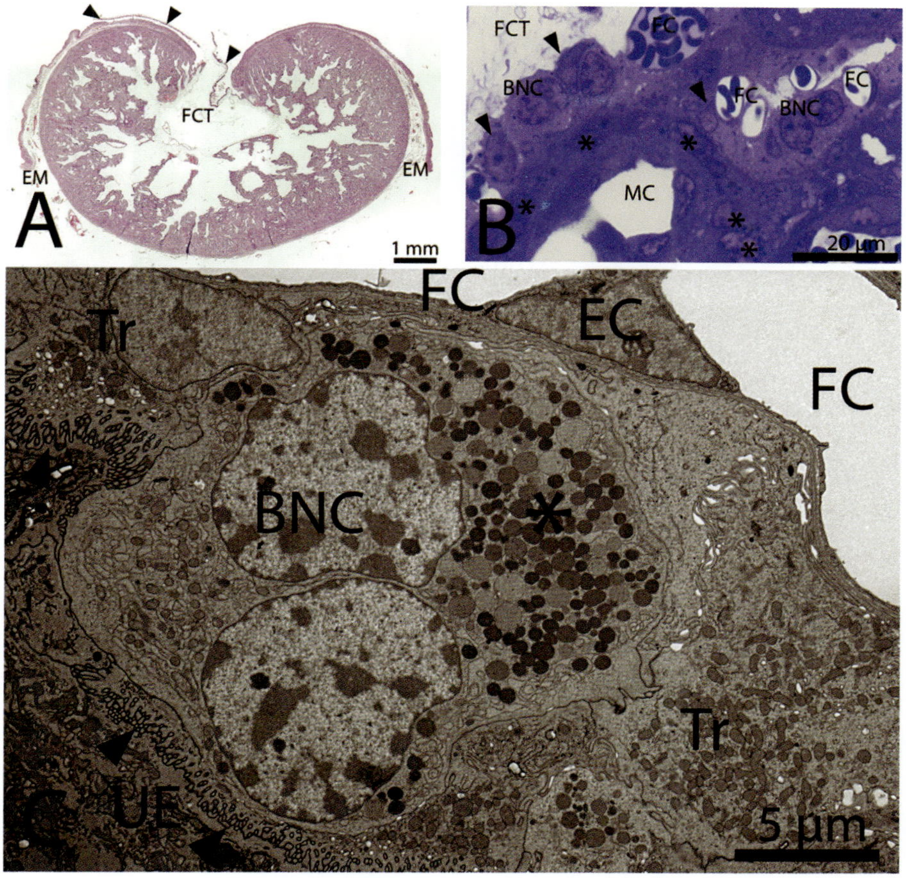

Figure 15-14 Structure of the ovine and caprine placenta. **A.** A caprine placentome shows a concave shape with allantochorion covering surface (partially visible, arrowheads), loosely attached to the endometrium (EM). **B.** Semithin section (methylene blue staining) shows caprine placentome with uninucleate trophoblast (arrowheads), binucleate trophoblast cell (BNC), and syncytial plaques in uterine epithelium, with multiple nuclei (asterisks). FCT, fetal connective tissue; FC, fetal capillary; MC, maternal capillary. **C.** Transmission electron micrograph of ovine placenta shows a binucleate trophoblast cell (BNC) surrounded by uninucleate trophoblast (Tr) cells. The BNC cytoplasm contains abundant secretory granules (asterisk), released into maternal CT after BNC fusion with uterine epithelium (UE). Feto-maternal contact area with interdigitating microvilli indicated by arrowheads. FC, fetal capillary; EC, endothelial cell.

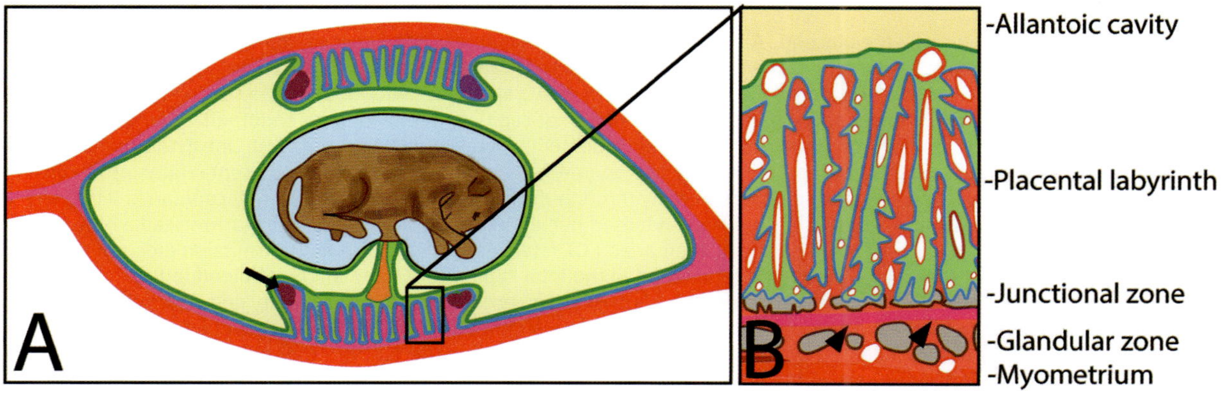

Figure 15-15 Schematic drawing of the carnivore (dog) placenta. **A.** The frondose chorion forms a circular girdle around the equator of the chorionic sac. The borders of the girdle show marginal hematomas (arrow), while the center mainly consists of the placental labyrinth (lamellar zone). Other chorion parts form the smooth chorion (chorion leave). **B.** In the placental labyrinth or lamellar zone, the lamellae of fetal (green and blue) and maternal (pink) tissue intertwine. In the junctional zone, the tips of the fetal lamellae protrude into superficial parts of the uterine glands. Placenta detaches at supraglandular layer (arrowheads) between the junctional and deep glandular zones during parturition.

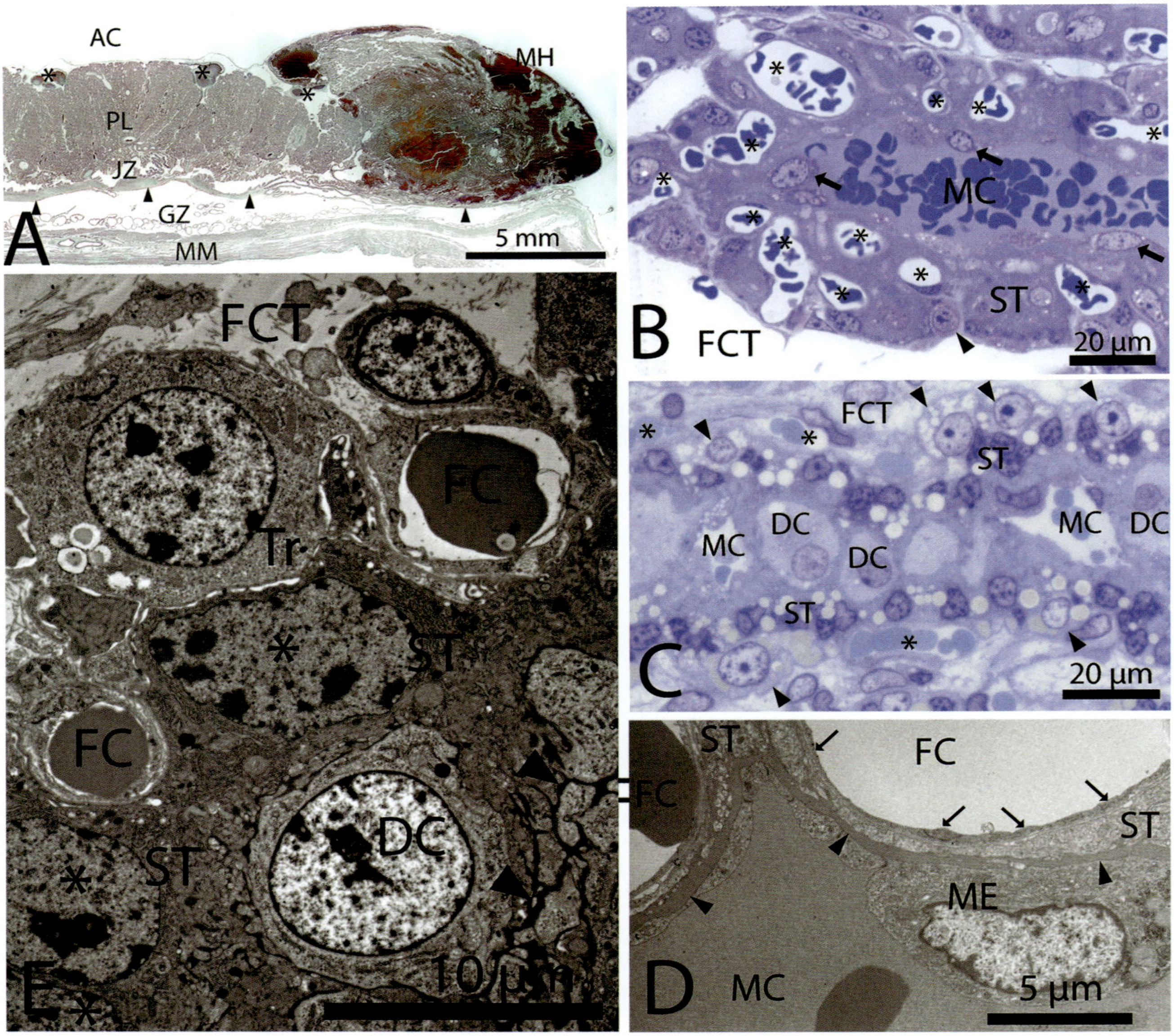

Figure 15-16 Structure of the carnivore placenta. **A.** Dog placenta at low magnification reveals marginal hematoma (MH) along one margin. The placental labyrinth (PL) or lamellar zone facilitates hemotrophic transfer. Supraglandular layer (arrowheads) separates the deep glandular zone (GZ) from the junctional zone (JZ). MM, myometrium; AC, allantoic cavity. **B.** Semithin section (methylene blue staining) of dog placental labyrinth (lamellar zone) shows a large maternal capillary (MC) with high endothelial lining (arrows). This maternal vessel is surrounded by syncytiotrophoblast (ST), deeply indented by fetal capillaries (asterisks). One cytotrophoblast cell is labeled (arrowhead). FCT, fetal connective tissue. **C.** Semithin section (methylene blue staining) of cat placental labyrinth (lamellar zone) showing a lamella of maternal tissue running horizontally through the center, composed of maternal capillaries (MCs) and large decidual cells (DCs). The syncytiotrophoblast (ST) has dark condensed nuclei. A few cytotrophoblast cells (arrowheads) have large euchromatic nuclei with distinct nucleoli. Asterisks: fetal capillaries. FCT, fetal connective tissue. **D.** Transmission electron micrograph of the interhemal barrier (dog) shows layers between fetal blood in the fetal capillary (FC) and maternal blood in the maternal capillary (MC). Layers are as follows: a thin fetal endothelium (arrows), basement membranes of capillary and trophoblast, syncytiotrophoblast, interstitial layer (arrowheads), and maternal capillary endothelium (ME). **E.** Transmission electron micrograph of dog syncytiotrophoblast (ST), deeply indented by fetal capillaries (FCs). The nuclei in the syncytiotrophoblast are depicted by asterisks. One cytotrophoblast cell (Tr) is located next to the fetal connective tissue (FCT). A decidual cell (DC) is adjacent to the interstitial layer (arrowheads), partially enveloping processes of decidual cells in the lower right corner.

The trophoblast layer is originally formed by discrete cells (cytotrophoblast). The fusion of some of these cells forms a syncytium (syncytiotrophoblast). The syncytium constitutes the major part of the lamellae and forms a continuous interhemal barrier (Figs. 15-16B to E). The cytotrophoblast is discontinuous, and the cells mainly occur along the mesenchymal parts of the lamellae (Figs. 15-16B, C, and E). The cytotrophoblast contains free ribosomes and a poorly developed ER. The syncytium possesses a conspicuous ER, numerous mitochondria, and dense bodies, which appear to be lysosomes. In queens, the syncytium contains numerous lipid droplets (Fig. 15-16C).

At parturition, the placenta separates from the endometrium through the junctional zone above the supraglandular layer (Fig. 15-16A).

Clinical Correlations

Placental Transfer of Antibodies

The provision of sufficient antibodies to the newborn is essential for its survival. Maternal antibodies are transferred from maternal blood through the hemochorial placenta (humans and rodents), but not through the epitheliochorial placenta, typical of most large domestic animals. Therefore, neonates of species with epitheliochorial placentae are totally dependent on the immunoglobulins in the colostrum, ingested immediately after parturition when the epithelium in the intestinal tract temporarily becomes permeable to these large molecules. The endothelial placenta of carnivores has a low to intermediate permeability for immunoglobulins, and puppies are born with immunoglobulin concentrations of 5 to 10% of the mothers. Failure to ingest adequate colostrum can lead to immunodeficiency in neonates, making them highly susceptible to infections.

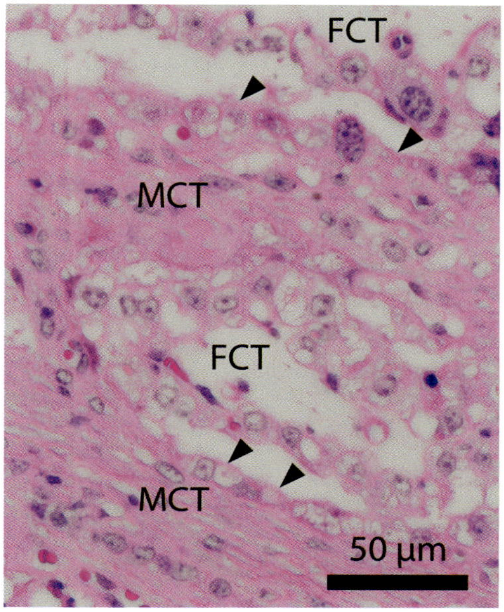

Figure 15-17 Bovine placentome (H&E-stained) postcalf expulsion. The cow later developed a retention of the fetal membranes. The septae of maternal connective tissue (MCT) are wide and the uterine epithelium (arrowheads) is still high. FCT, fetal connective tissue.

Retention of Fetal Membranes

A common complication (approximately 5%) of parturition in cattle is **retained afterbirth** (*retentio secundinarum*), in which the chorionic villi become trapped in the crypts and adhesion between fetal and maternal tissues remains high. Normally, the fetal membranes (chorion, allantois, and amnion) are expelled from the uterus within 12 hours after the calf is born. At a cellular level, the maternal (caruncular) epithelium flattens, and the number of fetal BNC decreases before parturition. In cases of retained afterbirth, the typical cellular processes associated with maturation prior to parturition fail to occur (Fig. 15-17). The fetal part of the placenta and the fetal membranes remain attached to the endometrial caruncles and typically putrefy and detach after several days. This severely impacts the health of the cows and may delay fertility.

Essentials

The mammalian placenta exhibits enormous structural variation between species.

The fetal side of the placental barrier is always formed by the trophoblast. This trophoblast shows many regional specializations across different species. In pigs and equids, the trophoblast mainly consists of uninucleate cytotrophoblast cells. Camelids, however, have large multinucleate trophoblast giant cells alongside the uninucleate trophoblast. Ruminants are characterized by the presence of BNCs, which fuse with maternal uterine cells. In carnivores, cytotrophoblast cells fuse to form a layer of multinucleated syncytiotrophoblast, directly interfacing with maternal tissue.

On the maternal side, the uterine epithelium is present as uninucleate cells in pigs, equids, and camelids. In ruminants, the uterine epithelium is modified due to the fusion of fetal BNC. In carnivores, the uterine epithelium is absent, and the trophoblast directly interfaces with the endothelium of maternal blood vessels.

Suggested Readings

Cornelis G, Heidmann O, Degrelle SA, et al. Captured retroviral envelope syncytin gene associated with the unique placental structure of higher ruminants. *Proc Natl Acad Sci USA* 2013;110:E828–E837.

Furukawa S, Kuroda Y, Sugiyama A. A comparison of the histological structure of the placenta in experimental animals. *J Toxicol Pathol* 2014;27:11–18.

Johnson GA, Bazer FW, Seo H. The early stages of implantation and placentation in the pig. *Adv Anat Embryol Cell Biol* 2021;234:61–89.

Kowalewski MP, Kazemian A, Klisch K, et al. Canine endotheliochorial placenta: morpho-functional aspects. *Adv Anat Embryol Cell Biol* 2021;234:155–179.

Pearson JM, Smith MC, Schlafer DH. Gross and histological description of the epidermal membrane found on normal neonatal piglets. *Lab Anim (NY)* 2015;44:445–447.

Père MC. Materno-foetal exchanges and utilisation of nutrients by the foetus: comparison between species. *Reprod Nutr Dev* 2023;43:1–15.

Wooding FBP. Current topic: the synepitheliochorial placenta of ruminants: binucleate cell fusions and hormone production. *Placenta* 1992;13:101–113.

Wooding FBP, Burton G. Comparative Placentation: Structures, Functions and Evolution. Springer, 2008.

16

Integument

Nancy A. Monteiro-Riviere

CHAPTER MENU

Dellmann's Textbook of Veterinary Histology, Seventh Edition. Edited by Marxa L. Figueiredo and John J. Turek.

Companion website: www.wiley.com/go/figueiredo/vethistology7e

Table 16-1 Functions of the Skin

Environmental barrier
Diffusion barrier
Metabolic barrier
Temperature regulation
Regulation of blood flow
Hair and fur
Sweating
Immunologic affector and effector axes
Mechanical support
Neurosensor/reception
Endocrine (e.g., vitamin D)
Apocrine/eccrine/sebaceous glandular secretion
Metabolism
Keratin
Collagen
Melanin
Lipid
Carbohydrate
Respiration
Biotransformation of xenobiotics

Skin is a complex, integrated, dynamic organ that has functions far beyond its role as a barrier to the environment (Table 16-1). The skin, or integument (derived from the Latin word meaning "to cover"), is the largest organ system of the body and consists of a superficial epidermis and an underlying dermis (Fig. 16-1).

In general, the basic architecture of the integument is similar in all mammals. However, differences in the thickness of the epidermis and dermis in various regions of the body exist between species and within the same species. Because dermatologic, cutaneous pharmacologic, and toxicologic studies use skin from different animal species and body sites, species differences in cutaneous structure must be taken into consideration.

Usually, the skin is thickest over the dorsal surface of the body and on the lateral surfaces of the limbs. It is thinnest on the ventral surface of the body and medial surfaces of the limbs. The surface of the skin may be smooth in some areas but has ridges or folds in other regions that reflect the contour of the underlying connective tissue (CT) layer (Fig.16-2, panels 2 and 3).

Epidermis

The **epidermis** is a keratinized stratified squamous epithelium derived from ectoderm and is the outermost layer of the skin (Figs. 16-1 and 16-2). In regions with a heavy protective coat of hair, the epidermis is thin; in nonhairy skin, such as that of the mucocutaneous junctions, the epidermis is thicker. Cells of the epidermis undergo an orderly pattern of proliferation, differentiation, and keratinization, the processes of which are not completely understood. During development, the epidermis can become specialized to form various skin appendages such as hair, sweat, and sebaceous glands; digital organs (hoof, claw, and digital pads); feathers; horn; and specialized glands.

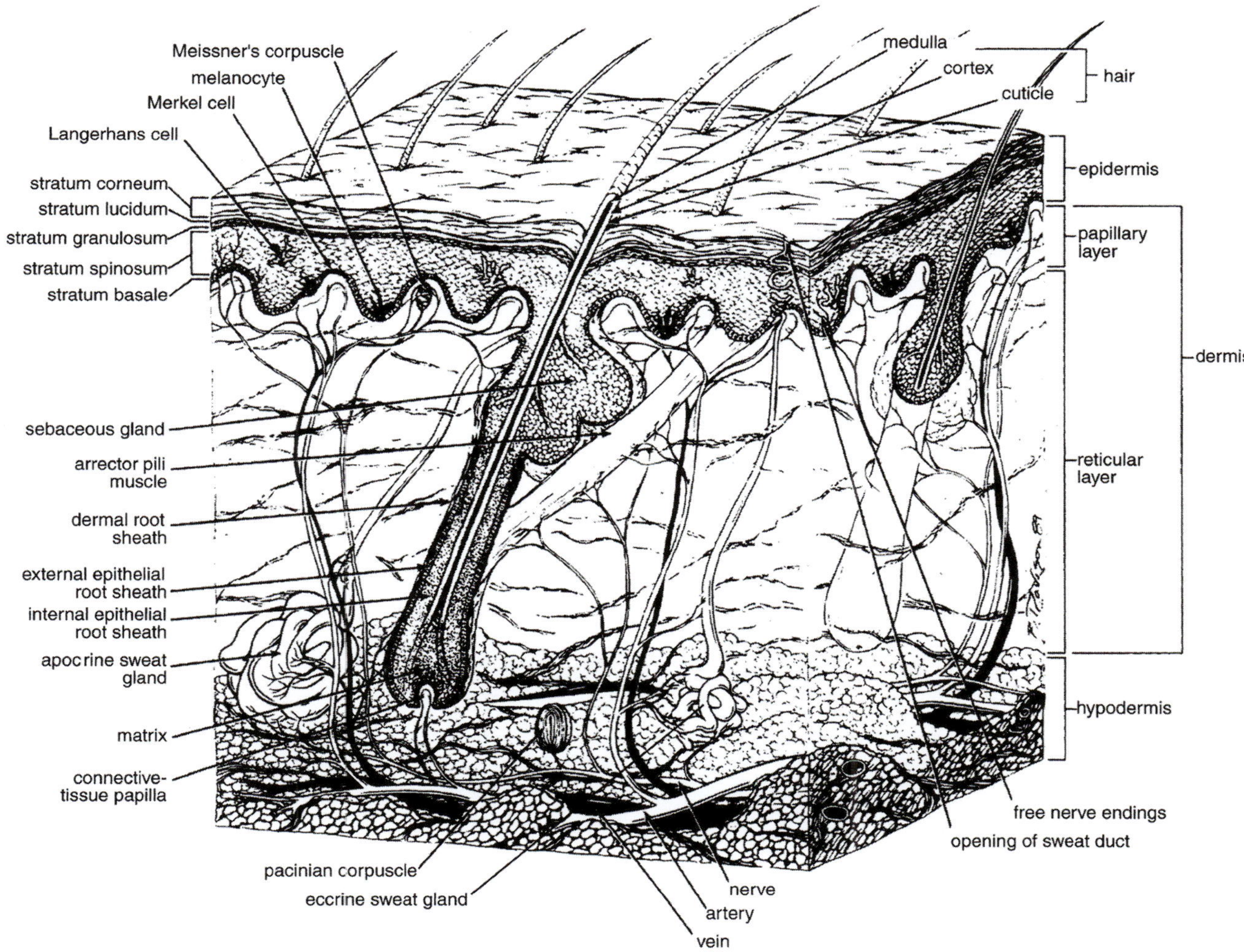

Figure 16-1 Schematic drawing representing the structure of the integument found in typical skin in various regions of the body. Right side of follicle depicts human skin showing the eccrine gland opening onto the surface of the skin, while the left side of the follicle shows the apocrine gland of animals depicting the duct penetrating the epidermis of the hair follicle just before it opens onto the surface of the skin. (Monteiro-Riviere, N.A. Comparative anatomy, physiology, and biochemistry of mammalian skin. In Hobson DW ed. Dermal and Ocular Toxicology. Fundamentals and methods. Boca Raton, FL: CRC Press 1991;1:3–74.)

The cells of the epidermis are categorized into two major groups: keratinocytes and nonkeratinocytes. The epidermal layers can be classified from the basement membrane to the outer surface as follows: stratum basale (basal layer), stratum spinosum (spinous or prickle layer), stratum granulosum (granular layer), stratum lucidum (clear layer), and stratum corneum (horny layer).

Epidermal Keratinocytes

Keratinocytes comprise about 85% of the epidermal cells and are classified into layers based on morphology. They vary in size and shape and differentiate as they migrate upward to form keratin.

Epidermal Nonkeratinocytes

Nonkeratinocytes are scattered throughout the epidermis and include melanocytes, tactile epithelioid cells, and intraepidermal macrophages.

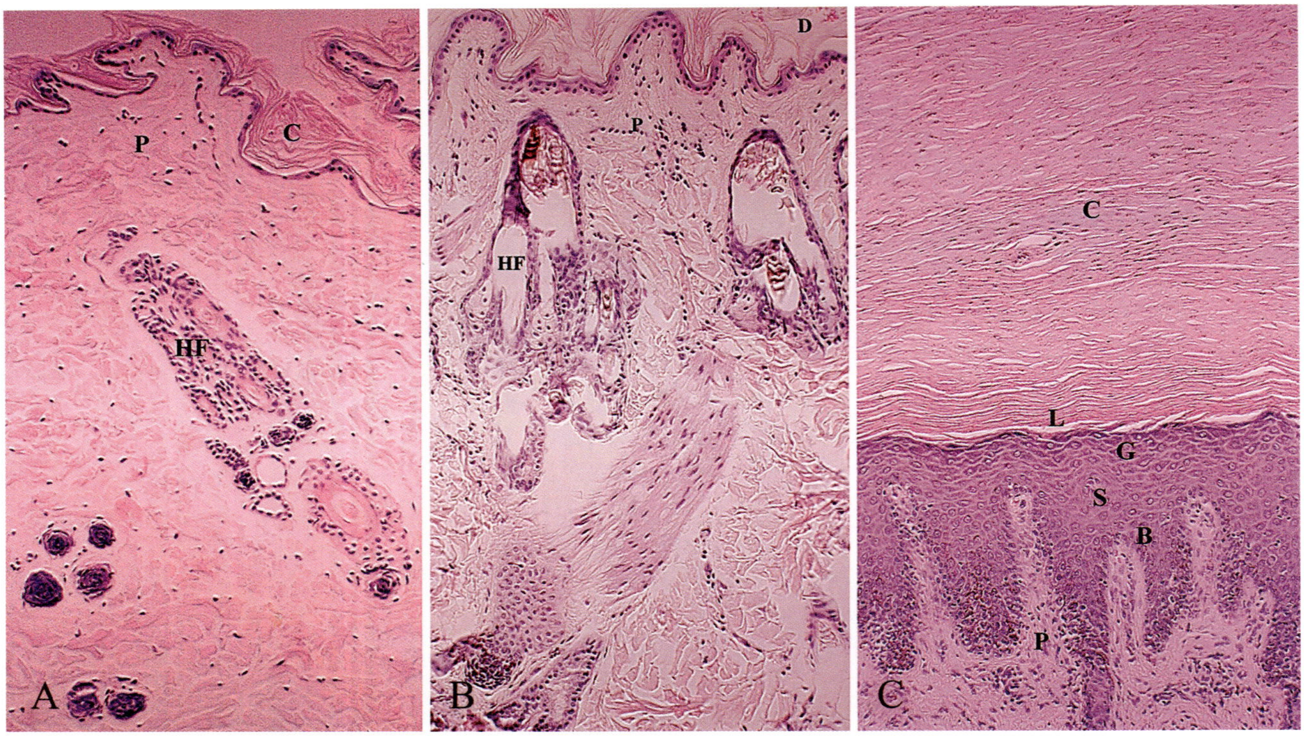

Figure 16-2 Skin (cat). **A.** Thin skin with one to two viable epidermal cell layers, abdomen. **B.** Skin with thin epidermis, lumbar region. **C.** Skin with thick stratum corneum and epidermis, foot pad. Stratum disjunctum (D), stratum corneum (C), stratum lucidum (L), stratum granulosum (G), stratum spinosum (S), stratum basale (B), superficial (papillary) layer of the dermis (P), and hair follicle cluster in dermis (HF). Hematoxylin and eosin (H&E) (×120).

Melanocytes

Melanocytes are derivatives of neural crest ectoderm and located in the basal layer of the epidermis (Fig. 16-1). They also occur in the external epithelial root sheath and hair matrix of hair follicles, in sweat gland ducts, and in sebaceous glands. Melanocytes have several dendritic processes that either extend between adjacent keratinocytes or run parallel to the basement membrane. The melanocyte has a spherical nucleus and contains typical organelles (ribosomes, endoplasmic reticulum, Golgi, etc.). The cytoplasm is clear except for pigment-containing ovoid granules, which are referred to as **melanosomes**. The melanosomes impart color to skin and hair. Dark brown pigment in skin is called **eumelanin**, while yellowish red pigment is called **pheomelanin**. The enzyme tyrosinase is needed to produce melanin within the melanocytes, and the reaction involves the following series of steps, in short: tyrosine → dopa → dopaquinone → melanin. Albino animals lack tyrosinase; therefore, they cannot produce melanin, even though they have a normal number of melanocytes. After melanogenesis, the melanosomes migrate to the tips of the dendritic processes of the melanocyte; the tips then become pinched off and are phagocytized by the adjacent keratinocytes. They remain as discrete membrane-bounded organelles or become aggregated and surrounded by a membrane to form a melanosome complex. Melanosomes are randomly distributed within the cytoplasm of the keratinocytes, although they often become localized over the nucleus, thereby forming a cap-like structure that presumably protects the nucleus from ultraviolet radiation (Fig. 16-3). Skin color is determined by several factors, such as the number, size, distribution, and degree of melanization of melanosomes.

Tactile Epithelioid Cells (Merkel Cells)

Tactile epithelioid cells, also known as Merkel cells, are located in the basal region of the epidermis in both hairless and hairy skin. Their long axis is usually parallel to the surface of the skin and, thus, perpendicular to the columnar basal epithelial cells above (Figs. 16-1 and 16-4). The nucleus is lobulated and irregular, and the cytoplasm is clear and lacks tonofilaments. These cells have a characteristic region of vacuolated cytoplasm near the dermis that has spherical electron-dense granules containing species-specific chemical mediators (e.g., serotonin, serotonin-like substances, vasoactive intestinal polypeptide, peptide histidine-isoleucine, and substance P). Tactile epithelioid cells are connected to adjacent keratinocytes by desmosomes. When associated with an axon, a tactile epithelioid cell–neurite complex or nonencapsulated tactile corpuscle is formed, and specialized areas of skin containing these complexes are known as **tactile hair discs** (Haarscheiben, hair discs, tactile pads, or tylotrich pads). The axon associated with a tactile epithelioid cell is myelinated, but as it approaches the epidermis, the axon loses its myelin sheath and terminates as a flat meniscus on the basal aspect of the cell (Fig. 16-4). Tactile epithelioid cells can release trophic factors that attract nerve endings into the epidermis and can stimulate keratinocyte growth. In addition, tactile epithelioid cells can function as slow adapting mechanoreceptors for touch.

Langerhans Cells

A specialized subset of dendritic cells located within the epidermis are **Langerhans cells** (LC), previously referred to as intraepidermal macrophages. They are found in adult pigs, cats, and dogs and are well characterized in rodents and humans. However, the specific phenotype (membrane receptors and antigens related to immune function) can vary between species. LC are found in the upper spinous layer of the epidermis (Figs. 16-1 and 16-5) and have been identified in the stratified squamous epithelium of the upper digestive tract, female genital tract, and ovine rumen. In addition, LC are considered bone marrow–derived leukocytes with an immunophenotype like the antigen-presenting monocyte macrophages. Dendritic cells in afferent dermal lymph vessels are referred to as "veiled cells," in lymph nodes "interdigitating cells." Further, they have been found in the lung in fibrotic disorders, mycosis fungoides, atopic dermatitis, and the nondermatologic disorder eosinophilic granulomatosis.

LC are usually not apparent in routine-stained sections but may appear as clear cells in the suprabasal epidermis. They can only be positively identified with special stains. At the ultrastructural level, these cells have an indented nucleus, and the cytoplasm contains typical organelles; they lack tonofilaments and desmosomes. A unique feature of this cell is distinctive rod- or racket-shaped cytoplasmic organelles known as **Birbeck granules**. These granules were found to contain the "lag" antigen with a C-type lectin receptor in LC,

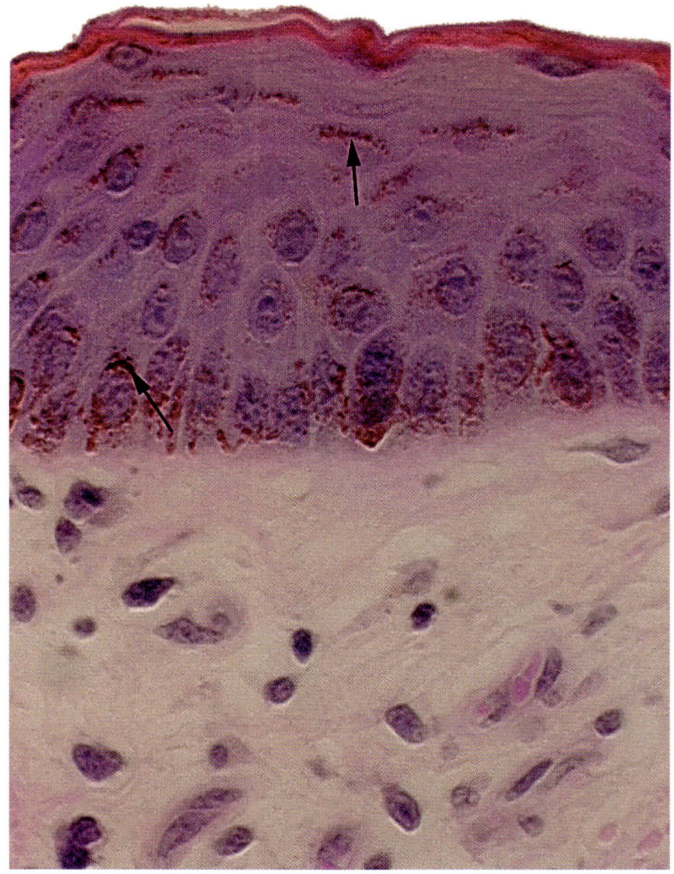

Figure 16-3 Melanin granules (arrows) highly concentrated in the stratum basale cell layer and forming apical caps in the upper layers of the horse abdominal skin. H&E (×800).

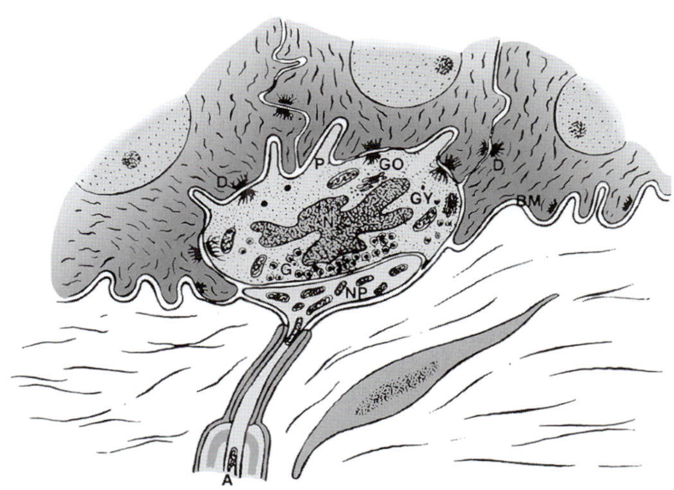

Figure 16-4 Schematic drawing of a tactile epithelioid cell–neurite complex from a foot pad of a cat. Irregular nucleus (N), Golgi (GO), desmosome (D) connecting to adjacent keratinocytes, glycogen (GY), cytoplasmic process (P), basement membrane (BM), Merkel cell dense core granules (G), axon (A), and nerve plate or disc (NP).

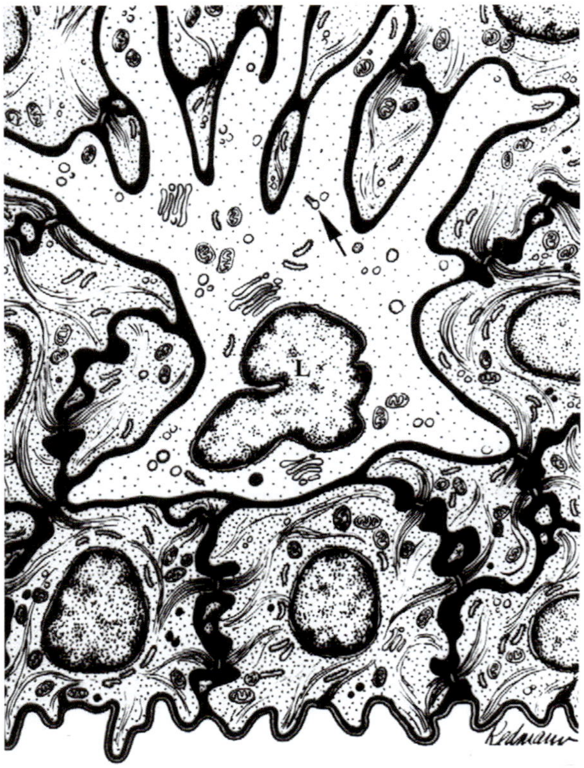

Figure 16-5 Schematic of a Langerhans cell (L). Heavy black areas represent the intercellular space. The racket shape granules (arrow) can be found in the dendritic processes. Note the indented nucleus and electron-lucent cytoplasm. (From Monteiro-Riviere NA. Ultrastructural evaluation of the porcine integument. In: Tumbleson ME, ed. Swine in biomedical research. New York: Plenum Press, 1986;1:641.)

therefore referred to as langerin, which is a constituent found in Birbeck granules. Since 1868, these dendritic cells have purported to have many different functions and are part of the mononuclear phagocyte system (monocyte-macrophage system). They are capable of presenting antigen to CD4+ T cells *in vivo*, can induce contact sensitivity, and what is known so far is that LC are prototypic antigen-presenting cells. It has been shown that tumor necrosis factor (TNF)-alpha plays a role in the exiting of LC from murine and human skin. Keratinocytes play a role in epidermal differentiation and move up the epidermis to be desquamated. LCs, with their dendritic processes, can also move up to pick up antigens or pathogens that entered or passed through the epidermal stratum corneum barrier. Cell movement is well known, but the molecular events are not fully understood.

Layers of the Epidermis

Stratum Basale

The **stratum basale** (stratum germinativum) consists of a single layer of columnar or cuboidal cells that rests on the basal lamina (Figs. 16-1 and 16-6). The cells are attached laterally to each other and to the overlying stratum spinosum cells by desmosomes and to the underlying basal lamina by hemidesmosomes. The nucleus is large and ovoid and occupies most of the cell. These basal cells are heterogeneous functionally. Some basal cells can act as stem cells, with the ability to divide and produce new cells, whereas others primarily serve to anchor the epidermis.

Stratum Spinosum

The succeeding outer layer is the **stratum spinosum**, or "prickle cell layer," which consists of several layers of irregular polyhedral cells (Figs. 16-2C and 16-7). Desmosomes connect these cells to adjacent stratum spinosum cells and to the stratum basale cells below. Tonofilaments are more prominent in this layer than in the stratum basale. The large intercellular space usually seen in this layer is a shrinkage artifact, which occurs during the preparation of the sample for light microscopic study. The uppermost layers of the stratum spinosum contain small membrane-bounded organelles known as **lamellar granules** (Odland bodies, lamellated bodies, or membrane-coating granules).

Stratum Granulosum

The third layer above the **stratum granulosum** consists of several layers of flattened cells lying parallel to the stratum corneum (Figs. 16-2C and 16-8). This layer contains irregularly shaped, nonmembrane-bounded, electron-dense **keratohyalin granules**. These granules contain profilaggrin, a structural protein and a precursor of filaggrin, and are believed to play a role in keratinization and barrier function. The stratum granulosum is not always present in all stratified squamous epithelia such as in the mucous membranes of the mouth (buccal mucosa). Another characteristic feature of the stratum granulosum is the presence of the **lamellar granules**. These granules are smaller than mitochondria and occur near the Golgi complex and smooth endoplasmic reticulum. Higher in the epidermis, these granules increase in number and size, move toward the cell membrane, and release their lipid contents by exocytosis into the intercellular space between the stratum granulosum and stratum corneum, thereby coating the cell membrane of the stratum corneum cells (Fig. 16-8). As one can now appreciate, the term "membrane-coating granule" is appropriate. The major components of lamellar granules are lipids (ceramides, cholesterol, fatty acids, and small amounts of cholesteryl esters) and hydrolytic enzymes (acid phosphates, proteases, lipases, and glycosidases). The content and mixture of lipids can vary between species.

Stratum Lucidum

The **stratum lucidum** (clear layer) is only found in specific areas of exceptionally thick skin and in hairless regions (e.g., plantar and palmar surfaces, and planum nasale) (Fig. 16-2C). It is a thin, translucent, homogeneous line between the stratum granulosum and stratum corneum. This stratum consists of several layers of fully keratinized, closely compacted, dense cells devoid of nuclei and cytoplasmic organelles. The cell cytoplasm contains protein-bound phospholipids and **eleidin**, which is a protein similar to keratin but has a different staining affinity.

Stratum Corneum

The **stratum corneum** is the outermost layer of the epidermis and consists of several layers of completely keratinized dead cells, which are constantly being shed. This layer appears clear and contains no nuclei or cytoplasmic organelles (Figs.16-1, 16-2C and 16-8). The most superficial layers of the stratum corneum that undergo constant desquamation are referred to as the **stratum disjunctum**. The stratum corneum varies in thickness in different areas (i.e., abdomen versus back) of the body and between species. On the palmar and plantar surfaces, where considerable abrasive action occurs, the stratum corneum is thickest (Fig. 16-2C). The stratum corneum cells are highly organized and stacked one upon another to form vertical interlocking columns with a flattened tetrakaidecahedron shape. This 14-sided polygonal structure provides a minimum surface-to-volume ratio, allowing for tight packing without gaps. This spatial arrangement, typical of hairy skin, helps one to understand that transepidermal water loss (TEWL) is a function of the integrity and permeability of this layer. The intercellular substance derived from the lamellar granules is present between the stratum corneum cells and helps to form the intercellular lipid component of a complex stratum corneum barrier, which prevents both the penetration of substances from the environment and the loss of body fluids. The keratinized cells are surrounded by a plasma membrane and a thick submembranous layer that contains a protein, **involucrin**. This protein is synthesized in the stratum spinosum and cross-linked in the stratum granulosum by an enzyme that makes it highly stable. Therefore, involucrin provides structural support to the cell, thereby allowing the cell to resist invasion by microorganisms and destruction, enabling it by environmental agents, but it does not seem to regulate permeability.

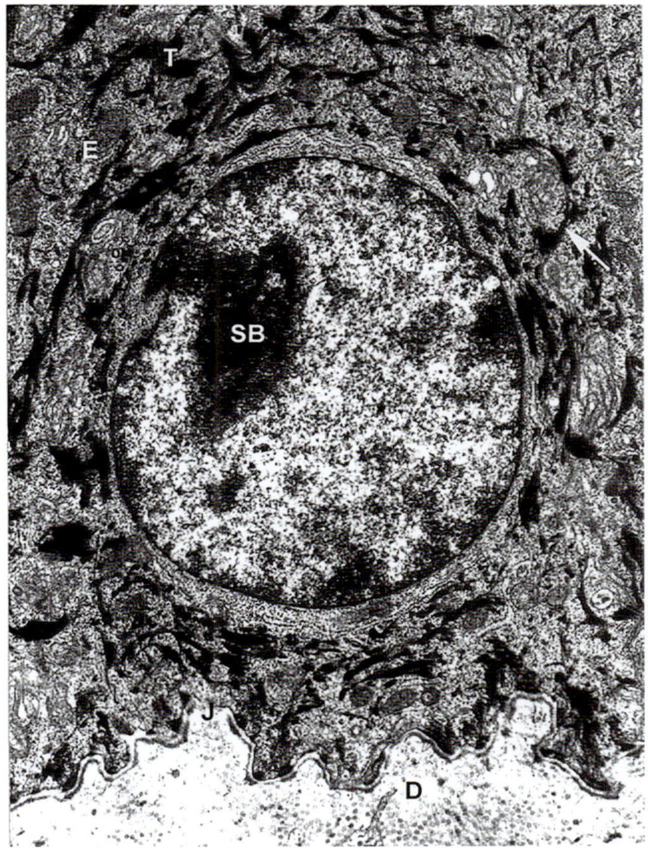

Figure 16-6 Transmission electron micrograph of pig skin. Area depicting the epidermis (E), dermis (D), epidermal–dermal junction (J), stratum basale cell (SB), tonofilaments (T), and desmosome attachments (arrow) (×10,700).

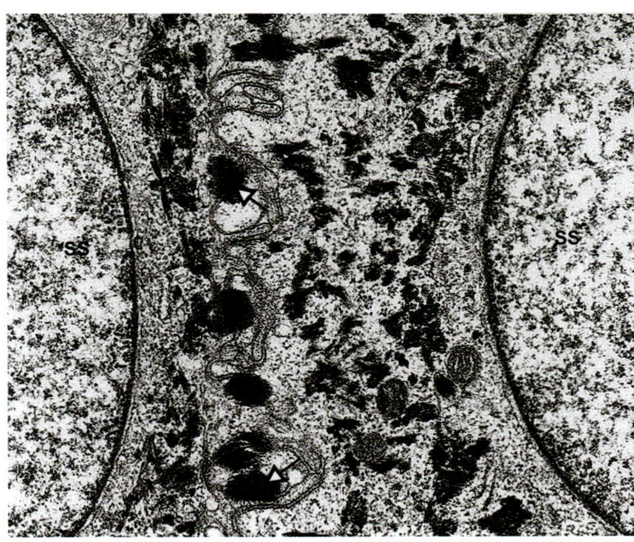

Figure 16-7 Transmission electron micrograph of the stratum spinosum of pig skin. Area shows the nuclei of two stratum spinosum (SS) cells attached by desmosomes (arrows) (×23,500).

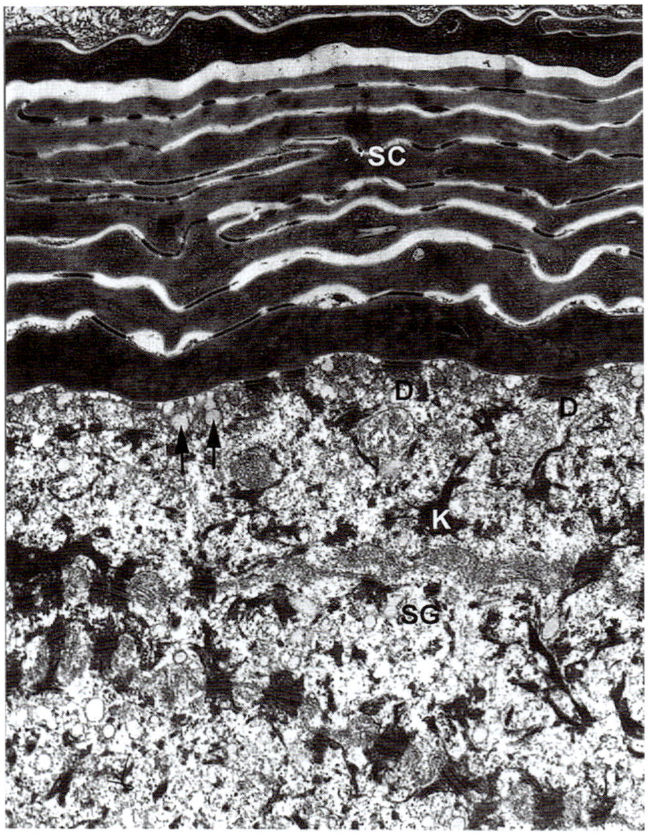

Figure 16-8 Transmission electron micrograph of the upper stratum granulosum (SG) and stratum corneum (SC) of pig skin. Membrane-coating granules or lamellar bodies (arrows) are present in the stratum granulosum, with some fusing to the plasma membrane to release their contents. Keratohyalin granules (K) and numerous desmosomes (D) are present (×14,900).

Keratinization

Keratinization is the process by which epidermal cells (keratinocytes) differentiate. After basal epithelial cells undergo mitosis, they migrate upward. During this migration, the cytoplasm volume increases, and differentiation products such as tonofilaments, keratohyalin granules, and lamellar granules are produced in large amounts. The tonofilaments and the amorphous material, keratohyalin, form a meshwork. As the cellular contents increase, the nuclei disintegrate, and the lamellar granules discharge their contents into the intercellular space, coating the cells. The remaining organelles such as mitochondria and ribosomes disintegrate, and the flattened cells become filled with filaments and keratohyalin, which then form bundles. The final product of this epidermal differentiation and keratinization process is the stratum corneum, which consists of protein-rich cells containing fibrous **keratin** and keratohyalin, surrounded by a thicker plasma membrane coated with an exterior lipid matrix. This forms the commonly known "brick and mortar" structure, where the lipid matrix acts as the mortar between the cells, which are the bricks.

Percutaneous Absorption

The ability of a chemical or drug to permeate the skin depends on numerous factors such as the vehicle and its components, disease state, hair follicle density, age, thickness, body site, blood flow, and the metabolism of the species. These factors can modulate chemical absorption and affect the skin barrier. Other components of chemical mixtures and vehicles, as well as products generated by the skin such as sweat, sebum, dead cells, and metabolic byproducts can alter the physicochemical properties of skin and influence the rate of a toxicant's penetration or toxicity. Numerous skin penetration studies do not consider these factors. For example, hair follicle growth cycle of the species and the body site are significant factors for hydrocortisone absorption. The challenge for researchers is to determine the key factors that have the greatest impact on a chemical's transdermal passage or toxicity. The ability of a chemical to traverse the skin is a primary determinant of its dermatotoxic potential. Understanding the skin layers is crucial to appreciate how a chemical can penetrate the stratum corneum, the rate-limiting barrier, to exert an effect on the lower cell layers. The quantitative prediction of the rate and extent of percutaneous penetration (into skin) and absorption (through skin) of topically applied chemicals is complicated by the biological complexity discussed above.

The skin is generally considered to be an efficient barrier preventing absorption (and thus systemic exposure) of most topically administered drugs. It is relatively impermeable to most ions and aqueous solutions; however, it is permeable to many lipophilic solids, liquids, and gases, suggesting the term barrier is inappropriate for these substances. Several agricultural workers have experienced acute dermal poisoning from direct exposure to pesticides, such as parathion during application, or from secondary exposure by contact with vegetation previously treated with such insecticides. In fact, percutaneous absorption of nicotine in tobacco workers led to the concept of the modern transdermal nicotine "patch" delivery systems. As discussed above, compared to most routes of drug absorption, the skin is by far the most diverse across species (e.g., sheep versus pig) and body sites (e.g., human forearm compared to scalp). The stratum corneum affords the greatest deterrent to absorption. Although the dead, keratinized cells are highly water retarding, they are also highly water absorbent (hydrophilic), a property that keeps the skin supple and soft as these cells absorb water on its way to being evaporated from the surface. This is the mechanism of action of most cosmetic moisturizers. Additionally, sebum appears to augment the water holding capacity of the epidermis but has no appreciable role in retarding the penetration of xenobiotics. Several studies have demonstrated that disruption of the stratum corneum removes all but a superficial deterrent to penetration. This is supported by "tape-stripping" experiments, where an adhesive (cellophane tape) is repeatedly applied to the skin to remove successive layers of the corneum. The skin ultimately loses its ability to retard penetration and compound flux increases greatly. This may be noninvasively assessed by measuring the skin's ability to prevent insensible evaporative water loss from the body to the environment by utilizing water as a marker of molecular transport across the epidermal barrier. This is performed by measuring TEWL with an instrument called an evaporimeter. TEWL greatly increases when the stratum corneum is either stripped, removed by extracting the intercellular barrier lipids with solvents such as acetone, or damaged in response to cutaneous toxicants.

As in most other epithelial tissues, the two other layers of the skin (dermis and subcutaneous tissue) offer little resistance to penetration. Once a substance has penetrated the outer stratum corneum, these tissues are rapidly traversed. This may not be true for highly lipid-soluble compounds because the dermis may function as an additional aqueous barrier preventing a chemical that has penetrated the epidermis from being absorbed into the blood.

Epidermal–Dermal Junction

The **epidermal–dermal junction** (or skin basement membrane zone) is a complex and highly specialized structure recognized with the light microscope (periodic acid-Schiff stain) as a thin, homogeneous band. When viewed with the transmission electron microscope, however, the epidermal–dermal junction consists of four components: (a) the cell membrane of the basal epithelial cell, which includes hemidesmosomes; (b) the lamina lucida (lamina rara); (c) the lamina densa (basal lamina); and (d) the sub-basal lamina (sublamina densa or reticular lamina) with a variety of fibrous structures (anchoring fibrils, dermal microfibril bundles, and microthread-like filaments) (Fig. 16-9). The basement membrane has a complex molecular architecture with numerous components that play a key role in adhesion of the epidermis to the dermis. The macromolecules, which are ubiquitous components of all basement membranes, include type IV collagen, laminin, entactin/nidogen, and heparan sulfate proteoglycans.

Other basement membrane components, such as bullous pemphigoid antigen (BPA), epidermolysis bullosa acquisita (EBA), fibronectin, GB3, L3d, and 19-DEJ-1, are specifically found in the epithelial basement membrane of the skin. The basal cell membrane of the epidermal–dermal junction is not always smooth. It may be irregular, forming fingerlike projections into the dermis. The basement membrane: (a) plays a role in maintaining epidermal–dermal adhesion, (b) acts as a selective barrier between the epidermis and dermis by restricting some molecules and permitting the passage of others, (c) influences cell behavior and wound healing, and (d) serves as a target for both immunologic (bullous diseases) and nonimmunologic injury (friction- or chemical-induced blisters).

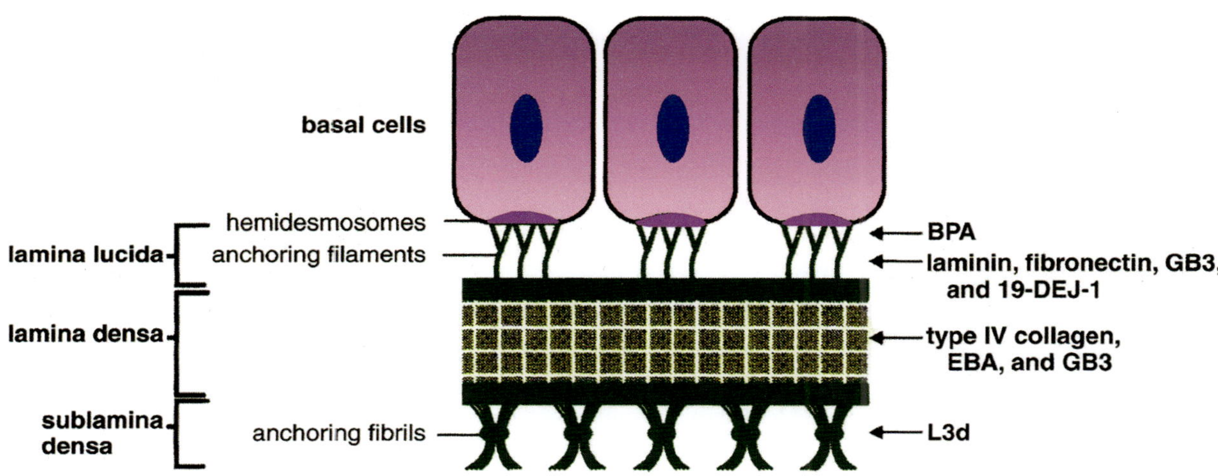

Figure 16-9 Schematic of the basement membrane of skin depicting the precise location of the macromolecular components. (From Monteiro-Riviere NA, Inman AO. Indirect immunohistochemistry and immunoelectron microscopy distribution of eight epidermal–dermal junction epitopes in the pig and in isolated perfused skin treated with bis (2chloroethyl) sulfide. *Toxicol Pathol* 1995;23:313).

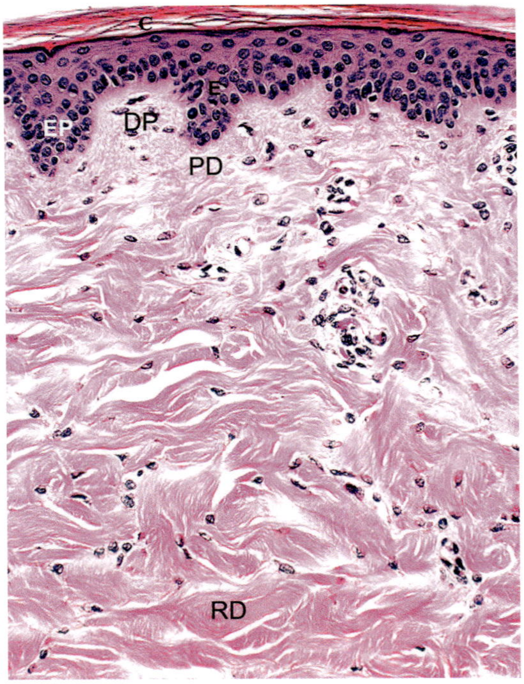

Figure 16-10 Pig skin from the abdomen. Epidermis (E), stratum corneum (C), superficial papillary dermis (PD), epidermal peg (EP), dermal papilla (DP), and deep reticular dermis (RD). H&E (×250).

Dermis

The **dermis**, or corium, lies beneath the basement membrane and extends to the hypodermis. This layer is of mesodermal origin and primarily consists of dense irregular CT with a feltwork of collagen, elastic, and reticular fibers embedded in amorphous ground substance. Predominant cell types of the dermis are fibrocytes, mast cells, and macrophages. Plasma cells, chromatophores, fat cells, and extravasated leukocytes are often found. The dermis is traversed by blood vessels, lymph vessels, and nerves. Sebaceous and sweat glands are also present, along with hair follicles and arrector pili muscles.

The dermis can be divided into a superficial papillary layer that blends into a deep reticular layer without a clear line of demarcation (Fig. 16-10). The **papillary layer** is the thinnest layer, consists of loose CT, is in contact with the epidermis, and conforms to the contour of the stratum basale. The papillary layer can protrude into the epidermis, thereby giving rise to the **dermal papilla**. When the epidermis invaginates into the dermis, **epidermal pegs** are formed. The **reticular layer** is thicker and consists of dense irregular CT, whereas CT cells are fewer in the deeper layers of the dermis.

In the dermis, smooth muscle fibers are located near hair follicles and are referred to as **arrector pili muscles**. In addition, dermal smooth muscle fibers are present in specialized areas such as the scrotum, penis, and teat. Skeletal muscle fibers of the cutaneous trunci penetrate the dermis and allow voluntary movement of the skin. Also, skeletal muscle fibers are associated with the large sinus hairs of the facial region.

Hypodermis

Beneath the dermis is a layer of loose CT, the **hypodermis** (subcutis), which is not part of the skin but rather the superficial fascia seen in gross anatomic dissections. The hypodermis anchors the dermis to the underlying muscle or bone. The loose arrangement of collagen and elastic fibers allows the skin flexibility and free movement over the underlying structures. Adipose tissue is present in this layer and may form small clusters of cells or large masses that create a cushion or pad of fat called the **panniculus adiposus** (Fig. 16-11). Pork bacon and fatback are derived from the panniculus adiposus. Large fat deposits (structural fat) in the hypodermis are characteristic of the carpal, metacarpal, and digital pads, where they act as shock absorbers.

Skin Appendages

Hair

In domestic mammals, hair covers the entire body, except the foot pads, hoofs, glans penis, mucocutaneous junctions, and teats of some species. **Hair** is a flexible, keratinized structure produced by a hair follicle. The distal or free part of the hair above the surface of the skin is the hair **shaft**. The part within the follicle is the hair **root**, which has a terminal, hollow knob called the hair **bulb**, which is attached to a dermal papilla.

The hair shaft is composed of three layers: an outermost cuticle, a cortex of densely packed keratinized cells, and, at its center, a medulla of loose cuboidal or flattened cells (Fig. 16-12). The **cuticle** is formed by a single layer of flat keratinized cells in which the free edges, which overlap like shingles on a roof, are directed toward the distal end of the shaft. The **cortex** consists of a layer of dense, compact, keratinized cells with their long axes parallel to the hair shaft. Nuclear remnants and pigment granules are present within the cells. Desmosomes hold the cells firmly together. Near the bulb, the cells are shorter and more oval-shaped, containing spherical nuclei. The **medulla** forms the center of the hair and is loosely filled with cuboidal or flattened cells (Fig. 16-12). In the root, the medulla is solid, whereas in the shaft, it contains air-filled spaces. The pattern of the surface of the cuticular cells, together with the cellular arrangement of the medulla, is characteristic for each species.

The hair or fleece of sheep is referred to as **fibers**. The three types of fibers are (a) wool fibers, tightly crimped fibers of small diameter lacking a medulla; (b) kemp fibers, coarse and with a characteristic medulla; and (c) coarse fibers of intermediate size relative to wool and kemp fibers. The various breeds of sheep produce wool with different characteristics, and these various kinds of fleece are used for different purposes.

Hair Follicles

Structure

The **hair follicle** is formed by growth of the ectoderm into the underlying mesoderm of the embryo. The epithelial downgrowth becomes canalized, and the surrounding cells differentiate into several layers or sheaths that surround the hair root. The follicle is embedded in the dermis, usually at an angle, and the bulb may extend as deep as the hypodermis (Figs. 16-11 and 16-13). The hair follicle consists of four major components: (a) internal epithelial root sheath, (b) external epithelial root sheath, (c) dermal papilla, and (d) hair matrix.

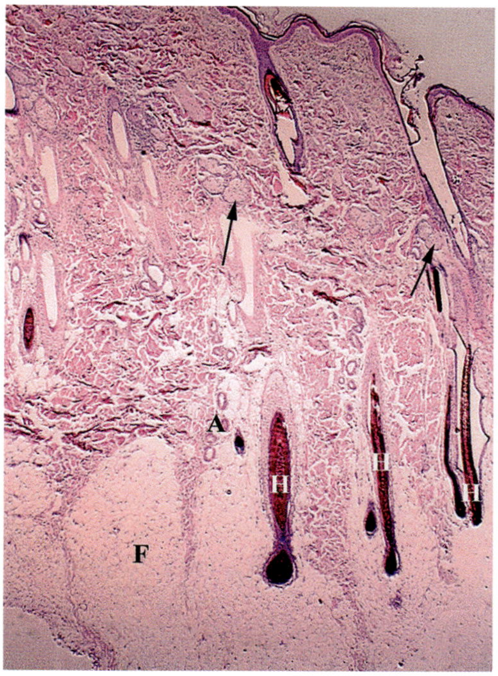

Figure 16-11 Hypodermis with three large primary hair follicles (H) extending into the subcutaneous fat (F) (dog). Note the sebaceous glands (arrows) and apocrine gland ducts (A). H&E (×35).

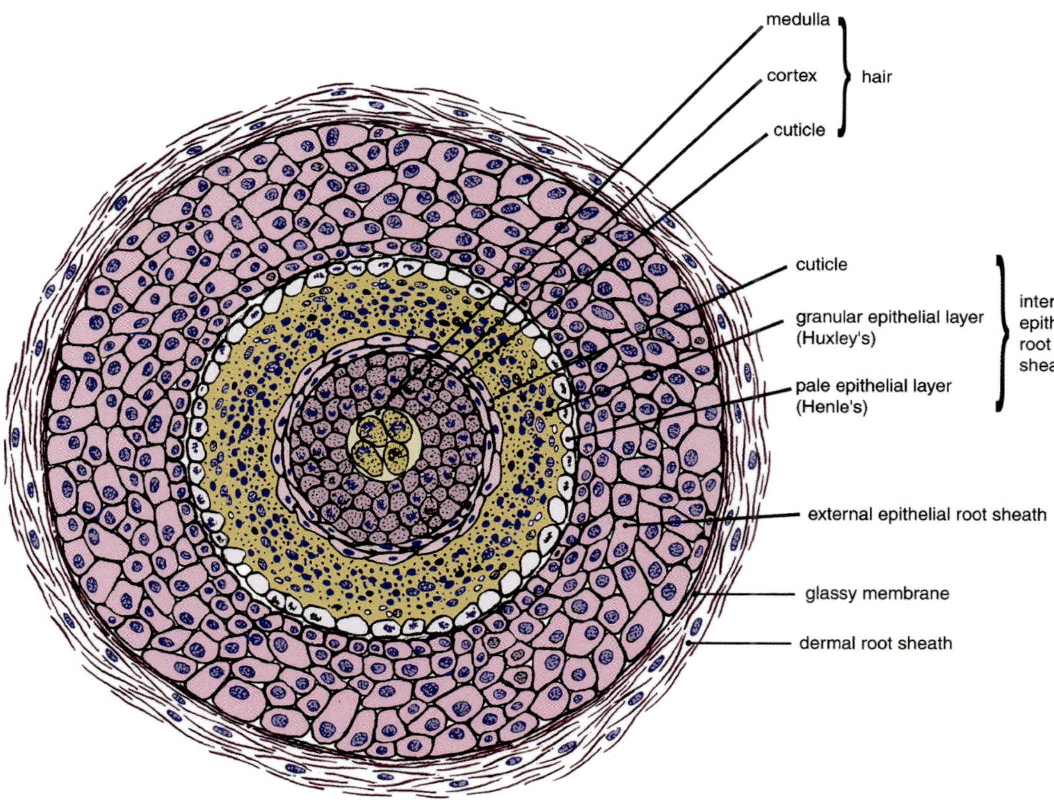

Figure 16-12 Schematic of a cross section of a hair follicle.

The innermost layer, next to the hair root, is the **internal epithelial root sheath**, which is composed of three layers: (a) internal root sheath cuticle, (b) middle granular epithelial layer (Huxley's layer), and (c) outer pale epithelial layer (Henle's layer) (Fig. 16-12). The **cuticle** of the internal epithelial root sheath is formed by overlapping keratinized cells like those of the cuticle of the hair, except that the free edges are oriented in the opposite direction or toward the hair bulb. This arrangement results in a solid implantation of the hair root in the hair follicle. The **granular epithelial layer** is composed of one to three layers of cells rich in trichohyalin (keratohyalin in hair) granules. The **pale epithelial layer** is the outermost layer of the internal epithelial root sheath and is composed of a single layer of keratinized cells. Immediately below the opening of the sebaceous glands, the internal epithelial root sheath of the large follicles becomes corrugated, forming several circular or follicular folds. The sheath then becomes thinner, and the cells fuse, disintegrate, and become part of the sebum.

The **external epithelial root sheath** is composed of several layers of cells similar to the epidermis in which it is continuous in the upper portion of the follicle. External to this layer is a homogeneous glassy membrane corresponding to the basal lamina of the epidermis (Fig. 16-12). The entire epithelial root sheath (internal and external) is enclosed by a **dermal root sheath** composed of collagen and elastic fibers richly supplied by blood vessels and nerves, especially in the dermal papilla.

The **dermal papilla** of the hair follicle is the region of CT directly underneath the hair matrix. The cells covering the dermal papilla and composing most of the hair bulb are the **hair matrix cells**. These are comparable to stratum basale cells of regular epidermis and give rise to the cells that keratinize to form the hair (Fig. 16-13). They differ from the keratinocytes of the surface epidermis with respect to the type of keratin produced. The surface keratinocytes produce a "soft" form of keratin that passes through a keratohyalin phase. The cells containing "soft" keratin have a high lipid content and a low sulfur content and desquamate when they reach the surface of the epidermis. In contrast, the matrix cells of the hair

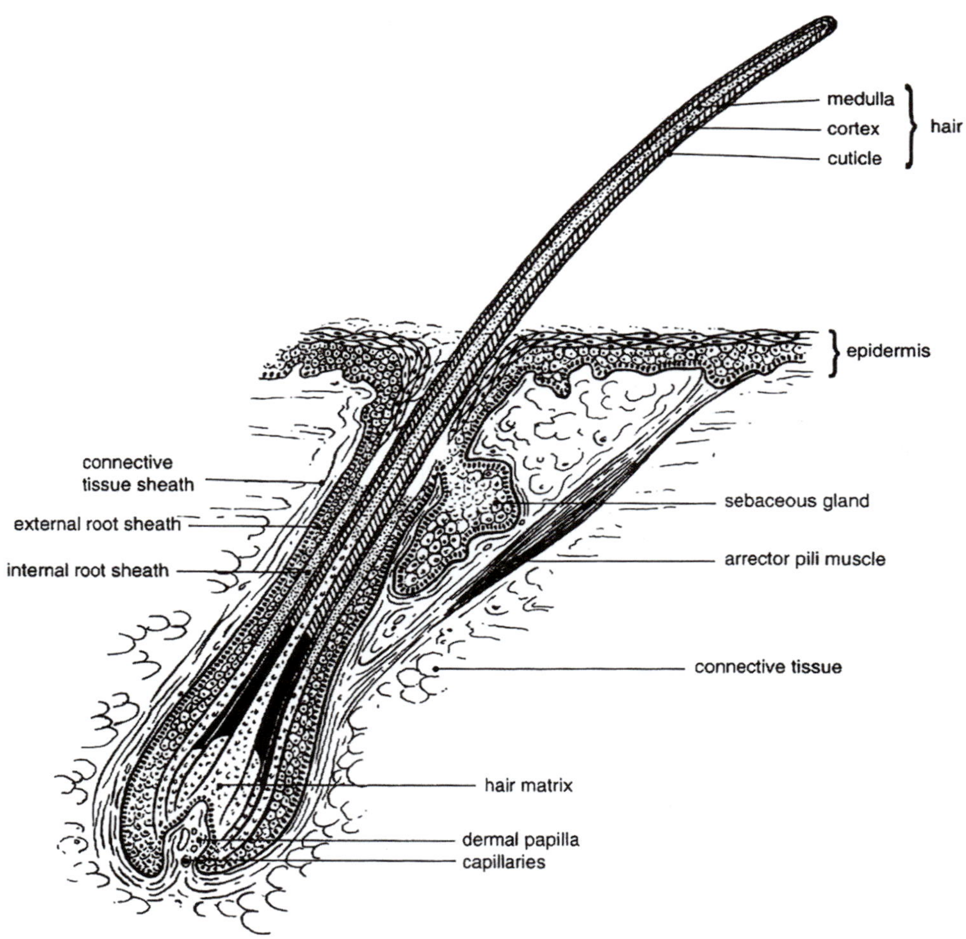

Figure 16-13 Schematic of a longitudinal section of a hair follicle.

follicle produce a "hard" keratin, which is also characteristic of horn and feather. The keratinocytes of the follicle do not go through a keratohyalin phase, do not desquamate, and have a low lipid and high sulfur content.

Hair pigment is derived from the epidermal melanocytes located over the dermal papilla. Gray hair results from the inability of melanocytes in the hair bulb to produce tyrosinase. Hair color is determined by the amount and distribution of pigment and by the presence of air, which appears white in reflected light. Silvery white hair is the result when the pigment has faded, and the medulla becomes filled with air.

Associated with most hair follicles are bundles of smooth muscle called the **arrector pili muscle**. This muscle attaches to the dermal root sheath of the hair follicle and extends toward the epidermis, where it connects to the papillary layer of the dermis (Figs. 16-13 and 16-14). These muscles are anchored by elastic fibers at their attachments and are innervated by autonomic nerve fibers. The arrector pili muscles are especially well developed along the back of dogs, where they cause the hair to "bristle" when they contract. The contraction of the arrector pili muscles during cold weather elevates the hairs, thus allowing minute air pockets to form in the coat. This dead-air space provides significant insulation that helps to maintain internal body temperature. The contraction of this muscle not only erects the hairs but also may play a role in emptying the sebaceous glands. In addition to the arrector pili muscle, the **interfollicular muscle** which spans the triad of hair follicles has been described in pigs (Figs. 16-14 and 16-15). It is located midway between the level of the sebaceous gland and the apocrine sweat gland. Upon contraction, the interfollicular muscle draws the three follicles close together and rotates the outer follicles of the triad into a new relationship. Adjustment of the hair follicle and hair may play a part in thermoregulation, sensory function, emptying of the skin glands, or self-defense.

Types of Hair Follicles

Hair follicles are classified into several types. A **primary hair follicle** has a large diameter, is rooted deep in the dermis, and is usually associated with sebaceous and sweat glands and an arrector pili muscle (Fig. 16-11). The hair that emerges from such a follicle is called a **primary hair** (guard hair). A **secondary follicle** is smaller in diameter than a primary follicle, and the root is nearer the surface. It may have a sebaceous gland but lacks a sweat gland and an arrector pili muscle. Hairs from these follicles are **secondary hair** or underhairs. Secondary hairs lack a medulla.

Follicles with only one hair emerging to the surface are called **single** or **simple follicles**. **Compound follicles**

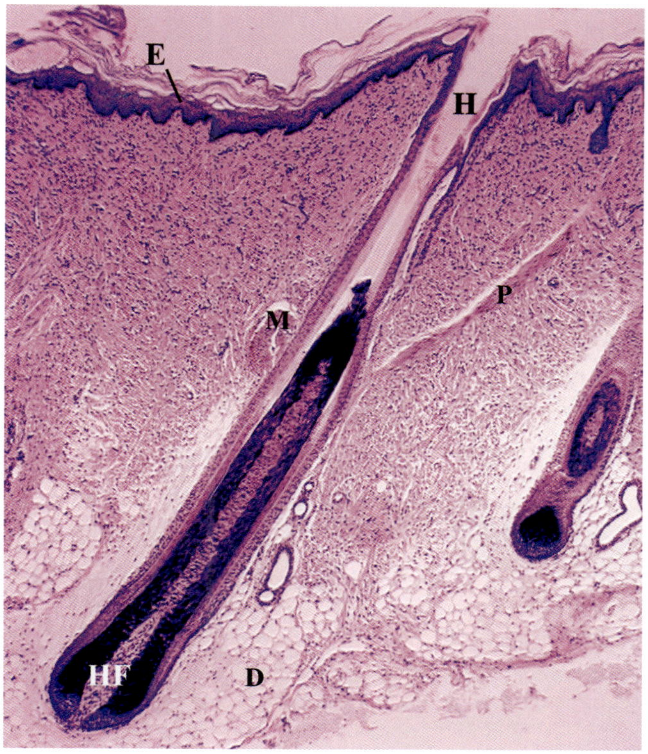

Figure 16-14 Longitudinal section of a hair follicle (HF) showing an attached arrector pili muscle (P), cross section of the interfollicular muscle (M), epidermis (E), hair (H), and hypodermis (D). Pig, H&E (×50). (From Stromberg MW, Hwang YC, Monteiro-Riviere NA. Interfollicular smooth muscle in the skin of the domesticated pig (*Sus scrofa*). *Anat Rec* 1981;201:455.)

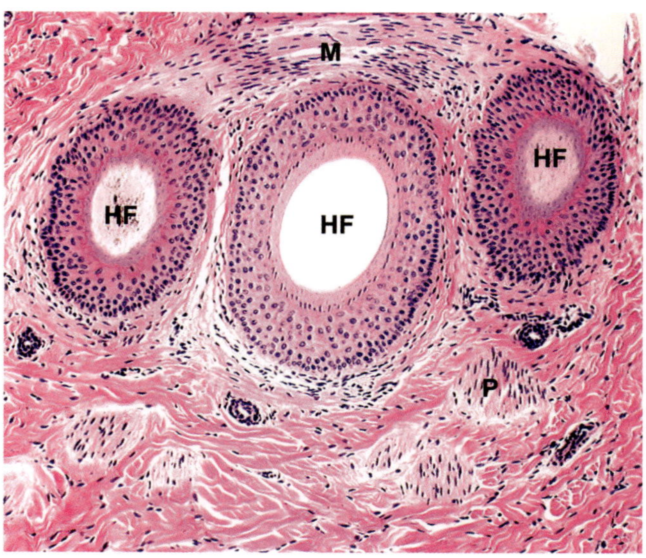

Figure 16-15 Hair follicle triad (pig). Note the hair follicles (HF) occurring in groups of three, typical of young pigs. The interfollicular muscle (M) and arrector pili muscle (P) can be seen. H&E (×100).

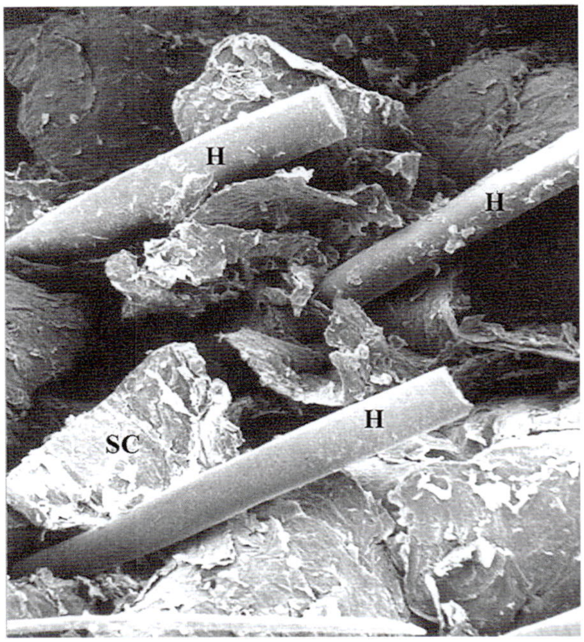

Figure 16-16 Scanning electron micrograph of pig skin depicting hairs (H) occurring in groups of three emerging from the stratum corneum. Note the flaky appearance of the stratum corneum (SC) cells (×60). (From Monteiro-Riviere NA. Comparative anatomy, physiology, and biochemistry of mammalian skin. In: Hobson DW, ed. Dermal and Ocular Toxicology: Fundamentals and Methods. Boca Raton, FL: CRC Press, 1991;1:3–74.)

are composed of clusters of several hair follicles located in the dermis. At the level of the sebaceous gland opening, the follicles fuse and the various hairs emerge through one external orifice. Compound hair follicles usually have one primary hair follicle and several secondary hair follicles.

Many differences exist in the arrangement of the hair follicles among the domestic animals. Horses and cattle have single hair follicles that are distributed evenly. Pigs have single follicles grouped in clusters of two to four follicles; clusters of three are most common in young pigs (Figs. 16-15 and 16-16). This cluster is usually surrounded by dense CT. The compound follicle of dogs consists of a single large primary hair and a group of smaller secondary underhairs (Fig. 16-17). A diversity of hair types is found among different breeds of dogs. For example, in the German Shepherd, a greater number of secondary hairs exist, whereas in the short-coat breeds like the rottweiler and terriers, a greater number of primary hairs are present. The arrangement of the follicles in cats consists of a single large primary (guard) hair follicle surrounded by clusters of two to five compound follicles (Fig. 16-18). Each compound follicle has three coarse primary hairs and 6 to 12 secondary hairs. The skin of sheep has hair-growing regions, such as the face, the distal

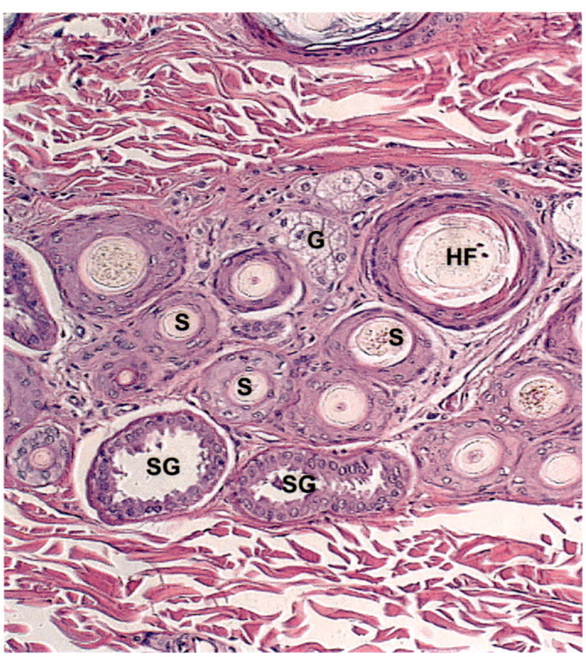

Figure 16-17 Compound hair follicle (dog). Primary hair follicle (HF), sebaceous gland (G), and sweat glands (SG). The other round structures are all secondary follicles (S). H&E (×150).

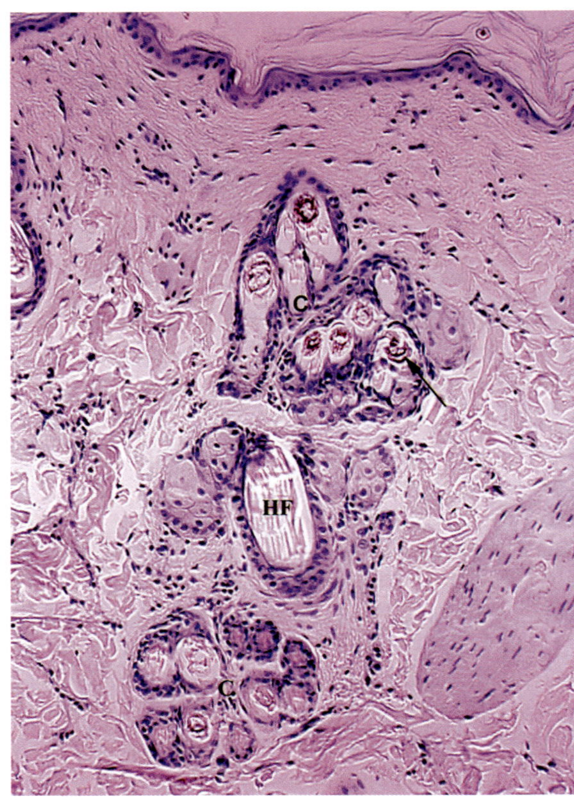

Figure 16-18 Hair follicle cluster (cat). Primary hair follicle (HF) surrounded by groups of compound follicle clusters (C) that contain primary and secondary hairs (arrow). H&E (×160).

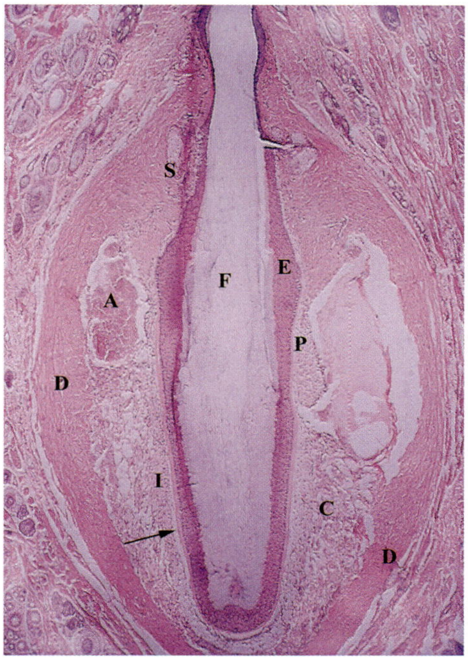

Figure 16-19 Sinus hair follicle (cat). Outer layer of the dermal root sheath (D), inner layer of the dermal root sheath (I), upper annular sinus filled with blood (nontrabecular) (A), cavernous blood sinus with trabeculae (C), glassy membrane (arrow), external epithelial root sheath (E), hair (F), sinus pad (P), and sebaceous glands (S) opening into the pilosebaceous canal. H&E (×50).

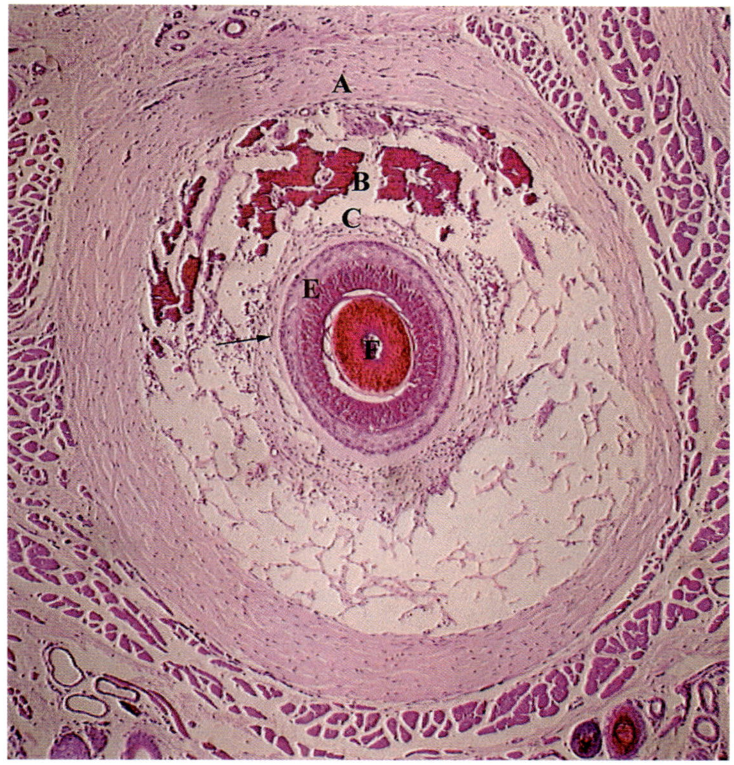

Figure 16-20 Cross section of a sinus hair follicle (cat). Outer layer of the dermal root sheath (A), lower cavernous blood sinus with trabeculae (B), inner layer of the dermal root sheath (C), glassy membrane (arrow), external epithelial root sheath (E), and hair (F). H&E (×60).

part of the limbs, and the pinna of the ear, and has wool-growing regions that cover most of the body. The hair-growing regions mostly contain single follicles, whereas the densely covered wool-growing regions have many compound follicles. The typical follicle cluster contains three single primary hair follicles and several secondary hair follicles. In goats, the single primary hair follicles occur in groups of three; three to six secondary hair follicles are associated with each group.

Sinus or **tactile hair follicles** of the head, e.g., the vibrissae (whiskers) of a cat, are highly specialized for tactile sense. They are very large single follicles characterized by a blood-filled sinus between the inner and outer layers of the dermal root sheath (Fig. 16-19). The sinus is divided into an upper annular sinus (nontrabecular, not separated by CT) and a lower cavernous sinus (trabecular, separated by CT) except in horses and ruminants, in which the annular sinus is traversed by fibroelastic trabeculae throughout its length. In pigs and carnivores, the inner layer of the dermal root sheath thickens in the upper portion of the sinus hair follicles, forming a sinus pad, and this pad is surrounded by an annular sinus free of trabeculae (Fig. 16-20). Skeletal muscles are attached to the outer layer of the dermal root sheath of the follicle, allowing some voluntary control of hair movement. Numerous nerve bundles penetrate the outer layer of the dermal root sheath and ramify in the trabeculae and inner layer of the dermal root sheath.

Hair Cycle

In the surface epidermis, the process of keratinization is continuous because of the uninterrupted production of new keratinocytes, but in the hair follicle, the matrix cells undergo periods of quiescence during which no mitotic activity occurs. When the matrix cell proliferation is reinstituted, a new hair is formed. This cyclic activity of the hair bulb allows for the seasonal change in the hair coat of domestic animals. Hair requires approximately 3 to 4 months to regrow after shaving for normal or short coats and up to 18 months for long coats. The length of time varies, depending on the growth stage of the hair follicle.

The period during which the cells of the hair bulb are mitotically active is called **anagen** (Fig. 16-21). After this growth phase, the hair follicles go through a regressive stage, referred to as **catagen**. During this period, metabolic activity slows

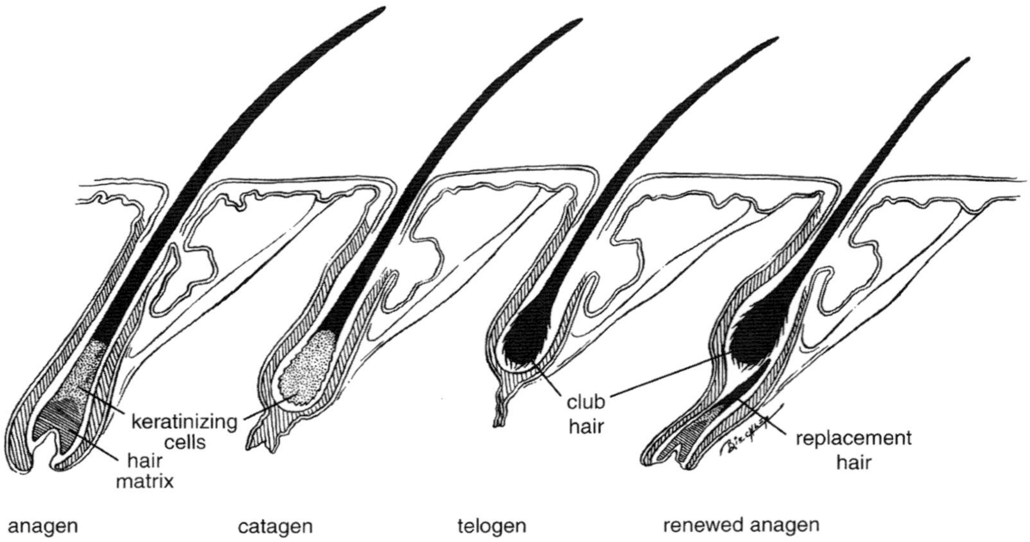

Figure 16-21 Schematic of the three main stages of hair follicle growth and replacement.

down, and the base of the follicle migrates upward in the skin toward the epidermal surface, until all that remains of the bulb is a flimsy, disorganized column of cells, or club hair. The hair follicle then enters **telogen**, a resting or quiescent phase in which growth stops and the base of the bulb is at the level of the sebaceous canal. After the resting phase, mitotic activity and keratinization start again in the renewed anagen phase and a new hair is formed. As the new hair grows beneath the telogen follicle, it gradually pushes the old hair upward toward the surface, where it is eventually shed. This intermittent mitotic activity and keratinization of the hair matrix cells constitute the **hair cycle**, which is controlled by several factors, including length of daily periods of light, ambient temperature, nutrition, and hormones, particularly estrogen, testosterone, adrenal steroids, and thyroid hormones.

Skin Glands

Sebaceous Glands

Sebaceous glands may be simple, branched, or compound alveolar glands that release their secretory product, sebum, by the holocrine mode. **Sebum**, an oily secretion containing a mixture of lipids and disintegrated cells, acts as an antibacterial agent and, in hairy mammals, as a waterproofing agent. The sebaceous glands are most frequently associated with hair follicles, into which their ducts empty to form the pilosebaceous canal of the hair follicle (Fig. 16-19). In certain hairless areas, such as the anal canal, the teat of horses, and the internal layer of the prepuce of some species, sebaceous glands empty directly onto the skin surface through a duct lined with stratified squamous epithelium. The secretory unit consists of a solid mass of epidermal cells, enclosed by a CT sheath that blends with the surrounding dermis. At the periphery of the glandular mass, a single layer of low cuboidal cells rests on a basal lamina (Fig. 16-22). Most of the mitotic activity takes place in this layer, and as the cells move inward, they enlarge, become polygonal, and accumulate numerous lipid droplets. The cells near the duct contain pyknotic nuclei, which are dense and shrunken due to chromatin condensation, typically seen in necrosis or apoptosis. The sebum passes into the lumen of the hair follicle through a short duct lined with stratified squamous epithelium. Many areas of the body of certain species have especially well-developed accumulations of sebaceous glands, some of which are associated with sweat glands. These sites include the infraorbital, inguinal, and interdigital regions of sheep; the base of the horn of goats; anal sacs of cats; and the prepuce and circumanal region of dogs; they are described later in this chapter. Some areas of the skin, such as the foot pads, hoofs, claws, and horn, lack sebaceous glands.

Sweat Glands

Based on their mode of release of the secretory product, sweat (sudoriferous) glands are classified into two types: apocrine and merocrine (eccrine). The apocrine type is the most extensively developed in domestic mammals. The structure of apocrine sweat glands varies considerably among species. It is uncertain whether the apocrine mode of secretion occurs in all sweat glands designated as apocrine and in all domestic species. Nevertheless, the term apocrine is retained, primarily for didactic reasons.

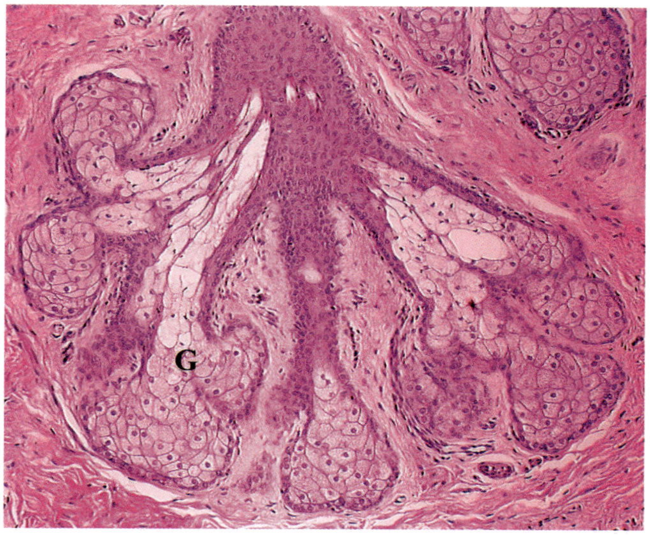

Figure 16-22 Multilobular sebaceous glands (G) of the labium (horse). H&E (×110).

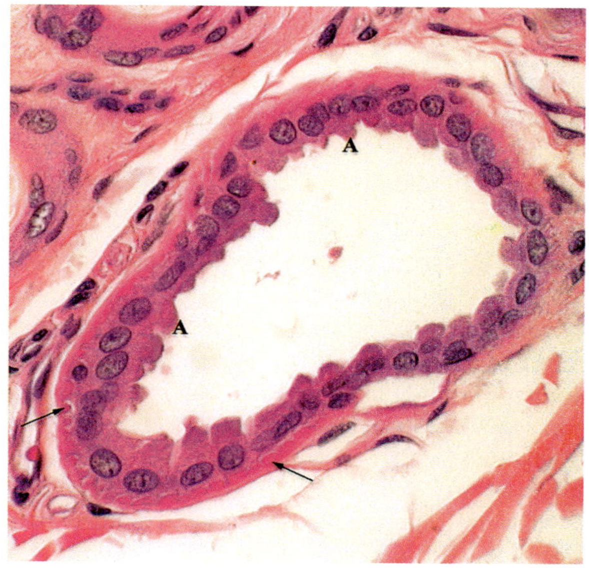

Figure 16-23 Apocrine sweat gland from a dog, illustrating myoepithelial cells (arrows) and apical secretory caps (A). H&E (×660).

The **apocrine sweat glands** are simple saccular or tubular glands with a coiled secretory portion and a straight duct (simple coiled tubular glands). The secretory portion has a large lumen lined with flattened cuboidal to low columnar epithelial cells, depending on the stage of their secretory activity (Fig. 16-23). The cytoplasm may contain glycogen, lipid, or pigment granules. The free surface of cells in apocrine sweat glands has varying cytoplasmic protrusions, indicative of secretory activity. Myoepithelial cells are located between the secretory cells and the basal lamina. The duct pursues a straight course toward the upper part of the dermis. It has a narrow lumen and two layers of flattened cuboidal cells. Most frequently, the duct penetrates the epidermis of the hair follicle, just before it opens onto the surface of the skin. The apocrine glands in the domestic animals are located throughout most of the skin. This characteristic contrasts with their distribution in humans, in which they are mainly in the axillary, pubic, and perianal regions. In horses, these glands secrete abundantly and produce visible sweat during exercise and at high temperatures. In other species, the secretion is scant and rarely perceptible. In dogs and cats, the glands may be tortuous or serpentine, and in ruminants, the lumen is dilated, giving the appearance of large saccules. Apocrine glands are least active in goats and cats. The function of apocrine glands is to produce a viscous secretion of lipids, proteins, and other organic compounds that contain a scent that is related to communications between species, probably as a sex attractant or as a territorial marker. Apocrine glands in several areas of the body are specialized in structure and function and are described later in this chapter.

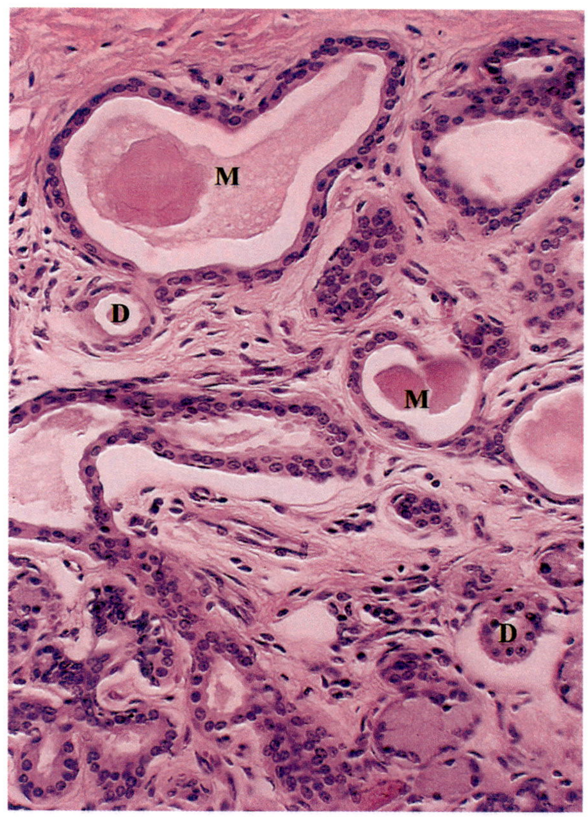

Figure 16-24 Merocrine sweat glands (M) and ducts (D) from the planum nasolabiale or nasolabial plane (cow). H&E (×300).

The **merocrine** (eccrine) **sweat glands** are found mainly in special skin areas, such as the foot pads of dogs and cats, the frog of horse hoofs, the planum rostrale of pigs, the carpal glands of swine, and the bovine planum nasolabiale (Fig. 16-24). They are simple tubular glands that open directly onto the skin surface rather than into hair follicles. The secretory portion is composed of cuboidal epithelium with two distinct cell types. **Dark cells** have more ribosomes than clear cells, and numerous mucin droplets occur in the apical part of the cell. In contrast, **clear cells** lack cytoplasmic basophilia, contain lipid inclusions, and produce aqueous sweat. At the base of these cells, there is an infolding of the plasma membrane, which suggests that they play a role in electrolyte transport. Intercellular canaliculi occur between adjacent clear cells and course from the lumen to the base of the epithelium. Myoepithelial cells surround the secretory units and aid in emptying the gland of secretion. The duct, which is composed of two layers of cuboidal epithelial cells, is relatively straight and opens directly onto the surface of the epidermis.

Blood Vessels, Lymph Vessels, and Nerves

Terminal branches of the cutaneous arteries give rise to three plexuses: (a) the deep or **subcutaneous plexus**, which in turn gives off branches to the (b) middle or **cutaneous plexus**, which provides branches to make up the (c) superficial or **subpapillary plexus** (Fig. 16-1). The reverse applies for venous return to the cutaneous veins. By this arrangement, all components of the skin are ensured an adequate blood supply. The superficial plexus also furnishes the capillary loops that extend into the dermal papillae when present. Lymph capillaries arise in the superficial dermis and form a network that drains into a subcutaneous plexus.

The nerve supply to the skin varies in different parts of the body. Small subcutaneous nerves give rise to a nerve plexus that pervades the dermis and sends small branches to the epidermis. Several kinds of endings are present: free afferent nerve endings in the epidermis and dermis (encircle hair follicles); free efferent endings in the hypodermis (at arrector pili muscles, glands, and blood vessels); nonencapsulated tactile corpuscles (Merkel cells); and encapsulated tactile (Meissner's) corpuscles (see Chapter 4). Lamellar (Pacinian) corpuscles have been observed in the frog of the equine hoof, the digital cushion of the dog and cat, and the anal sac wall of the cat.

Special Structures of the Integument

External Ear

The pinna (auricle) of the ear is covered on both sides by thin skin containing sweat and sebaceous glands and hair follicles (Fig. 16-25). The convex surface of the pinna usually has more hair follicles per unit area than the concave surface. Blood vessels traverse perforations in the elastic cartilage that forms the core of the pinna. Trauma to or even bending of the cartilage can damage the blood vessels and may cause subcutaneous hematomas in ears of dogs.

The lumen of the external auditory meatus is irregular in contour, the result of several permanent skin folds. The skin that lines the canal contains small hair follicles, sebaceous glands, and **ceruminous glands**. Ceruminous glands are simple coiled tubular apocrine sweat glands. The ceruminous glands open either into hair follicles or onto the surface. They increase in number in the lower third of the meatus. The combination of sebum, ceruminous gland secretion, and the desquamating stratified squamous epithelium forms the **cerumen** or ear wax. The external auditory meatus is supported by elastic cartilage in the outer portion and by bone near the tympanic membrane.

Eyelids

The outermost covering of both upper and lower eyelids consists of typical skin containing sweat and sebaceous glands and hair follicles (Fig. 16-26). The cilia, also known as eyelashes, and their associated sebaceous glands (glands of Zeis) are numerous in the upper lid of all species except in cats. In the lower eyelid, the cilia are fewer in number in ruminants and horses and are generally absent in cats, dogs, and pigs. Tactile hairs may be present on or near the eyelids. The inner surface of the eyelids, the palpebral conjunctiva, is a mucous membrane and contains lymphatic tissue at its base (conjunctival fornix). Its epithelial covering varies with the area and species from stratified squamous epithelium near the edge of the eyelid to various combinations of columnar, cuboidal, polyhedral, and squamous cells. As a result, it is variously described as stratified squamous, stratified cuboidal, stratified columnar, and transitional or pseudostratified. Goblet cells are often present (Fig. 16-27).

The most characteristic feature of the eyelids is the **tarsal glands** (meibomian glands), which are better developed in the upper lid (Fig. 16-28). They are multilobular sebaceous glands with a central duct, which opens at the margin of the eyelid. These glands are most highly developed in cats and poorly developed in swine. The tarsal glands are surrounded by the

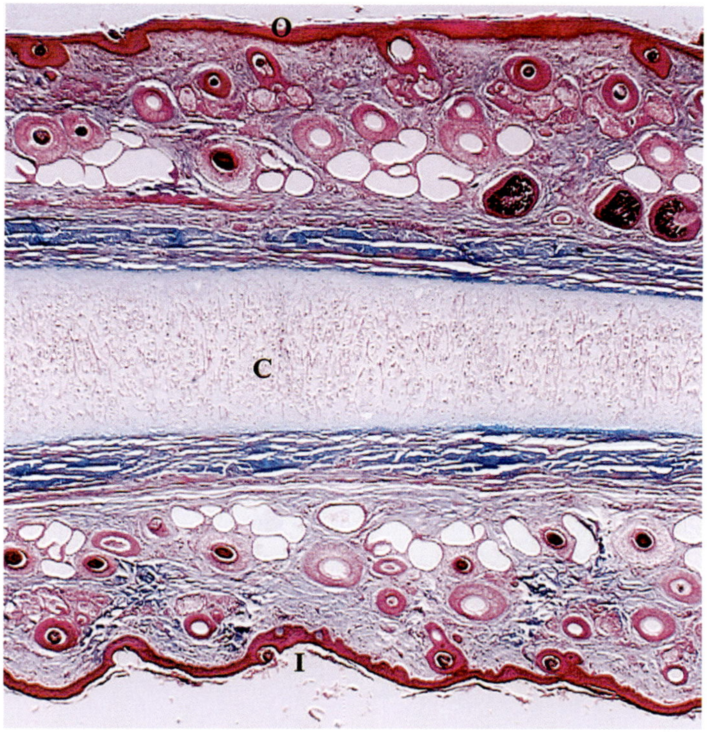

Figure 16-25 Auricula of the ear (cow). Outer surface (O), inner surface (I), and auricular elastic cartilage (C). Masson's trichrome (×30).

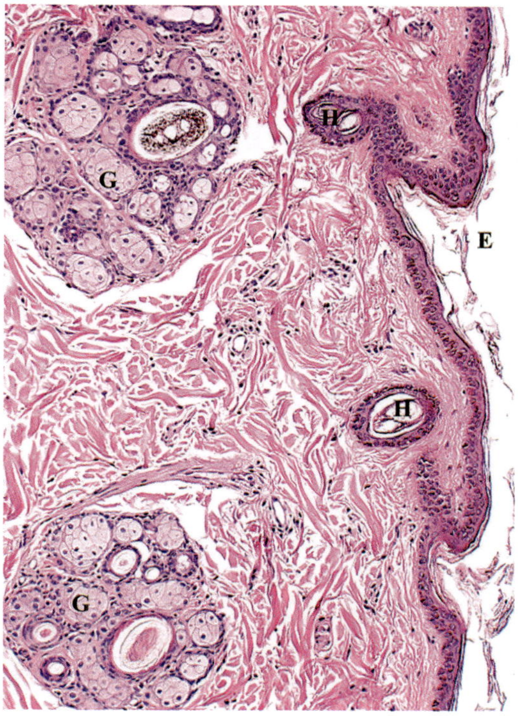

Figure 16-26 Upper eyelid (dog). Anterior or skin surface (E). Numerous hairs (H) and sebaceous glands (G) are present. H&E (×50).

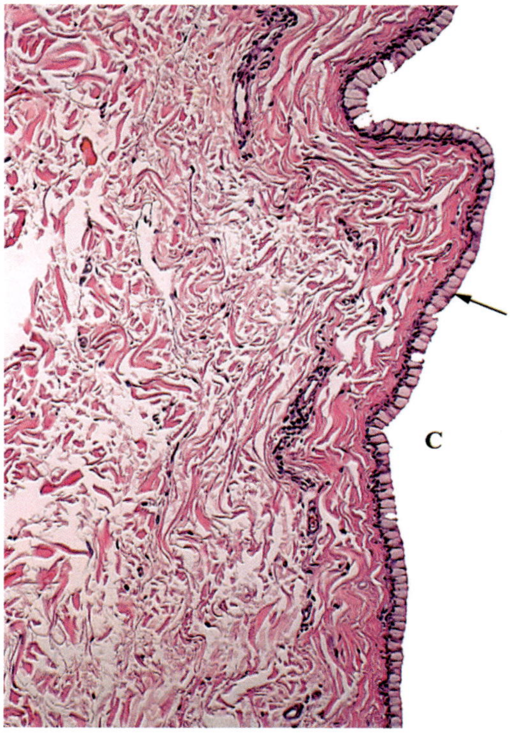

Figure 16-27 Upper eyelid (dog). Posterior or conjunctival surface (C) with pseudostratified epithelium with many goblet cells (arrow). H&E (×150).

tarsal plate, a compact layer of collagen and elastic fibers. Skeletal muscle fibers from the orbicular muscle (orbicularis oculi) penetrate the eyelid, and scattered bundles of smooth muscle fibers are also present.

Apocrine sweat glands, referred to as **ciliary glands** (glands of Moll), open rostrally to the tarsal glands and near the cilia or into the follicles of the cilia. Unlike ordinary sweat glands, the terminal portions of ciliary glands are only slightly coiled, and the gland lumina are more dilated. They are lined by typical cylindric secretory and myoepithelial cells. Their structure and location are similar in all domestic animals, but their function is obscure.

Infraorbital Sinus

The infraorbital sinus of sheep, located medially and rostrally to the eye, is lined with thin skin that contains few hairs, large sebaceous glands that form a continuous layer around the sinus, and a few peripherally located apocrine sweat glands. The secretions of these glands are responsible for the sticky, yellow fatty substance on the skin.

Nose

The skin around the external openings (nares) of the nasal cavity is slightly modified in each species. The planum nasolabiale of cattle has a smooth, thick keratinized epidermis (Fig. 16-29), whereas the

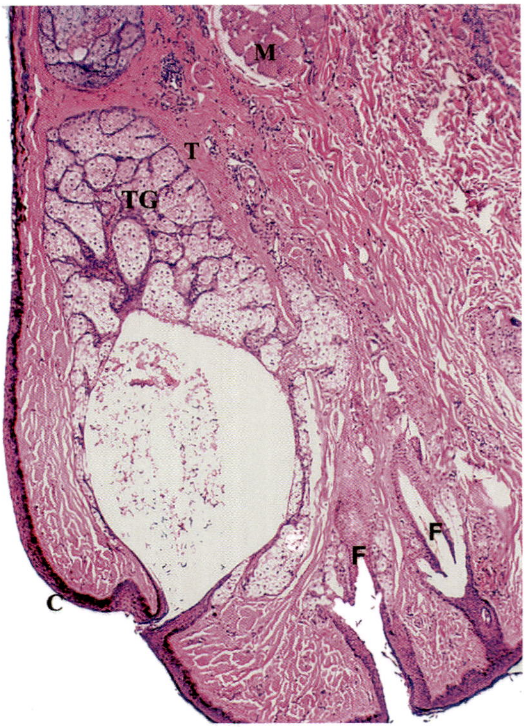

Figure 16-28 Tarsal gland in the upper eyelid (dog). Multilobular sebaceous tarsal gland (TG) in longitudinal section surrounded by the tarsal plate (T), skeletal muscle (M), and hair follicles (F). The conjunctival surface (C) is nonkeratinized stratified squamous epithelium. H&E (×40).

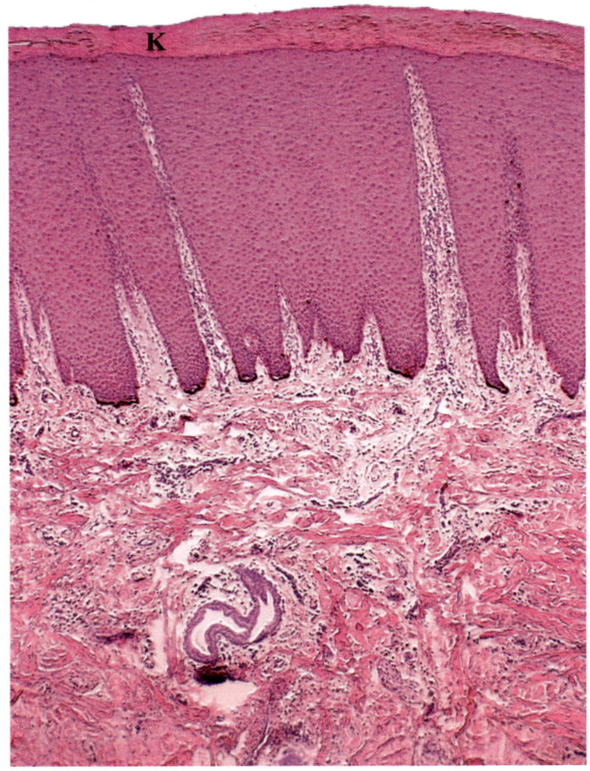

Figure 16-29 Planum nasolabiale (cow). Note the thickened keratinized (K) stratified squamous epithelium. H&E (×50).

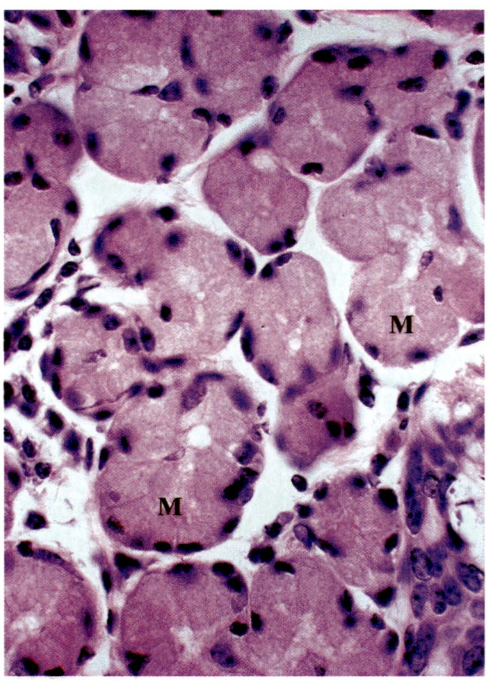

Figure 16-30 Merocrine (mucous) glands (M) of the nasolabial region (cow). H&E (×780).

planum nasale of dogs and cats is composed of a thick, keratinized epidermis with distinct elevations and grooves. These characteristics provide the basis for identification by nose printing, similar to fingerprinting. Neither sweat nor sebaceous glands are associated with the planum nasale. The skin around the nostril of horses is usually thin and contains fine hairs and numerous sebaceous glands. The planum rostrale of pigs has tactile (sinus) hairs distributed over the surface and numerous large merocrine sweat glands. The planum nasale of small ruminants and the planum nasolabiale of large ruminants contain no hair follicles but have large serous merocrine glands (Fig. 16-30) with the same morphologic characteristics as salivary glands. The secretion from these glands aids in keeping the nasolabial plane moist.

Mental Organ

The **mental organ** of pigs consists of a large spherical mass of apocrine and sebaceous glands with a few tactile hairs located midway between the jaws behind the angle of the chin. Tactile (Meissner's) corpuscles and nerve fibers are present in the dermis and, therefore, are believed to play a role in transmitting mechanical stimuli.

Submental Organ

The **submental organ** of cats, located in the intermandibular space, is composed of sebaceous gland lobules, each containing a central collecting space. These lobules are surrounded by skeletal muscles. Cats rub this gland on specific items during olfactory marking and the sebaceous scent is transferred to the rubbed object.

Carpal Glands

The **carpal glands** of pigs are accumulations of numerous lobules of densely packed merocrine sweat glands on the medial surface of the carpus. They open to the skin surface through three to five diverticula lined with stratified squamous epithelium. Each lobule is drained by a duct lined with a bilayered cuboidal epithelium, which pursues a tortuous course through the dermis and epidermis and then opens into a diverticulum.

Interdigital Sinus

The **interdigital sinus** of sheep is located between the digits just above the hoofs. The opening of the sinus is at the dorsal tip of the interdigital space. The skin of the sinus contains a few hair follicles, associated sebaceous glands, and numerous large apocrine glands collectively referred to as the **interdigital glands**.

Inguinal Sinus

The **inguinal sinus** of sheep is a cutaneous diverticulum in the inguinal region of both sexes that contains scattered small hair follicles, sebaceous glands, and apocrine glands.

Scrotum

Generally, scrotal skin is thinner than skin on other parts of the body. Sebaceous and apocrine sweat glands are present but differ in size and number in various species. Boars have only a few small apocrine sweat glands in the scrotal skin, whereas stallions have both large sebaceous glands and well-developed apocrine sweat glands. The amount of pigment varies with species and breed. Short, fine hair is characteristic of scrotal skin of all species. The **tunica dartos** is a unique layer of smooth muscle and fibroelastic CT within the subcutaneous tissue of the scrotum. These muscle fibers play an important role in the regulation of testicular temperature.

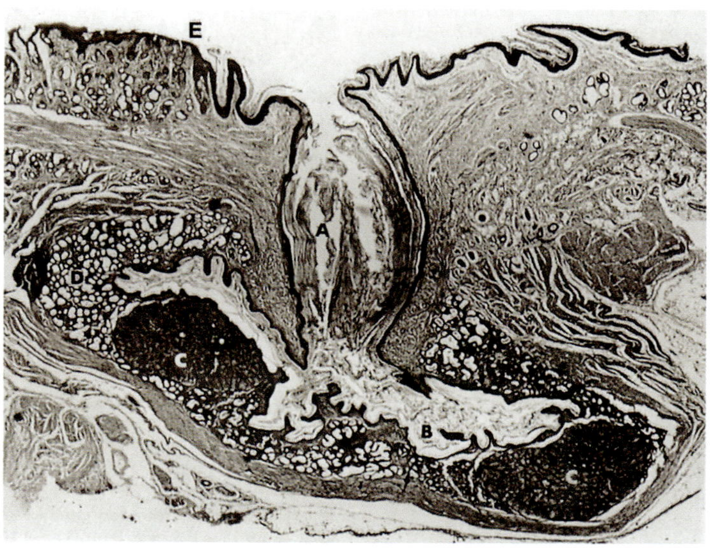

Figure 16-31 Anal sac and associated glands (cat). Duct (A) and lumen (B) of the anal sac filled with keratinized epithelial fragments and secretory material. Sebaceous gland masses (C), apocrine anal sac glands (D), and linea anocutanea (E). H&E (×17). (Greer MB, Calhoun ML. The anal sacs of the domestic cat- *Felis domesticus*. *Am J Vet Res* 1966;27:773.)

Anal Sacs

The **anal sacs** (sinus paranales) of domestic carnivores are paired cutaneous diverticula, the ducts of which open into the anal canal at the level of the anocutaneous line (Fig. 16-31). The ducts and sacs are lined by keratinized stratified squamous epithelium. The **glands of anal sacs** are modified sweat glands located beneath the epithelium, empty into the lumen of the anal sac. Both sebaceous and apocrine sweat glands are present in the wall of the anal sac in cats (Fig. 16-32), but dogs have only large apocrine sweat glands. The anal sac duct of dogs is prone to occlusion, which

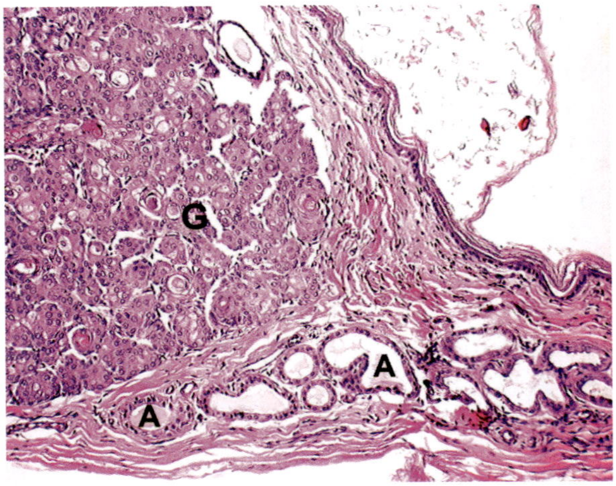

Figure 16-32 Higher magnification of the anal sac (cat). Note the large apocrine glands (A) and sebaceous glands (G). H&E (×100).

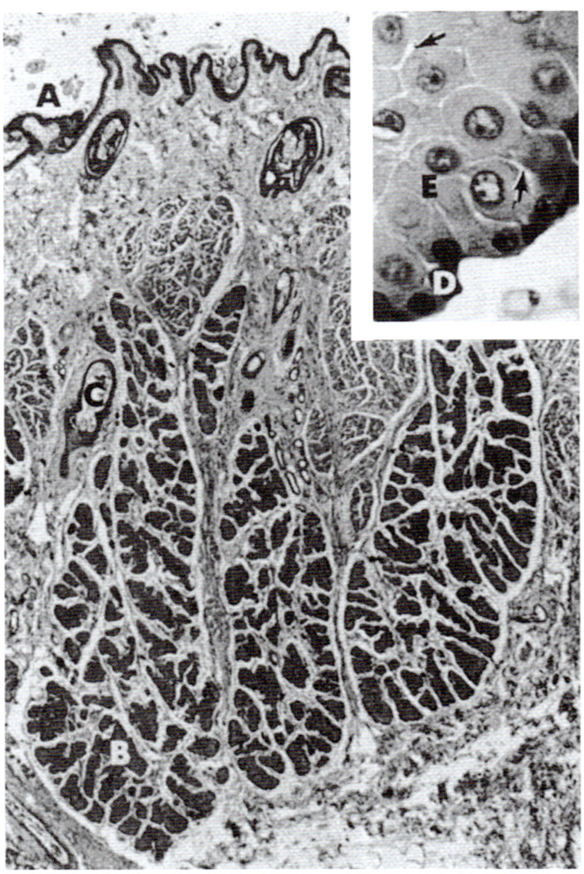

Figure 16-33 Circumanal glands (dog). Cutaneous zone (A), hepatoid circumanal gland (B), and ducts (C). H&E (×20). Inset: Peripheral cells (D), nonsebaceous gland cells (E), and intercellular canaliculi (arrows). H&E (×480).

results in anal sac engorgement with secretory material and detritus. The infection that frequently follows this occlusion necessitates either the expression of the content of the sac or the surgical removal of the sac. This problem is rare in cats, probably because the sebaceous glands within the sac wall add enough lipid to the secretory material, reducing the risk of duct blockage. The secretion of these glands is a brownish and oily fluid that may function in social recognition in dogs and can have a pungent odor with impaction and infection. Clinically, apocrine gland adenocarcinomas are malignant and one of the most common tumors of dogs but rarely found in cats.

Circumanal Glands

The **circumanal glands** of dogs are lobulated, modified sebaceous glands located around the anus in the cutaneous zone (Fig. 16-33). They extend from the mucocutaneous junction peripherally for approximately 1 to 3 cm in all directions. Similar glands have been described in the skin of the prepuce, tail, loin, and groin. These glands are present shortly after birth, increase in size throughout adult life, and tend to atrophy at senility. The superficial portion of the circumanal glands consists of typical sebaceous glands, whereas the deep portion is ductless and composed of solid, compact masses of polygonal cells arranged in lobules. The cells have granular eosinophilic cytoplasm and intercellular canaliculi (Fig. 16-33). The term **hepatoid** has been used to describe the glandular parenchyma of each lobule as it closely resembles packed liver cells. A precise function for these glands has not been determined; however, they may be involved in the metabolism of a steroid hormone. The circumanal glands are clinically important because they rank third in frequency as a site of canine tumors.

Supracaudal Gland

The **supracaudal gland** (tail gland or preen gland), located in an oval circumscribed area on the dorsum of the tail (3 to 9 cm from the base of the tail) in dogs and cats, is an accumulation of large sebaceous glands that empty into single hair follicles (Fig. 16-34). The apocrine sweat glands in this region are rudimentary. Well-developed arrector pili muscles appear as large bundles of smooth muscle. The epidermis above this gland is extremely thin, and the structure of this gland is like the superficial portion of the circumanal glands. The secretion may aid in olfactory recognition, and it can cause a matting of the hair of the region, especially if the glands are overactive. In cats, it is commonly known as stud tail. This matting can present a problem in show cats because the appearance of the hair coat of the tail is affected.

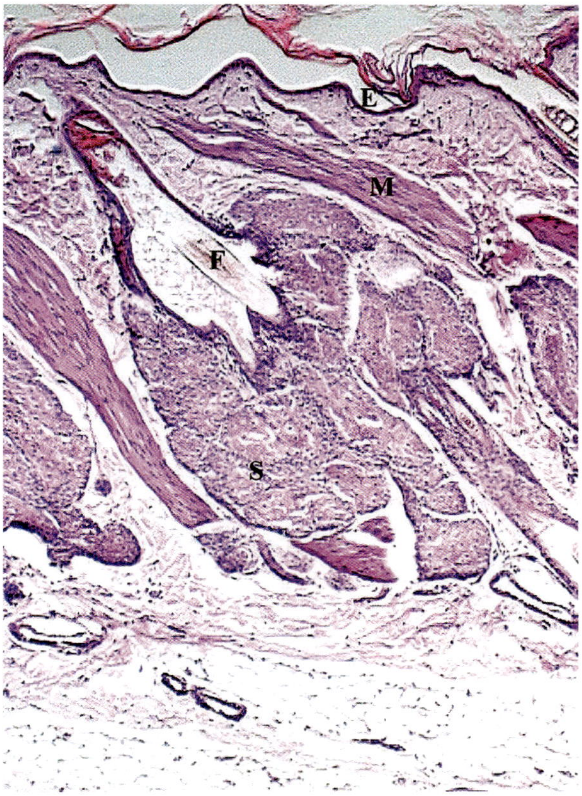

Figure 16-34 Supracaudal gland, tail region (cat). Thin epidermis (E), sebaceous glands (S) and ducts opening into hair follicles (F), and large bundles of smooth muscle (M). H&E (×80).

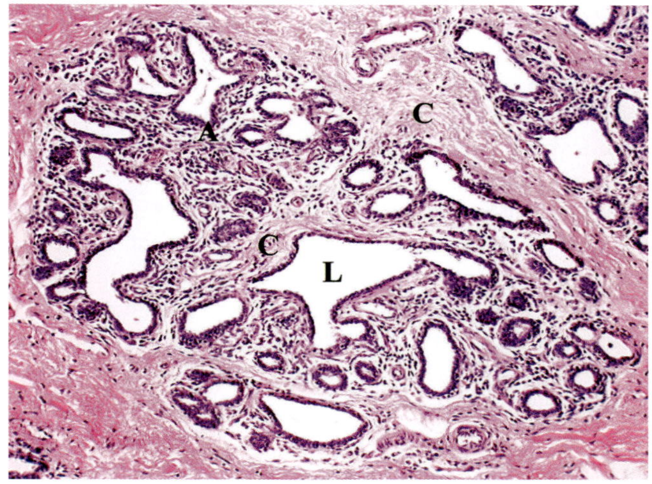

Figure 16-35 Nonlactating mammary gland (cow). Gland lobules with alveoli (A), large irregular openings represent intralobular ducts (L), and loose CT (C). H&E (×100).

Mammary Gland

Knowledge of the microscopic anatomy of the mammary gland is important to the understanding of mastitis in large animals and mammary tumors in small animals. Mastitis is inflammation of this gland and is one of the most common and economically significant clinical diseases in cows. In response to bacterial infection, inflammatory changes occur in the gland with an influx of many blood-borne neutrophils.

The mammary gland is a compound tubuloalveolar gland (Fig. 16-35). Groups of tubuloalveolar secretory units form lobules separated by CT septa.

Alveoli

Secretory alveoli of the mammary gland are spherical to ovoid in shape with a large lumen (Figs. 16-35 and 16-36). Continuous milk production enlarges the lumen, and adjacent alveoli may fuse partially (Fig. 16-36). Shortly after milking, as the alveolus begins a new secretory cycle, the lumen is partially collapsed and irregular in outline.

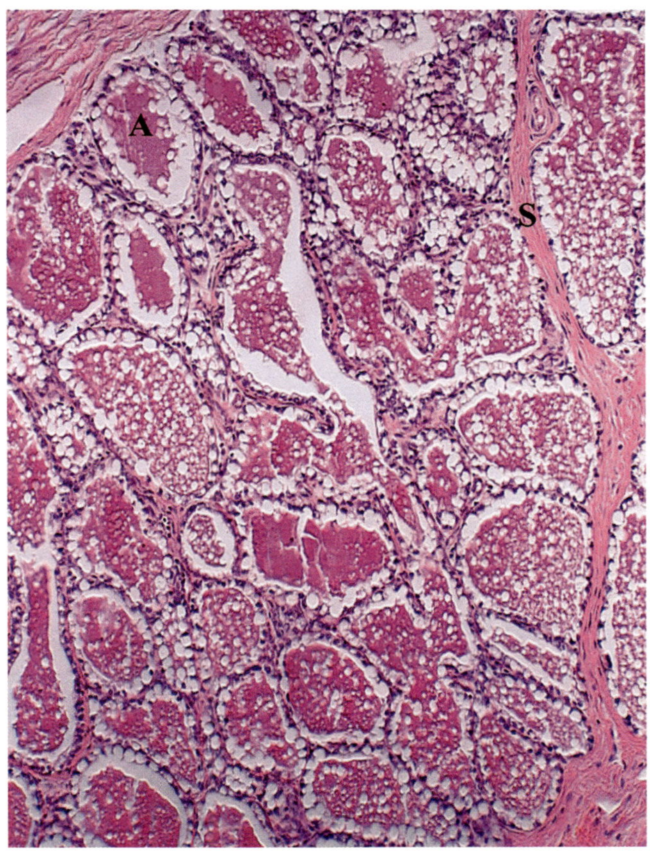

Figure 16-36 Lactating mammary gland filled with colostrum (sheep). Alveolus (A) and interlobular septum (S). H&E (×120).

Clusters of alveoli form lobules within the gland. Not all lobules are in the same secretory phase simultaneously. Some lobules may complete their secretory cycle and fill with milk before others begin. Therefore, a single histologic section may contain lobules in various stages of activity. Usually, all of the secretory alveoli within a lobule are in approximately the same secretory phase.

The epithelium of the alveoli varies markedly in height during the various stages of secretory activity. During active secretion, the basal portion of the columnar epithelial cells contains a well-developed rough endoplasmic reticulum. The spherical nuclei are located near the center of the cell. Lipid droplets, in close association with mitochondria, and vesicles, filled with micelles of milk protein, occur throughout the cell apex. As the secretory cycle continues, the lipid droplets move toward the cell surface that protrudes into the alveolar lumen. The lipid droplets are released from the cell, surrounded by varying amounts of cytoplasm and plasmalemma. The protein-filled vesicles also move toward the cell surface, where they are released by exocytosis. Milk is thus produced by both apocrine and merocrine secretion. At the end of the secretory cycle, the epithelial cells are low cuboidal in shape.

Myoepithelial cells, surrounding the alveolar epithelial cells, contract in response to oxytocin released from the neurohypophysis. The contraction forces the milk from the secretory units into the duct system. This phenomenon is called **milk letdown**.

Interstitium

The interstitial tissue of the mammary gland provides important structural support for the secretory units and contains the blood vessels, lymph vessels, and nerves. Each secretory unit is surrounded by loose CT with an extensive plexus of blood and lymph capillaries. Plasma cells and lymphocytes are common, particularly at parturition when the immunoglobulin-rich colostrum is secreted. The interlobular CT is thick and contains the lobular ducts and larger blood and lymph vessels.

Ducts

The duct system begins with an **intralobular duct** (Fig. 16-35), which drains into a **lobular duct**. The lobular duct, in turn, drains into a **lobar lactiferous duct**, which is the primary excretory duct for a lobe. The intralobular duct epithelium is simple cuboidal. Spindle-shaped myoepithelial cells may be associated with these ducts. Lobular ducts are lined proximally by a simple cuboidal epithelium and, more distally, by two layers of cuboidal cells. Longitudinal smooth muscle fibers become associated with these ducts as they merge with other lobular ducts to form the large lactiferous ducts. The two-layered cuboidal epithelium continues in these larger ducts, and smooth muscle becomes more prominent. Sacculations result from variations in the diameter of the lumen. The constrictions between these sacculations may have an annular fold containing smooth muscle. Several lactiferous ducts empty into a **lactiferous sinus** (gland sinus) at the base of the teat.

Teat

The **teat**, or nipple, contains the terminal part of the duct system. The lactiferous sinus is continuous with the **teat sinus** (teat cistern cavity of the teat), which is lined by stratified cuboidal epithelium. The lamina propria of the teat sinus may contain small clusters of mammary gland tissue. Smooth muscle bundles, oriented parallel to the long axis of the teat, are prominent in some species, and form the boundary between the teat mucosa and the surrounding dermis of the skin. Numerous blood vessels in the dermis form a vascular stratum that becomes engorged with blood during the milking or suckling process; thus, the overlying skin of the teat is stretched, resulting in a smooth surface. After milking, when the blood has drained from the teat vessels and the longitudinal smooth muscle has contracted, the teat surface returns to its typical corrugated appearance.

An annular fold of the mucosa extends into the opening between the lactiferous sinus and teat sinus. The size of this opening is somewhat variable from one animal to another. Occasionally, trabeculae of CT may extend across the opening, resulting in the reduction of milk flow from the lactiferous sinus to the teat sinus. These trabeculae are called “spiders,” and frequently, veterinarians must cut them surgically.

The teat sinus empties into one or more **papillary ducts** (teat canal or streak canal) leading to the external surface of the teat. A single papillary duct is present in ruminants while multiple papillary ducts open separately onto the teat surface of other species. Horses have 2 papillary ducts, pigs have 2 or 3, cats have 4 to 7, and dogs have 7 to 16. The papillary duct is lined with stratified squamous epithelium. Circularly oriented bundles of smooth muscle in the mucosa form a sphincter to hold the milk in the teat sinus above the duct until it is forced out by milking or suckling.

The skin of the teat in cows and sows is composed of a thick, keratinized stratified squamous epithelium and dermis without hair follicles, and sweat or sebaceous glands. However, in some domestic species such as sheep and goats, the teat may contain fine hairs and sweat and sebaceous glands.

Mammary Gland Involution

After the lactation period or sudden arrest of suckling or milking, glandular involution begins. The alveoli are distended by accumulated milk and no further secretion occurs until they are emptied. It was once believed that if the secretory product were not removed for several days, the epithelial cells would degenerate and the residual milk in the lumen would be absorbed gradually. However, recent research has suggested less loss of mammary epithelial cells than previously believed. Characteristically, the involuted mammary gland has more interstitial tissue than glandular elements, and isolated clusters of branched tubules with a few small alveoli are all that remain of the parenchyma (Fig. 16-35). The alveoli are lined by a low cuboidal epithelium with prominent underlying myoepithelial cells. The CT septa are thicker, and fat cells may occur singly or in clusters. Lymphocytes and plasma cells are present in significant amounts. Small, dark-staining bodies of casein (corpora amylacea) may be found in the alveoli, ducts, or interstitial tissue.

Digital Organs and Horn

The digital organ consists of a keratinized epidermis, underlying dermis, and a hypodermis of variable thickness. Hard keratin, or horn, forms the keratinized portion of the hoofs of horses, ruminants, and pigs, as well as the claws of carnivores. The dermis (corium) contains blood vessels and nerves. The hypodermis is absent in some regions of the digit (hoof wall, sole, and claw), but in the ground contact region, the hypodermis is modified to form the digital cushion, located deep to the dermis. Bones or phalanges and their ligaments and tendons form the supportive structure of the digit.

Equine Hoof

The epidermis of the skin on the equine limb continues distally as the **periople**, a ring of epidermis that produces soft, nonpigmented tubular, and intertubular horn above the coronary border of the hoof. Toward the back of the foot, the periople widens into a broad keratinized layer or **bulb** (heel). From the periople, the epidermis angles internally to line the **coronary groove**. Finally, **epidermal laminae** extend vertically from the coronary groove to the ground surface of the hoof.

The dermis of the hoof is usually referred to as the **corium**. **Perioplic corium** is continuous with **coronary corium**, anchoring epidermal structures (periople and coronary epidermis) to underlying tissues. The **laminar corium** interdigitates with the epidermal laminae and fills the space between the laminae and the distal phalanx. The corium is composed of bundles of coarse collagen fibers and a massive network of large arteries and veins without valves. This vascular bed helps to dampen the compressive forces transmitted from the hard inflexible hoof to the phalanx.

The keratinized portion of the equine hoof is composed of three main parts. The wall (paries) is that portion that is visible when the foot is placed on the ground. The sole (solea) forms the greatest part of the ventral surface of the foot; the frog (cuneus ungulae) is a wedge-shaped structure that projects into the sole.

Wall

The **wall** of the hoof is composed of three layers (Fig. 16-37). From the outside inward, they are the **stratum externum** (tectorium), the **stratum medium**, and the **stratum internum** (lamellatum). Each of these is structurally distinct and separately described in the following paragraphs.

The **stratum externum** is a thin layer of tubular and intertubular horn, which is a continuation of the stratum corneum of the perioplic epidermis. This layer covers the outer surface of the hoof wall.

The **stratum medium** consists of tubular and intertubular "hard" horn and is the main supportive structure of the wall (Fig. 16-38). The **horny tubules** are solid rods and oriented parallel to the outer surface of the hoof. Their keratinized cells have a highly ordered arrangement. The cross-sectional profiles of the tubules may be circular, oval, or wedge-shaped. They have a central region (**medulla**) of loose keratinized cells similar to the medulla of a hair shaft and a peripheral cortex of more compact keratinized cells. The **cortex** of the tubule has three zones (Fig. 16-39). The **inner zone** contains keratinized cells oriented around the medulla in tight coils; the cells of the **middle zone** form loose spirals; and the cells of the **outer zone** form another layer of tight coils. This coiled, spring-like arrangement of the cells of tubular horn helps dampen the compression of the hoof when it strikes a hard surface. The **intertubular horn** fills the spaces between the tubular horn.

The stratum medium is produced by the stratum basale and stratum spinosum of the epidermis lining the coronary groove. This epidermis covers the **coronary corium**, which is a bed of vascularized CT with long papillae. The germinal cells covering the tips of the papillae give rise to loose cells of the medulla of the tubule, whereas those over the sides and base of the papillae

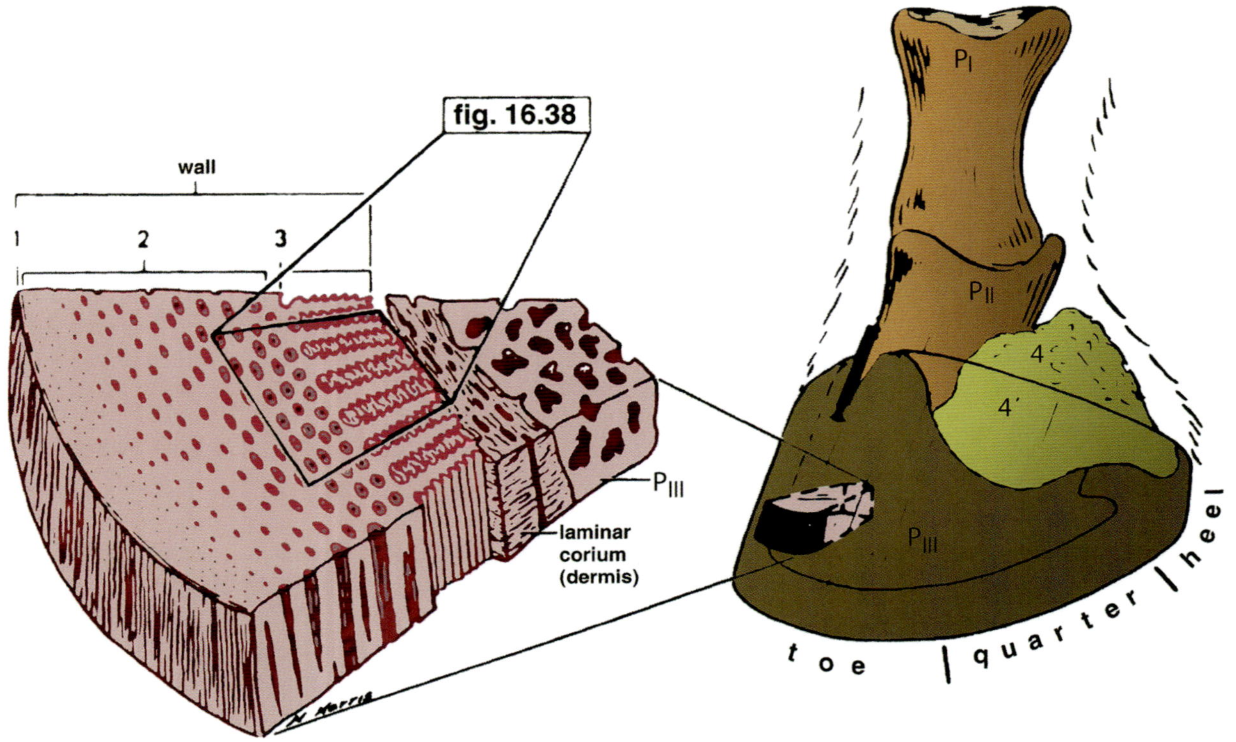

Figure 16-37 Equine foot (dorsolateral view). The wall of the hoof is composed of three layers: stratum externum (1), stratum medium (2), and stratum internum (3). Also shown are the proximal (PI), medial (PII), and distal (PIII) phalanges, and cartilage of the hoof (4) and (4′). (From Stump JE. Anatomy of the normal equine foot, including microscopic features of the laminar region. *J Am Vet Med Assoc* 1967;151:1588.)

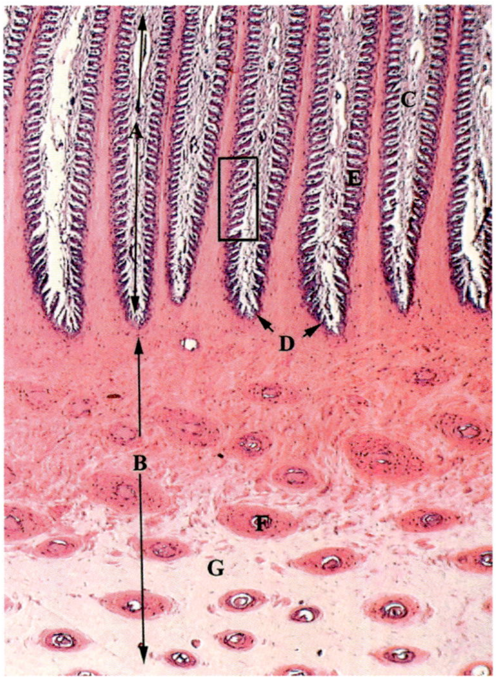

Figure 16-38 Wall of hoof (horse) from the area marked in Figure 16-37. Stratum internum (A), stratum medium (B), primary dermal lamina (C), primary epidermal lamina (D), secondary epidermal and dermal laminae (E), tubular horn (F), and intertubular horn (G). Area in box is Figure 16-40. H&E (×40).

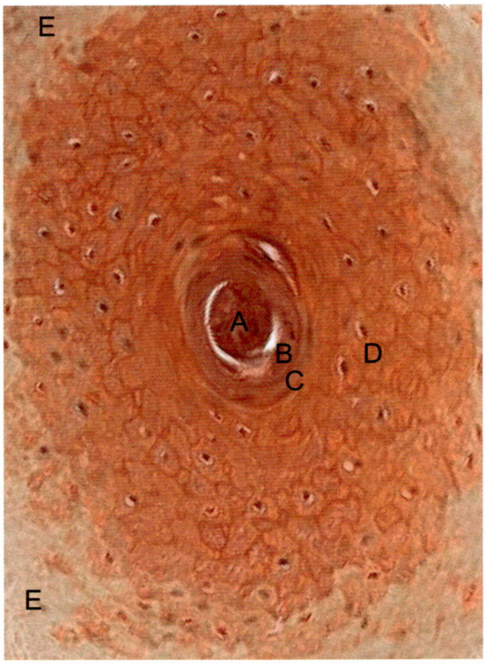

Figure 16-39 Stratum medium showing the cellular arrangement of tubular horn, hoof (horse). Medulla (A), inner zone of cortex (B), middle zone of cortex (C), outer zone of cortex (D), and intertubular horn (E). H&E (×250).

proliferate to form the keratinized cells of the cortex. The germinal cells covering the interpapillary part of the coronary corium give rise to the intertubular horn. The layers of the intertubular horn consist of hard keratin that helps hold the tubules together. The hypodermis deep to the coronary corium is referred to as the coronary cushion. It is composed of dense collagen fibers and numerous large blood vessels.

The **stratum internum** (lamellatum) consists of approximately 600 vertically oriented, keratinized primary epidermal laminae extending inward from the stratum medium, with which they are continuous (Fig. 16-38). One hundred to 200 secondary laminae project at acute angles from each primary lamina (Fig. 16-40). These secondary laminae interdigitate with similar laminae of the lamellar corium and form a complex epidermal–dermal association that anchors the keratinized hoof to the underlying CT. The **primary epidermal laminae** are part of the stratum corneum (hard keratin) produced by the stratum germinativum, which is located between the proximal ends of the dermal laminae at the deep edge of the coronary groove. The cells keratinize as they move downward toward the ground surface of the hoof, accompanying the lengthening stratum medium. The **secondary epidermal laminae** are cellular and composed of stratum germinativum. The stratum basale of each secondary epidermal lamina rests on the CT of each **secondary dermal lamina**, forming the interdigitation between the two laminae. The central core of each secondary epidermal lamina is composed of stratum spinosum, one to three cell layers in thickness, that attaches to the sides of the keratinized primary epidermal lamina (Fig. 16-40). The germinal cells of the secondary epidermal laminae multiply throughout the length of the laminae only at a rate to keep up with the downward growth of the horny primary laminae. The wall grows in length at the rate of 6.4 mm per month; 9 to 12 months are required for the hoof to grow from the coronary border to the ground at the toe region. Growth is accomplished by the distal sliding of the stratum medium and primary epidermal laminae over the stationary secondary epidermal laminae. The interdigitation between the nonpigmented wall laminae with the pigmented tubular and intertubular horn of the sole is referred to as the **white line**.

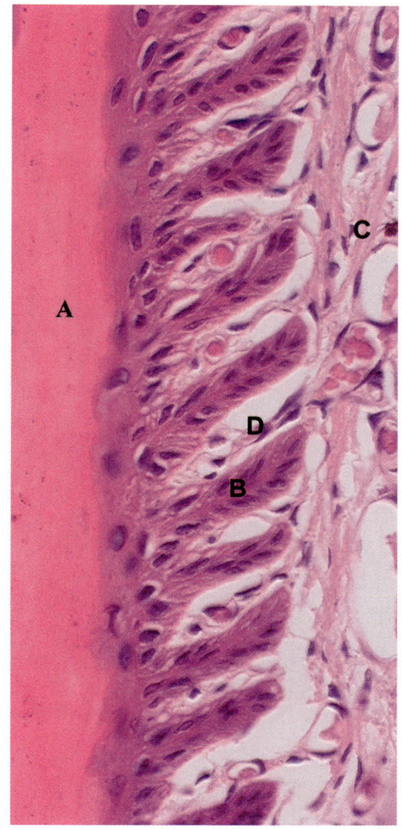

Figure 16-40 Secondary laminae, hoof (horse). See area marked in Figure 16-38. Primary epidermal lamina of the wall (A), secondary epidermal lamina (B), primary dermal lamina (C), and secondary dermal lamina (D). H&E (×725).

Knowledge of the structure of the tissues of the hoof is important to the understanding of the pathophysiology of laminitis, the most devastating clinical disease syndrome of the equine hoof. A disturbance in the physical and physiological (nutritional blood supply) influences on various parts of the hoof results in inflammation of the laminae, often resulting in separation of the hoof from the digit and loss of the horse.

Sole

The epidermis of the **sole** produces tubular and intertubular horn. Its superficial layers are not firmly attached and can be peeled off in the form of small flakes. The corium (dermis) of the sole bears long papillae, the epidermal covering of which gives rise to the tubular horn of the sole. In addition, the corium blends with the periosteum of the ventral surface of the distal phalanx.

Frog

The epidermis of the **frog** produces tubular and intertubular horn that is softer than that of the wall and sole. The corium (dermis) of the frog forms small, short papillae. The corium blends with the **digital cushion**, which is a wedge-shaped mass of collagen and elastic fibers among masses of fat that acts as a shock absorber. Branched coiled merocrine sweat glands chiefly occur in the part that overlies the central sulcus of the frog.

Ruminant and Swine Hoofs

The hoofs of ruminants and pigs are similar to those of horses, with a few exceptions. The stratum internum and corresponding laminar corium consist of only primary laminae (Fig. 16-41). The sole consists of a narrow rim next to the angle of inflection of the wall. There is no frog, but a prominent bulb of soft, thin horn that is continuous with the skin makes up a large part of the ventral surface of the hoof.

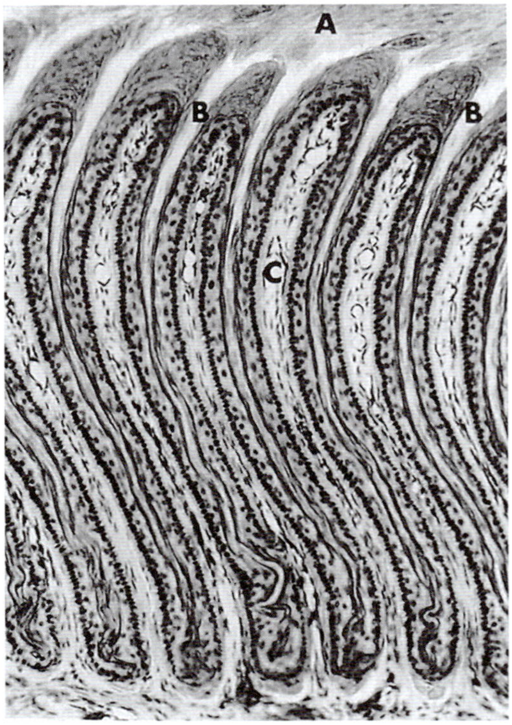

Figure 16-41 Stratum internum, hoof (sheep). Stratum medium (A), primary laminae (B), and laminar corium with numerous capillaries (C). H&E (×120).

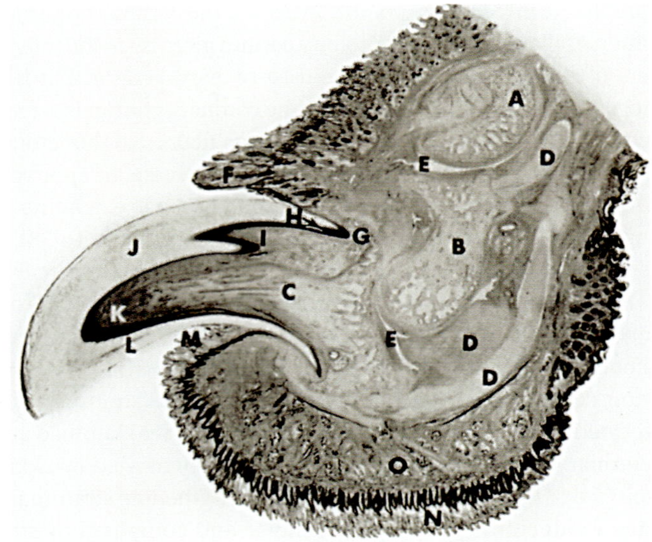

Figure 16-42 Claw (dog). Proximal phalanx (A), middle phalanx (B), distal phalanx (C), tendons (D), joint cavities with accompanying joint capsules and articular cartilages (E), fold of skin overlying claw (F), ungual crest (G), nonkeratinized epidermal layers of the claw (H), dorsal ridge (I), stratum corneum of the claw epidermis (J), dermis (K), sole (L), limiting furrow (M) between the sole and digital pad (N), and dermis of the digital pad with clusters of coiled merocrine sweat glands and fat (O). H&E (×4). (From Adam WS, Calhoun ML, Smith EM, et al. Microscopic Anatomy of the Dog: A Photographic Atlas. Springfield, IL: Charles C. Thomas, 1970.)

Claw

The **claws**, or nails, of dogs and cats are specialized structures that are continuous with the epidermis and dermis of the skin of the foot. Claws consist of shields of hard keratin that cover the distal phalanges and possess both a wall and a sole (Fig. 16-42).

The **wall** or **claw plate** covers the coronary corium and the wall corium. It is thickest in the area of the dorsal ridge and gradually thins out along the side. Its thin ventral margins extend beyond the junction of the wall with the sole. The epidermis of the dorsal ridge forms a few short laminae that interdigitate with similar dermal laminae.

The epidermis of the **sole** is thick and produces a softer form of keratin than that of the wall. A stratum granulosum and a stratum lucidum are present.

The dermis of the claw is composed of dense irregular CT that forms a thick ridge over the dorsal surface of the distal phalanx. It is rich in blood vessels and prone to hemorrhage if the nail is cut too short.

The **claw fold** is a fold of skin, like the periople of the hoof, that covers the claw plate for a short distance on its dorsal and lateral margins. As the plate grows, it carries with it a thin layer of keratinized cells. This layer of cells is produced by the epidermis of the inner surface of the claw fold.

Digital Pads

The **digital pads** of the dog and cat are covered by a thick hairless epidermis that contains all epidermal cell layers, including a stratum lucidum. The surface is smooth in the cat (Fig. 16-43) and roughened by keratinized conical/rounded papillae in the dog (Fig. 16-44). The dermis has prominent papillae that interdigitate with the epidermal pegs and contains coiled merocrine sweat glands that extend into the digital cushion, the hypodermis. Subcutaneous masses of adipose tissue are separated and enclosed by collagen and elastic fibers.

Chestnut and Ergot

The equine **chestnut** and **ergot** have a thick epidermis composed of tubular and intertubular horn interdigitating with long dermal papillae (Fig. 16-45). Arrector pili muscles, glands, and hairs are absent in both of these structures.

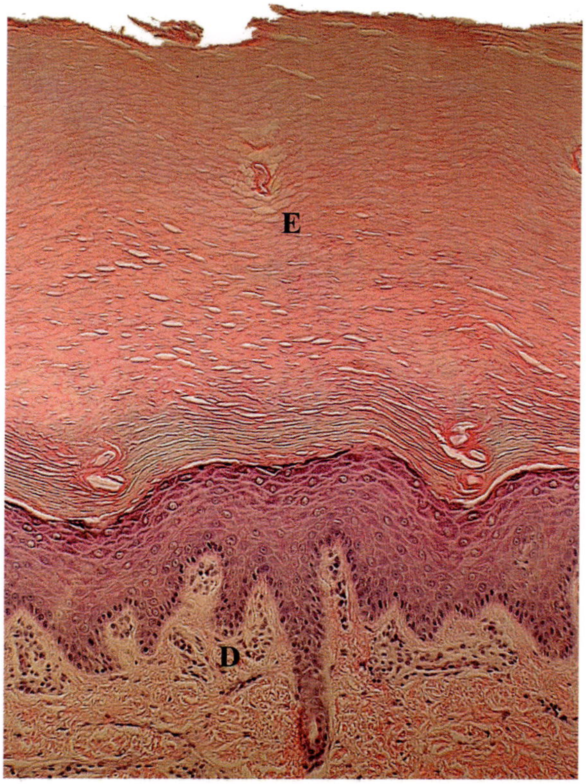

Figure 16-43 Foot pad (cat). The keratinized epidermis (E) is smooth and the dermis (D) is papillated. H&E (×130).

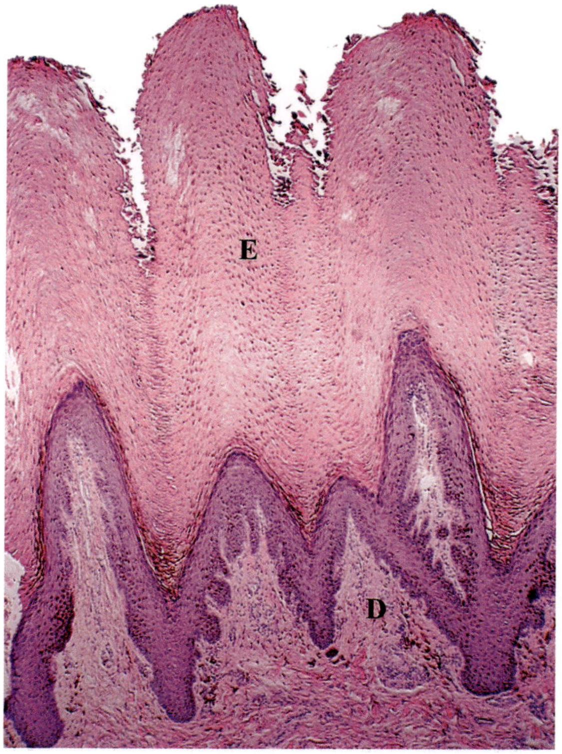

Figure 16-44 Foot pad (dog). The keratinized epidermis (E) is rough in the dog and the dermis (D) is papillated. H&E (×50).

Horn

Horns of the ruminant species are actually coverings of the cornual processes of the frontal bone of the skull. The horns consist of a hard keratinized epidermis, a dermis, and a hypodermis.

The epidermis has a thick stratum corneum composed of hard tubular and intertubular horn. A thin outermost layer of soft keratin, the **epikeras**, forms at the root of the horn and is similar to the epidermis of the periople. It desquamates as keratinized scales, similar to the stratum externum of the hoof. The dermis is papillated and, together with the thin hypodermis, fills the space between the epidermis and the periosteum of the bone.

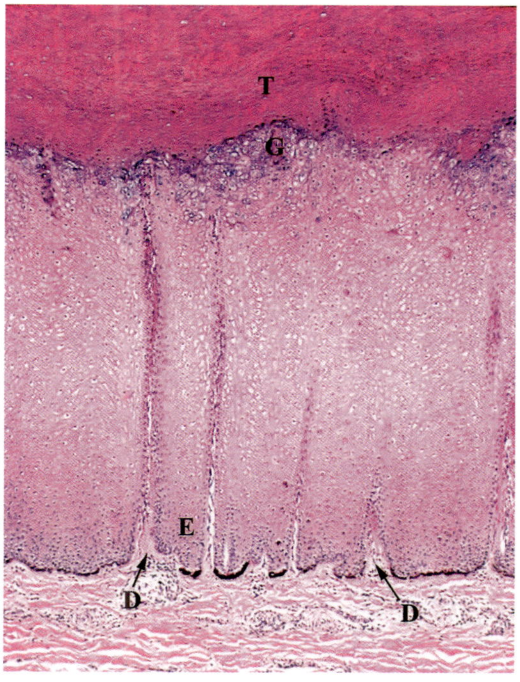

Figure 16-45 Chestnut (horse). Epidermal papillae (E), stratum granulosum (G), dermal papillae (D), and horny tubules (T). H&E (×25).

Avian Integument

The avian **epidermis** is composed of keratinized stratified squamous epithelium that is similar to but thinner than that of mammals (Fig. 16-46). The epidermis of feathered skin consists of only a few cell layers (Fig. 16-47), whereas unfeathered skin is much thicker. The terminology of the epidermal cell layers is different from that in mammals. The avian layers include a **stratum basale**, a **stratum intermedium** (actually stratum spinosum), a **stratum transitivum** (actually stratum granulosum but lacks keratohyalin granules), and a **stratum corneum**. The term **stratum germinativum** is also used

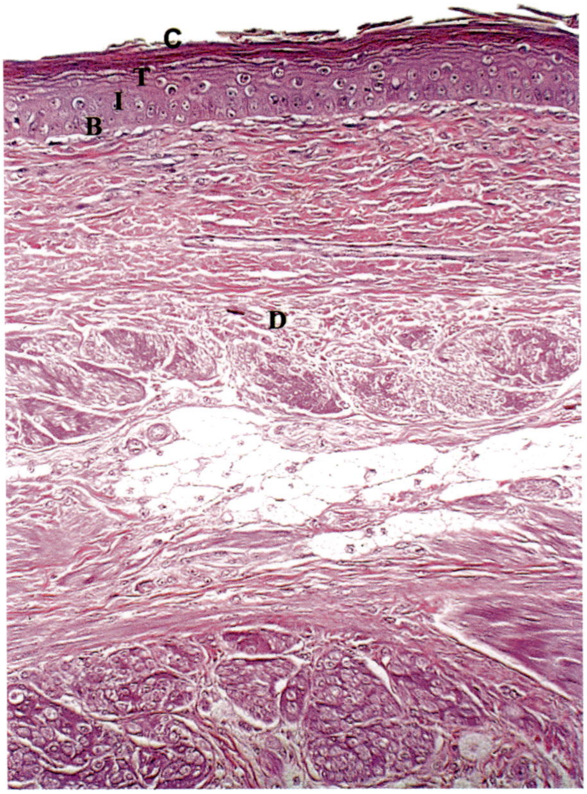

Figure 16-46 Unfeathered chicken skin. Note the stratum basale (B), stratum intermedium (I), stratum transitivum (T), and stratum corneum (C) cell layers. The dermis (D) and subdivided layers can be seen. H&E (×250).

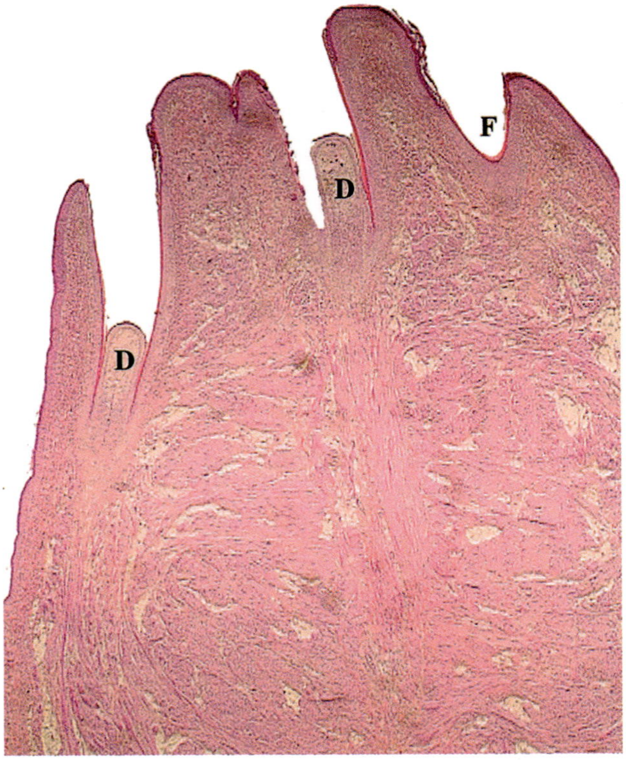

Figure 16-47 Feathered chicken skin. Note two developing follicles (D) and a mature follicle (F). H&E (×35).

to represent all the cell layers except for the stratum corneum. The avian integument is sometimes referred to as an organ of lipogenesis because of the extensive amount of lipid found in the epidermal cells in most avian species. The epidermis synthesizes triacylglycerols, phospholipids, wax esters, free fatty acids, monoglycerols, and diacylglycerols.

The skin of birds, unlike that of mammals, is completely aglandular, with the exception of the **uropygial gland** or preen gland (Figs. 16-48 and 16-49). This gland is a bilobed structure (Fig. 16-48) that lies dorsally at the base of the tail and opens through a papilla onto the surface of the skin. This gland is analogous to the sebaceous gland in mammals because it produces a fatty and oily substance that is released by the holocrine mode of secretion and regulated by hormonal influences (Fig. 16-49). The combination of both the uropygial gland sebum and the lipid from the epidermal cells acts as an antibacterial agent, prevents the feather keratin from drying out, and acts as a waterproofing agent.

Feathers are structurally similar to hair, are of epidermal origin, and develop within a follicle (Fig. 16-47). The feather primarily consists of keratin and remains in the follicle until it is plucked or molted and then a new feather develops in its place. Interfollicular muscles are common in birds and believed to play a significant role in governing the radiated heat load by adjusting the angle of the feather.

The dermis is subdivided into the **stratum superficiale** (superficial layer); **stratum profundum** (deep layer), which includes the **stratum compactum** (dense layer) and the **stratum laxum** (loose CT containing fat, large vessels, smooth muscle, and follicles); and **lamina elastica** (elastic lamina of the dermis). In addition, several smooth muscles with elastic tendons are associated with each feather follicle, and cutaneous striated muscles function in voluntary movement of the skin in response to stimuli.

The avian plantar skin does not possess all cell layers like the plantar skin of dogs and cats (Fig. 16-50). Skin from this region lacks a true stratum granulosum and has a thick smooth surface consisting of ridges of keratin.

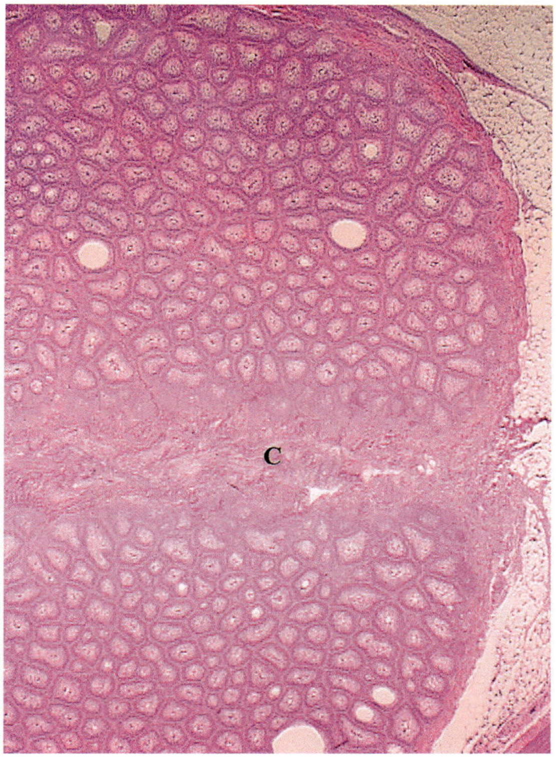

Figure 16-48 Uropygial gland. Note the bilobed structure separated by CT (C). H&E (×35).

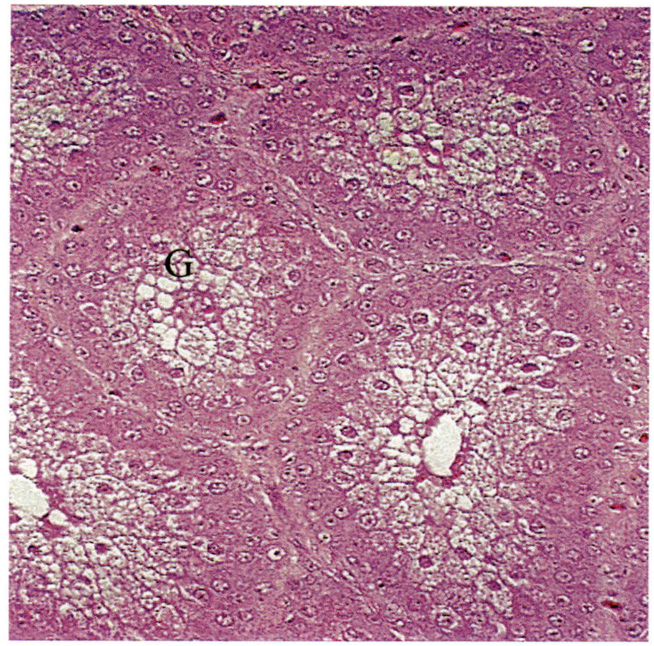

Figure 16-49 Higher magnification of the uropygial gland in Figure 16-48. Note the large sebaceous glands (G). H&E (×350).

The comb, paired wattles, and ear lobes consist of a double layer of skin with numerous blood vessels in the dermis. During mating, the vessels become congested, thereby giving a bright red appearance to the comb and wattles.

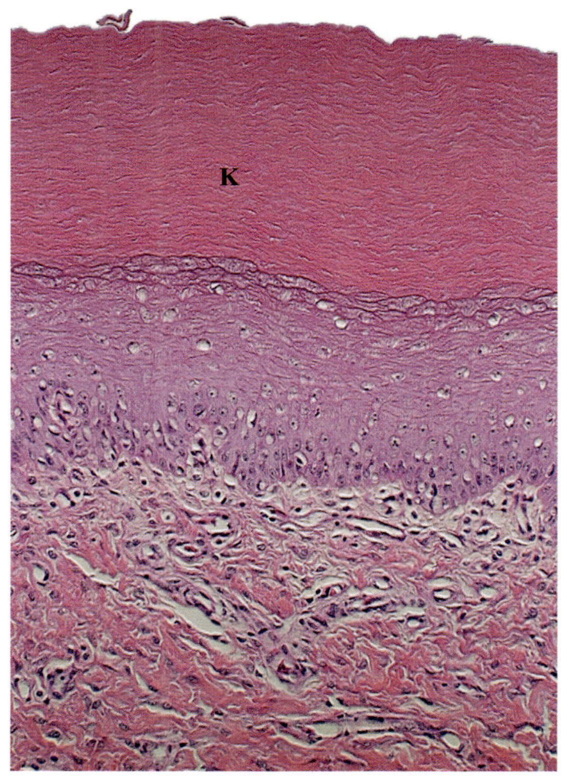

Figure 16-50 Avian plantar skin. Note that the thickened keratinized region (K) is smooth. H&E (×250).

Clinical Correlations

Dermatophytosis is one of the most common skin fungal infections in animals, and it is contagious and zoonotic to humans. Fungal hyphae can infect any of the cornified components of the skin, including the stratum corneum, hair shafts, and claws. Hair shaft infection by dermatophyte fungi *Microsporum canis* in a dog (Fig. 16-51A) causes hair shaft loss and leads to alopecia as a main presenting clinical sign. Typically, infected hair shafts trigger inflammation of the hair follicle, called folliculitis, to cause alopecia. Infection of the stratum corneum causes an increased production and reduced desquamation of this layer, and this results in increased scale on the skin surface. This is another major type of skin lesion associated with dermatophytosis. Fungal organisms are often visualized on histology sections with special histochemical stains such as Periodic Acid-Schiff (Fig. 16-51B). Dermatophyte fungi in skin lesions produce arthrospores (Fig. 16-51A and B) that are shed into the animal's environment and can infect other animals and humans.

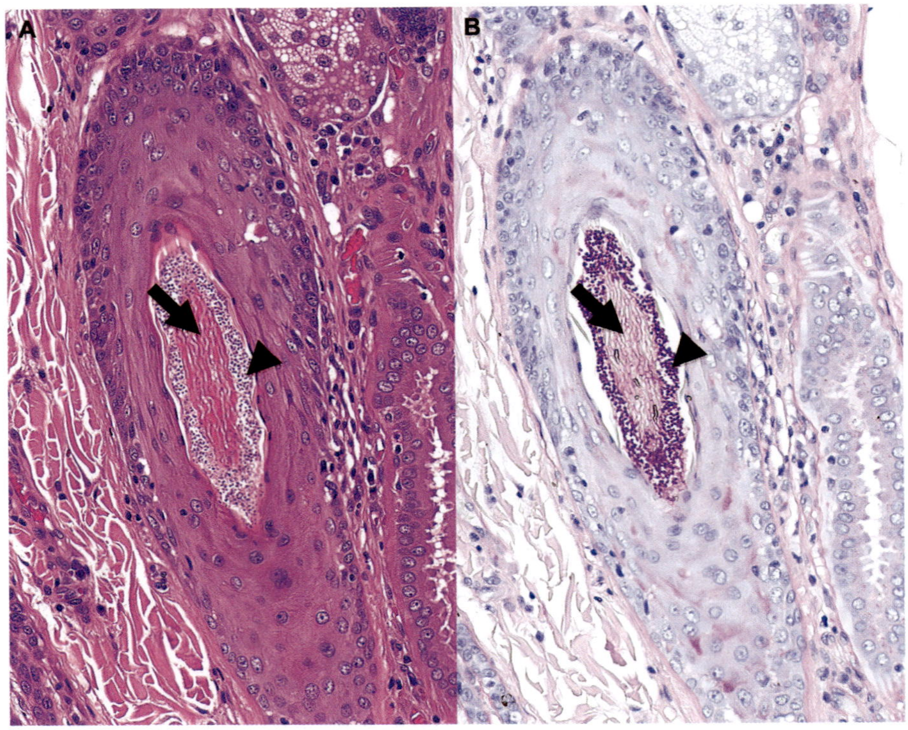

Figure 16-51 Haired skin of a dog with dermatophytosis due to *Microsporum canis*. **A.** Histological section of a hair follicle containing numerous linear fungal hyphae in a hair shaft (arrow), and the hair shaft is surrounded by many small round arthrospores (arrowhead) in the hair follicle lumen. H&E. 200X. **B.** The serial histological section of the hair follicle in image A shows positive Periodic Acid-Schiff staining highlighting the walls of dermatophyte fungal hyphae (arrow) and arthrospores (arrowhead) with a magenta color (×200). (Dr Keith Linder, Zoetis Reference Labs.)

Essentials

1) Skin is one of the largest organs of the body and its primary function is to act as a barrier to the external environment.
2) Skin serves as an important route of entry to topically applied drugs and a multiple of environmental toxins.
3) Normal anatomical structure within skin may contribute to and affect its barrier function. Other functions of skin include mechanical support, being a substrate for hair follicles, sebaceous and sweat glands, serving as a neurosensory organ for touch and temperature, providing protection from ultraviolet light via melanin, metabolism, and being intimately involved in the immunological and endocrine systems.
4) The structure and function of skin is overviewed from multiple perspectives based on function and due to its anatomical complexity, which is seen when comparing to different species.
5) Keratinized epidermis forms the basis of the numerous structures such as fur, foot pads, scales, and feathers. Hard keratin or horn forms the keratinized portion of the hoofs of horses, ruminants and pigs, and the claws of carnivores. These skin-derived structures visibly differentiate veterinary species.

Suggested Readings

Adam WS, Calhoun ML, Smith EM, et al. Microscopic anatomy of the dog: A Photographic Atlas.

Anderson RR. Mammary gland. In: Larson BL, ed. Lactation. Ames, IA: Iowa State University Press, 1985: 3.

Briggaman RA. Epidermal–dermal junction: structure, composition, function and disease relationships. In: Moshnell AN, ed. Dermatology, Part II. Evanston, IL: Dermatology Foundation, 1990: 1.

Budras KD, Hullinger RL, Sack WO. Light and electron microscopy of keratinization in the laminar epidermis of the equine hoof with reference to laminitis. *Am J Vet Res* 1989;50:1150.

Cameron R. Integumentary system: skin, hoof and claw. *Diseases of swine*. 2012:256–7.
Elias PE. Epidermal lipids, barrier function, and desquamation. *J Invest Dermatol* 1983;80:44s.
Greer MB, Calhoun ML. The anal sacs of the domestic cat- *Felis domesticus. Am J Vet Res* 1966;27:773.
Hodges RD. The integumentary system. In: The Histology of the Fowl. New York: Academic Press, 1974: 1.
Jenkinson DM, Elder HY, Bovell DL. Equine sweating and anhidrosis Part 1–equine sweating. *Veterinary Dermatology*. 2006;17(6):361–92.
Lavker RM, Sunt TT. Heterogeneity in basal keratinocytes: morphological and functional correlations. *Science* 1982;215:1239.
Lucas AM, Stettenhein PR. Avian Anatomy. Integument. Agricultural Handbook 362, Part II. Washington, DC: U.S. Department of Agriculture, 1972.
Marcarian HQ, Calhoun ML. The microscopic anatomy of the integument of the adult swine. *Am J Vet Res* 1966;27:765.
Menton DN. A liquid film model of tetrakaidecahedral packing to account for the establishment of epidermal cell columns. *J Invest Dermatol* 1976;66:283.
Monteiro-Rivere NA, Stromberg MW. Ultrastructure of the integument of the domestic pig (*Sus scrofa*) from one through fourteen weeks of age. *Anat Histol Embryol* 1985;14:97.
Monteiro-Riviere NA. Ultrastructural evaluation of the porcine integument. In: Tumbleson ME, ed. Swine in Biomedical Research. Vol. 1. New York: Plenum Press, 1986: 641.
Monteiro-Riviere NA. Comparative anatomy, physiology, and biochemistry of mammalian skin. In: Hobson DW, ed. Dermal and Ocular Toxicology: Fundamentals and Methods. Vol. 1. Boca Raton, FL: CRC Press, 1991: 3.
Monteiro-Riviere NA. Integument. In: Pond WG, Mersmann HJ, eds. Biology of the Pig. Vol. 14. Ithaca, NY: Cornell University Press, 2001: 653.
Monteiro-Riviere NA, Inman AO. Indirect immunohistochemistry and immunoelectron microscopy distribution of eight epidermal–dermal junction epitopes in the pig and in isolated perfused skin treated with bis (2-chloroethyl) sulfide. *Toxicol Pathol* 1995;23:313.
Monteiro-Riviere NA, Bristol DG, Manning TO, et al. Interspecies and interregional analysis of the comparative histologic thickness and laser Doppler blood flow measurements at five cutaneous sites in nine species. *J Invest Dermatol* 1990;95:582.
Monteiro-Riviere NA, Inman AO, Mak V, et al. Effect of selective lipid extraction from different body regions on epidermal barrier function. *Pharm Res* 2001;18:992.
Romani N, Brunner PM, Stingl G. Changing views of the role of the Langerhans cells. *J Invest Dermatol* 2012;132:872.
Smith JL, Calhoun ML. The microscopic anatomy of the integument of the newborn swine. *Am J Vet Res* 1964;24:165.
Stettenheim PR. The integumentary morphology of modern birds—an overview. *American Zoologist*. 2000;40(4):461–77.
Stromberg MW, Hwang YC, Monteiro-Riviere NA. Interfollicular smooth muscle in the skin of the domesticated pig (*Sus scrofa*). *Anat Rec* 1981;201:455.
Stump JE. Anatomy of the normal equine foot, including microscopic features of the laminar region. *J Am Vet Med Assoc* 1967;151:1588.
Talukdar AH, Calhoun ML, Stinson AW. Sweat glands of the horse: a histologic study. *Am J Vet Res* 1970;31:2179.
Webb AJ, Calhoun ML. The microscopic anatomy of the skin of mongrel dogs. *Am J Vet Res* 1954;15:274.
Wolff-Schreiner EC. Ultrastructural cytochemistry of the epidermis. *Int J Dermatol* 1977;16:77.

17

Sensory Organs

Cornelia W. Peterson

CHAPTER MENU

Dellmann's Textbook of Veterinary Histology, Seventh Edition. Edited by Marxa L. Figueiredo and John J. Turek.

Companion website: www.wiley.com/go/figueiredo/vethistology7e

The Eye

The eye is a spherical organ responsible for photoreception, the process by which light energy is absorbed by specialized nerve cells, the photoreceptors, and relayed to the optic nerve and brain to be processed as vision. The eye is located within the bony orbit, along with extraocular muscles, glandular tissue, and supporting CTs. The lacrimal apparatus, the eyelids, and the third eyelid provide protection to the eye. Structurally, the globe consists of three basic layers or tunics.

The three layers or tunics of the eye are (Fig. 17-1) (a) the **fibrous** outer tunic, which includes the transparent cornea covering the anterior 1/6th of the globe, and the white collagenous sclera covering the posterior 5/6th of the globe; (b) the **vascular** middle tunic, also referred to as the uvea, composed of the iris, the ciliary body, and the choroid, from anterior to posterior; and (c) the **neuroepithelial** inner tunic, which includes the retina containing sensory photoreceptor neurons, along with epithelium covering the ciliary body and the posterior surface of the iris.

The **anterior chamber** is located between the cornea and the iris. The **posterior chamber** is located between the iris and the vitreous body and contains the lens. Both the anterior and posterior chambers are filled with aqueous humor. **The vitreous cavity or chamber**, located between the posterior aspect of the lens and the anterior aspect of the retina, is filled with the vitreous body.

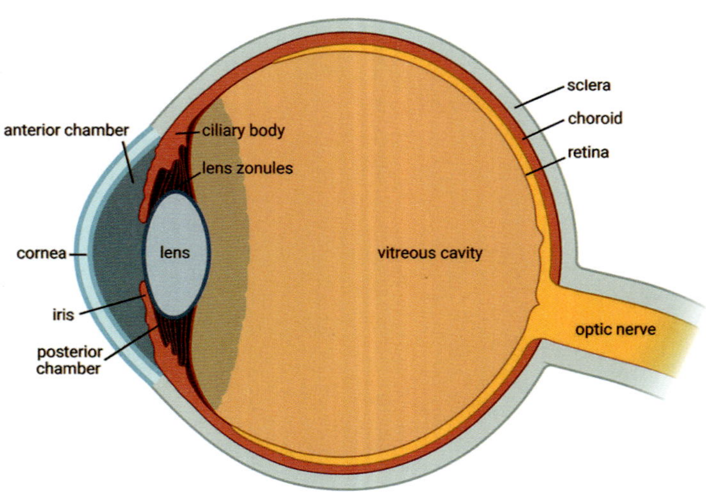

Figure 17-1 Schematic drawing of a sagittal section through the eye.

Fibrous Tunic

Cornea

The transparent **cornea**, along with its associated tear film, provides the highest refractive power of all the ocular structures due to the regular arrangement of collagenous fibrils. In addition to its refractive capacity, the cornea also functions to provide a physical barrier against environmental trauma and microbial organisms.

The cornea is composed of five layers: (a) surface epithelium, (b) subepithelial basement membrane, (c) substantia propria or stroma, (d) corneal endothelial basement membrane (Descemet's membrane), and (e) corneal endothelium.

Surface Epithelium

The **surface epithelium** is nonkeratinized stratified squamous, with layers of basal cells, polygonal or wing cells, and flattened superficial squamous cells ranging from 4 to 12 cells thick. Basal epithelial cells form a single layer that rests on the epithelial basement membrane. The transdifferentiation of basal epithelial cells results in a mitotic product of two wing cells, which then move apically toward the anterior and middle layers of the epithelium. The superficial cells possess apical microvilli and microplicae, which secrete a prominent glycocalyx that interacts with and stabilizes the tear film. The epithelial cells are held together through tight junctions and desmosomes and are adherent to the underlying basement membrane through hemidesmosomes. There are numerous free nerve endings present among the epithelial cells.

The regenerative capability of injured corneal epithelium is pronounced; mitotic divisions, along with cell movements, ensure a rapid return of injured epithelium to its normal structure.

Subepithelial Basement Membrane

The **subepithelial basement membrane**, or basal lamina, is formed by the organized secretion of collagens, primarily types IV and VII, and proteoglycans by the basal epithelial cells. Frequently, this layer can be distinguished with light microscopy (Fig. 17-2). It should not be confused with the **anterior limiting lamina** (Bowman's membrane), which is the condensed anteriormost layer of the substantia propria found in many nondomestic veterinary species. The integrity of the subepithelial basement membrane is a critical factor in both the extent and rate of corneal wound healing responses.

Substantia Propria (Stroma)

The corneal **substantia propria**, or stroma, consists of hundreds of layers or lamellae of predominantly type I collagen and constitutes approximately 90% of the corneal thickness (Fig. 17-2). The precise arrangement of parallel collagen fibrils within each lamella permits the transmission of virtually all light through the cornea without scattering. Interspersed among these collagenous lamellae are sensory nerve fibers, proteoglycans, glycosaminoglycans, and the resident cell type, the keratocyte (Fig. 17-2). Keratocytes can differentiate to fibroblasts and myofibroblasts to promote the migration and proliferation required for wound healing, often seen with sight-threatening scar formation.

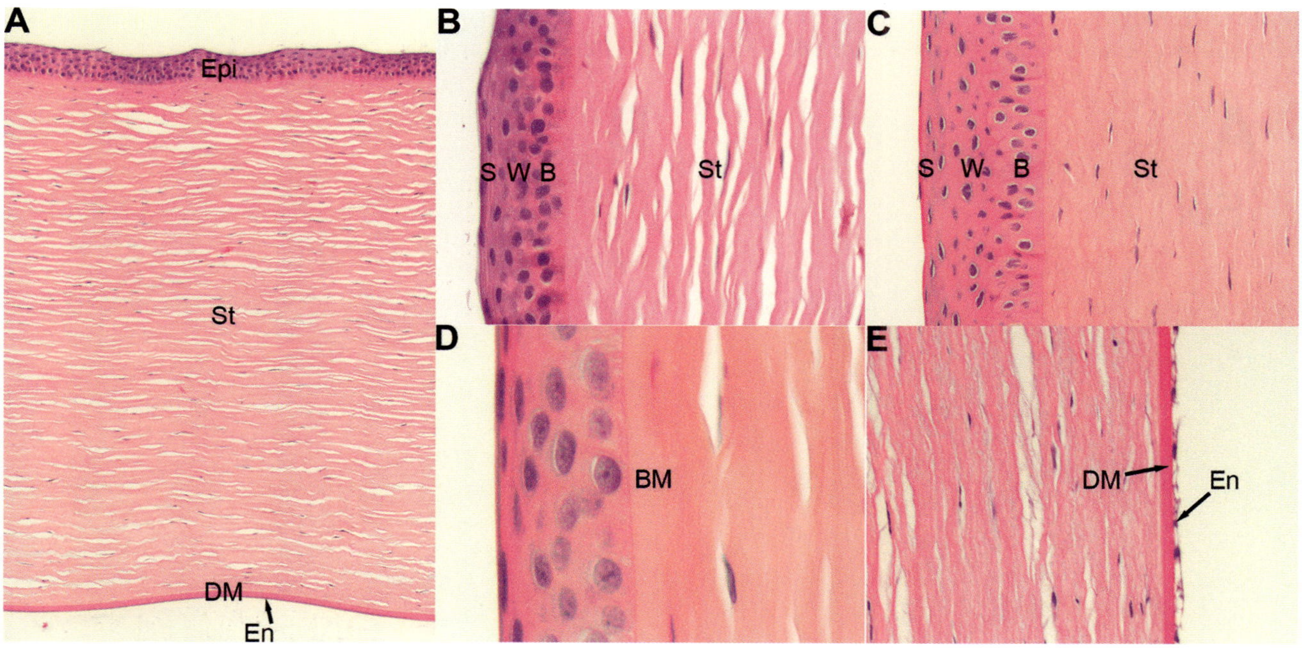

Figure 17-2 Cornea. **A. Canine cornea**. Corneal epithelium (Epi), stroma (St), Descemet's membrane (DM), and endothelium (En). Hematoxylin and eosin (H&E) (×100). **B. Canine cornea**. The corneal epithelium is a nonkeratinized stratified squamous epithelium with basal cells (B), intermediate wing (W) cells, and flattened superficial squamous cells (S), and is separated from the stroma by a basement membrane. H&E (×200). **C. Caprine cornea**. The corneal epithelium of large animals is thicker than that of small animals with an increased number of intermediate wing (W) cells. **D. Nonhuman primate cornea**. The anteriormost stroma is condensed and acellular, forming the Bowman's membrane (BM). H&E (×400). **E. Canine cornea**. The corneal endothelium (En) is supported by a variably thick basement membrane (Descemet's membrane [DM]). H&E (×200).

Corneal Endothelial Basement Membrane (Descemet's Membrane)

The **corneal endothelial basement membrane** (Descemet's membrane) appears as a highly refractile, thick amorphous layer with light microscopy and can be further demonstrated with a Periodic Acid-Schiff stain (Fig. 17-2). Ultrastructurally, this lamina consists of three regions: an anterior unbanded zone containing type V and VI collagens, an anterior banded zone with type IV and VIII collagens, and a posterior unbanded zone, with type III and IV collagens. The posterior limiting lamina is continually produced throughout life by the corneal endothelium, resulting in a thicker membrane in aging animals.

Corneal Endothelium

The **corneal endothelium** (Fig. 17-2) is a simple squamous epithelium arranged in a hexagonal mosaic covering the posterior surface of the cornea. The endothelial cells are rich in mitochondria to generate adenosine triphosphate (ATP) for the cellular pumps responsible for maintaining corneal hydration and transparency. Defects in the endothelium result in edema and opacification of the cornea. The regenerative ability of the posterior epithelium is limited and varies with species and age.

Sclera

The **sclera** is comprised of dense irregular connective tissue (CT) that protects the eye and maintains its shape and intraocular pressure (Fig. 17-3). Species variations include scleral cartilage in some fish, amphibians, and birds, and bony ossicles in some avian species. Scleral thickness varies across different parts of the eye and among species. The sclera is thinnest at the equator of the globe and thickest at the limbus (the junction of the cornea and sclera) in dogs and cats, and around the optic nerve in ungulates. Collagen fibers predominate in the sclera, but elastic fibers, fibrocytes, and melanocytes also are interlaced among them, becoming more numerous in the deeper aspects of the posterior sclera that border the choroid.

The orbital fasciae, located external to the sclera, consist of the following components: the thin CT periorbita, which is connected to the external or dural sheath of the optic nerve; the fasci bulbi, also called Tenon's capsule, a collagenous tissue that encircles the globe; and the epimysium of the extraocular muscles. The extraocular muscle tendons firmly attach to the sclera through an interweaving of tendon and scleral fibers. The optic nerve axons exit the eye through numerous perforations in a sieve-like area of the posterior sclera referred to as the **lamina cribrosa** (Fig. 17-3).

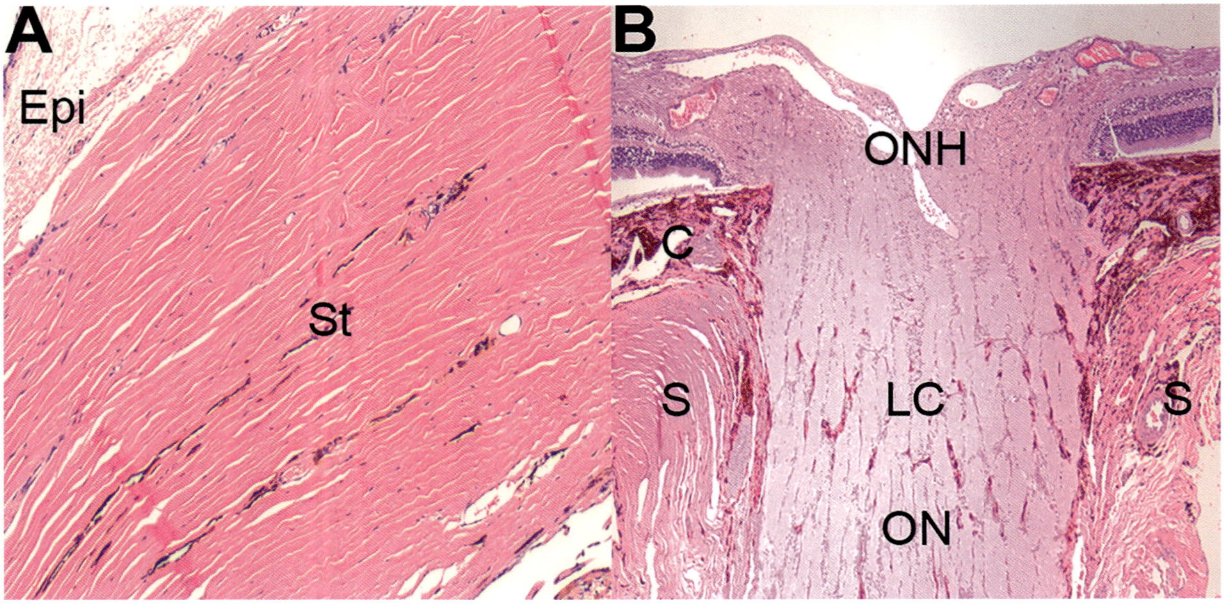

Figure 17-3 Feline sclera. **A. Anterior** aspect of the sclera featuring a superficial episclera (Epi), comprised of vascularized loose CT, and the scleral stroma (St), comprised of dense collagenous tissue. H&E (×100). **B. Posterior** aspect of the sclera (S) is interrupted by numerous foramina called the lamina cribrosa (LC), through which axons pass from the optic nerve head (ONH), penetrate the choroid (C), and leave the globe as the optic nerve (ON). H&E (×40).

Corneoscleral Junction (Limbus)

At the **corneoscleral junction** or limbus, the sclera overlaps the cornea. The corneal epithelium gradually transitions into secretory conjunctival epithelium, which rests on a lamina propria of loose CT. The characteristically layered collagen fibers of the corneal stroma assume a more irregular arrangement, become associated with elastic fibers, and are continuous with the equatorial bundles of the sclera. The posterior limiting lamina of the endothelium terminates at the limbus near the apex of the trabecular meshwork (Fig. 17-4).

The vascular supply to the cornea is found exclusively at the level of the limbus; the normal cornea is completely devoid of blood vessels. Corneal nerves originate from a dense marginal nerve fiber plexus at the same level as the blood vessels or from the ciliary plexus of the vascular tunic.

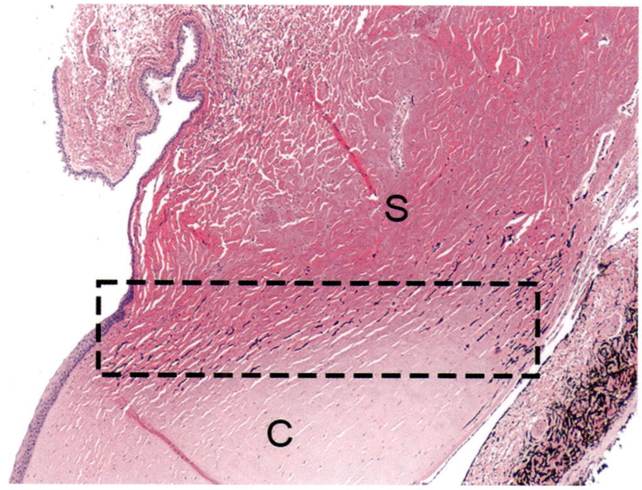

Figure 17-4 Canine limbus. The corneoscleral junction, or limbus (boxed region), marks the transition between the cornea (C) and sclera (S). The stratified squamous corneal epithelium and dense regular CT of the corneal stroma transition to a secretory conjunctival epithelium and dense irregular CT of the scleral stroma. H&E (×40).

Vascular Tunic

The **vascular tunic**, or uvea, comprises three portions: the mesenchymal components of the iris, the ciliary body, and the choroid.

Iris

The iris is located anterior to the lens and separates the anterior and posterior chambers of the eye, which are continuous through a central aperture, the **pupil**. The iris extends from the ciliary body to the pupil margin and consists of a stroma of pigmented, highly vascularized loose CT, **sphincter** and **dilator muscles that regulate pupil size**, and a bilayered epithelium on its posterior aspect.

Iridial Stroma

The anterior surface of the iris lacks epithelium. Its anteriormost aspect, facing the anterior chamber, is comprised of a thin condensation of fibroblasts arranged over dense aggregates of melanocytes, which form the **anterior border layer** (Fig. 17-5). This layer lacks both a basement membrane and blood vessels but is rich in proteoglycans. Depressions or crypts frequently penetrate deep into the underlying stroma, especially at the pupillary margin, and often communicate with the anterior chamber.

The deeper and more vascularized layer of the stroma consists of trabeculae or radial columns of collagen fibers and fibroblasts, supported by highly vascularized loose CT containing many melanocytes. Other nonpigmented cells within the iris stroma include immune cells such as lymphocytes, macrophages, and mast cells.

The arterial vessels originate from the major arterial circle at the periphery of the iris and radiate centripetally, into the stroma, forming capillary beds in the vicinity of the pupillary margin. These stromal capillaries are nonfenestrated, and the tight junctions between the endothelial cells aid in maintaining the blood–aqueous barrier.

Iris color is determined by the amount and type of pigmentation within the pigment-containing cells of the anterior border layer and stroma, as well as the density of pigment within melanocytes.

Iridial Muscles

Two iridial muscles, the sphincter and dilator muscles, regulate pupil size. Both muscles originate from neuroepithelial (pigmented epithelial) cells. In mammalian companion animals, these muscles are smooth, while in avian species, they are striated and may be controlled voluntarily.

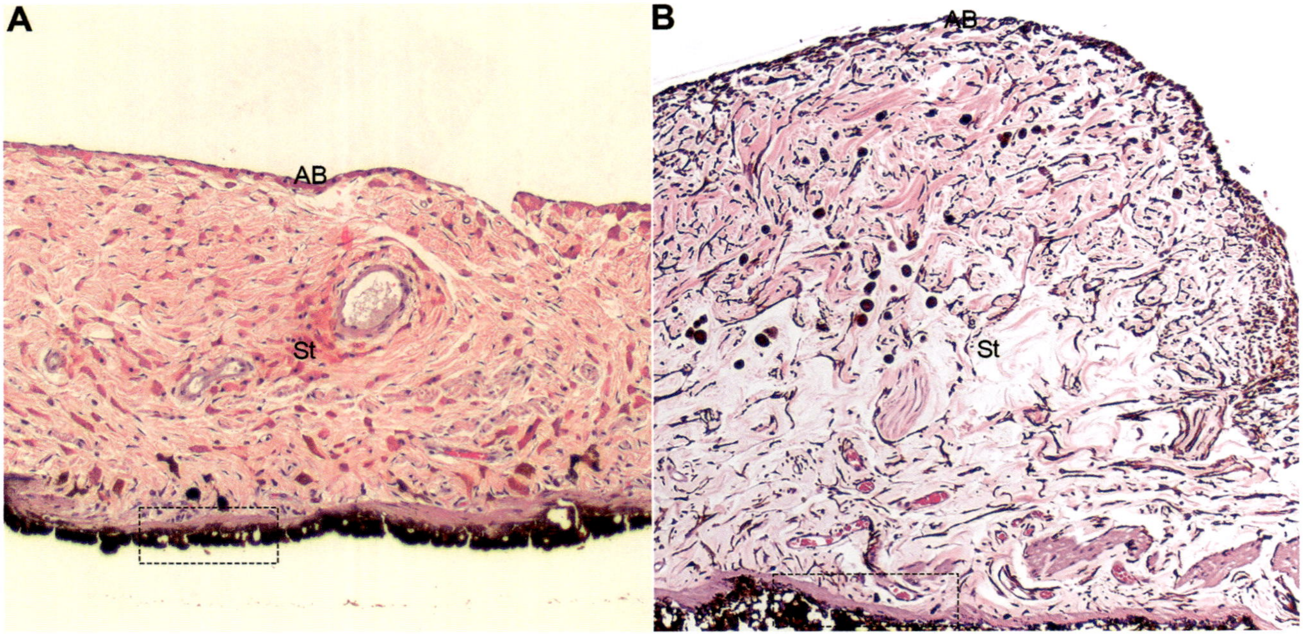

Figure 17-5 Iris. **A. Feline iris.** The anterior border layer (AB) faces the anterior chamber and is superficial to the stroma (St), the thickest layer containing many blood vessels and melanocytes. The posterior aspect of the iris is covered by a bilayered epithelium (boxed region). H&E (×100). **B. Equine iris.** The same features, including the anterior border layer (AB), stroma (St), and bilayered epithelium on the posterior aspect (boxed region), are present, with an increased abundance of darkly pigmented melanocytes within the stroma compared to the cat. H&E (×100).

The **sphincter muscle** is composed of a network of smooth muscle cells, circularly arranged near the pupillary margin. The fibers encircle the pupil in animals with circular pupils (dogs, pigs, primates, and avians). The muscle fibers are oriented dorsoventrally around the pupil in animals with slit-like pupils (cat) or horizontally around the pupil in ruminants and horses. The collagen fiber bundles of the iris stroma form arches that pass through the muscle network, enabling the muscle fibers to directly interact with them. The sphincter muscle receives parasympathetic innervation through CN III (the oculomotor nerve), which originate from the Edinger–Westphal nucleus and synapse in the ciliary ganglion. Contraction of the sphincter muscle results in the reduction of the pupillary aperture (miosis).

The **dilator muscle** originates and partially differentiates from the anterior aspect of the bilayered epithelial layer on the posterior iris (Fig. 17-6). The basal portions of the anterior epithelial cells possess the structural characteristics of smooth muscle cells, extending from the mid-end of the sphincter muscle to the iris root, while the apical portions retain typical pigmented epithelial cell features. The dilator muscle is innervated by sympathetic postganglionic neurons located in the cranial cervical ganglion. Contraction of the dilator muscle results in the dilation of the pupillary aperture (mydriasis).

Iridial Epithelium

The **anterior iris epithelium**, discussed above, is oriented with its basal aspect and elongated contractile smooth muscle processes facing the iris stroma, while its apical processes face the apical aspect of the posterior iris epithelium. The heavily pigmented **posterior iris epithelium** (Fig. 17-6) consists of a single layer of columnar cells that are continuous with the nonpigmented epithelial layer of the ciliary processes. Frequently, the epithelial cells are separated by wide intercellular spaces, but the apical aspects of both the anterior and posterior iris epithelia are joined by desmosomes. On its posterior (inner) surface, the epithelium is covered by a thin basement membrane, the internal limiting membrane of the iris.

In ungulates, several dark aggregates of pigmented tissue, called **corpora nigra** (iridial granules or granulae iridica), are found at the dorsal and ventral pupillary margins. The corpora nigra originating from the dorsal pupillary margin are much larger than those from the ventral margin. This tissue consists of focal proliferations of the two epithelial layers that project into the anterior chamber at the dorsal and ventral pupillary margins (Fig. 17-7).

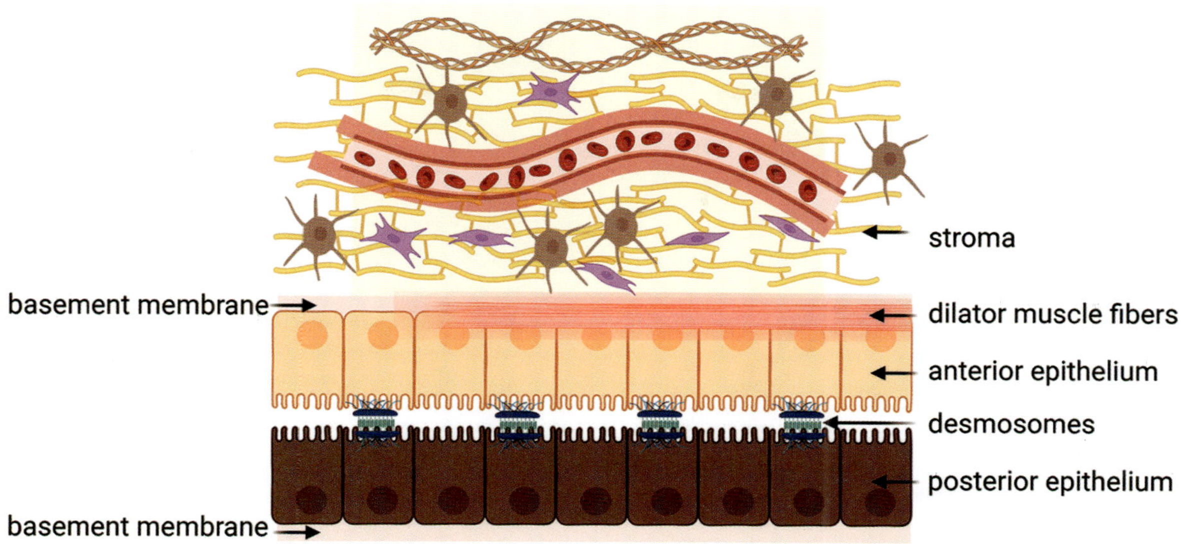

Figure 17-6 Iris epithelia. The bilayered iris epithelium on the posterior aspect is comprised of an anterior cuboidal epithelium with myoepithelial components forming the myofibrils of the dilator muscle and the posterior cuboidal epithelium arranged apex to apex with the anterior epithelium.

Ciliary Body

The **ciliary body** is directly continuous with both the iris and choroid (Fig. 17-1). In cross section, the ciliary body is triangular, with the anterior base beginning at the iris root and the apex extending posteriorly to the ora serrata, marking the transition between the ciliary body and peripheral retina. Externally, the ciliary body lies against the sclera, while internally it contacts the aqueous humor of the posterior chamber.

Anteriorly, the ciliary body projects **ciliary processes** into the posterior chamber (Fig. 17-8). Collectively, these processes form the region of the ciliary body referred to as the **pars plicata**. The ciliary processes increase the surface area for the production of aqueous humor and also serve as the origin for zonular fibers, which attach to and anchor the lens. The posterior portion of the ciliary body is flat and smooth and is referred to as the **pars plana**. Histologically, the ciliary body consists of ciliary epithelium, a stromal layer, and ciliary musculature.

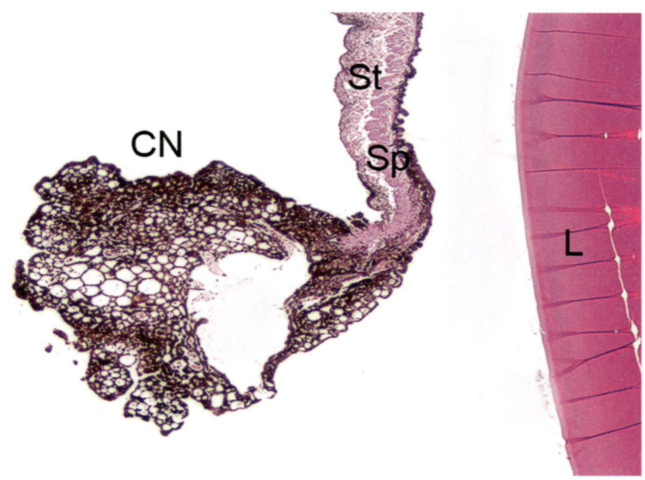

Figure 17-7 Equine corpora nigra. The proliferation of iridial epithelia, or corpora nigra (CN), projects into the anterior chamber at the pupillary margin anterior to the lens (L). This section of iris also demonstrates the iridial stroma (St) and the sphincter muscle (Sp) in the mid to posterior iris encircling the pupillary aperture. H&E (×20).

Ciliary Epithelium

The ciliary body is covered by two layers of cuboidal epithelial cells of neuroepithelial origin. These epithelial layers are joined apex to apex by cell junctions, with the basement membranes facing outward, similar to the arrangement described in the iris epithelia (Fig. 17-9).

The outer **pigmented epithelial layer** of the ciliary body is continuous with the retinal pigmented epithelium (RPE). It consists of heavily pigmented, simple cuboidal epithelium (Fig. 17-9), supported by basement membranes adjacent to the stroma. These cells have deep basal invaginations of the plasma membrane.

The inner **nonpigmented epithelial layer** consists of cuboidal or columnar cells with its own basement membrane, which separates it from the posterior chamber. This epithelium is continuous with the neurosensory layers of the retina and the posterior pigmented epithelium of the iris. The cells possess numerous deep plasmalemmal invaginations and

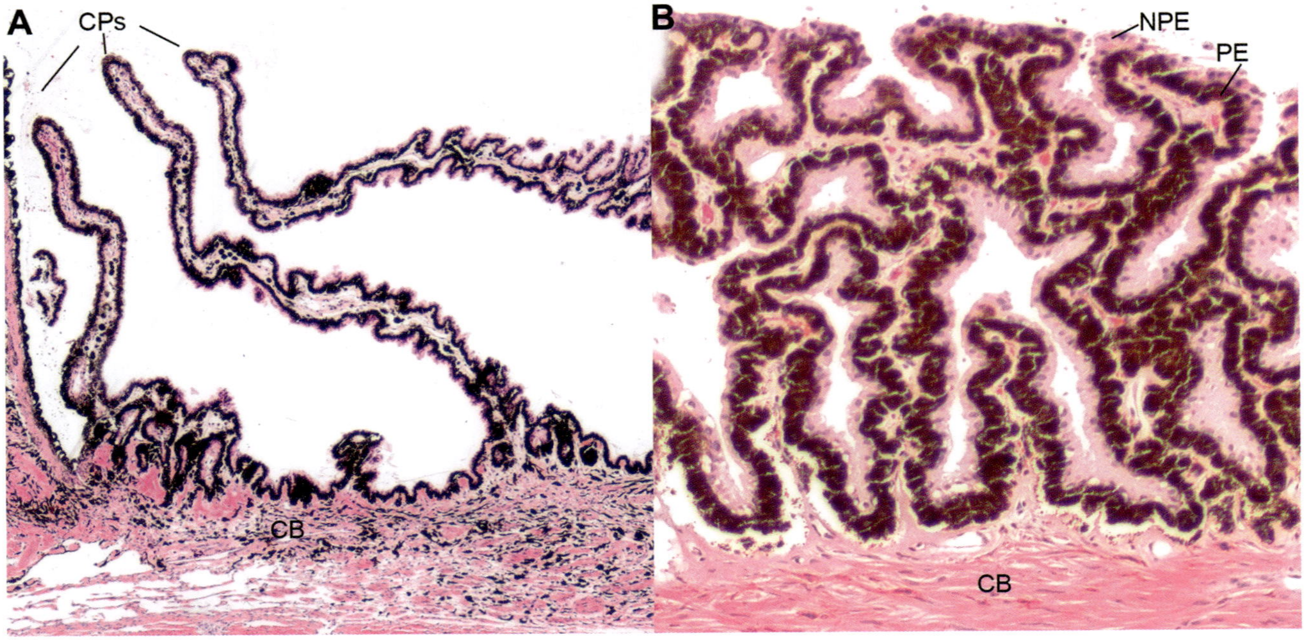

Figure 17-8 Ciliary body. **A. Canine ciliary body**. The ciliary body (CB) lies internal to the sclera and projects numerous ciliary processes (CPs) into the posterior chamber. H&E (×40). **B. Ovine ciliary body**. The ciliary processes are covered by a bilayered epithelium comprised of an inner nonpigmented epithelium (NPE) and an outer pigmented epithelium (PE). H&E (×100).

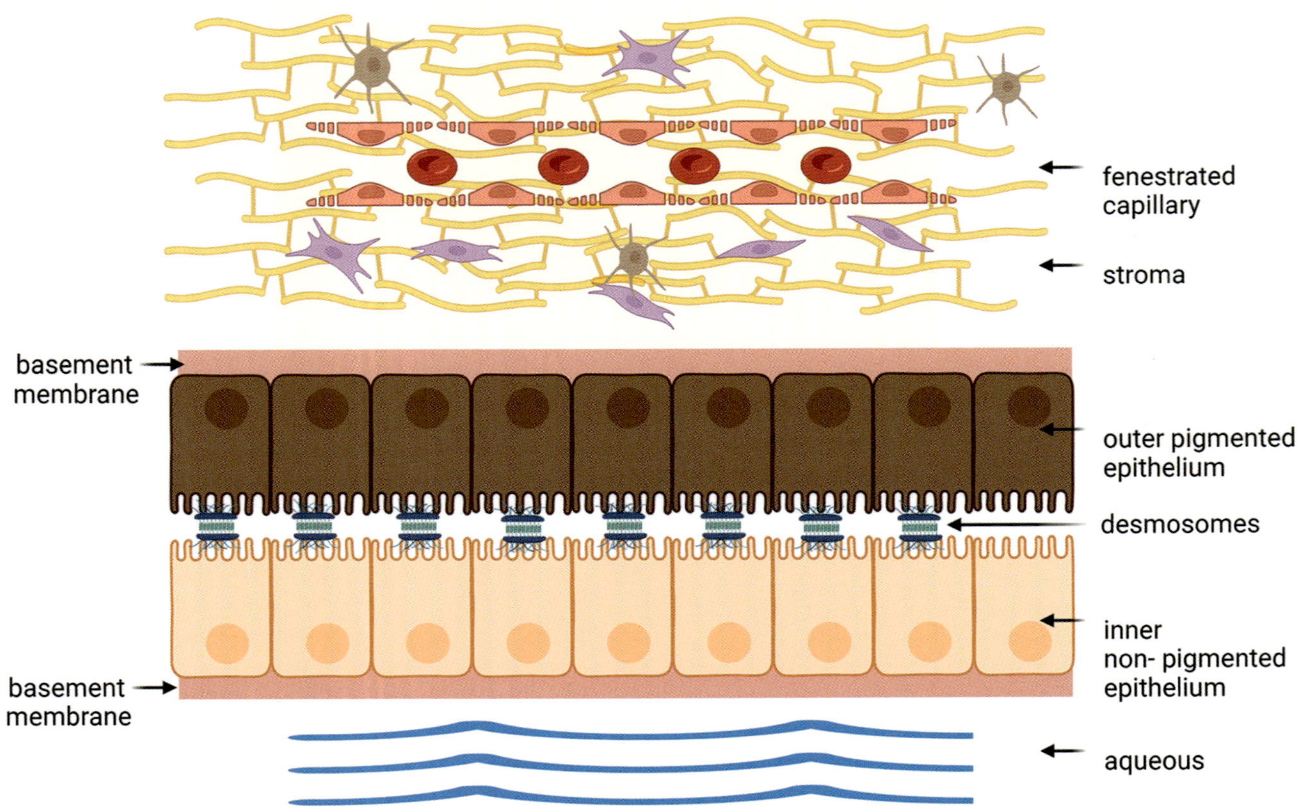

Figure 17-9 Ciliary epithelia. The bilayered ciliary epithelium covering the ciliary processes is comprised of an inner nonpigmented epithelium and an outer pigmented epithelium arranged apex to apex.

associated mitochondria. Extensive rough endoplasmic reticulum and Golgi complexes are present in the cell apices. The lateral surfaces of the epithelial cells are joined by tight junctions, contributing to the blood–aqueous barrier.

Ciliary Stroma

The ciliary body and the ciliary processes have a stromal core of loose CT permeated by a dense network of capillaries. Blood vessels originate from the anterior and posterior ciliary arteries, which together form the major arterial circle that supplies the ciliary body and processes.

Ciliary Muscle

The ciliary muscle is located peripherally in the ciliary body and consists of smooth muscle fibers oriented longitudinally, radially, and circularly from external to internal. Muscle fibers originate from the corneal stroma, the CT of the trabecular meshwork of the iridocorneal angle, and the sclera, and attach posteriorly to the choroid. Contraction of the ciliary muscle during accommodation reduces tension of the zonular fibers of the lens, and the lens becomes more convex, whereas relaxation has the opposite effect.

Aqueous Humor

The aqueous humor is a thin, clear fluid similar in appearance to blood plasma but with considerably lower protein content. It is derived as a serum ultrafiltrate from the hydrostatic pressure gradient across fenestrated capillaries within the ciliary stroma. This ultrafiltrate is modified by the ciliary epithelium and then subsequently secreted into the posterior chamber. The enzyme carbonic anhydrase (necessary to the formation of aqueous humor) is localized in the nonpigmented epithelium of the ciliary processes. The transport of aqueous humor is selective in that certain molecules are excluded from transepithelial passage. The aqueous humor flows from the posterior chamber through the pupil into the anterior chamber, where it drains via the iridocorneal angle (described below). Aqueous humor serves to provide nutrition to and remove waste from anterior segment structures, maintains intraocular pressure, and contributes to the optical properties of the eye.

Iridocorneal Angle

The **iridocorneal angle**, also called the filtration or drainage angle (Fig. 17-10), is a region located at the periphery of the anterior chamber where the corneoscleral junction, the ciliary body, and the iris converge. Structurally, it consists of a meshwork that comprises the pectinate ligament, trabecular meshwork, and trabecular (aqueous) veins. Aqueous humor from the anterior chamber percolates through these structures before draining into the blood vessels of the angle.

Pectinate Ligament

The **pectinate ligament** consists of numerous long, thin primary and accessory strands extending between the corneoscleral junction and the base of the iris (Fig. 17-10). Each strand comprises a core of collagen fibrils covered by endothelium, which is continuous with the corneal endothelium. The spaces between the strands of the pectinate ligament are known as the **spaces of Fontana**, through which aqueous humor exits the anterior chamber.

Trabecular Meshwork

The **uveal trabecular meshwork** is continuous with the pectinate ligament and forms a dense network of flattened, arborizing, perforated sheets of endothelial-covered collagen fibrils (Fig. 17-10). This meshwork gradually becomes the structurally identical but more tightly meshed, rope-like **corneoscleral trabecular meshwork** adjacent to the cornea and sclera.

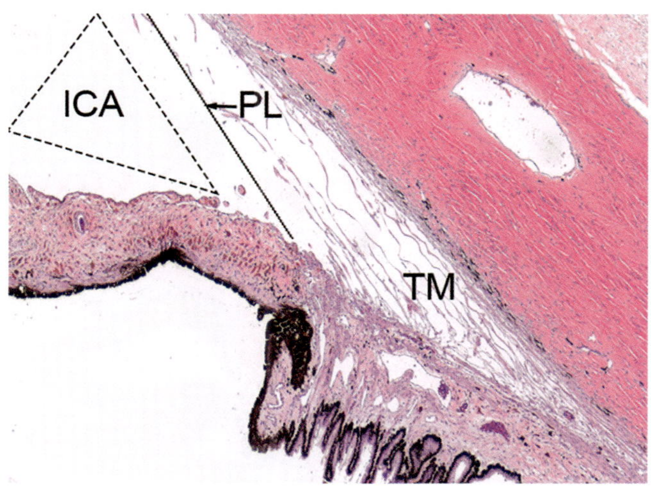

Figure 17-10 Feline iridocorneal angle. The drainage or iridocorneal angle (ICA) is the triangular area located at the level of the limbus and iris root. The pectinate ligament (PL) is comprised of long collagenous strands that extend across the ICA and is continuous with the more posterior trabecular meshwork (TM). H&E (×40).

Venous Drainage

Aqueous humor is removed from the eye by two methods: conventional or nonconventional (uveoscleral) outflow. In most species, conventional outflow predominates. With **conventional outflow**, the aqueous humor drains through the spaces of Fontana in the pectinate ligament into the trabecular meshwork, where it accumulates in the **aqueous collecting veins**. Aqueous then passes into the **scleral venous plexus**, consisting of two to four large vessels located posterior to the limbus in the sclera. The aqueous humor then passes into the vortex veins and joins the blood circulation. The canal of Schlemm, a circular channel lined with endothelium and present in human and nonhuman primate eyes, is absent in domestic mammals. The **nonconventional outflow** consists of the percolation of aqueous humor through the uvea into the supraciliary and suprachoroidal spaces, followed by entry into the adjacent sclera.

Choroid

The **choroid** is a thick, highly vascularized layer that extends from the anterior stroma of the ciliary body to the optic nerve head posteriorly (Figs. 17-11 and 17-12). The external surface of the choroid is connected to the sclera, while internally, its basement membrane is intimately attached to the RPE. The choroid is subdivided into five layers.

Suprachoroid

The **suprachoroid** is the most external layer of the choroid and is the transition between the sclera and the choroid. It consists of bundles of collagen with fewer elastic fibers, along with fibrocytes and numerous melanocytes.

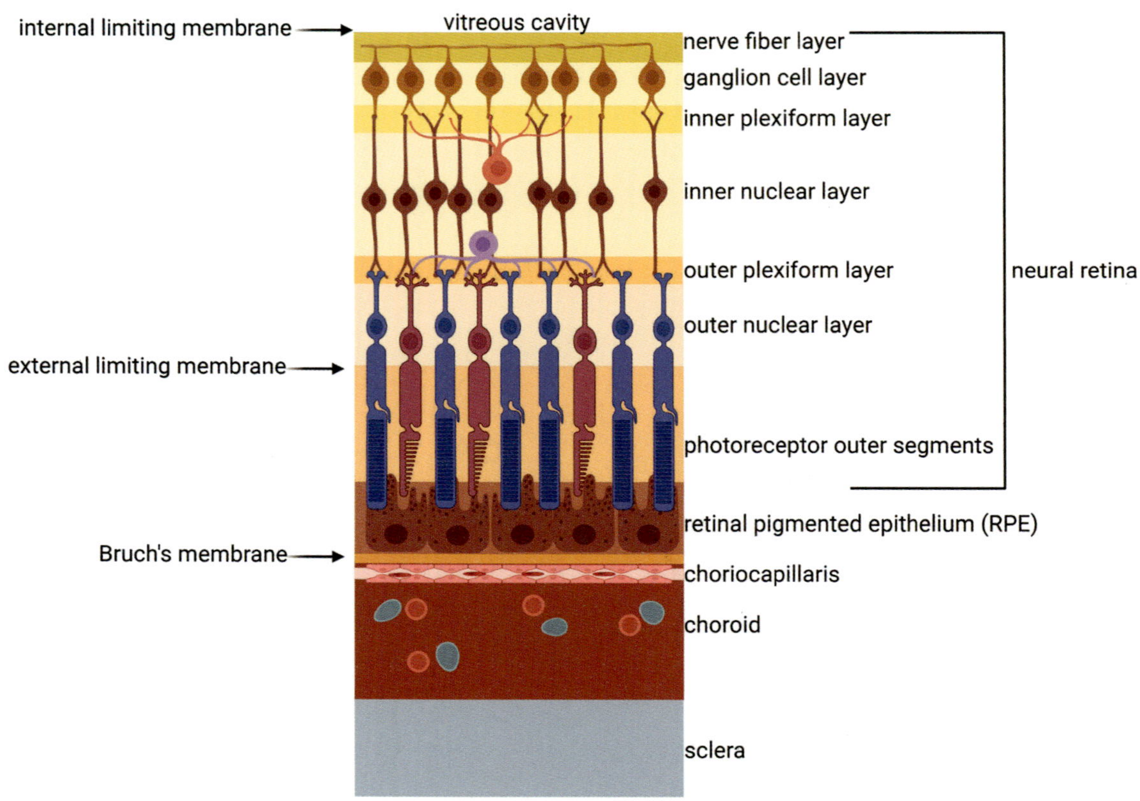

Figure 17-11 Schematic drawing of the retina and choroid. The neural retina is composed of nine layers. The inner limiting membrane abuts the vitreous cavity. The nerve fiber layer contains ganglion cell axons, and the ganglion cell layer contains ganglion cell bodies. The remaining layers include neuronal synapses and cell bodies. The photoreceptor layer has rod and cone outer segments. The retinal pigmented epithelium is external to the neural retina, supported by Bruch's membrane, and adjacent to the choriocapillaris layer of the choroid. The choroidal stroma lies between the choriocapillaris and the sclera. Radial glial (Müller) cell nuclei (purple and/or red cells) are interspersed among other nuclei. The external limiting membrane is formed by junctions between radial glial cells and photoreceptors. The outer nuclear layer contains photoreceptor nuclei. The outer plexiform layer consists of photoreceptor axon terminals forming synapses with horizontal and bipolar cell processes.

Choroidal Stroma

The **choroidal stroma** consists of numerous large arteries and veins. These vessels are surrounded by CT containing collagen and elastic fibrils, fibroblasts, leukocytes, and melanocytes, similar to those found in the suprachoroid. These vessels provide a major source of oxygen and nutrients to the retina.

Tapetum Lucidum

A layer of medium caliber vessels and CT lies internal to the choroidal stroma. The dorsal portion of this layer contains the **tapetum lucidum**, which acts as a light-reflecting layer, supposedly increasing light perception under conditions of poor illumination. In herbivores, the tapetum is fibrous, consisting of intermingling collagen fibers and a few fibrocytes. In carnivores, the tapetum is cellular, consisting of a varying number of layers of flat polygonal cells that appear brick-like in cross section (Figs. 17-12 and 17-13). The thickness of the tapetum varies, being multilayered at its center (up to 15 cell layers thick in dogs and 35 cell layers thick in cats) and thinning to a single cell at its periphery. The tapetum is absent in swine and camelids.

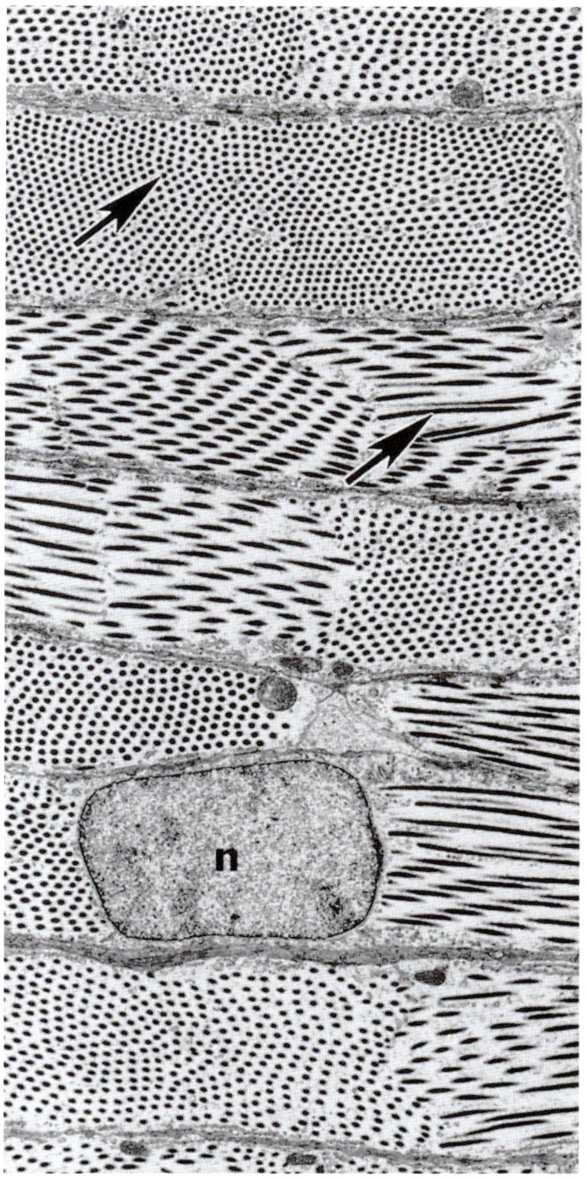

Figure 17-12 Feline tapetum lucidum. Electron micrograph of the feline tapetum lucidum illustrating the brick-like arrangement of cells and bundles of parallel rods (arrows), oriented in various directions with their long axes perpendicular to the angle of incident light, and an atapetal cell nucleus (n) (×3780). (Courtesy of E.J. King.)

Choriocapillaris

The **choriocapillaris** is a dense network of capillaries immediately adjacent to Bruch's membrane (Fig. 17-11). The capillary endothelium is fenestrated, and endothelial nuclei and pericytes are located only toward the choroidal (external) side of the capillaries. Capillaries provide nutrients to the pigmented epithelium and photoreceptors (rods and cones).

Bruch's Membrane

Bruch's membrane is a trilaminar or pentalaminar structure containing the basement membranes of both the choriocapillaris and RPE in species with and without a tapetum,

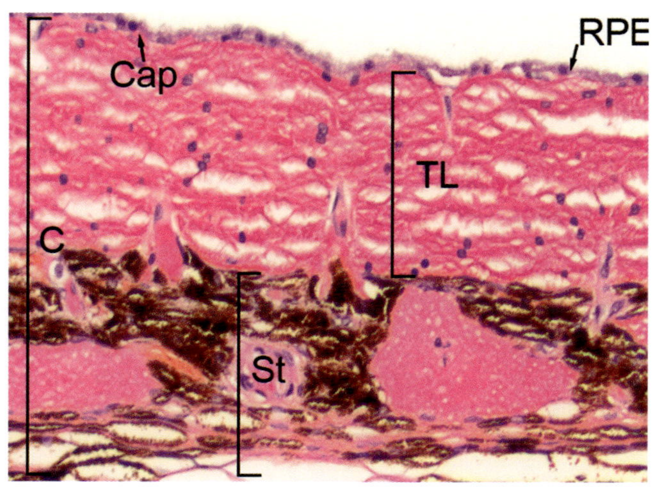

Figure 17-13 Feline choroid. The choroid (C) is located between the retina and sclera. It is highly vascularized and contains many pigmented cells. The choriocapillaris (Cap) lies external to the RPE and internal to the tapetum lucidum (TL). The tapetum is nonpigmented in the dorsal (tapetal) region. The choroidal stroma (St) extends from the outer aspect of the tapetum to the suprachoroid. The suprachoroid (not pictured) is the outermost layer of the choroid, adjacent to the sclera. H&E (×200).

respectively. The extracellular matrix of pentalaminar complexes contains an additional layer of collagen and an intervening band of elastic fibrils. The complex contributes to the blood–retinal barrier by physically separating the blood in the choriocapillary vessels from the RPE.

Neuroepithelial Tunic—Retina

The neuroepithelial tunic, or retina, consists of the neural retina, responsible for the sensory functions of the eye, and the RPE.

Except at the optic disk, the neural portion of the retina consists of the following layers (Figs. 17-11 and 17-14): (a) internal limiting membrane, (b) nerve fiber layer, (c) ganglion cell layer, (d) inner plexiform layer, (e) inner nuclear layer, (f) outer plexiform layer, (g) outer nuclear layer, (h) external limiting membrane, and (i) photoreceptor outer segments. The RPE lies external to the photoreceptors.

The **RPE** is a layer of flat, polygonal to low cuboidal cells resting on a basement membrane (Figs. 17-11 and 17-13). Capillaries of the choriocapillaris frequently deeply indent these cells. The basal aspect of the RPE cells is characterized by deep infoldings of the plasma membrane with numerous associated mitochondria. The apical aspects are connected by both zonulae adherens and occludens. Numerous melanin granules are present, except in the cells that overly the tapetum, when the RPE is nonpigmented. Microvillous apical processes partially surround the outer segments of the photoreceptors (Figs. 17-11 and 17-14). This arrangement allows the RPE to transport nutrients and metabolites from the choriocapillaris to the photoreceptors and to phagocytize and degrade the shed rod and cone outer segments.

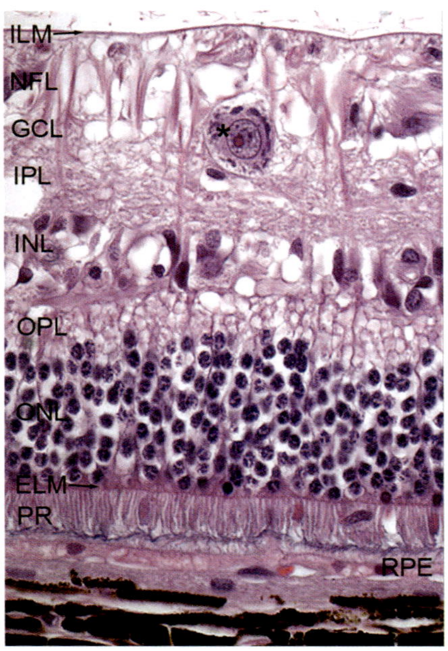

Figure 17-14 Canine tapetal retina. Layers of the retina include the internal limiting membrane (ILM); nerve fiber layer (NFL); ganglion cell layer (GCL; asterisk: ganglion cell); inner plexiform layer (IPL); inner nuclear layer (INL); outer plexiform layer (OPL); outer nuclear layer (ONL); external limiting membrane (ELM); photoreceptor outer segments (PR); and retinal pigment epithelium (RPE), which shares a basement membrane complex with the choriocapillaris (Cap). Note that the RPE is not pigmented in the region of the retina where it overlies the tapetum. H&E (×40).

The photoreceptors, called **rods** and **cones** due to the morphology of their inner segments, are the first neurons of the visual pathway. The rods are responsible for vision in dim light, whereas the cone cells function in bright light and are responsible for color vision; thus, nocturnal animals possess fewer cones compared to diurnal species. The photoreceptor nuclei comprise the outer nuclear layer, and their outer segments constitute the photoreceptor layer of the retina. Each photoreceptor outer segment is connected to the inner segment by a cilium. In rods, the **outer segment** consists of stacks of membranous disks enclosed by the cell membrane, whereas in cones, the disks are occasionally open to the extracellular space. Molecules of **visual pigments** (rhodopsin in rods and iodopsins in cones) are present in the membranes. The oldest, most external disks are regularly shed from the photoreceptors, then phagocytized and degraded by the RPE cells. New disks are continually added to the inner ends of the outer segments. The **inner segment** includes two portions (ellipsoid and myoid) that contain the numerous intracellular organelles necessary for phototransduction.

The **external limiting membrane** is formed by intercellular junctions spanning between the extracellular processes adjoining **radial glial (Müller) cells** and the photoreceptors. The microvilli of the radial glial cells project peripherally between the inner segments of rods and cones (Fig. 17-11).

The **outer nuclear layer** contains the photoreceptor nuclei (Fig. 17-11). The **outer plexiform layer** is composed of the axon terminals of the photoreceptors—spherules for rods and pedicles for cones—forming synapses with the processes of the horizontal cells and the dendrites of bipolar cells (Fig. 17-11).

Several layers of nuclei form the **inner nuclear layer** (Fig. 17-11), which comprises bipolar, horizontal, amacrine, and radial glial cells. Most of the nuclei of this layer belong to rod and **cone bipolar cells**, the second neurons in the visual pathway, with fewer belonging to horizontal and amacrine cells. The nuclei of radial glial (Müller) cells are interspersed among these other nuclei.

The radial glial cells are elongated, fibrous astrocytes that span between the internal and external limiting membranes (Fig. 17-11), providing mechanical support and nutrition to the retina.

The **inner plexiform layer** forms another synaptic layer, important for synapses between bipolar cells and ganglion cells (Fig. 17-11).

The **ganglion cell layer**, composed of large neurons (perikaryal), represents the third neurons of the visual pathway (Fig. 17-14). The axons of ganglion cells form a separate layer, the **nerve fiber layer** (Figs. 17-11 and 17-14). These axons converge and exit at the **optic disk** (papilla) of the retina to form the **optic nerve (CN II)**.

The **internal limiting membrane** is synthesized and secreted by the expanded foot processes of the Müller cells, which form a true basement membrane at the posterior face of the vitreous body.

The **area centralis retinae** is a small round or oval area of the retina located dorsally and laterally to the optic disk. This area differs from the remainder of the retina in that it has an increased number of cones, a thickened inner plexiform layer, a higher density of ganglion cells, a thinner nerve fiber layer, and the absence of large blood vessels. The area centralis retinae is where vision is most acute and corresponds to the macular region in primates.

The retinal vascular pattern greatly varies among species. In the **holangiotic** pattern (cats, dogs, cattle, pigs, and sheep), blood vessels are present in the nerve fiber layer. Wide capillaries are found at the periphery of the retina, and venules and arterioles are present toward the optic disk. Numerous capillaries also are present in the inner nuclear, ganglion cell, and nerve fiber layers. In the **paurangiotic** pattern (horses), retinal vessels only radiate a short distance from the optic disk. In the **merangiotic** retina (rabbits), the vessels migrate medially and laterally along myelinated optic nerve fibers within medullary rays. **Anangiotic** retinas (birds and reptiles) are devoid of blood vessels and instead possess vascular structures that project into the vitreous, called the pecten and conus papillaris, respectively.

Refractive Media

Lens and Zonular Fibers

The **lens** is a transparent, biconvex structure that is situated between the iris and the vitreous body in the posterior chamber, suspended by the zonular fibers from the ciliary body (Figs. 17-15 and 17-16). It consists of the lens capsule, lens epithelium, and lens fibers.

The lens is entirely surrounded by the **lens capsule** (Figs. 17-15 and 17-16), which consists of several layers of fibrillar collagen alternating with type IV collagen, forming a basement membrane. The capsule is thicker on the anterior lens surface than on the posterior surface.

Beneath the anterior lens capsule is the **lens epithelium** (Figs. 17-15 and 17-16), a layer of simple cuboidal epithelial cells. The basal region of the cells faces outward toward the lens capsule, while the apical region is oriented toward the lens fibers. At the equator, the cells elongate and differentiate into **lens fibers**, which make up the bulk of the lens (Figs. 17-15 and 17-16). Fully differentiated lens fibers are U-shaped prism-shaped cells that extend toward the anterior and posterior poles of the lens. They lack a nucleus and are virtually devoid of organelles. Lens fibers interdigitate extensively, especially where fibers from opposite sides of the equator meet to form lens sutures (Fig. 17-15), and they are interconnected through gap junctions and desmosomes. Through continuous differentiation of lens epithelial cells and the addition of fibers, the lens continues to grow throughout life.

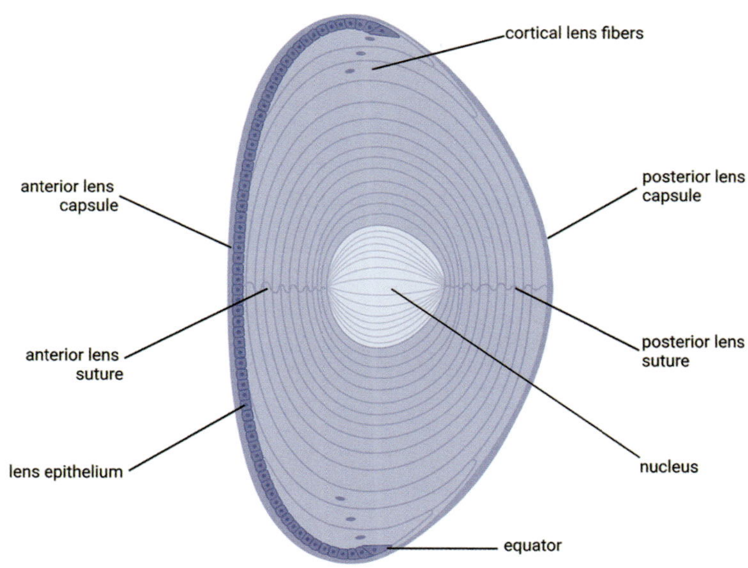

Figure 17-15 Schematic drawing of the lens. Lens fibers extend from the equator toward the anterior and posterior aspects where they interdigitate and form two sutures.

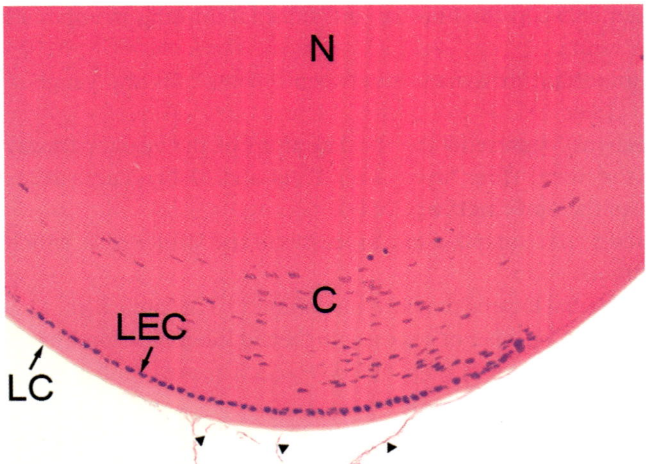

Figure 17-16 Murine lens. The lens capsule (LC) covers the anterior lens epithelium (LEC), beneath which are the lens fibers forming the cortex (C) and surrounding the nucleus (N). Remnant zonular fibers are attached to the lens capsule near the equator (arrowheads) H&E (×200).

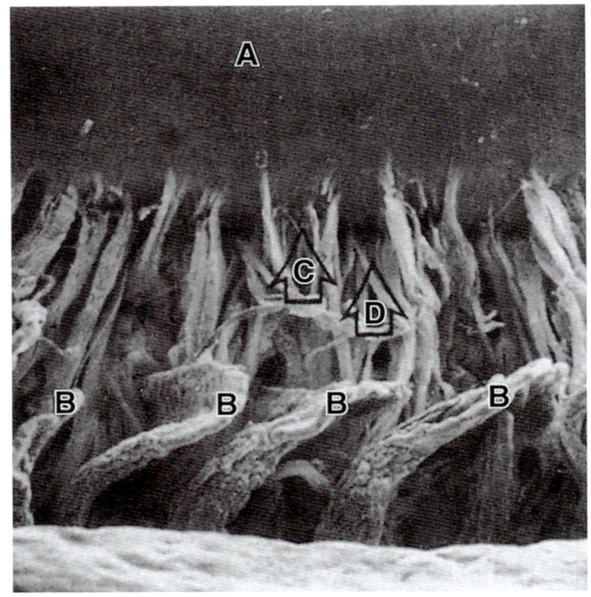

Figure 17-17 Scanning electron micrograph illustrating a posterior view of ciliary processes and attachment of zonular fibers to the lens (cat). Posterior lens (A), ciliary process (B), posterior zonular fibers (C), and anterior zonular fibers (D). Note that the zonular fibers extend from the bases of the ciliary processes and converge at their attachment points on the lens. (From Gelatt KM. Textbook of Veterinary Ophthalmology. Philadelphia: Lea & Febiger, 1981.)

The **zonular fibers** originate from the basement membrane of the inner nonpigmented ciliary epithelium (Fig. 17-17). The fibers are composed of noncollagenous glycoproteins similar to elastic fibers (see Chapter 3) and attach to the lens capsule by fusing with its outermost layers.

When the ciliary muscle contracts during accommodation, the zonular fibers slacken. This action allows the elastic lens fibers to shorten, causing the lens to assume a more spherical shape, which focuses the image on the retina. During ciliary muscle relaxation, the zonular fibers tense, causing the lens to become more discoid and reducing its axial thickness.

Vitreous Body

The vitreous body occupies the vitreous, or posterior chamber, which is the space between the lens and the retina, or about two thirds of the volume of the globe (Fig. 17-1). Vitreous is a hydrogel containing 99% water, with the remaining 1% primarily composed of hyaluronic acid and widely spaced collagen fibrils. The vitreous adheres tightly to the optic disk (papilla) and the ora serrata. Also, it attaches to the internal limiting membrane of the retina and the posterior part (pars plana) of the ciliary body. In most domestic mammals, the vitreous body also is attached firmly to the posterior lens capsule through the hyaloideocapsular ligament.

Accessory Organs

Eyelids

The **eyelids, or palpebrae**, are movable folds of haired skin and conjunctiva that meet in the medial and lateral aspects of the orbit in regions called the canthi (singular: canthus). Eyelids protect the eye by reducing the palpebral fissure (the gap between the upper and lower eyelids). The eyelids contain several sebaceous glands, chiefly the Meibomian glands, which contribute the lipid portion of the tear film (Figs. 17-18 and 17-21). Also, there are fewer glands of Zeis associated with the cilia (eyelashes) and the sebaceous glands of the pilosebaceous units on the surface of the haired skin. Modified apocrine sweat glands, called the glands of Moll, are also present within the eyelid skin. The structure of skin and adnexal structures is described in Chapter 16.

Third Eyelid and Conjunctiva

The **third eyelid** (nictitating membrane) is a conjunctival fold fortified by hyaline (ruminants and dogs) or elastic (horses, pigs, and cats) cartilage. It originates adjacent to the inferionasal aspect of the globe, positioned between the cornea and the lower eyelid. The conjunctiva (Fig. 17-19) consists of a secretory epithelium covering a CT substantia propria. The **conjunctival epithelium** is a pseudostratified columnar, transitioning to stratified squamous near the eyelid margin where it meets the haired skin (Fig. 17-18). The conjunctiva is divided into three components: *bulbar* (covering the anterior aspect of the globe over the sclera and limbus), *palpebral* (covering the inner aspect of the eyelids), and *forniceal* (covering the fornix between the palpebral and bulbar aspects). Goblet cells are scattered throughout the conjunctiva, with the highest densities found in the lower nasal to middle fornix region in dogs (Fig. 17-19). These cells produce the inner mucinous layer of the tear film (Fig. 17-21). Underlying the conjunctival epithelium is a substantia propria of highly vascularized loose CT rich in fibrocytes, lymphocytes, and plasma cells, with some mast cells and macrophages also present. Also, this layer may contain solitary and aggregated lymphatic nodules.

The **gland of the third eyelid** surrounds the base of the shaft of the T-shaped cartilage plate (Fig. 17-20). It is similar in structure to the lacrimal gland and likewise contributes aqueous secretion to the tear film. In horses and cats, it is serous; in cattle and dogs, seromucous; and in pigs, mucous. Frequently, acinar cells secrete lipid.

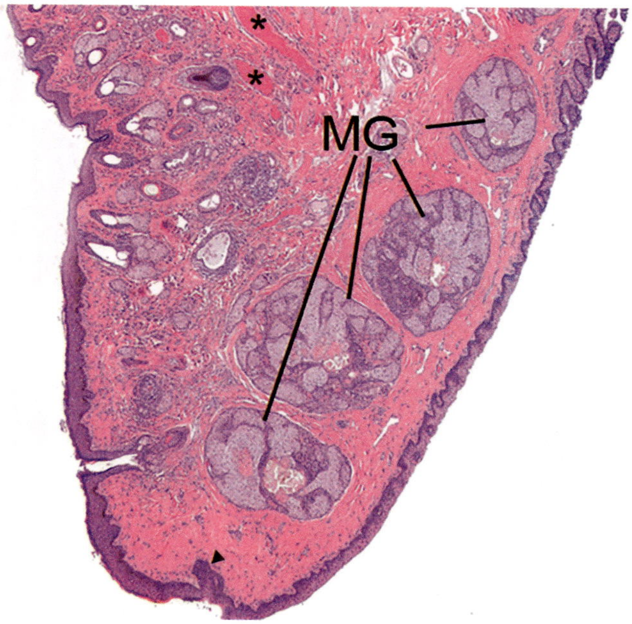

Figure 17-18 Canine eyelid. The eyelid is composed of a haired skin surface (left side of image) transitioning to an internal conjunctival surface (right side of image) at the eyelid margin (arrowhead). Numerous lobules of large Meibomian glands (MG) are composed of acini of sebaceous cells that secrete lipid contents at the eyelid opening to prevent evaporation of the aqueous portion of the tear film. A few bundles of orbicularis oculi myofibers, which aid in closing the eyelids, are seen in cross sections (asterisks). H&E (×20).

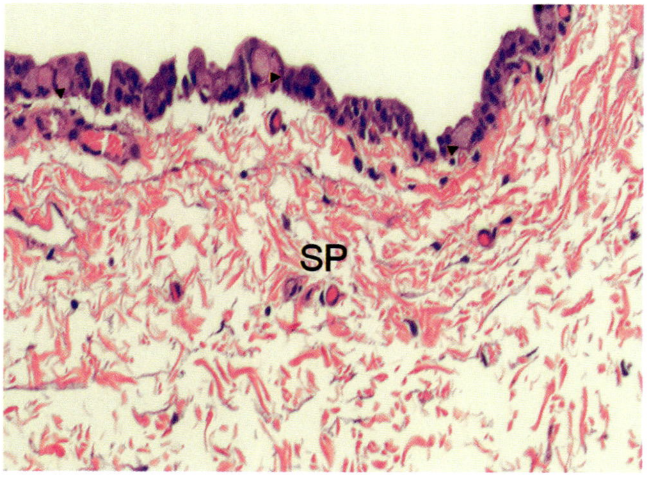

Figure 17-19 Canine conjunctiva. The pseudostratified columnar epithelium contains multiple goblet cells (arrowheads) and is supported by a vascularized, loose CT stroma (SP: substantia propria). H&E (×200).

Lacrimal Apparatus

The **lacrimal gland** is a compound gland comprised of acini surrounded by myoepithelial cells, which aid in secretion (Fig. 17-21). It is serous in cats and seromucous in dogs and ungulates. The intercalated and secretory ducts are lined by simple and stratified cuboidal epithelia, respectively, while the lacrimal ductules are lined by stratified cuboidal epithelium.

The gland of the third eyelid (described above) is also part of the lacrimal apparatus. Together, the lacrimal gland and the gland of the third eyelid produce approximately 60% and 35%, respectively, of the aqueous portion of the tear film.

Excess tears accumulate in the lacrimal lake, a widening of the conjunctiva located medially and lined by stratified squamous and columnar epithelium. From the lacrimal lake, tears ears enter the **lacrimal puncta**, which open into the **lacrimal canaliculi**, two small caliber ducts lined by stratified squamous epithelium, before emptying into the lacrimal sac and its continuation, the nasolacrimal duct.

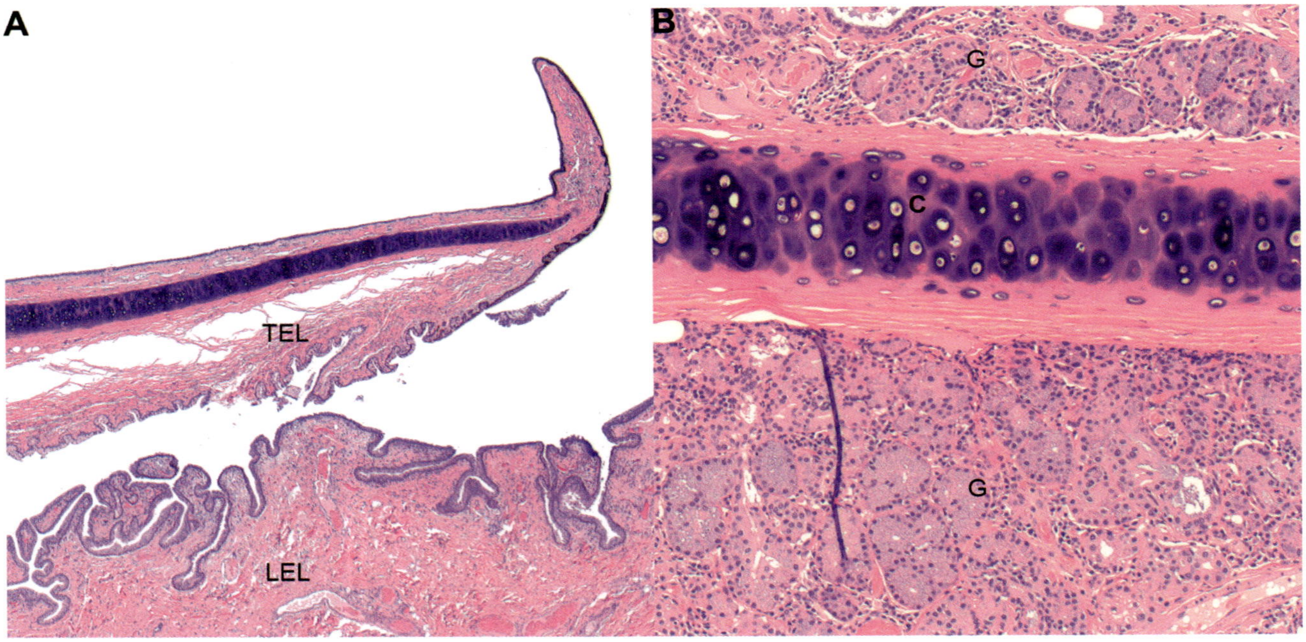

Figure 17-20 Canine nictitating membrane. **A.** The nictitating membrane, or third eyelid (TEL), is a fold of tissue containing a cartilaginous core located between the lower eyelid (LEL) and the cornea. H&E (×20). **B.** The gland (G) of the third eyelid surrounds the base of the T-shaped cartilage (C) and is comprised of lobules of secretory tissue that contributes a proportion of the aqueous component of the tear film. H&E (×100).

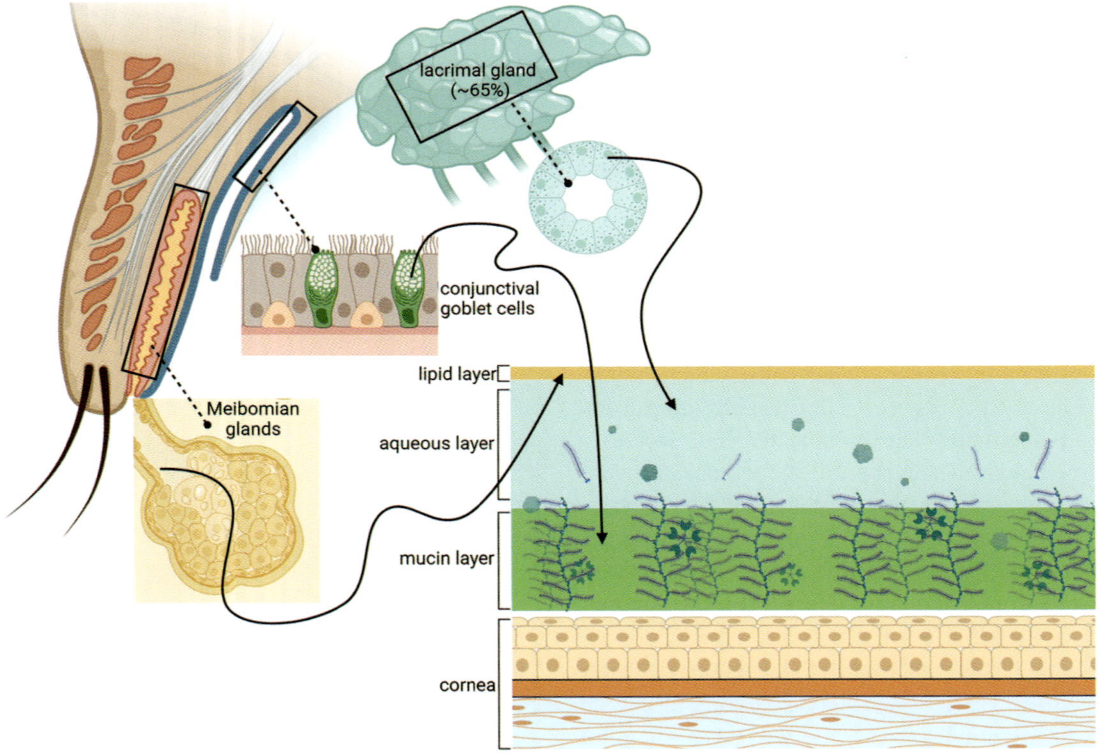

Figure 17-21 Schematic drawing of the tear film. The Meibomian glands produce the outermost lipid component of the tear film, which helps prevent evaporative loss. The lacrimal gland, and to a lesser extent, the gland of the third eyelid, produces the middle aqueous portion of the tear film. The conjunctival goblet cells produce the inner mucin layer of the tear film, which is stabilized on the ocular surface by a glycocalyx secreted by the superficial corneal epithelium.

The **nasolacrimal duct** is lined by stratified columnar epithelium with goblet cells, or transitional epithelium in pigs. The duct begins with an ampullar widening, **the lacrimal sac**, whose lamina propria contains lymphatic tissue. Toward the distal end of the duct, simple branched tubuloacinar mucous (or seromucous in sheep and goats) glands are present.

Species Variations

Many ocular anatomic and histologic variations occur among species. In mammals, differences include globe and corneal size and shape; corneal and scleral thickness; optic nerve penetration scleral site; pupil shape and orientation; type and distribution of melanin granules; extent of ciliary muscle development; lenticular shape, relative size, and color; retinal thickness and vascular pattern; tapetal presence and location; choroidal thickness; and lacrimal gland morphology.

The differences between mammalian eyes and those of other vertebrates are much more striking. For example, eyes of birds vary greatly in shape, and their sclerae contain cartilage and, in many species, bony ossicles. Avian species also have skeletal rather than smooth muscle within the iris and ciliary body, with some species having ciliary processes attaching directly to an annular lens pad. Several other differences exist between mammalian eyes and those of other vertebrates, and the reader is referred to the suggested reading list for additional information.

The Ear

The ear is composed of three divisions: the external ear, the middle ear, and the internal (inner) ear. Structured for sound collection, the external ear is composed of the auricle and the external acoustic meatus. The middle ear consists of the tympanic membrane, tympanic cavity, and three auditory ossicles plus their associated muscles and ligaments. The air-filled tympanic cavity of the middle ear is connected to the nasopharynx by the auditory tube. Sound conduction is the primary function of the middle ear. The inner ear, consisting of the membranous labyrinth enclosed within the osseous (bony) labyrinth of the petrous temporal bone, plays a role in both hearing and equilibrium.

External Ear

The microscopic description of the auricle, or pinna, and the external acoustic meatus is included in Chapter 16.

Middle Ear

Tympanic Membrane

The thin **tympanic membrane** delimits the external acoustic meatus from the tympanic cavity (Fig. 17-22). This membrane is covered externally by stratified squamous epithelium and internally by simple squamous epithelium continuous with that of the tympanic cavity. Between these two epithelial sheets is a CT layer composed of a central region of circularly arranged collagen fibers and a peripheral region of radially arranged collagen fibers. Ventrally, at the site where the manubrium of the malleus attaches to the tympanic membrane, the CT is somewhat thicker, referred to as the **tense** part, and contains blood vessels and nerves that course along the manubrium and spread radially. Collagen fibers are sparse to absent in the dorsal portion of the membrane, referred to as the **flaccid** part.

Tympanic Cavity

The air-filled tympanic cavity contains three small bones, the auditory ossicles, and their muscles and ligaments (Fig. 17-22). The cavity is lined with squamous or simple cuboidal epithelium, which covers the ossicles. The epithelium rests on a thin layer of CT. A few epithelial cells are ciliated, particularly those on the floor of the cavity.

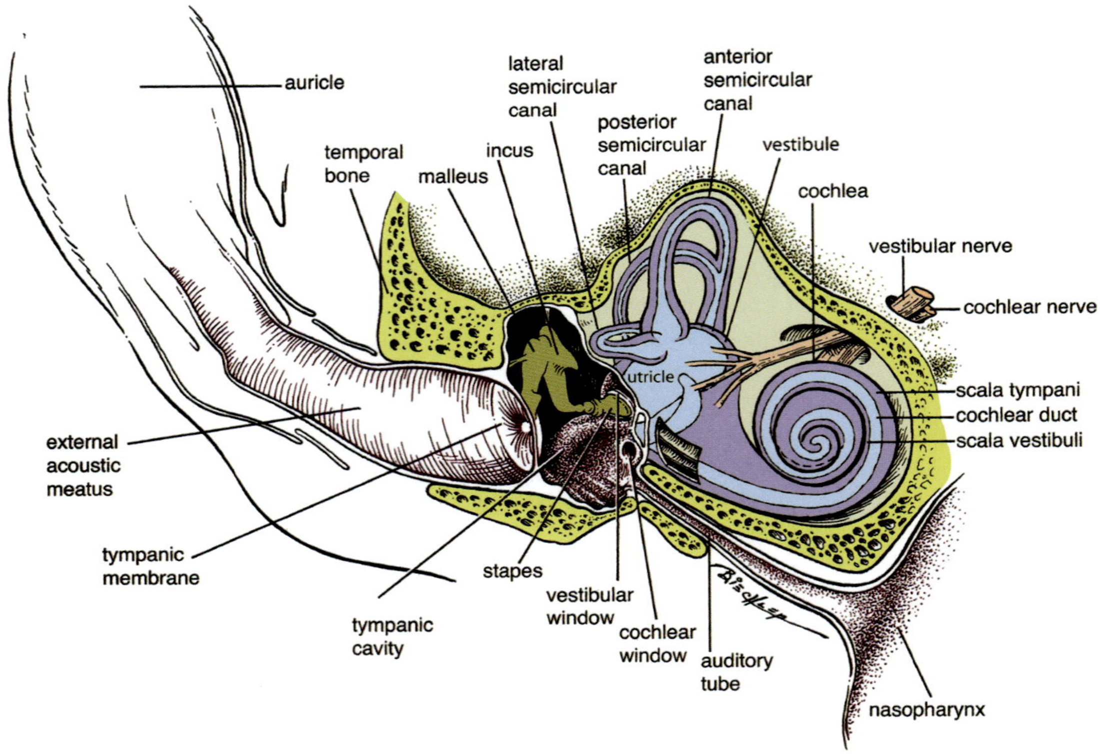

Figure 17-22 Schematic drawing of the right ear (dog), rostral aspect. The external ear consists of the auricle and external acoustic meatus. The middle ear contains the tympanic membrane; auditory ossicles (malleus, incus, and stapes); tympanic cavity; auditory tube with connection to the nasopharynx; cochlear window; and the vestibular window, where the footplate of the stapes is located. The internal ear houses the bony labyrinth (bone cut away for easier viewing of the membranous labyrinth) comprising the anterior, lateral, and posterior semicircular canals, each with an osseous ampulla; vestibule; cochlea with the scala vestibule and the scala tympani; and membranous labyrinth (dotted lines) comprising the anterior, lateral, and posterior semicircular ducts (each with a membranous ampulla), and utricle, saccule, and the cochlear duct. Moreover, the vestibulocochlear nerve (CN VIII), comprising the vestibular nerve and the cochlear nerve, is depicted entering the cranial cavity through the temporal bone.

Auditory Ossicles and Muscles of the Middle Ear

The three **auditory ossicles** (malleus, incus, and stapes) traverse the middle ear, connecting the tympanic membrane to the membrane of the vestibular (oval) window of the internal ear (Fig. 17-22).

These compact bones transmit vibrations across the middle ear cavity. The manubrium of the malleus is firmly attached to the tympanic membrane, and the small hooklike process on the neck of the malleus serves as an attachment for the tendon of the tensor tympani muscle. The head of the malleus articulates with the incus, which, in turn, articulates with the stapes. Ligaments hold these synovial articulations in place.

Muscles of the middle ear (tensor tympani and stapedius) are skeletal muscles and function to dampen ossicle movement, protecting the structures of the inner ear from excessive vibration. The stapedius muscle attaches to the rostral crus of the stapes, and the footplate (base) of the stapes is attached to the vestibular (oval) window by an annular ligament.

Auditory Tube

The **auditory tube** connects the tympanic cavity to the nasopharynx (Fig. 17-22). The tube is lined by ciliated pseudostratified columnar epithelium (with goblet cells) resting on loose CT. The lamina propria of the tube is thin and lacks glands in the osseous region of the tube; it becomes thicker in the cartilaginous region and assumes adnexal structures including seromucous glands and lymphatic nodules. Aggregated lymphatic nodules (the tubal tonsil) are present near the proximal opening in pharynx. The auditory tube is surrounded either by bone distally, near the tympanic membrane, and/or by an incomplete cartilaginous tube proximally, toward the pharynx (Fig. 17-22). Hyaline cartilage is present in the proximal portion of the tube near the bone, but the tissue transitions to elastic cartilage toward the pharynx.

In the horse, the auditory tube expands ventrally to form the **guttural pouch**. The pouch has the same histologic features as the pharyngeal portion of the auditory tube but lacks cartilaginous support.

The function of the auditory tube is to ensure equal air pressure on both sides of the tympanic membrane. Usually, the auditory tube is closed, but it opens during yawning and swallowing.

Internal Ear

The structural divisions of the inner ear comprise the bony labyrinth and the membranous labyrinth. The functional divisions of the internal ear are the vestibular apparatus and the auditory apparatus.

Bony Labyrinth

The **bony labyrinth** is a system of canals and cavities within the petrous temporal bone. Bone of the labyrinth is very dense and lamellar.

The cavities of the labyrinth include the vestibule, three semicircular canals, and the cochlea (Fig. 17-22). The **vestibule** is a small oval space which spans between the cochlea and the semicircular canals located near the medial wall of the tympanic cavity. Three **semicircular canals** (anterior, posterior, and lateral) lie at right angles to each other, and all communicate with the vestibule. The cochlea is a bony tube wound in a helical shape. The **spiral canal** of the cochlea makes several turns around a central axis comprised of spongy bone, called the **modiolus**. The modiolus is a cone-shaped hollow osseous structure in which the cochlear nerve and its spiral ganglion are located. The number of coils varies among veterinary species (e.g., dog, 3¼; cat, 3; horse, 2¼; pig, 4; guinea pig, 4½; cow, 3¼). The base of the modiolus forms the rostral part of the internal acoustic meatus, where the cochlear nerve and blood vessels enter the cochlea. The bony canal is partially divided by a hollow bony projection, the osseous **spiral lamina**, which contains the branches of the cochlear nerve coursing to the spiral organ. The lamina is widest at the cochlear window and narrows toward the apex of the cochlea.

The canals and cavities of the bony labyrinth are lined by periosteum. A clear fluid, **perilymph**, fills the **perilymphatic space** between the periosteum and the membranous labyrinth (Figs. 17-23 and 17-24). Perilymph has similar ionic composition to cerebrospinal fluid and plasma, with sodium as the main cation. Perilymph flows from the subarachnoid space through the cochlear canaliculus into the cavities of the bony labyrinth. The **vestibular aqueduct**, a space surrounding the endolymphatic duct, also contains perilymph.

Membranous Labyrinth

The membranous labyrinth comprises the semicircular ducts, utricle, saccule, cochlear duct, endolymphatic duct, and endolymphatic sac (Fig. 17-23). The membranous labyrinth is lined by squamous epithelium and filled with a fluid called **endolymph**, which is more viscous than perilymph. Endolymph is produced by the epithelium of the vestibule and stria vascularis (described later) and contains a similar protein composition, higher levels of potassium, and lower to levels of sodium when compared to perilymph. The CT underlying the epithelium of the membranous labyrinth forms fine trabeculae (Fig. 17-24). The trabeculae span the adjacent perilymphatic space and anchor the suspended membranous labyrinth to the periosteum of the bony wall. The periosteum and the spaces between the trabeculae are lined by flattened mesothelial cells.

Semicircular Ducts

The **semicircular ducts** lie within the semicircular canals (Fig. 17-22). One end of each duct is dilated as an **ampulla**. The ducts are lined by squamous epithelium. Connection of the ducts with the utricle is shown in Figure 17-23.

Utricle and Saccule

The medial wall of the vestibule contains two depressions in which the **utricle** (caudodorsal) and the **saccule** (rostroventral) are housed (Fig. 17-23). Two portions of the **utriculosaccular duct** extend from the utricle and saccule, respectively, and converge to form the **endolymphatic duct**, which terminates as the **endolymphatic sac**. Part of the endolymphatic

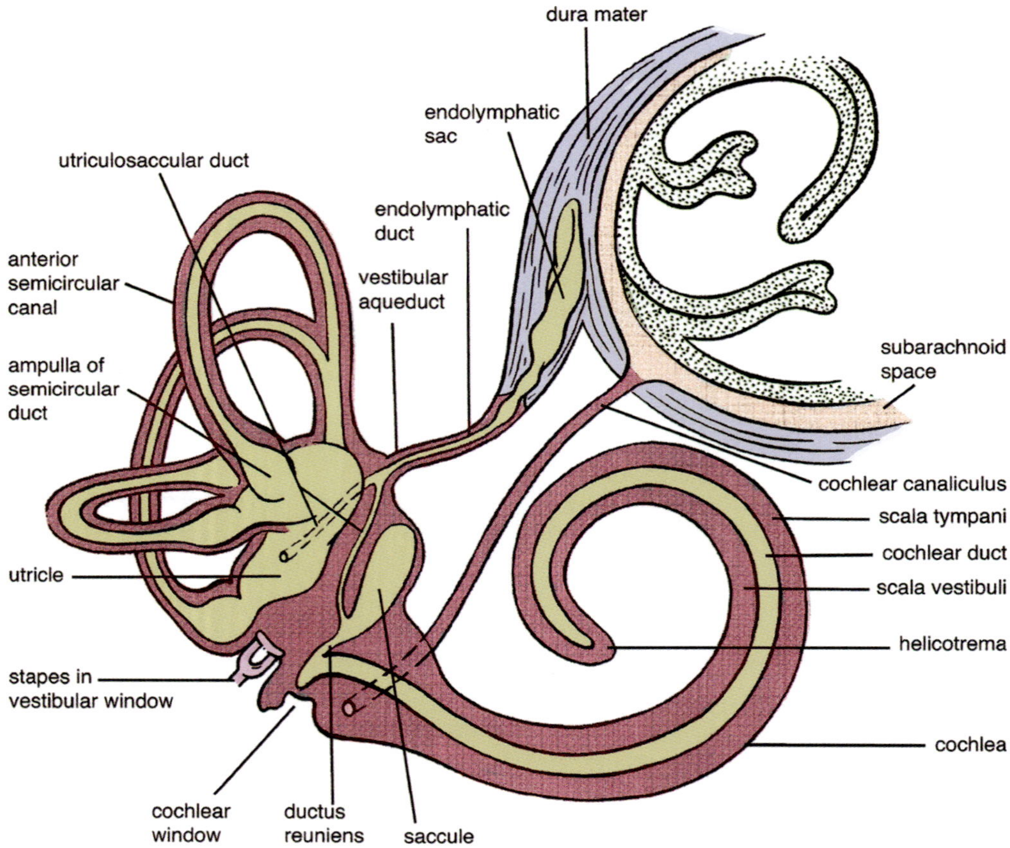

Figure 17-23 Schematic drawing of the right internal ear with its connections to the cranial cavity, intradural space, and subarachnoid space (rostral aspect). The cochlea with its contents is drawn uncoiled to show the helicotrema, where there is an open connection between the scala vestibuli and scala tympani. Note especially that the cochlear canaliculus connects with the subarachnoid space, which contains cerebrospinal fluid (CSF), and the scala tympani. Perilymph fills the space between the membranous labyrinth and the bony labyrinth. The other connection to the cranial cavity is the vestibular aqueduct, which houses portions of the endolymphatic duct and endolymphatic sac. Structures of the membranous labyrinth containing endolymph are shown in tan. Dura mater, the utriculosaccular duct, ductus reuniens, saccule, utricle, and stapes in the vestibular window are also indicated.

duct and the endolymphatic sac lie within the vestibular aqueduct. The remaining portion of the endolymphatic sac lies between two laminae of the dura. The function of the sac is to regulate endolymphatic pressure and volume.

Cochlear Duct

The **cochlear duct** is connected to the saccule by a small duct, the **ductus reuniens**, and ends as a blind sac at the apex of the cochlea. The triangular cochlear duct lies between two additional compartments of the cochlea (Fig. 17-25). The dorsal compartment, or **scala vestibuli**, extends from the region of the **vestibular** (oval) **window** to the apex of the cochlea, where it becomes confluent with the ventral compartment, the **scala tympani**, through an opening called the **helicotrema** (Fig. 17-23). The scala tympani terminates at the **cochlear** (round) **window**. The cochlear duct is separated from the scala vestibuli by the **vestibular membrane** and from the scala tympani by the **basilar membrane** (Figs. 17-25 to 17-30). Scant collagen fibers form the vestibular membrane, which is covered by squamous epithelium on both surfaces (Figs. 17-27 and 17-28). Basement membranes separate the epithelia from the CT. The basilar membrane is attached to the outer osseous cochlea by the **spiral ligament** and extends to the **spiral lamina** of the modiolus. The membrane is composed of collagen fibers embedded in homogeneous ground substance; it increases in thickness as it progresses from the cochlear window toward the helicotrema. The width of the basilar membrane increases continuously from the cochlear window, where it is narrowest, to the helicotrema, where it is widest. The basilar membrane is covered by squamous epithelium on the surface facing the scala tympani, while the **spiral organ** (organ of Corti) is present on the cochlear duct surface.

Stria Vascularis

The third wall of the triangular-shaped cochlear duct contains the **stria vascularis**, which contributes to the production and ion regulation of endolymph (Figs. 17-25 to 17-30). Stratified cuboidal cells of the stria rest directly on a layer of CT without an intervening basal lamina (Fig. 17-28). Three epithelial cell types (basal, intermediate, and marginal cells) appear similar with electron microscopy. While epithelium in general is considered to be avascular, many capillaries are present between the epithelial cells of the stria vascularis (Fig. 17-27). At the junction of the stria vascularis and spiral organ, the stratified epithelium changes abruptly to simple cuboidal. This transitional region is called the **spiral prominence** (Fig. 17-27).

Vestibular Apparatus

The **vestibular apparatus** is responsible for equilibrium and is composed of the semicircular ducts, saccule, and utricle. Within these structures are specialized neuroepithelial areas, the crista ampullaris, macula utriculi, and macula sacculi, which function to detect motion and maintain equilibrium.

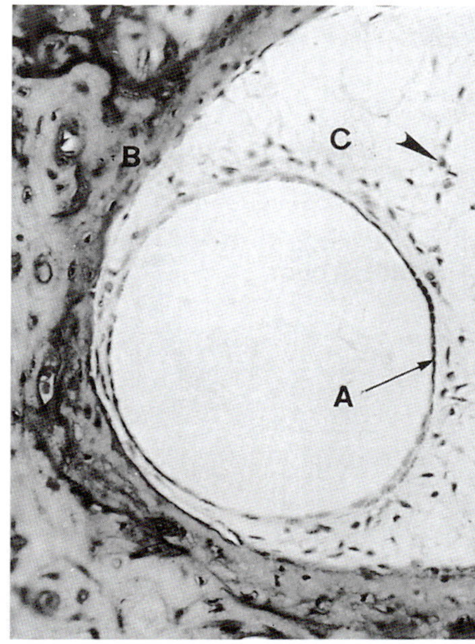

Figure 17-24 Feline semicircular canal. The semicircular duct, an epithelium-lined membranous tube (A), lies within the semicircular canal of the osseous labyrinth (B). The perilymphatic space (C) contains delicate CT trabeculae (arrowhead). The spaces between the trabeculae are lined with mesothelium. H&E (×400).

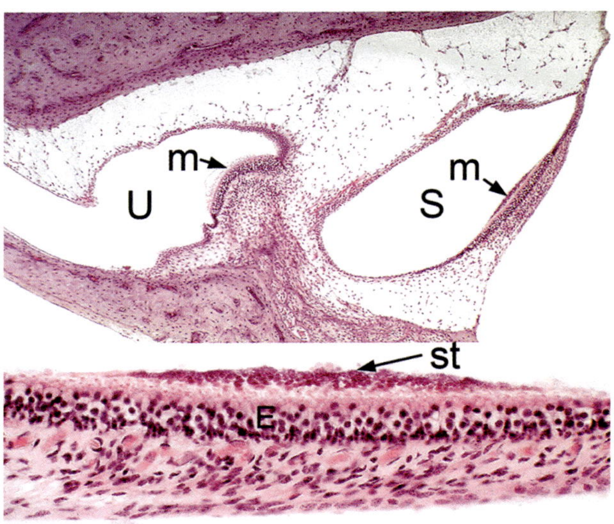

Figure 17-25 Guinea pig inner ear. Top: The utricle (U) and saccule (S) both have foci of neurosensory epithelium (m) called macula utriculi and macula sacculi, respectively (top). H&E (×63). (Image by W.E. Haensly.) Bottom: The macula sacculi in the saccule (S) wall is composed of neurosensory epithelium (E) with type I and type II sensory cells, plus supporting cells. Each macula is covered by a statoconial membrane (st) made of gelatinous material with embedded calcium carbonate crystals (bottom). Hair bundles of the sensory cells penetrate this membrane. When endolymph moves in the utricle or saccule, the statoconial membrane triggers neural impulses from the hair cells of both maculae. As in the crista ampullaris, these impulses are carried by the vestibular nerve to the brain. H&E (×160). (Image by W.E. Haensly.)

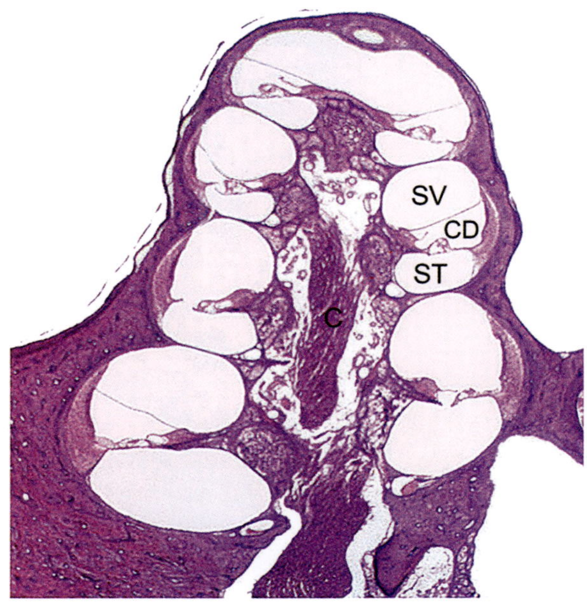

Figure 17-26 Guinea pig cochlea. The cochlea is a bony tube wound in the shape of a spiral. The spiral canal within the bone makes several turns around an axis, the modiolus. Blood vessels and the cochlear nerve (C) enter through the modiolus. The cochlear canal is subdivided by three compartments, the scala vestibuli (SV), cochlear duct (CD), and scala tympani (ST). H&E (×25). (Image by W.E. Haensly.)

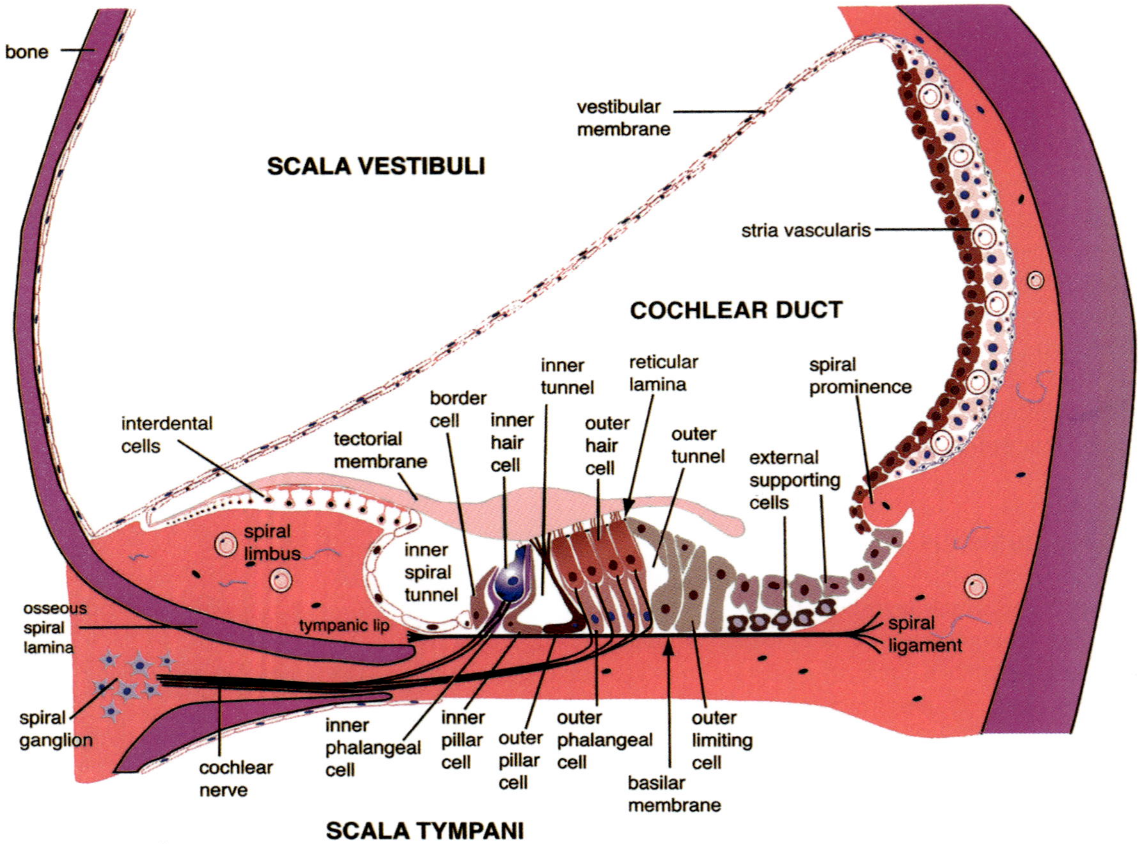

Figure 17-27 Schematic representation of the structure of the scala vestibuli, cochlear duct, and scala tympani. Note the structure of the spiral organ, which includes many cell types that lie under the tectorial membrane above the basilar membrane. Other major structures include the stria vascularis, vestibular membrane, spiral ligament, cochlear nerve, and spiral ganglion. At the junction of the stria vascularis and spiral organ, the stratified epithelium changes abruptly to simple cuboidal. This transitional region is called the spiral prominence.

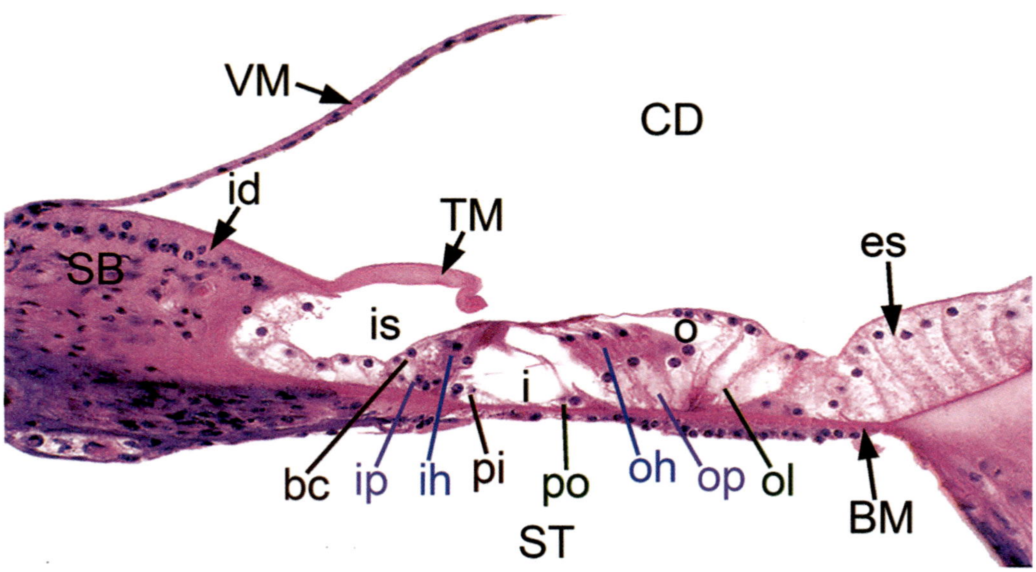

Figure 17-28 Guinea pig cochlea. The cochlear duct (CD) contains the spiral organ (organ of Corti). A portion of the vestibular membrane (VM) that forms one wall of the cochlear duct is present in this image. The spiral organ rests on the basilar membrane (BM) within the cochlear duct above the scala tympani (ST). Sensory cells of the organ transform mechanical energy of sound into electrical energy. The sensory cells include the outer hair cells (oh) and inner hair cells (ih). Supporting cells surround the sensory cells and include border cells (bc), inner (pi) and outer (po) pillar cells, inner (ip) and outer (op) phalangeal cells, outer limiting cells (ol), and external supporting cells (es). Inner and outer pillar cells form a triangular space, the inner tunnel (i). Outer limiting cells are separated from the outer phalangeal cells by the outer tunnel (o). The tectorial membrane (TM) contacts the tips of the tallest stereocilia of the outer hair cells. Interdental cells (id) lie above the spiral limbus (SB) and secrete the gel-like substance of the tectorial membrane. The inner spiral tunnel (is) lies beneath the membrane. H&E (×250). (Image by W.E. Haensly.)

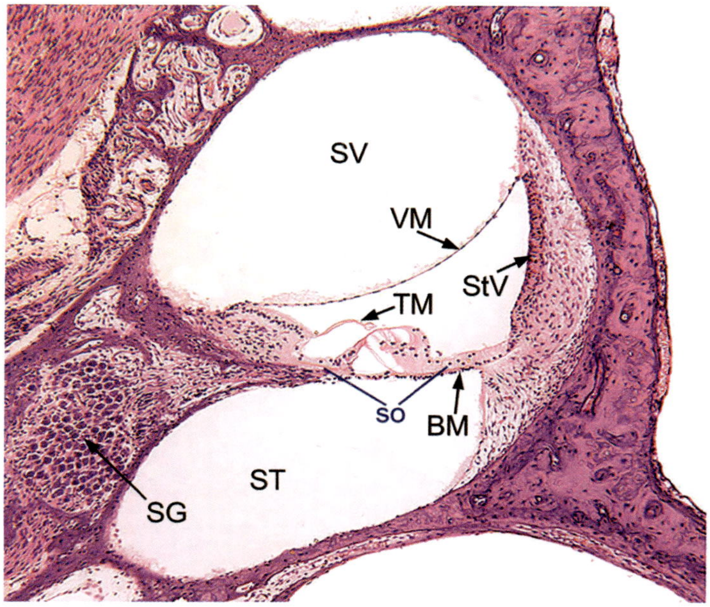

Figure 17-29 A section through one turn of the cochlea with the modiolus to the left. The vestibular membrane (VM) separates the scala vestibule (SV) from the cochlear duct. The tectorial membrane (TM) lies over cells of the spiral organ (so), which are located above the basilar membrane (BM). Nerve fibers from the spiral ganglion (SG) innervate the hair cells of the spiral organ. The vascularized stria vascularis (StV) region of the cochlear duct produces endolymph. H&E (×75). (Image by J. Eurell.)

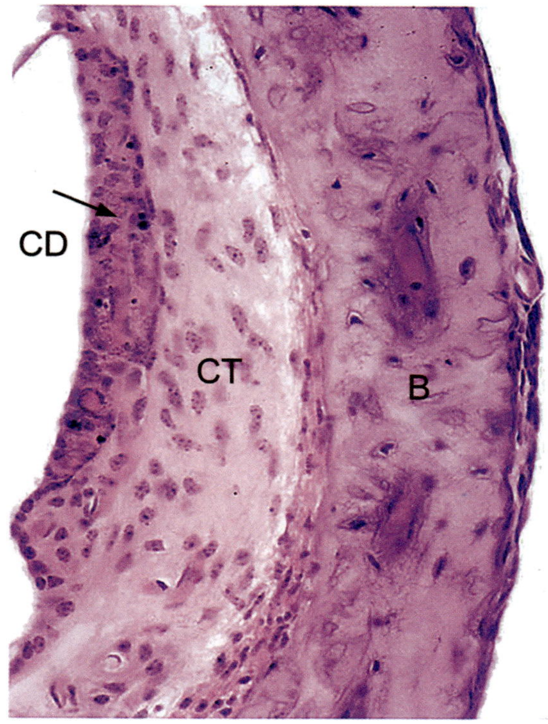

Figure 17-30 Guinea pig cochlea. The third wall of the triangular-shaped cochlear duct (cd) contains the stria vascularis, which contributes to the production of endolymph and regulates its unique ion content. Stratified cuboidal cells (arrow) form an epithelium that contains numerous capillaries. The epithelium rests directly on CT without an intervening basement membrane. The bony labyrinth (B) of the cochlea supports this region of the membranous labyrinth. H&E (×400). (Image by W.E. Haensly.)

Crista Ampullaris

The membranous ampulla of each semicircular duct contains a **crista ampullaris**, which is sensitive to rotary movements (angular acceleration and deceleration) (Fig. 17-31). The crista ampullaris is composed of a ridge of sensory epithelium resting on thickened CT, which projects into the lumen of the ampulla.

Sensory epithelium of the crista ampullaris consists of hair cells and supporting cells (Figs. 17-31 and 17-32). Two types of hair cells (types I and II) are recognized based on their ultrastructural morphology. Stereocilia present on the hair cells project into an overlying gelatinous **cupula**, and the orientation of the stereocilia provides the hair cells with the functional polarization responsible for neural transmission of equilibrium that occurs with rotation of the head. The **supporting cells** of the epithelium are tall and columnar with microvilli. They synthesize the matrix of the cupula and therefore contain numerous secretory vesicles.

Maculae of the Utricle and Saccule

Two receptor organs, the **macula utriculi** and **macula sacculi**, lie perpendicular to each other, located on the lateral wall of the utricle and the floor of the saccule, respectively.

The sensory epithelium of both maculae rests on loose CT containing blood vessels and nerves (Fig. 17-25). The cells of the sensory epithelium of the maculae are essentially the same as those of the crista ampullaris, that is, type I and II sensory cells and supporting cells (Figs. 17-25 and 17-34).

Hair bundles of the sensory cells of the maculae penetrate an overlying gelatinous mass with calcium carbonate crystals called **statoconia** (otoliths). Together, the hair bundles, gelatinous material, and statoconia form the **statoconial** (otolithic) **membrane**.

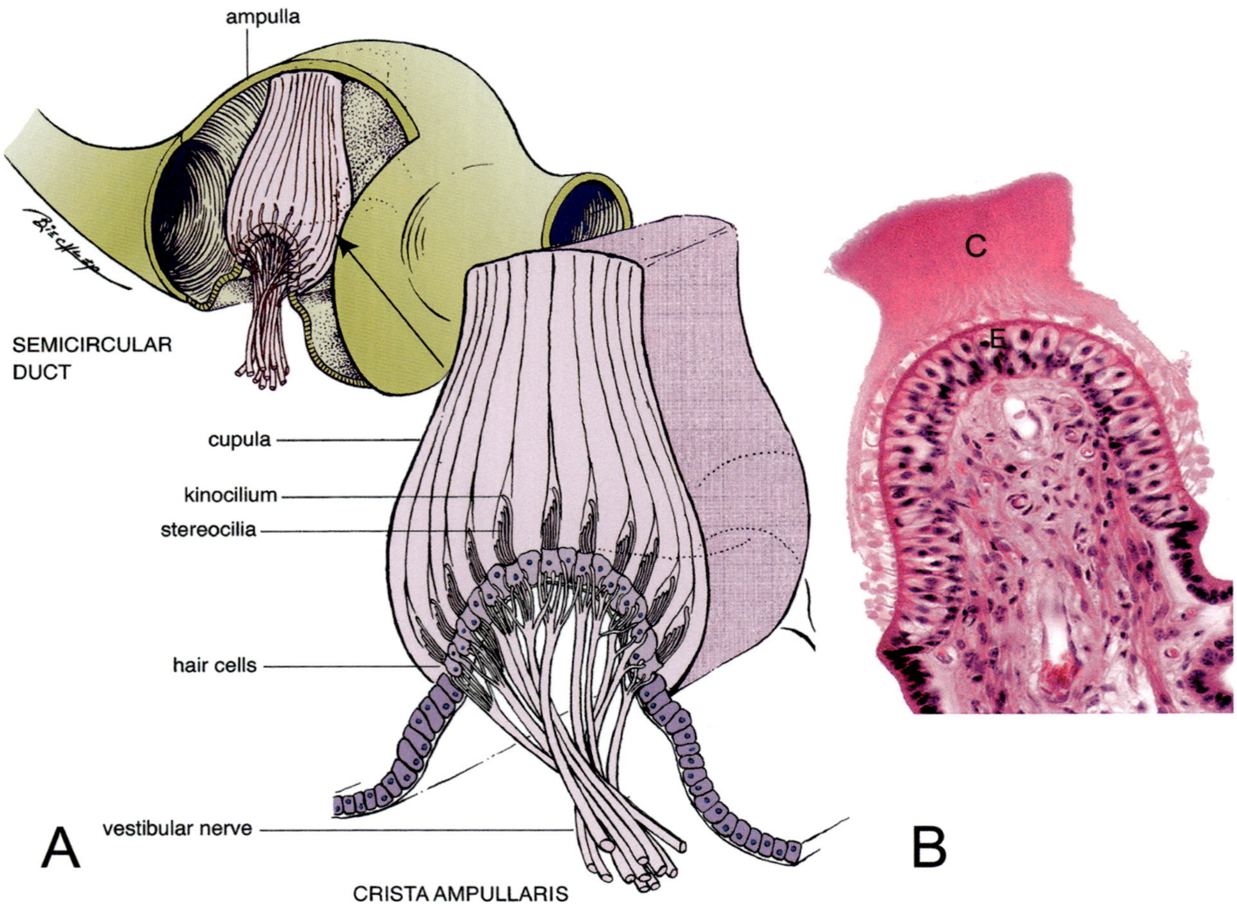

Figure 17-31 **A.** Schematic drawing of the ampulla of the semicircular duct, open to show the crista ampullaris within. The enlarged drawing of the crista shows the hair cells beneath the cup-shaped gelatinous cupula. Each hair cell has one kinocilium and several stereocilia of different lengths on the apical surface. Processes of the vestibular nerve contact the basal region of the hair cells. **B.** Guinea pig inner ear. The membranous ampulla of each semicircular duct contains a crista ampullaris. The crista ampullaris contains a ridge of sensory epithelium (E). Sensory hair cells project into an overlying gelatinous cupula (C). H&E (×400). (Image by W.E. Haensly.)

Auditory Apparatus

The auditory apparatus comprises the organ of hearing, which includes the scala tympani, scala vestibuli, and cochlear duct. Within the cochlear duct is the epithelial spiral organ, which functions in hearing.

Spiral Organ (Organ of Corti)

The sensory portion of the spiral organ is a complex structure that rests on the cochlear duct side of the basilar membrane (Figs. 17-35 and 17-36). This receptor organ has three major components: (a) the sensory cells that transform mechanical energy of sound vibrations into electrical energy, (b) a supportive structure for the sensory cells, and (c) the afferent and efferent nerve terminals of the cochlear nerve, a branch of CN VIII (Fig. 17-33).

Sensory Cells

The sensory cells are arranged in two groups, both containing sterocilia: the outer hair cells, arranged in three to four rows, and a single row of inner hair cells. The outer hair cells are morphologically polarized, much like the vestibular hair cells.

The longest stereocilia are embedded in the tectorial membrane. At the base of the outer hair cells, a few afferent nerve endings and many efferent terminals containing vesicles are present. The stereocilia of the inner hair cells are not embedded in the tectorial membrane; however, the longest stereocilia do touch it. Tip links connect the stereocilia of inner hair cells in a fashion similar to that seen in outer hair cells. In contrast to outer hair cells, many afferent nerve endings and a few efferent terminals are present at the base of the inner hair cells.

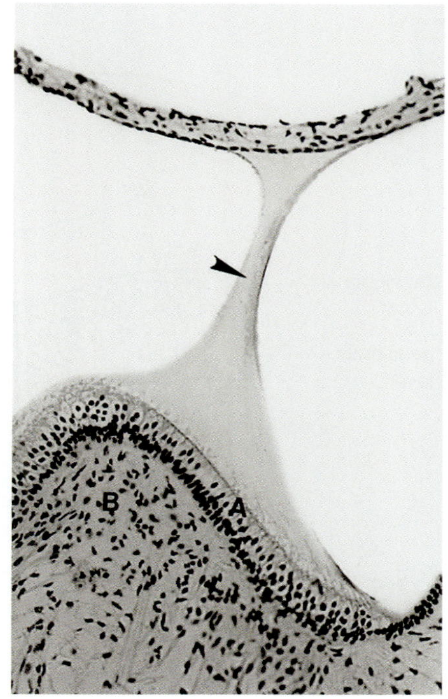

Figure 17-32 Guinea pig crista ampullaris. The sensory and supporting cells (A) and the underlying CT (B) form the crista ampullaris within the ampulla. The gelatinous cupula (arrowhead) on top of the epithelium extends across the lumen of the ampulla to the opposite wall. H&E (×400).

Supporting Cells

The supporting cells of the spiral organ include the border cells, inner and outer pillar cells, inner and outer phalangeal cells, outer limiting cells, and external supporting cells (Fig. 17-35).

The columnar **border cells** rest on the **tympanic lip** of the spiral limbus, forming a single row on the inner side of the inner hair cells. The **inner and outer pillar cells** line a prominent triangular space, the **inner tunnel** (Corti's tunnel). The **inner and outer phalangeal cells** are supportive cells that rest on the basilar membrane and extend upward to cradle the base of the hair cells and then send long cytoplasmic processes toward the surface. Inner hair cells are almost totally enveloped by inner phalangeal cells, while the outer hair cells are only partially surrounded by outer phalangeal cells. The free surface of phalangeal cells and hair cells, with its massive terminal web and intercellular junctions, forms the **reticular lamina**, which holds the apical part of the hair cells rigid. The outer limiting cells and the external supporting cells complete the cellular component of the spiral organ.

Tectorial Membrane

Overlying the spiral organ is the **tectorial membrane**, a gelatinous structure containing glycoprotein and extending from the spiral limbus over the hair cells (Figs. 17-28 and 17-29). The lower surface of this membrane rests on the tips of the tallest stereocilia in each bundle of the inner hair cells, whereas the tallest stereocilia of the outer hair cells are embedded in the membrane. **Interdental cells**, located where the tectorial membrane attaches to the spiral limbus, secrete the gel-like substance of the membrane.

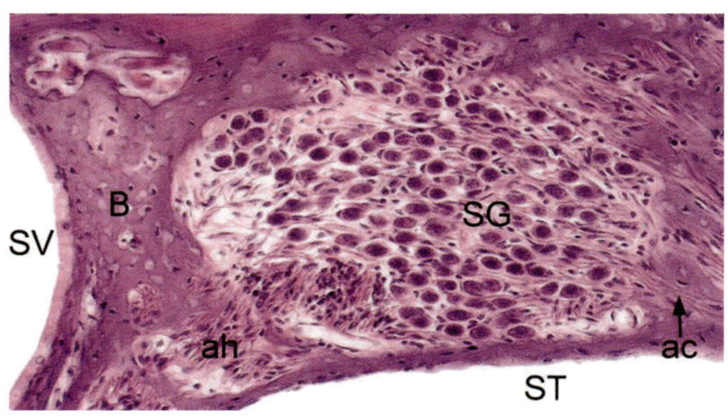

Figure 17-33 Guinea pig cochlea. Bipolar neurons in the spiral ganglion (SG) project axons (ah) to either the inner or outer hair cells of the spiral organ. In the opposite direction, the axons (ac) project toward the brain as the cochlear nerve (a branch of the vestibulocochlear nerve [CN VIII]). The ganglion is found in the bony modiolus (B) that is the central axis of the spiraling cochlea. Scala tympani (ST) and scala vestibuli (SV). H&E (×250). (Image by W.E. Haensly.)

Spiral Ganglion

Bipolar neurons in the **spiral ganglion** at the base of the modiolus project to either the inner hair cells (type I spiral ganglion cells) or the outer hair cells (type II spiral ganglion cells) of the spiral organ (Fig 17-33). The spiral ganglion neurons project in the opposite direction to form the cochlear nerve, a branch of the vestibulocochlear nerve (CN VIII) that propagates electric potentials toward the cochlear nuclei in the brain stem.

Loss of hearing may be related to any condition that interferes with the conduction of sound through the structure of the ear. External or internal ear infections, changes in the bones of the middle ear, or conditions that affect nerve impulse transmission can all affect hearing (Fig. 17-36).

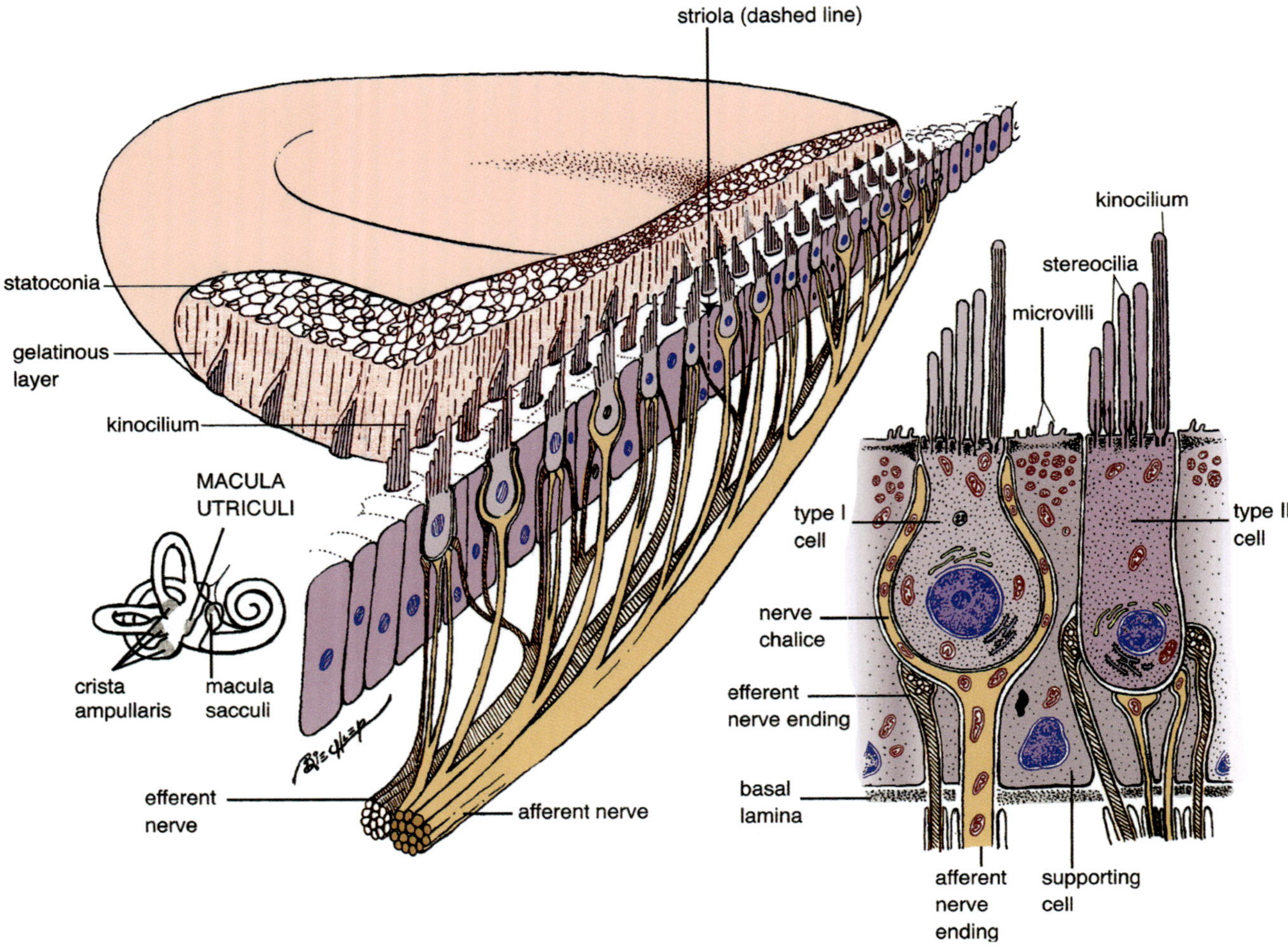

Figure 17-34 Schematic drawing of the membranous labyrinth. The lower left drawing of the membranous labyrinth indicates the location of the macula utriculi, macula sacculi, and cristae ampullaris. The larger schematic drawing of the macula utriculi illustrates the sensory epithelium. The statoconial membrane has been cut away to better illustrate the underlying cells. The numerous stereocilia and single kinocilium of each sensory cell form a cone-like arrangement; each kinocilium faces the striola, represented as a dashed line. Note the change in the morphologic polarization of the sensory cells at the striola. Afferent nerve fibers are solid orange, while efferent nerve fibers are hatched orange. In the lower right corner, a schematic drawing illustrates the general structure of the vestibular sensory epithelium. The type I hair cell has a constricted neck and a rounded base and is almost completely surrounded by a nerve chalice. The cylindrical type II cell is innervated by two types of bud-shaped nerve endings: sparsely vesiculated afferent (orange) and richly vesiculated efferent (orange-hatched). (Colorized, modified, and redrawn after Lindemann H.H. Anatomy of the otolith organs. *Adv Otorhinolaryngol* 1973;20:405.)

Clinical Correlations

Numerous ophthalmic diseases will present routinely to the veterinary clinician in general or emergency practice, including inflammatory (keratitis) and ulcerative corneal diseases, glaucoma (characterized by degeneration and atrophy of the neural tissue of the eye, often as a sequel to elevated intraocular pressure), inflammation within the anterior chamber (anterior uveitis), and blunt or penetrating trauma to the globe. As the cornea is readily visible to owners, veterinary clinicians should become familiar with common corneal pathologies, including keratoconjunctivitis sicca, or canine "dry eye" (Fig. 17-37).

Among the most common presentations in small animal medicine is otitis externa (inflammation of the external ear), which is commonly associated with underlying allergic dermatitis. When complicated by bacterial and/or yeast infection, the inflammation can extend to the middle or inner ear (otitis media and interna). Due to the course of the facial nerve (CN VII) and the postganglionic portion of the sympathetic nerve within or adjacent to the tympanic bulla, deep seeded ear infections may result in facial nerve paralysis or oculosympathetic paresis (Horner's syndrome, Fig. 17-38).

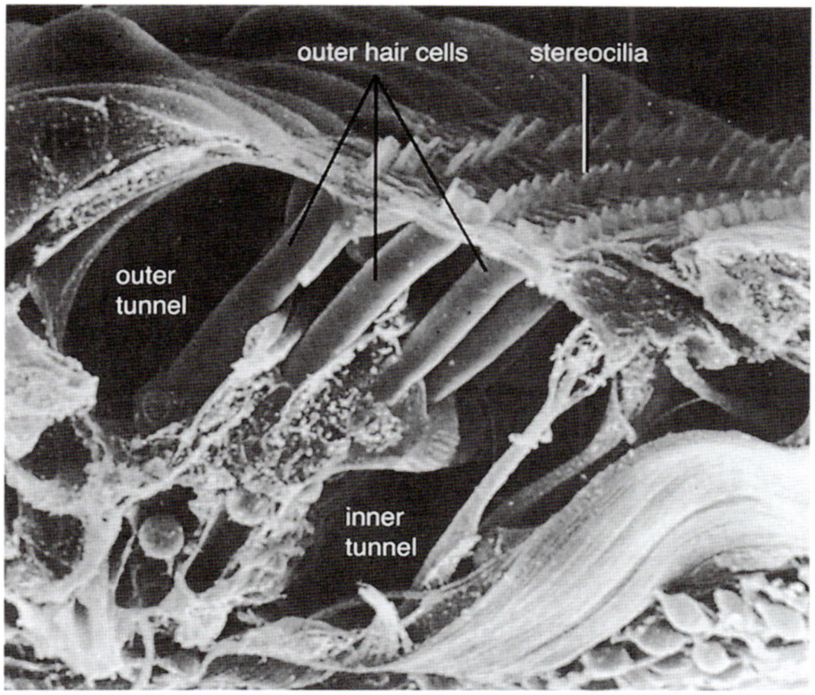

Figure 17-35 Scanning electron micrograph of the spiral organ. Outer hair cells with rows of stereocilia on their apical surface are shown in this image of a portion of the spiral organ. (From Weiss L, ed. Cell and Tissue Biology, a Textbook of Histology. 6th Ed. Baltimore: Urban & Schwarzenberg, 1988:1118.)

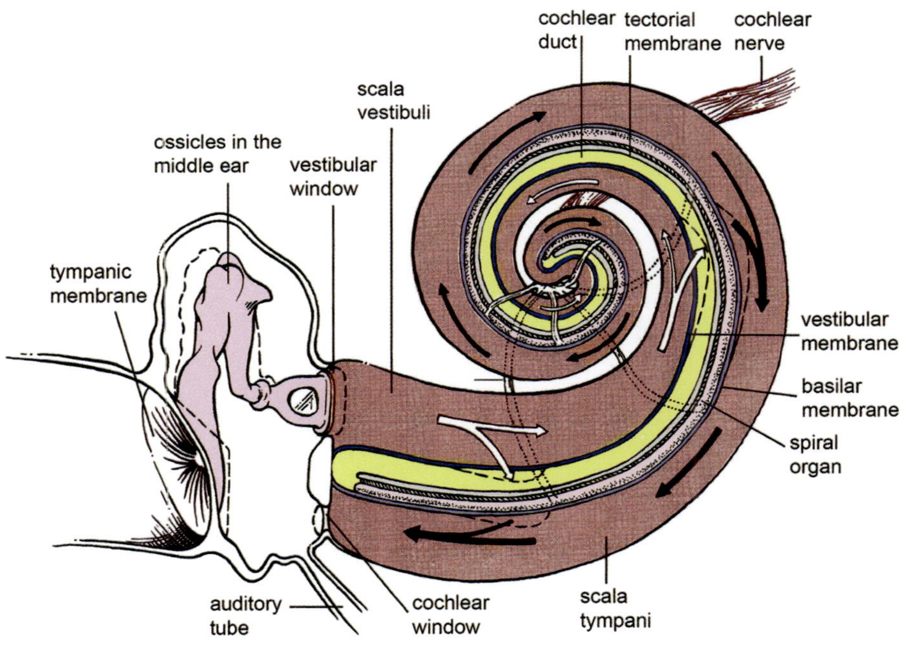

Figure 17-36 Schematic diagram of the events of sound transmission in the ear. The cochlea has been uncoiled to more easily visualize the process. Sound waves impinge on the tympanic membrane, causing it to vibrate. The ear ossicles vibrate as a unit; the range of position of ear ossicles is indicated by dashed lines. The footplate of the stapes moves in and out of the vestibular window, causing changes in fluid pressure within the scala vestibuli. Perilymph (red) fills the scala vestibuli and scala tympani, while endolymph (yellow) fills the cochlear duct. The thickness of the white arrows in the scala vestibuli and the black arrows in the scala tympani indicates increased (thick arrow) or decreased (thin arrow) fluid pressure. Because fluid is incompressible, pressure changes cause distortion of the vestibular and basilar membranes. Deflection of the basilar membrane pushes the hair cells of the spiral organ into the overlying tectorial membrane, generating neural impulses in the cochlear nerve. Short sound waves (high frequency and high pitch) affect the base of the cochlea, while long waves (low frequency and low pitch) affect the apex of the cochlea. Waves may also travel around the helicotrema at the apex of the cochlea. Impact of the waves on the secondary tympanic membrane covering the cochlear window causes it to move in and out in opposite phases to the vestibular window.

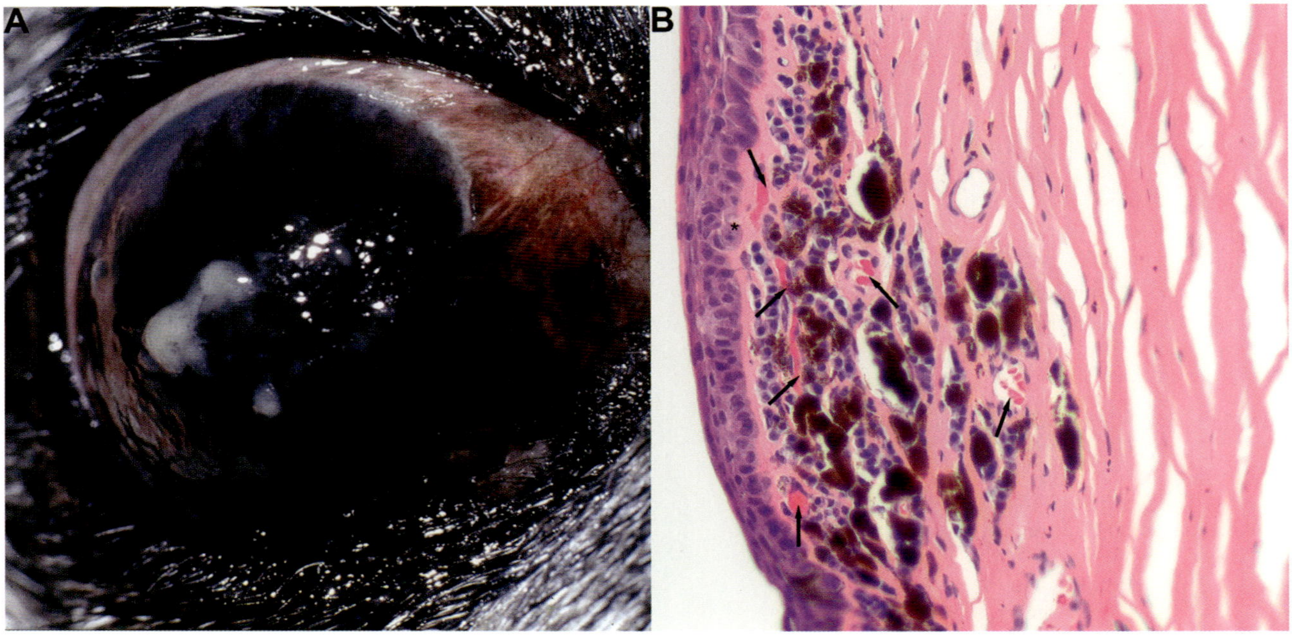

Figure 17-37 Canine "dry eye." Numerous ophthalmic diseases will present routinely to the veterinary clinician in general or emergency practice, including inflammatory and ulcerative corneal diseases, glaucoma, inflammation within the anterior chamber, and blunt or penetrating trauma to the globe. Pictured here is a 13-year-old pug with chronic inflammation, dark brown to black pigmentation, and recurrent ulceration of both corneas, accompanied by mucoid discharge. (A: Courtesy of Dr David Wilkie.) These findings are consistent with Keratoconjunctivitis Sicca or "dry eye," an immune-mediated condition affecting the lacrimal gland, which results in decreased production of the aqueous portion of the tear film. Histological examination also highlights the chronic corneal changes in this animal, including vascularization of the anterior corneal stroma (arrows), severe pigmentation (brown), mixed inflammation, and basal epithelial apoptosis (cell death, asterisk) (B: H&E ×200).

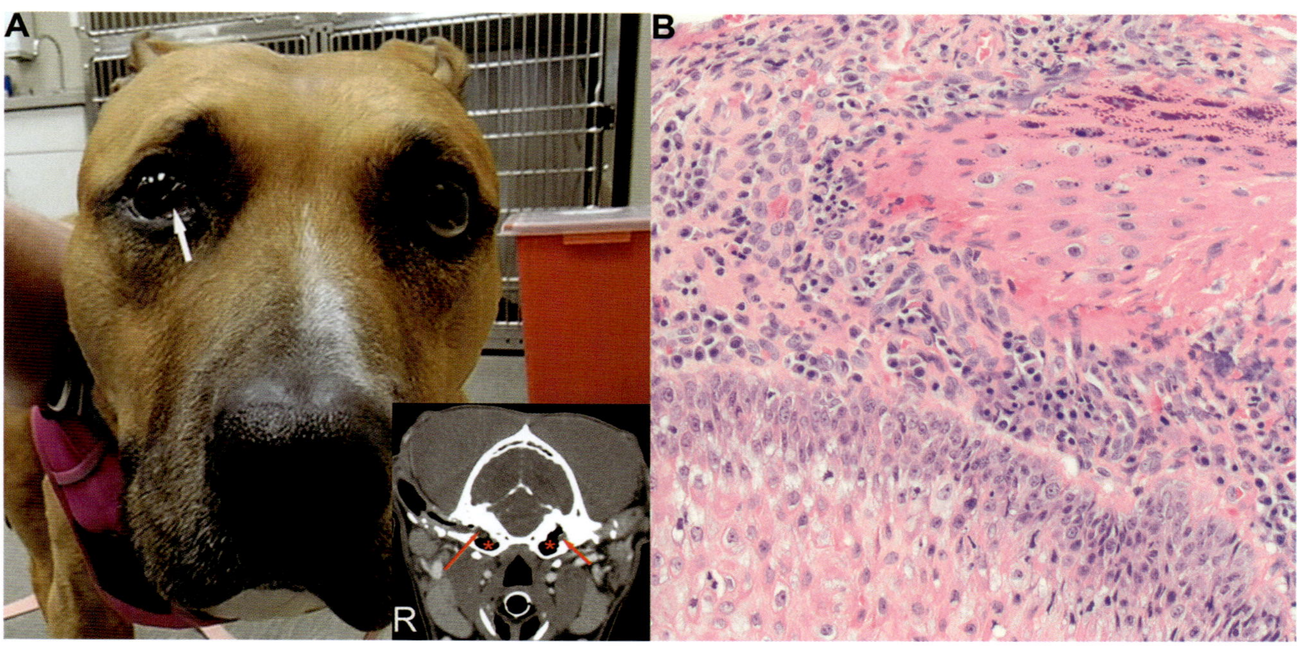

Figure 17-38 Canine otitis media with Horner's syndrome. Otitis externa is commonly associated with underlying allergic dermatitis. Pictured is an 11-year-old mixed breed dog with Horner's syndrome of the right eye. Horner's syndrome includes miosis, enophthalmos, ptosis, and elevation of the third eyelid (arrow) due to loss of sympathetic tone to the eye. The inset demonstrates the skull CT scan with this animal with soft tissue material (arrows) within the external ear canals bilaterally, which extends into the tympanic bullae of the middle ears (asterisks). (A: Courtesy of Dr Jacob Stewart Leslie.) The histology, obtained from a total ear canal ablation, shows marked thickening of the epithelium lining the tympanic bulla with increased numbers of lamellar keratin and moderate infiltration of the mucosa and lumen by neutrophils, lymphocytes, and plasma cells (B: H&E ×200).

Essentials

Eye	Ear
Fibrous tunic • Cornea: surface epithelium, stroma, Descemet's membrane, and endothelium • Corneoscleral junction (limbus) • Sclera: episcleral and stroma	External ear • Pinna • External acoustic meatus
Vascular tunic • Iris: anterior border layer, stroma, anterior epithelium (with sympathetic dilator muscle), posterior epithelium, and parasympathetic sphincter muscle • Ciliary body: epithelium (inner nonpigmented and outer pigmented) and aqueous humor production • Iridocorneal angle: pectinate ligament, trabecular meshwork, and venous drainage • Choroid: suprachoroid, stroma, tapetum lucidum, choriocapillaris, and Bruch's membrane	Middle ear • Tympanic membrane • Auditory ossicles: malleus (manubrium, neck, and head), incus, and stapes • Muscles: tensor tympani and stapedius • Tympanic cavity • Auditory tube (guttural pouch) • Cochlear (round) window • Vestibular (oval) window
Neuroepithelial tunic • Neural retina: inner limiting membrane, nerve fiber layer, ganglion cell layer, inner plexiform layer, inner nuclear layer, outer plexiform layer, outer nuclear layer, external limiting membrane, and photoreceptors • RPE Refractive media • Lens: capsule, epithelium, cortex, nucleus, equator, and sutures • Vitreous body Accessory organs • Eyelids: haired skin, conjunctiva (epithelium, stroma), and Meibomian glands • Third eyelid: cartilage and gland • Lacrimal apparatus: lacrimal gland, lacrimal lake, lacrimal puncta, lacrimal canaliculi, lacrimal sac, and nasolacrimal duct	Inner ear • Bony labyrinth: Cochlea: scala vestibuli (vestibular membrane), cochlear duct (organ of Corti, tectorial membrane, and spiral canal), scala tympani (basilar membrane), scala vascularis, and modiolus (spiral ganglion) Vestibule Semicircular canals Perilymphatic space • Membranous labyrinth: semicircular duct: ampulla (crista ampullaris) Utricle Saccule Endolymphatic duct Endolymphatic sac

Suggested Readings

Couloigner V, Teixeira M, Sterkers O, et al. The endolymphatic sac: its roles in the inner ear. *Med Sei (Paris)* 2004;20(3):304.

Dubielzig RR. Veterinary Ocular Pathology, a Comparative Review. Philadelphia, PA: Elsevier, 2010.

Flock Å. The ear. In: Weiss L, ed. Cell and Tissue Biology. A Textbook of Histology. 6th Ed. Baltimore: Urban & Schwarzenberg, Inc., 1988.

Forrester JV, Dick AD, McMenamin PG, et al. The Eye, Basic Sciences in Practice. 5th Ed. Philadelphia, PA: Elsevier, 2021.

Friedmann I, Ballantyne J. Ultrastructural Atlas of the Inner Ear. London: Butterworths & Co., 1984.

Kumar A, Roman-Auerhahn MR. Anatomy of canine and feline ear. In: Gotthelf LN, ed. Small Animal Ear Diseases: An Illustrated Guide. 2nd Ed. Philadelphia, PA: Elsevier, 2005.

Levin LA, Nilsson SFE, Ver Hoeve J, et al. Adler's Physiology of the Eye. 11th Ed. Philadelphia, PA: Elsevier-Saunders, 2011.

Lindeman HH. Anatomy of the otolith organs. *Adv Otorhinolaryngol.* 1973;20:405–33. doi: 10.1159/000393113. PMID: 4267996.

Meekins JM, Rankin AJ, Samuelson DA. Ophthalmic anatomy. In: Gelatt KN, ed. Veterinary Ophthalmology. 6th Ed. Hoboken, NJ: Wiley-Blackwell, 2021.

Njaa BL, Sula MJ. Collection and preparation of dog and cat ears for histologic examination. *Vet Clin North Am Small Anim Pract* 2012;42(6):1127–1135.

Osborne MP, Comis SD, Pickles JO. Morphology and cross linkage of stereo-cilia in the guinea-pig labyrinth examined without the use of osmium as a fixative. *Cell Tissue Res* 1984;237:43.

Raphael Y, Altschuler RA. Structure and innervation of the cochlea. *Brain Res Bull* 2003;60:397.

Schuknecht HF. Anatomy. In: Schuknecht HF, ed. Pathology of the Ear. 3rd Ed. Philadelphia, PA: Elsevier, 2010.

Singh B. Special senses. In: Dyce KM, Sack WO, CJG W, eds. Dyce, Sack, and Wensing's Textbook of Veterinary Anatomy. 5th Ed. Philadelphia, PA: Elsevier, 2018.

Weiss, Leon. Cell and Tissue Biology: A Textbook of Histology. 6th ed. Baltimore: Urban & Schwarzenberg, 1988. Print.

Yanoff M, Sassani JW. Ocular Histology, a Text and Atlas. 9th Ed. Philadelphia, PA: Elsevier, 2024.

Index

Dellmann's Textbook of Veterinary Histology, Seventh Edition. Edited by Marxa L. Figueiredo and John J. Turek.

Companion website: www.wiley.com/go/figueiredo/vethistology7e

b

f

g

h

j

k

r